HPV Infections: Diagnosis, Prevention and Treatment

HPV Infections: Diagnosis, Prevention and Treatment

Edited by Frank Reese

AMERICAN
MEDICAL PUBLISHERS
www.americanmedicalpublishers.com

American Medical Publishers,
41 Flatbush Avenue,
1st Floor, New York,
NY 11217, USA

Visit us on the World Wide Web at:
www.americanmedicalpublishers.com

ISBN: 978-1-63927-222-8

Cataloging-in-Publication Data

HPV infections : diagnosis, prevention and treatment / edited by Frank Reese.
p. cm.
Includes bibliographical references and index.
ISBN 978-1-63927-222-8
1. Papillomavirus diseases--Infections. 2. Papillomaviruses. 3. Papillomavirus diseases--Diagnosis.
4. Papillomavirus diseases--Prevention. 5. Papillomavirus diseases--Treatment. I. Reese, Frank.
RC168.P15 H68 2022
616.911--dc23

Table of Contents

Preface

The infection caused by the DNA virus human papillomavirus is known as human papillomavirus infection. A variety of causes that lead to this infection have been identified. Some of these are smoking, early age sexual intercourse, many sexual partners and poor immune system functioning. Some of the clinical symptoms related to this infection are warts and precancerous lesions. These lesions increase the risk of cervix, vagina, mouth, vulva and anus cancer. Various diagnostic techniques have been used for its identification. These include cervical testing and mouth testing. The use of HPV vaccines and early cervical cancer detection are some of the prevention techniques that have been identified by this discipline. This book contains some of the path-breaking studies related to HPV infections. It discusses the fundamental as well as modern approaches to the diagnosis, prevention and treatment of HPV infection. This book will provide comprehensive knowledge to the readers.

This book has been the outcome of endless efforts put in by authors and researchers on various issues and topics within the field. The book is a comprehensive collection of significant researches that are addressed in a variety of chapters. It will surely enhance the knowledge of the field among readers across the globe.

It gives us an immense pleasure to thank our researchers and authors for their efforts to submit their piece of writing before the deadlines. Finally in the end, I would like to thank my family and colleagues who have been a great source of inspiration and support.

Editor

1

Genotype distribution characteristics of multiple human papillomavirus in women from the Taihu River Basin, on the coast of eastern China

Jing-fen Lu*, Guo-rong Shen, Qiong Li, Xu Chen, Chun-fang Ma and Tong-hua Zhu

Abstract

Background: There is limited data on the genotype distribution of human papillomavirus (HPV) in the Taihu River Basin, home to 1.29 million people on the coast of eastern China. This study evaluated the prevalence and genotypes among different female age groups in this region.

Methods: Twenty-six HPV strains (low-risk HPV 6, 11, 40, 42, 44, 61, 73 and high-risk HPV 16, 18, 26, 31, 33, 35, 39, 45, 51, 52, 53, 55, 56, 58, 59, 66, 68, 82, and 83) were detected using Tellgenplex™ HPV technology in samples obtained from three clinical hospitals located in different regions of the Taihu Lake Basin.

Results: The results showed that 1855 samples (20.97% of all samples) were found to be HPV-positive. Of these, 1375 samples (15.55% of all samples) were found to have a single HPV infection. Age-specific prevalence showed two peaks, one that corresponded to the group of 21–30 year-old women and the other peak that corresponded to the group of women over 51 years old. The three most prevalent genotypes were HPV52 (19.95%, 370/1855), HPV16 (13.48%, 150/1855), and HPV58 (11.32%, 210/1855). Mixed strains HPV58 + HPV33 and HPV58 + HPV52 were most commonly found in females infected with multiple HPV types.

Conclusions: This investigation reveals that HPV infection in the Taihu River Basin varied significantly among different age groups. The most prevalent genotypes are included in the nonavalent vaccine, V503, however this vaccine is not licensed for use in mainland China. The most frequently occurring genotypes should be considered in the development of next-generation HPV vaccines for optimal protection of public health.

Keywords: Human papillomavirus, Cervical cancer, Genotypes, Distribution

Background

Cervical cancer (CC) is a major cause of morbidity and mortality among women in China, and also represents an important global public health problem. Persistent infection by high-risk human papillomavirus (hrHPV) is required for the development of pre-invasive and invasive carcinogenesis [1, 2]. To date, more than 200 different viral types have been identified, and 40 of these types can infect the mucosa of the anogenital tract [3]. To some extent, improved detection of hrHPV may reduce the risk for the development of CC and associated deaths [4].

Early studies demonstrated that the distribution of HPV genotypes in CC varies with geographic location [2, 5, 6]. Hence, an accurate assessment of the regional genotype distribution is very important for effective strategies to prevent CC. Several studies have assessed the prevalence of HPV strains in mainland China, such as studies focused on Yunnan and Shanghai [7, 8] and a study that examined the HPV distribution in 37 cities in China [9]. However, there is limited data on the genotype distribution in the Taihu River Basin, which is a largely agricultural and industrial coastal area in eastern China. HPV genotyping detection is used to study

* Correspondence: petiteberyl@163.com
Department of Clinical laboratory, Wujiang First People's Hospital, Suzhou, People's Republic of China

HPV strain-specificity to facilitate the implementation, monitoring, and evaluation of vaccination programs. The American Society for Colposcopy and Cervical Pathology (ASCCP) guideline indicated that cervical screening should start at the age of 21, and screening using both the HPV test and the Pap test should be performed every 5 years for women 30–65 years in age [10]. The aim of this study was to determine the distribution of HPV genotypes in the Taihu River Basin to facilitate a better understanding of the HPV virus and to predict the efficacy of a HPV vaccine.

Methods

Study population

The purpose of this investigation was to obtain data on the prevalence of HPV genotypes, including age-specific prevalence differences and the distribution of multiple HPV genotypes. This investigation analyzed samples obtained from 3 clinical hospitals located in different regions of the Taihu River Basin. From November 2013 and June 2015, a total of 9012 women aged 21–70 years old (14,280 subjects were invited, but 5268 patients did not participate in the screening for various reasons) attended a gynecological outpatient clinic and expressed interest in cervical cancer screening. Participants met the following selection criteria: a) had not had sexual intercourse, had not used vaginal medications, and had not washed in the previous 48 h; b) not currently pregnant; c) with no history of total uterus or cervix resection; d) a permanent resident of the region; and e) agreed to undergo the HPV test and participate in this study.

Specimen collection

The cervico-vaginal cells at the transformation zone of the uterine cervix were collected from all participants by a gynecologist using a standard cytobrush according to the standard sampling procedure at the recruitment sites. Cells were resuspended in 3 ml sample transport medium (STM) for the Tellgenplex™ HPV DNA Test (Tellgen Life Science, Shanghai, China) and stored at 4 °C. According to the kit instructions, samples can be stored in STM for 1 month at 2–8 °C and 6 months at −20 °C. We stored all samples at 4 °C for 1 week prior to testing to obtain the most accurate results.

Ethics statement

This investigation was approved by the Ethical Committee of Wujiang First Hospital affiliated with Nantong University (permit number: 201405). All the specimens and their corresponding information were obtained with written informed consent from the participants involved in the project.

HPV Genotyping

The Tellgenplex™ HPV DNA Test uses one multiplex PCR test combined with Luminex technology to identify the 26 most common HPV types (−6, −11, −16, −18, −26, −31, −33, −35, −39, −40, −42, −44, −45, −51, −52, −53, −55, −56, −58, −59, −61, −66, −68, −73, −82, and −83). The procedure includes DNA extraction, PCR amplification, and bead-coated hybridization and was performed according to the manufacturer's guidelines [9, 11]. Each assay required 10–20 pg/ml HPV DNA as template. Females who were negative for β-globin were excluded from analyses.

Statistical analysis

All statistical analyses were performed using SPSS version 19.0 (IBM, Armonk, NY, USA). All genotypes from single and multiple infections were computed individually. A multiple-type infection was defined as one that was positive for at least 2 types. These data were also stratified by age (21–30 years, 31–40 years, 41–50 years, 51–60 years, and 61–65 years).

Results

Distribution characteristics of HPV genotypes

Among the 9012 individuals included in this study, 29 specimens were found to be negative for β-globin, and 138 cases could not be grouped because the analysis was restricted to women 21–65 old. Therefore, 8845 subjects (the median age was 42 and the quartile range was 32–47 years) were included in the analysis. As shown in Fig. 1, the overall prevalence of HPV was 20.97% (1855/8845), and 15.55% (1375/8845) of positive samples were found to have a single HPV infection, more than the number of subjects with a multiple infection. Among the study participants, 1430 had hrHPV infections, accounting for approximately 77% of the positive samples. The top 4 high-risk genotypes, 52, 16, 58, and 18, were detected in 19.95%, 13.48%, 11.32%, and 9.43% of positive specimens, respectively. HPV52 was the most prevalent type in subjects with a single HPV infection (260/1855 = 14.02%). Among the 480 individuals infected with multiple HPV types, 380 had dual infections (380/480 = 79.17%), and 100 subjects were infected by at least three HPV types (100/480 = 20.83%). The four most prevalent high-risk HPV types for subjects infected with multiple strains were HPV16, 52, 58, and 18, with frequencies of 6.20%, 5.93%, 4.58%, and 4.58% of positive samples, respectively.

Prevalence of HPV infection in different age groups

Among the age groups, the HPV infection prevalence ranged from 16.3% for women aged 31–40 years to 25% for those 51–60 yeas old (Fig. 2a, b). The frequency of hrHPV types also differed among these age groups.

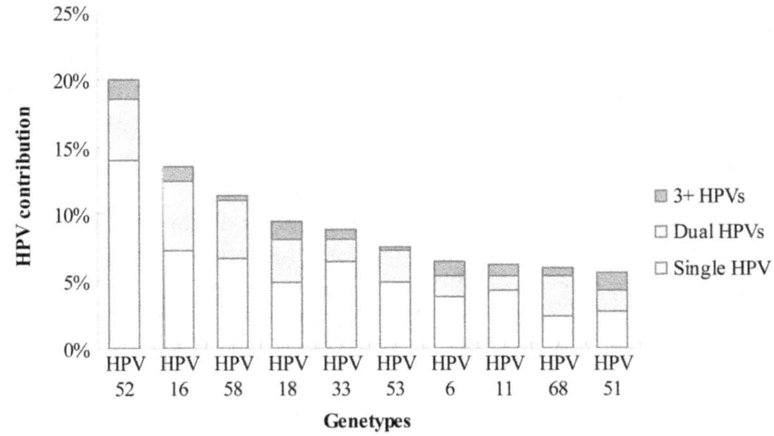

Fig. 1 The top 10 HPV positive genotypes and their contribution

Similar to the overall prevalence of HPV, the highest overall prevalence of hrHPV was found in women 51–60 years old (16.67%, 75/450), and the lowest hrHPV prevalence was found in women 31–40 years old (12.17%, 280/2300; Fig. 2b). The prevalence for single and dual HPV infections exhibited two peaks, one for the group 21–30 years old and the other for the group 51–60 years old (Fig. 2a).

Discussion

HPV infection is the most common sexually transmitted infection. The majority of HPV infections are temporary, especially among young women, but CC usually develops after 10 years of persistent hrHPV infection [12]. Regular gynecological screening and treatment of precancerous lesions are less effective strategies for the prevention

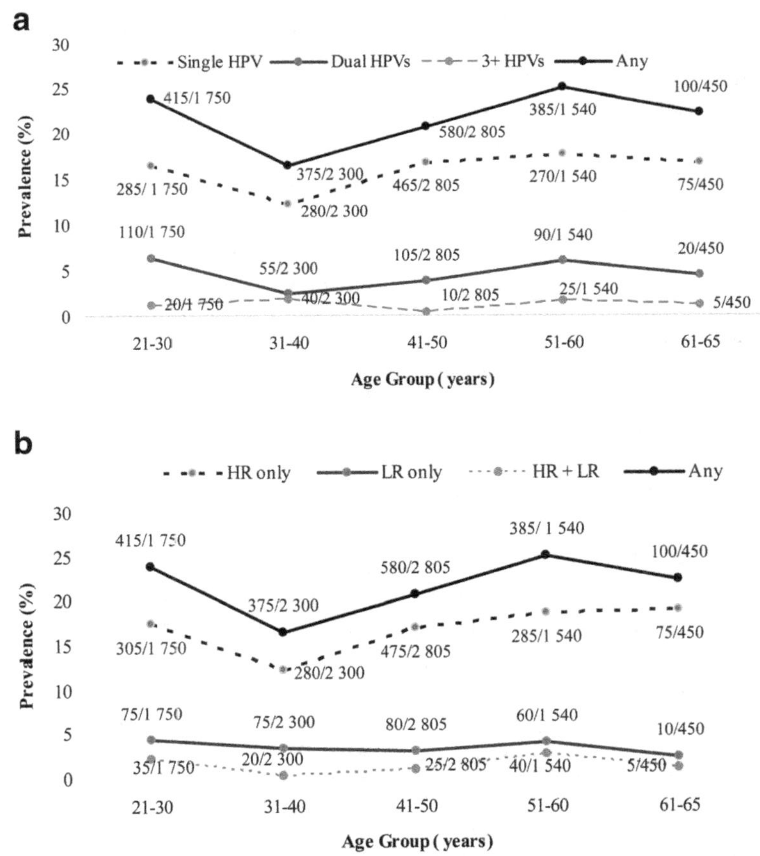

Fig. 2 a Relative contribution of single and multiple HPV infections by age at diagnosis. **b** Relative contribution of high- and low-risk HPV infection by age at diagnosis

of adenocarcinoma [13]. Fortunately, adenocarcinoma should be controllable by HPV vaccines [14]. Two different prophylactic HPV vaccines have been licensed and are now available in most countries except Mainland China. Obtaining a current dataset for a particular region will enable the development of optimal and effective screening and vaccination programs.

In this study, a rate of 20.97% HPV infection was observed in patients ranging from 21 to 65 years old. Most patients had a single infection. Of these HPV-positive patients, 77.09% were hrHPV infections, and there were two peaks in this analysis corresponding to women 21–30 years old and 51–60 years old. HPV is a sexually transmitted disease, and the higher rate of infection in younger, single women may be because these women may have more frequent sexual intercourse, particularly with more than one partner. Older women also show a higher rate of infection due to effects of physiological and immunological disorders associated with hormone fluctuations during the menopausal transition. These two peaks were also observed in the frequency analysis of multiple infections. Additionally, the frequency of dual and 3+ HPV infections was highest in individuals over 50 years old. These trends are consistent with the results of other researches that reported a second peak for the prevalence of multiple infections in females who are ≥50 or 60 years of age [8, 9, 12].

Of the three most dominant HPV genotypes, HPV 52, HPV 16, and HPV 58, 70.3%, 54%, and 59.5%, respectively, were single-infections and the remaining cases of these genotypes were present together with other HPVs. Wang et al. [15] reported that infections with multiple genotypes had higher risk of the development and progression of CC, but this does not necessarily mean that the cancerous stage requires multiple infections. Because cervical precursor lesions need years to develop into CC, multiple types may facilitate growth during the precancerous Cervical Intraepithelial Neoplasia (CIN) stages, but the oncogenic capability of the latter stages may not be controlled by multiple genotypes. In this present study, the top most frequent combinations of genotypes were HPV58 + HPV33 (32 cases) and HPV58 + HPV52 (25 cases) (Additional file 1: Table S1.). Both HPV52 and HPV58 are more prevalent in Eastern Asia, and the linking of HPV58 to cervical cancer was 1.8 higher than for HPV52 [16]. Further comparative analysis showed that HPV16, 52, and 58 are the three top hrHPV types in the Chinese reports, but the relative prevalence rates varied widely and other genotype distributions also differed regionally in Mainland [7, 17–19]. Therefore, infection with HPV58 or 52 in this region should be given the same attention as HPV16 and 18 infections. Fortunately, the V503 nonavalent vaccine appears to be safe and effective in the prevention of persistent infection and precancerous lesions associated with hrHPV types −16, −18, −31, −33, −45, −52, and −58, as well as genital warts that are related to lrHPV 6 and 11 infection [20]. This would cover 70.18% (965/1375) of single infections and 51.46% (247/480) of multiple infections in this area. However, this vaccine is not licensed in mainland China.

This analysis of HPV genotype distribution in the Taihu River Basin in China has potential limitations. First, this study determined the distribution of the prevalence of HPV genotypes in women aged 21–65 years who attended a cervical screening, however, the absence of cytological data of cervical pre-cancer or cancer remains a major concern. Second, there was no sampling of tissue specimens in this study. Comparison of HPV detection rates between cervical scraping and biopsy methods may help to clarify the pathological mechanism of HPV infection and the evolution of CC. Overall, this study provides a description of the genotype-specific prevalence in women from the Taihu River Basin on the coast of eastern China.

Conclusions

Lifestyle and health are dramatically affected by economic conditions, cultural habits, and changing population dynamics. Therefore, it is urgent to pay attention to changes in the prevalence of HPV infection, particularly at a regional level. In the Taihu River Basin, the coast of eastern China, we found that the three top genotypes were HPV 52 (19.95%), HPV 16 (13.48%), and HPV 58 (11.32%). Mixed strains HPV58 + HPV33 and HPV58 + HPV52 were most frequently found in women with multiple infections. Considering the specific genotypes present in this geographic location, a cost-effective vaccine, such as the nonavalent vaccine V503, may provide optimal prevention of cervical cancer in this area.

Abbreviations

CC: Cervical cancer; CIN: Cervical intraepithelial neoplasia; HPV: Human papillomavirus; hr-: High-risk; lr-: Low-risk

Acknowledgements

Special thanks to the staff for their help in carrying out this study. We also thank the staff of the sciworks language service for medical writing services. Research support: Social development plan, soft science research project of Wujiang area in Suzhou, Jiangsu Province, China (grant number WS201302).

Funding

This present study was financially supported by the Social Development Plan and Soft Science Research Project of Wujiang Area in Suzhou, Jiangsu Province, China (grant number WS201302).

Authors' contributions

QL, CFM, THZ, XC coordinated and performed all sample analyses. JFL and GRS drafted and revised the manuscript. All authors read and approved the final manuscript.

Competing interests
The authors have declare that they have no competing interests.

Consent for publication
Not applicable.

References
1. de Sanjose S, Quint WG, Alemany L, Geraets DT, Klaustermeier JE, Lloveras B, et al. Human papillomavirus genotype attribution in invasive cervical cancer: a retrospective cross-sectional worldwide study. Lancet Oncol. 2010;11(11): 1048–56.
2. Al Moustafa AE, Ghabreau L, Akil N, Rastam S, Alachkar A, Yasmeen A. High-risk HPVs and human carcinomas in the Syrian population. Front Oncol. 2014;4(1):68.
3. Padalko E, Ali-Risasi C, Mesmaekers S, et al. Comparative analysis of cervical cytology and human papillomavirus genotyping by three different methods in a routine diagnostic setting. Eur J Cancer Prev. 2015;24(5):447–58.
4. Villiers EMD. Cross-roads in the classification of papillomaviruses. Virology. 2013;445(1–2):2–10.
5. Li N, Franceschi S, Howell-Jones R, Snijders PJ, Clifford GM. Human papillomavirus type distribution in 30,848 invasive cervical cancers worldwide: Variation by geographical region, histological type and year of publication. Int J Cancer. 2011;128(4):927–35.
6. Roteli-Martins CM, de Carvalho NS, Naud P, Teixeira J, Borba P, Derchain S, et al. Prevalence of human papillomavirus infection and associated risk factors in young women in Brazil, Canada, and the United States: a multicenter cross-sectional study. Int J Gynecol Pathol. 2011;30(2):173–84.
7. Li Z, Liu F, Cheng S, et al. Prevalence of HPV infection among 28,457 Chinese women in Yunnan Province, southwest China. Sci. Rep. 2016;6:21039.
8. Singh S, Zhou Q, Yu Y, Xu X, Huang X, Zhao J, et al. Distribution of HPV genotypes in Shanghai women. Int J Clin Exp Pathol. 2015;8(9):11901.
9. Wang R, Guo XL, Wisman GBA, et al. Nationwide prevalence of human papillomavirus infection and viral genotype distribution in 37 cities in China. BMC Infect Dis. 2015;15(1):257.
10. Smith RA, Manassaram-Baptiste D, Brooks D, Doroshenk M, Fedewa S, Saslow D, et al. Cancer screening in the United States, 2015: a review of current American Cancer Society guidelines and current issues in cancer screening. CA Cancer J Clin. 2015;65(1):30–54.
11. Wei W, Shi Q, Guo F, Zhang BY, Chen C, Zhang NS, et al. The distribution of human papillomavirus in tissues from patients with head and neck squamous cell carcinoma. Oncol Rep. 2012;28(5):1750–6.
12. Jing L, Zhong X, Zhong Z, et al. Prevalence of human papillomavirus infection in Guangdong Province, China: a population-based survey of 78,355 women. Sex Transm Dis. 2014;41(12):732–8
13. Chew GK, Cruickshank ME, Rooney PH, Miller ID, Parkin DE, Murray GI. Human papillomavirus 16 infection in adenocarcinoma of the cervix. Br J Cancer. 2005;93(11):1301–4.
14. Stokley S, Jeyarajah J, Yankey D, et al. Human papillomavirus vaccination coverage among adolescents, 2007-2013, and postlicensure vaccine safety monitoring, 2006-2014-United States. MMWR. 2014;63(29):620–4.
15. Wang L, Wu B, Li J, et al. Prevalence of human papillomavirus and its genotype among 1336 invasive cervical cancer patients in Hunan province, central south China. J Med Virol. 2014;87(3):516–21.
16. Chan P K, Ho W C, Chan M C, Wong M C, Yeung A C, Chor J S, et al. Meta-Analysis on Prevalence and Attribution of Human Papillomavirus Types 52 and 58 in Cervical Neoplasia Worldwide 2014.
17. Bi Q, Zhang L, Zhao Z, Mu X, Zhang M, Wang P. Human papillomavirus prevalence and genotypes distribution among female outpatients in Qingdao, East China. J Med Virol. 2015;87(12):2114–21.
18. Hong H, He TF, Ni HX, Zhang S, Xu GZ. Prevalence and genotype distribution of HPV infection among women in Ningbo, China. Int J Gynecol Obstet. 2015;131(1):96–9.
19. Xue H, Lin X, Li T, Yan X, Guo K, Zhang Y. Prevalence and genotype distribution of human papillomavirus infection in asymptomatic women in Liaoning province, China. J Med Virol. 2015;87(7):1248–53.
20. Chatterjee A. The next generation of HPV vaccines: nonavalent vaccine V503 on the horizon. Expert Rev. Vaccines. 2014;13(11):1279.

2

The prevalence of human papillomavirus infections and associated risk factors in men-who-have-sex-with-men in Cape Town, South Africa

Etienne E. Müller[1*], Kevin Rebe[2,3,4], Tobias F. Chirwa[5], Helen Struthers[2,3,4], James McIntyre[2,3,6] and David A. Lewis[7,8]

Abstract

Background: We investigated the prevalence of human papillomavirus (HPV) infection and associated behavioural risk factors in men-who-have-sex-with-men (MSM) attending a clinical service in Cape Town, South Africa.

Methods: MSM were enrolled at the Ivan Toms Centre for Men's Health in Cape Town. A psychosocial and sexual behavioral risk questionnaire was completed for each participant and urine, oro-pharyngeal and anal swabs were collected for HPV testing using the Linear Array HPV Genotyping Test. Logistic regression analyses were performed to determine sexual risk factors associated with HPV infection at the three anatomical sites.

Results: The median age of all 200 participants was 32 years (IQR 26-39.5), of which 31.0 % were black, 31.5 % mixed race/coloured and 35.5 % white. The majority of the participants (73.0 %) had completed high school, 42.0 % had a tertiary level qualification and 69.0 % were employed. HPV genotypes were detected in 72.8 % [95 % CI: 65.9–79.0 %], 11.5 % [95 % CI: 7.4–16.8 %] and 15.3 % [95 % CI: 10.5–21.2 %] of anal, oro-pharyngeal and urine specimens, respectively. Prevalence of high-risk (HR)-HPV types was 57.6 % [95 % CI: 50.3–64.7 %] in anal samples, 7.5 % [95 % CI: 4.3–12.1 %] in oro-pharyngeal samples and 7.9 % [95 % CI: 4.5–12.7 %] in urine, with HPV-16 being the most common HR-HPV type detected at all sites. HPV-6/11/16/18 was detected in 40.3 % [95 % CI: 33.3–47.6 %], 4.5 % [95 % CI: 2.1–8.4 %] and 3.2 % [95 % CI: 1.2–6.8 %] of anal, oro-pharyngeal and urine samples, respectively. Multiple HPV types were more common in the anal canal of MSM while single HPV types constituted the majority of HPV infections in the oropharynx and urine. Among the 88 MSM (44.0 %) that were HIV positive, 91.8 % [95 % CI: 83.8–96.6 %] had an anal HPV infection, 81.2 % [95 % CI: 71.2–88.8 %] had anal HR-HPV and 85.9 % [95 % CI: 76.6–92.5 %] had multiple anal HPV types. Having sex with men only, engaging in group sex in lifetime, living with HIV and practising receptive anal intercourse were the only factors independently associated with having any anal HPV infection.

Conclusions: Anal HPV infections were common among MSM in Cape Town with the highest HPV burden among HIV co-infected MSM, men who have sex with men only and those that practiced receptive anal intercourse. Behavioural intervention strategies and the possible roll-out of HPV vaccines among all boys are urgently needed to address the high prevalence of HPV and HIV co-infections among MSM in South Africa.

Keywords: HPV, Anal, Oro-pharyngeal, Urine, MSM, Risk factors, South Africa

* Correspondence: etiennem@nicd.ac.za
[1]Centre for HIV and Sexually Transmitted Infections, National Institute for Communicable Diseases, National Health Laboratory Service, Johannesburg, South Africa
Full list of author information is available at the end of the article

Background

Human papillomavirus (HPV) is the most common sexually transmitted viral infection worldwide and is associated with occurrence of warts (condylomas) and a variety of cancers in both men and women [1]. The outcome of HPV infection depends on the specific HPV type/s present and can range from asymptomatic infection to severe squamous cell malignancies. Low-risk HPV types (such as types 6 and 11) are associated with anogenital warts and mild dysplasia, while high-risk types (such as 16 and 18) are associated with high-grade dysplasia and cancers of the cervix, vulva, vagina, urethra, penis, anus and oropharynx [1]. HPV is an independent risk factor for the acquisition of HIV [2]. HIV infection is also associated with an increased risk of acquiring new HPV infections and a reduction in the rate of HPV clearance [3]. South Africa has one of the highest HIV prevalence rates globally with an estimated prevalence of 12.2 % in the general population in 2012 [4]. HIV is especially prevalent among men-who-have-sex-with-men (MSM), with estimated prevalence rates of 22.3 %, 26.8 % and 48.2 % in Cape Town, Johannesburg and Durban, respectively [5]. Unprotected receptive anal intercourse is up to sixteen times more likely to transmit HIV than unprotected vaginal sex, placing MSM at higher risk of acquiring and transmitting HIV [6]. A meta-analysis of 53 studies reported HPV co-infection in 89 % - 93 % of HIV-infected MSM [7].

HPV infection in men is an important concern due to its association with anal, urethral, penile and oropharyngeal cancers. In South Africa, relatively little is known about the incidence rates of these cancers in men, and although these cancers are less common than cervical cancer, their association with HPV infection make them amenable to similar preventative measures as those for cervical cancer. The risk of developing invasive anal cancer was 17 times higher among MSM than in men-who-have-sex-with-women (MSW) and the risk doubled in HIV-infected MSM [8]. A number of studies reported anal HPV prevalence rates of 30–70 % in HIV-negative MSM and 71–100 % in HIV-positive MSM [9–12]. Oral HPV infection is less common in adults than anogenital HPV infection but is still strongly associated with HIV infection, high-risk sexual practices, especially engaging in oro-genital sex and having a high number of sexual partners [13, 14]. HPV can also be found in the urinary tract, indicating HPV infection in either the distal or proximal urethra, prostate and/or urinary bladder [15]. There are currently three HPV vaccines available that were designed to prevent HPV-associated cancer to certain HR-HPV genotypes. These HPV vaccines include the bivalent Cervarix® HPV vaccine (GSK Aspen) (targeting HPV types 16 and 18), the quadrivalent Gardasil® HPV vaccine (MSD) (targeting HPV types 6, 11, 16 and 18) as well as the 9-valent Gardasil® 9 HPV vaccine (MSD) (targeting HPV types 6, 11, 16, 18, 31, 33, 45, 52 and 58).

Epidemiological research has remained very limited among the MSM population in South Africa and as a result there are currently no HPV prevalence data for MSM. Due to high HIV prevalence rates among MSM in South Africa, this group has been identified by the South African Department of Health for targeted healthcare interventions and HIV prevention programs [16]. This study will therefore aim to investigate the prevalence of HPV genotypes at different anatomical sites (anus, oropharynx and urine) in a sample of 200 MSM seeking care at a dedicated men's clinic in Cape Town, South Africa.

Methods

Population and sample selection

This study is a secondary analysis of data collected during a cross-sectional study of symptomatic and asymptomatic STIs among MSM in Cape Town, South Africa [17]. A convenience sample of 200 sequential MSM were enrolled by Health4Men (Anova Health Institute) at the Ivan Toms Centre for Men's Health (ITCMH) in Cape Town during 2011 and 2012. These MSM were mostly asymptomatic (71.0 %) for STIs and attended the ITCMH for HIV, sexual health and/or mental health care and for commodities such as condoms and lubricants. The inclusion criteria for study participation included being 18 years of age or older, having sex with other men within one year prior to recruitment, understanding the study procedures, risks and benefits and willingness to give informed consent. Study participants attended two study-related visits two weeks apart. During the first visit participants were assessed for STI symptoms and examined for STI and HIV-related clinical conditions. All participants completed a researcher administered study questionnaire and provided a self-collected urine specimen and clinician collected rectal and oro-pharyngeal swab. These specimens were tested for *Neisseria gonorrhoeae* and *Chlamydia trachomatis* using the RNA-based Aptima Combo 2 assay (Hologic-Gen-Probe, San Diego, CA, USA.) and stored at −70 °C for HPV testing. At the follow-up visit, results were relayed to all participants and diagnosed conditions were treated according to the South African Department of Health's first-line comprehensive management and control of STIs protocol [18]. All 200 participants gave permission for their specimens to be used for future research. Ethical approvals for this study were obtained from the Human Research Ethics Committee (Medical) of the University of the Witwatersrand [protocol M120454] and the Bioethics Department at the University of Cape Town [protocol 419/2011].

Psychosocial and sexual behavioural data collection

Socio-demographic and sexual behavior characteristics were collected by designated study staff for the primary study through personal interviews using a standardized questionnaire. Circumcision status was confirmed during clinical examination. A sexual partner matrix (SPM) for the last 10 sexual encounters in the past 12 months (or less if the participant had less than 10 sexual encounters in the past 12 months) was completed for each participant. The SPM recorded the gender of each partner and condom use during sexual practices that included receptive and insertive anal intercourse, oral sex and oro-anal sex. Vaginal intercourse was recorded for men who had sexual encounters with female partners in the past 12 months.

HPV detection and genotyping

HPV testing was performed at the STI Section, Centre for HIV and STIs, National Institute for Communicable Diseases (NICD), in Johannesburg. Three archived specimens for each of the 200 enrolled MSM participants were analysed, which included a first-void urine specimen, an oro-pharyngeal swab and an anal swab, which were all previously stored at −70 °C at the STI Section, Centre for HIV and STIs, NICD.

Genomic DNA was extracted from urine and swab specimens using the MagNAPure Compact Automated DNA Extractor (Roche) and used for HPV genotyping. The Linear Array (LA) HPV Genotyping Test (Roche Molecular Systems, Inc., Branchburg, NJ, USA) was used to determine the HPV genotype distribution in these 600 specimens. The LA test amplified the target HPV DNA for 37 anogenital HPV genotypes, which included 24 low risk HPV types (6, 11, 26, 40, 42, 53, 54, 55, 61, 62, 64, 66, 67, 69, 70, 71, 72, 73, 81, 82, 83, 84, IS39 and CP6108) and 13 high risk HPV types (16, 18, 31, 33, 35, 39, 45, 51, 52, 56, 58, 59 and 68). HPV-52 was only recorded positive in the absence of HPV types 33, 35 and 58 due to the combined probe used for these 4 types in the LA assay. The β-globin gene was amplified as a control for cell adequacy, extraction and amplification. Samples with a negative β-globin result and a positive HPV DNA result were considered valid and adequate for analyses.

Detection of HIV and other STIs

Laboratory detection of HIV, syphilis, gonorrhea and chlamydia infection at the urethral, anal and oro-pharyngeal sites were previously determined for the primary study [17]. Syphilis testing was done on site using the SD Bioline rapid syphilis test and HIV serostatus was determined using both the SD Bioline HIV 1/2 3.0 test (Standard Diagnostics, Korea) and the Alere Determine HIV-1/2 kit (Alere Medical, Japan). Specimens were previously analysed for gonorrheal and chlamydial infection at the STI Section, NICD, using the Aptima 2 Combo assay (Hologic-Gen-Probe, San Diego, CA, USA.).

Data confidentiality

Individual specimens and questionnaire data were delinked from all personal identifiers and each participant was assigned with a unique random HPV study number to ensure anonymity. There were no documents in existence linking original study numbers with HPV study numbers. The HPV genotyping results obtained were therefore not relayed to any patients and the results were only used for research purposes.

Variables and definitions

The main outcome variables consisted of type-specific HPV prevalence, any HPV type, HR-HPV types and multiple HPV types. A participant was considered to have a HR-HPV infection if he tested positive for one or more HR- HPV genotypes, irrespective of the participant being co-infected with one or more LR-HPV genotypes. Multiple HPV was defined in participants with two or more HR or LR HPV genotypes. Socio-demographic variables of interest included age, gender, ethnicity, dwelling location, level of education, job status and income. For the purpose of this study MSM consisted of MSM not having sex with women (MSM only) and men who had sex with both men and women (MSMW). Additional sexual behaviours included last sex with men and women, number of male and female partners in the past 12 months, having a main partner, sex at sex-on-site venues in past 12 months, sex with a partner met on the internet in past 12 months, engaging in group sex in past 12 months and lifetime, sharing sex toys, participating in transactional sex, sex while under the influence of alcohol and drugs, lubrication used during sex and having an STI diagnosed in the past 12 months.

Statistical analyses

HPV prevalence and questionnaire data were entered and analysed using both Epi Info version 7 (USDHHS, Centers for Disease Control and Prevention) and STATA SE version 14.0 (Stata Corporation, College Station, Texas, USA). Descriptive statistics included frequency tables for categorical variables such as level of education, HR-HPV and multiple HPV and summary measures i.e. mean and standard deviation (SD) or median and interquartile range (IQR) for continuous variables such as age. Factors associated with HPV infection, comparing differences between MSM only and MSMW and differences between HIV-positive and HIV-negative participants were assessed with Pearson chi-square test and Fisher's exact test for categorical variables and Student's *t*-test for continuous variables. Factors with a *p*-value of ≤ 0.05 in the univariate logistic regression analyses were included in the multiple logistic regression model to determine possible associations with outcome variables. The HPV outcome variables included HPV prevalence rates in this selected study population for any HPV, HR-HPV and multiple HPV at the 3 anatomical sites and their 95 % confidence intervals (CI); crude odds ratios (COR) and adjusted odds ratios (AOR) and its 95 % CI were calculated.

Results

Demographic and behavioural characteristics

Baseline characteristics, sexual behaviour and STI risks for the 200 participants have been published [17]. Briefly, the median age of all 200 participants was 32 years (IQR 26–39.5) with three-quarters (150) under 40 years of age. A total of fifteen participants (7.5 %) identified as transgender women (TGW; male to female). All three major South African racial groups were equally represented with 62 (31.0 %) black, 63 (31.5 %) mixed race/coloured and 71 (35.5 %) white participants. Baseline and sexual behavioural characteristics of men who have sex with men only (MSM only) and men who have sex with men and women (MSMW) are summarised in Table 1.

The majority of MSM participants (155; 77.5 %) indicated that they had sex with men only while 45 (22.5 %) had sex with both men and women in the preceding 12 months. More than a third of all participants (77; 38.5 %), reported transactional sex (paid and/or received money for sex) in the past year. Significantly more MSMW reported participating in transactional sex in the past year ($p < 0.001$) and having had sex while under the influence of drugs in their lifetime ($p = 0.004$). More than half (52.3 %) of all MSM only participants were HIV positive while only 15.6 % of MSMW had an HIV infection ($p < 0.001$).

Insertive and receptive anal sex in the last 12 months were reported by 143 (71.5 %) and 140 (70.0 %) participants, respectively. Among MSMW, insertive anal sex was more commonly practised than receptive anal sex (86.5 % vs 33.3 %), while MSM only reported more receptive anal sex than insertive anal sex (80.6 % vs 67.1 %). Compared to MSM only, significantly more MSMW practised insertive anal sex ($p = 0.010$) and less receptive anal sex ($p < 0.001$). MSM only participants practised significantly more receptive oral sex (95.5 % vs 57.8 %) and insertive oro-anal sex (43.2 % vs 22.2 %) in the last 12 months. The SPM analysis revealed that 36 (80.0 %) MSMW participants had a female partner among their last 10 sexual partners. Performing vaginal intercourse was reported by 34 (94.4 %) of these MSMW participants, performing anal sex on women was less common (15/36; 41.7 %), while performing and receiving oral sex with women was reported by 29 (80.6 %) and 22 (61.1 %) participants, respectively. Performing and receiving oro-anal sex with women was only reported by 7/36 (19.4 %) participants.

HIV and STI prevalence

As previously reported, 47 (23.5 %) participants reported having an STI diagnosis within the previous year, mostly with a single STI episode (80.9 % of cases) [17]. Eighty eight (44.0 %) participants were HIV positive with the majority (74.1 %) having CD4 counts below 500 cells/μl. Twenty two (11.0 %) participants tested positive for syphilis antibodies. *Neisseria gonorrhoeae* and *Chlamydia trachomatis* infections were detected in 32 (16 %) and 23 (11.5 %) MSM, respectively.

HPV prevalence and genotype distribution

As shown in Tables 2 and 3, a total of 191 anal swabs (95.5 %), 200 oro-pharyngeal swabs (100 %) and 190 urines (95 %) had a valid HPV DNA result and were ncluded in the analysis; test strips lacking human beta globin DNA detection were reported as invalid. An overall HPV prevalence of 75 % (150/200) [95 % CI: 68.4–80.8 %] was observed for all patients, irrespective of the site of HPV positivity. HPV genotypes were detected in 139/191 (72.8 %) [95 % CI: 65.9–79.0 %], 23/200 (11.5 %) [95 % CI: 7.4–16.8 %] and 29/190 (15.3 %) [95 % CI: 10.5–21.2 %] of anal, oro-pharyngeal and urine specimens, respectively. The mean number of HPV types observed in anal, oro-pharyngeal and urine specimens were 4.47, 1.74 and 1.41 HPV types in HPV-positive MSM, respectively. Multiple HPV types were observed in 113/191 (59.2 %) [95 % CI: 51.8–66.2 %] of anal specimens, 7/200 (3.5 %) [95 % CI: 1.4–7.1 %] of oro-pharyngeal specimens and 7/190 (3.7 %) [95 % CI: 1.5–7.4 %] of urine specimens (Fig. 1). The most HPV types observed in an anal specimen was 15, followed by 6 HPV types in an oro-pharyngeal specimen and 4 HPV types in a urine specimen.

For anal specimens, a total of 110 (57.6 %) [95 % CI: 50.3–64.7 %] were HR-HPV positive. HR-HPV types were less prevalent in the pharynx and urine, with 15 (7.5 %) [95 % CI: 4.3–12.1 %] oro-pharyngeal specimens and 15 (7.9 %) [95 % CI: 4.5–12.7 %] urine specimens testing positive for HR-HPV. HPV types 16 and 18, the only HR-HPV types included in both the bivalent and quadrivalent HPV vaccines, were detected in 55 (28.8 %) [95 % CI: 22.5–35.8 %] anal specimens, 6 (3.0 %) [95 % CI: 1.1–6.4 %] oro-pharyngeal specimens and 3 (1.6 %) [95 % CI: 0.3–4.5 %] urine specimens. The prevalence rates of all HPV genotypes included in the quadrivalent HPV vaccine (HPV-6/11/16/18) were 77 (40.3 %) [95 % CI: 33.3–47.6 %], 9 (4.5 %) [95 % CI: 2.1–8.4 %] and 6 (3.2 %) [95 % CI: 1.2–6.8 %] in anal, oro-pharyngeal and urine samples, respectively. HPV types included in the new 9-valent HPV vaccine (HPV-6/11/16/18/31/33/45/52/58) were detected in 110 (57.6 %) [95 % CI: 50.3–64.7 %], 12 (6.0 %) [95 %

Table 1 Baseline and sexual behavioural characteristics stratified according to men who have sex with men only (MSM only) and men who have sex with men and women (MSMW)

Variable	No. (%) of men			*p*-value
	MSM only (*n* = 155)	MSMW (*n* = 45)	Totals (*n* = 200)	
Age [years(IQR)]	33 (26–40)	28 (24–37)	32 (26–39.5)	0.025
Gender				
Male	140 (90.3)	45 (100.0)	185 (92.5)	0.030
Transgender	15 (9.7)	0 (0.0)	15 (7.5)	
Ethnicity				
Black	48 (31.0)	14 (31.1)	62 (31.0)	<0.001
Coloured	38 (24.5)	25 (55.6)	63 (31.5)	
White	65 (41.9)	6 (13.3)	71 (35.5)	
Other	4 (2.6)	0 (0.0)	4 (2.0)	
Education				
Completed high school	122 (78.7)	33 (73.3)	145 (72.5)	<0.001
Tertiary qualification	73 (47.1)	11 (24.4)	84 (42.0)	
Transactional sex				
No	112 (72.3)	11 (24.4)	123 (61.5)	<0.001
Yes, paid money for sex	17 (11.0)	7 (15.6)	24 (12.0)	
Yes, received money for sex	21 (13.5)	15 (33.3)	36 (18.0)	
Yes, paid and received money for sex	5 (3.2)	12 (26.7)	17 (8.5)	
Sex while under the influence of drugs				
Yes	73 (47.1)	32 (71.1)	105 (52.5)	0.004
No	82 (52.9)	13 (28.9)	95 (47.5)	
HIV serostatus				
Positive	81 (52.3)	7 (15.6)	88 (44.0)	<0.001
Negative	74 (47.7)	38 (84.4)	112 (56.0)	
Frequency of insertive anal sex				
Yes	104 (67.1)	39 (86.7)	143 (71.5)	0.010
No	51 (32.9)	6 (13.3)	57 (28.5)	
Frequency of receptive anal sex				
Yes	125 (80.6)	15 (33.3)	140 (70.0)	<0.001
No	30 (19.4)	30 (66.7)	60 (30.0)	
Frequency of receptive oral sex				
Yes	148 (95.5)	26 (57.8)	174 (87.0)	<0.001
No	7 (4.5)	19 (42.2)	26 (13.0)	
Performing oro-anal sex (rimming)				
Yes	67 (43.2)	10 (22.2)	77 (38.9)	0.011
No	88 (56.8)	35 (77.8)	123 (61.5)	

CI: 3.1–10.3 %] and 10 (5.3 %) [95%CI: 2.6–9.5 %] anal, oro-pharyngeal and urine specimens, respectively.

The most common HPV types detected in anal specimens were HPV-16 (42; 22 %), HPV-6 (39; 20.4 %) and HPV-51 (31; 16.2 %). In oro-pharyngeal specimens, the most common HPV types detected were HPV-16 (6; 3.0 %), HPV-72 (4; 2.0 %), followed by HPV-35 and HPV-51 (both 3; 1.5 %). The most prevalent HPV types in urine were HPV-16, HPV-45, HPV-55, HPV-59, HPV-61, HPV-62, HPV-66 and HPV-70 (all 3; 1.6 %). The HPV type specific prevalence rates in anal, oro-pharyngeal and urine specimens are summarised in Fig. 2.

HPV and HIV co-infections

A total of 88 (44.0 %) participants tested HIV-positive in this study. Among the 85 HIV-positive participants with

Table 2 HPV and HIV-co-infection at 3 anatomical sites among MSM in Cape Town, South Africa

HPV type classification	ANAL (n = 191)				ORO-PHARYNGEAL (n = 200)				URINE (n = 190)			
	Total (%)	HIV- (n = 106)	HIV+ (n = 85)	*P*-value	Total (%)	HIV- (n = 112)	HIV+ (n = 88)	*P*-value	Total (%)	HIV- (n = 107)	HIV+ (n = 83)	*P*-value
No type	52 (27.2)	45 (42.4)	7 (8.2)	<0.001	177 (88.5)	104 (92.9)	73 (83.0)	0.029	161 (84.7)	91 (85.1)	70 (84.3)	0.892
Any type	139 (72.8)	61 (57.6)	78 (91.8)	<0.001	23 (11.5)	8 (7.1)	15 (17.1)	0.029	29 (15.3)	16 (14.3)	13 (14.8)	0.892
Single type	26 (13.6)	21 (19.8)	5 (5.9)	0.005	16 (8.0)	6 (5.4)	10 (11.4)	0.120	22 (11.6)	14 (12.5)	8 (9.1)	0.461
Multiple types	113 (59.2)	40 (37.7)	73 (85.9)	<0.001	7 (3.5)	2 (1.8)	5 (5.7)	0.136	7 (3.7)	2 (1.8)	5 (5.7)	0.131
LR-HPV	126 (66.0)	50 (47.2)	76 (89.4)	<0.001	14 (7.0)	4 (3.6)	10 (11.4)	0.032	19 (10.0)	8 (7.5)	11 (13.3)	0.188
HR-HPV	110 (57.6)	41 (38.7)	69 (81.2)	<0.001	15 (7.5)	6 (5.4)	9 (10.2)	0.194	15 (7.9)	9 (8.4)	6 (7.2)	0.764
HPV-6/11	50 (26.2)	19 (17.9)	31 (36.5)	0.003	3 (1.5)	1 (0.9)	2 (2.3)	0.425	3 (1.6)	0 (0.0)	3 (3.6)	0.047
HPV-16/18	55 (28.8)	19 (17.9)	36 (42.4)	<0.001	6 (3.0)	3 (2.7)	3 (3.4)	0.763	3 (1.6)	2 (1.9)	1 (1.2)	0.715
HPV-6/11 /16/18	77 (40.3)	30 (28.3)	47 (55.3)	<0.001	9 (4.5)	4 (3.6)	5 (5.7)	0.474	6 (3.2)	2 (1.9)	4 (4.8)	0.248
HPV-31 /33/45	50 (26.2)	14 (13.2)	36 (42.4)	<0.001	3 (1.5)	0 (0.0)	3 (3.4)	0.048	5 (2.6)	3 (2.8)	2 (2.4)	0.866
HPV-6/11/16 /18/31/33/45	98 (51.3)	36 (34.0)	62 (72.9)	<0.001	11 (5.5)	4 (3.6)	7 (8.0)	0.177	10 (5.3)	5 (4.7)	5 (6.0)	0.679

valid anal HPV results, 78 (91.8 %) were co-infected with any anal HPV ($p < 0.001$), 73 (85.9 %) had multiple anal HPV types ($p < 0.001$), 76 (89.4 %) had LR-HPV ($p < 0.001$) and 69 (81.2 %) were co-infected with HR-HPV ($p < 0.001$) (Table 2). Quadrivalent HPV vaccine types 6, 11, 16 and 18 were detected in 47 (55.3 %) anal specimens of HIV-positive participants ($p < 0.001$), and increased to 62 (72.9 %) with the addition of cross-protection HPV types 31, 33 and 45 ($p < 0.001$). Having any oro-pharyngeal HPV infection (15/88; 17.1 %) and having a LR-HPV oro-pharyngeal infection (10/88; 11.4 %) were significantly associated with being HIV-positive ($p = 0.029$ and $p = 0.032$ respectively). Multiple anal HPV types were detected more frequently in HIV-positive MSM (85.9 % vs 37.7 % in HIV-negative MSM). The mean number of HPV types detected in HPV-positive anal samples was 5.7 (range 1–15) in HIV-positive participants and 2.9 (range 1–10) in HIV-negative participants ($p < 0.001$).

HPV according to sex partner status

Significant differences in anal HPV prevalence were observed between men who had sex with men only (MSM only) and men who had sex with men and women (MSMW) (Table 3). MSMW were less likely to have any

Table 3 HPV infection among MSM only and MSMW at 3 anatomical sites among MSM in Cape Town, South Africa

HPV type classification	ANAL (n = 191)				ORO-PHARYNGEAL (n = 200)				URINE (n = 190)			
	Total (%)	MSM only (n = 150)	MSMW (n = 41)	*P*-value	Total (%)	MSM only (n = 155)	MSMW (n = 45)	*P*-value	Total (%)	MSM only (n = 145)	MSMW (n = 45)	*P*-value
No type	52 (27.2)	22 (14.8)	30 (73.2)	<0.001	177 (88.5)	133 (85.8)	44 (97.8)	0.027	161 (84.7)	123 (84.8)	38 (84.4)	0.950
Any type	139 (72.8)	128 (85.3)	11 (26.8)	<0.001	23 (11.5)	22 (14.2)	1 (2.2)	0.027	29 (15.3)	22 (15.2)	7 (15.6)	0.950
Single type	26 (13.6)	22 (14.7)	4 (9.8)	0.416	16 (8.0)	15 (9.7)	1 (2.2)	0.105	22 (11.6)	18 (12.4)	4 (8.9)	0.519
Multiple types	113 (59.2)	106 (70.7)	7 (17.1)	<0.001	7 (3.5)	7 (4.5)	0 (0.0)	0.147	7 (3.7)	4 (2.8)	3 (6.7)	0.224
LR-HPV	126 (66.0)	117 (78.0)	9 (22.0)	<0.001	14 (7.0)	13 (8.4)	1 (2.2)	0.154	19 (10.0)	15 (10.3)	4 (8.9)	0.776
HR-HPV	110 (57.6)	102 (68.0)	8 (19.50	<0.001	15 (7.5)	15 (9.7)	0 (0.0)	0.030	15 (7.9)	10 (6.9)	5 (11.1)	0.359
HPV-6/11	50 (26.2)	48 (32.0)	2 (4.9)	<0.001	3 (1.5)	3 (1.9)	0 (0.0)	0.347	3 (1.6)	3 (2.1)	0 (0.0)	0.331
HPV-16/18	55 (28.8)	52 (34.7)	3 (7.3)	<0.001	6 (3.0)	6 (3.9)	0 (0.0)	0.180	3 (1.6)	2 (1.4)	1 (2.2)	0.692
HPV-6/11 /16/18	77 (40.3)	73 (48.7)	4 (9.8)	<0.001	9 (4.5)	9 (5.8)	0 (0.0)	0.098	6 (3.2)	5 (3.5)	1 (2.2)	0.681
HPV-31 /33/45	50 (26.2)	48 (32.0)	2 (4.9)	<0.001	3 (1.5)	3 (1.9)	0 (0.0)	0.347	5 (2.6)	2 (1.4)	3 (6.7)	0.053
HPV-6/11/16 /18/31/33/45	98 (51.3)	94 (62.7)	4 (9.8)	<0.001	11 (5.5)	11 (7.1)	0 (0.0)	0.066	10 (5.3)	6 (4.1)	4 (8.9)	0.212

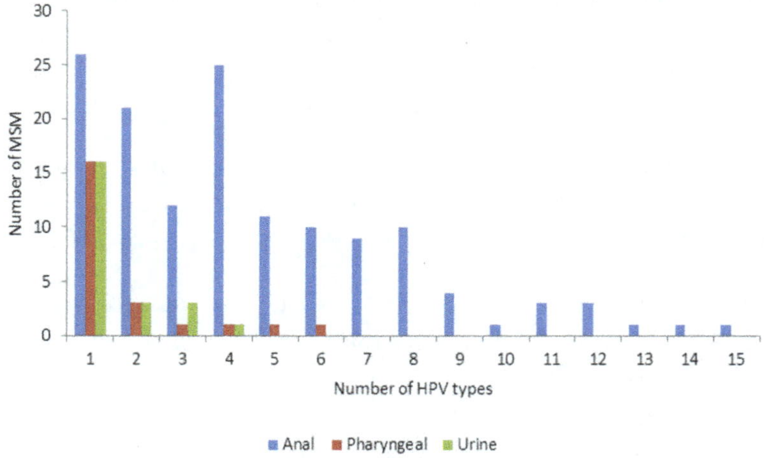

Fig. 1 Number of HPV types in anal, oro-pharyngeal and urine specimens obtained from MSM participants in Cape Town

anal HPV (85.3 % vs.26.8 %; $p < 0.001$), multiple anal HPV (70.7 % vs. 17.1 %; $p < 0.001$), anal LR-HPV (78.0 % vs. 22.0 %; $p < 0.001$), anal HR-HPV (68.0 % vs. 19.5 %; $p < 0.001$), anal HPV-6/11/16/18 (48.7 % vs. 9.8 %; $p < 0.001$) and anal HPV-6/11/16/18/31/33/45 (62.7 % vs. 9.8 %; $p < 0.001$). Individuals who had sex with men only were more likely to have any oro-pharyngeal HPV infection (14.2 % vs. 2.2 %; $p = 0.027$) and to have an oro-pharyngeal HR-HPV infection (9.7 % vs 0.0 %; $p = 0.030$). No significant differences were observed between MSM only and MSMW with regards to the prevalence of HPV in urine specimens.

Risk factors associated with HPV infections

Univariate and multiple logistic regression analyses were performed to assess potential and independent associations between participant characteristics/sexual risk factors and HPV infection in this population (Table 4). In univariate analysis having any anal HPV infection was significantly associated with receiving an income ($p = 0.044$), having sex with men only ($p < 0.001$), engaging in group sex in their lifetime ($p = 0.002$), being HIV positive ($p < 0.001$) and practising receptive anal sex ($p < 0.001$). Having a HR-HPV infection in the anal canal was significantly associated with living outside the city ($p = 0.050$), transgender identity ($p = 0.031$), having sex with men only ($p < 0.001$), engaging in group sex in their lifetime ($p = 0.006$), sharing sex toys in last year ($p = 0.042$), being HIV positive ($p < 0.001$), practising receptive anal sex ($p < 0.001$) and having a gonococcal co-infection ($p = 0.043$). Multiple anal HPV infections were detected more frequently in participants that identified as transgender ($p = 0.022$), having sex with men only ($p < 0.001$), being HIV positive ($p < 0.001$), practising receptive anal sex ($p < 0.001$) and having a gonococcal co-infection ($p = 0.028$). Compared to other ethnicities, coloured MSM had significantly less anal HPV infections overall ($p = 0.023$), including HR-HPV ($p = 0.003$) and multiple HPV types ($p = 0.013$). Individuals who participated in transactional sex had fewer multiple anal HPV infections ($p = 0.010$). In multiple logistic regression analyses, having sex with men only (AOR: 10.9, 95 % CI:

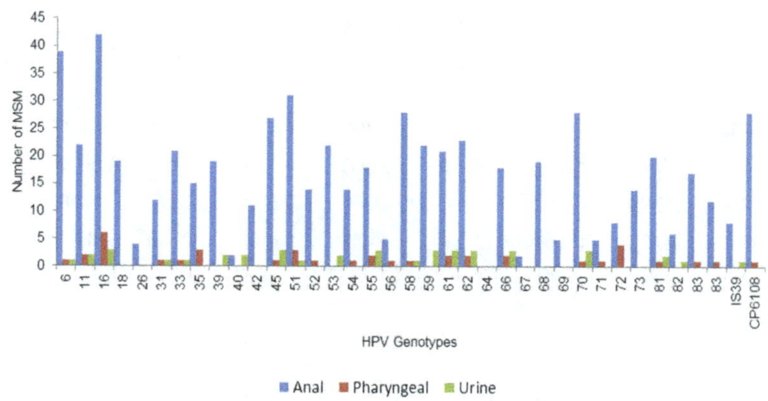

Fig. 2 HPV type-specific prevalence rates in anal, oro-pharyngeal and urine specimens obtained from MSM participants in Cape Town

Table 4 Univariate and multivariate logistic regression analyses for factors associated with any-, high-risk and multiple anal HPV infections

Risk factor	Any HPV					HR-HPV					Multiple HPV				
	No (%)	COR (95 % CI)	*p*	AOR (95 % CI)	*p*	No (%)	COR (95 % CI)	*p*	AOR (95 % CI)	*p*	No (%)	COR (95 % CI)	*p*	AOR (95 % CI)	*p*
Gender															
Male	124 (89.2)	Ref				97 (88.2)	Ref				99 (87.6)	Ref			
Transgender (MTF)	15 (10.8)	1.0				13 (11.8)	5.3 (1.16–24.16)	0.031			14 (12.4)	10.9 (1.40–84.63)	0.022		
Ethnicity															
Black	46 (33.1)	Ref		Ref		40 (36.4)	Ref		Ref		39 (34.5)	Ref			
Coloured	35 (25.2)	0.4 (0.18–0.88)	0.023	0.5 (0.15–1.42)	0.177	24 (21.8)	0.3 (0.15–0.67)	0.003	0.4 (0.13–0.96)	0.042	26 (23.0)	0.4 (0.19–0.82)	0.013		
White	55 (39.6)	1.2 (0.50–2.83)	0.685	0.5 (0.17–1.74)	0.303	45 (40.9)	0.9 (0.44–1.95)	0.847	0.5 (0.19–1.46)	0.219	47 (41.6)	1.2 (0.54–2.42)	0.717		
Other	3 (2.2)	0.9 (0.08–8.85)	0.890	0.2 (0.01–2.14)	0.162	1 (0.9)	0.2 (0.02–1.62)	0.121	0.0 (0.00–0.55)	0.016	1 (0.9)	0.2 (0.02–1.75)	0.137		
Residence															
City/suburbs	96 (69.1)	Ref				73 (66.4)	Ref				76 (67.3)	Ref			
Informal settlement	33 (23.7)	1.6 (0.72–3.73)	0.236			28 (25.5)	1.8 (0.88–3.73)	0.108			28 (24.8)	1.7 (0.80–3.42)	0.171		
Outside city	10 (7.2)	1.0				9 (8.2)	8.1 (1.00–65.96)	0.050			9 (8.0)	7.5 (0.92–60.49)	0.060		
Income status															
No income	24 (17.3)	Ref				18 (16.4)	Ref				20 (17.7)	Ref			
Income	115 (82.7)	2.1 (1.02–4.44)	0.044			92 (83.6)	1.9 (0.94–3.85)	0.072			93 (82.3)	1.6 (0.80–3.23)	0.187		
Sexual behaviour															
Sex partners															
Men and women	11 (2.9)	Ref		Ref		8 (7.3)	Ref		Ref		7 (6.2)	Ref		Ref	
Men only	128 (92.1)	15.9 (6.95–36.24)	<0.001	10.9 (3.88–30.81)	<0.001	102 (92.7)	8.8 (3.75–20.41)	<0.001	4.6 (1.63–12.74)	0.005	106 (93.8)	11.7 (4.82–28.39)	<0.001	5.5 (1.92–15.51)	0.001
Engaged in group sex in lifetime															
No	40 (28.8)	Ref		Ref		30 (27.3)	Ref		Ref		34 (30.1)	Ref			

Table 4 Univariate and multivariate logistic regression analyses for factors associated with any-, high-risk and multiple anal HPV infections *(Continued)*

Shared sex toys in past 12 months															
No	111 (79.9)	Ref				85 (77.3)	Ref				88 (77.9)	Ref			
Yes	28 (20.1)	1.9 (0.75–4.98)	0.172			25 (22.7)	2.4 (1.03–5.36)	0.042			25 (22.1)	2.2 (0.95–4.97)	0.064		
Transactional sex															
No	92 (66.2)	Ref				74 (67.3)	Ref				79 (69.9)	Ref			
Paid and/or received money	47 (33.8)	0.6 (0.29–1.05)	0.072			36 (32.7)	0.6 (0.34–1.10)	0.100			34 (30.1)	0.5 (0.25–0.82)	0.010		
HIV serostatus															
Negative	61 (43.9)	Ref		Ref		41 (37.3)	Ref		Ref		40 (35.4)	Ref		Ref	
Positive	78 (56.1)	8.2 (3.46–19.50)	<0.001	4.1 (1.52–11.22)	0.006	69 (62.7)	6.8 (3.50–13.36)	<0.001	4.0 (1.82–8.65)	<0.001	73 (64.6)	10.0 (4.86–20.74)	<0.001	6.9 (3.10–15.42)	<0.001
Receptive anal intercourse with men															
Never practised	24 (17.3)	Ref				14 (12.7)	Ref		Ref		14 (12.4)	Ref		Ref	
Practised	115 (82.7)	7.7 (3.77–15.61)	<0.001	3.3 (1.36–8.09)	0.009	96 (87.3)	11.0 (4.97–24.21)	<0.001	4.3 (1.80–10.13)	0.001	99 (87.6)	11.3 (5.13–24.95)	<0.001	4.2 (1.79–9.65)	0.001
Anal gonorrhoea															
Negative	125 (89.9)	Ref				98 (89.1)	Ref				100 (88.5)	Ref			
Positive	14 (10.1)	1.0				12 (10.9)	4.8 (1.05–22.25)	0.043			13 (11.5)	10.0 (1.28–78.19)	0.028		

3.88–30.81, $p < 0.001$), engaging in group sex in lifetime (AOR: 4.7, 95 % CI: 1.79–12.43, $p = 0.002$), being HIV-positive (AOR: 4.1, 95 % CI: 1.52–11.22, $p = 0.006$) and practising receptive anal intercourse (AOR: 3.3, 95 % CI: 1.36–8.09, $p = 0.009$) were the only factors associated with having any anal HPV infection after adjusting for confounders and other variables found significant in the univariate analysis. Coloured ethnicity was associated with significantly less anal HR-HPV infections (AOR: 0.4, 95 % CI: 0.13–0.96, $p = 0.042$) while having sex with men only (AOR: 4.6, 95 % CI: 1.63–12.74, $p = 0.005$), engaging in group sex in lifetime (AOR: 3.1, 95 % CI: 1.35–7.07, $p = 0.006$), being HIV-positive (AOR: 4.1, 95 % CI: 1.89–8.83, $p < 0.001$) and practicing receptive anal intercourse (AOR: 4.3, 95 % CI: 1.80–10.13, $p < 0.001$) were all associated with having a greater likelihood of infection by a HR-HPV type. Having multiple anal HPV infections were independently associated with having sex with men only (AOR: 5.5, 95 % CI: 1.92–15.51, $p = 0.001$), being HIV-positive (AOR: 6.9, 95 % CI: 3.10–15.42, $p < 0.001$) and practising receptive anal intercourse (AOR: 4.2, 95 % CI: 1.79–9.65, $p = 0.001$). Age group, education, job status, partner status, number of male sexual partners in the past 12 months, sex at sex-on-site venues, sex with a partner met through the internet, engaging in group sex in the past 12 months, alcohol and drug use during sex, having had a STI in the past 12 months, syphilis serostatus and having an anal chlamydial infection were not significantly associated with the three HPV outcomes in the anal canal. Further, no risk factors were independently associated with oro-pharyngeal HPV infections or with HPV detected in the urine.

Discussion

This study reports HPV prevalence and risk factors associated with HPV infections at three different anatomical sites among high-risk MSM in Cape Town. We found a high prevalence of HR-HPV (57.6 %) in the anal canal of study participants. HPV genotypes were less frequently detected in the pharynx (11.5 %) and urine (15.3 %) of study participants. Previous studies have shown that anal HPV infection is more common among MSM than heterosexual men (MSW), and that anal HPV prevalence rates can be 4–10 times higher in MSM compared to MSW [19, 20]. The high prevalence of anal HPV infection observed in this study is similar to anal HPV prevalence rates for high-risk MSM reported in Peru, Italy and Thailand but higher than anal HPV prevalence rates reported in countries such as Australia and Puerto Rico [9, 21–24].

MSM who are HIV-positive have an increased risk of anal HPV infection and anal cancer. HPV prevalence rates of 89–93 % have been reported among HIV-positive MSM in a recent systematic review and meta-analysis of 53 studies [7]. The incidence of anal cancer among HIV-positive MSM is more than 80-fold higher than that observed in the general population [25]. HIV infection has been shown to increase susceptibility to persistent HPV, increasing the risk of acquiring new HPV infections and reactivation of latent HPV infections [12]. Persons who are at high risk for HIV acquisition may be at higher risk of HPV infection due to the same high risk sexual practises [11]. As shown in Table 2, HIV-positive MSM had significantly more anal HPV infections overall (91.8 % HIV-infected vs. 57.6 % HIV-uninfected), including LR-HPV, HR-HPV, multiple HPV types and HPV vaccine types (HPV-6/11/16/18 + 31/33/45). The most common LR-HPV and HR-HPV types detected in the anal specimens of all MSM as well as HIV-positive MSM were HPV-6 and HPV-16 respectively, followed by high risk types HPV-58, HPV-45 and HPV-51. HPV-16 was also the most common HR-HPV type found in HIV-positive MSM from Thailand, USA, China, Spain and Canada [9, 12, 26–28].

Multiple anal HPV infections are commonly described among MSM, especially HIV-positive MSM [8, 26–28]. Having more than one HPV type detected was more common in the anal canal of MSM while single HPV infections were more frequently detected in the pharynx and urine. In this study, multiple HPV types were detected in the anal specimens of 59.2 % of all MSM, 81.3 % of all HPV-positive MSM and 85.9 % of HIV-positive MSM. Among an HIV-positive MSM cohort in Canada (HIPVIRG cohort study), the majority of participants (90.9 %) were infected with multiple HPV types in the anal canal, ranging between 0 and 18 HPV types (mean 5 HPV types) [12]. More recently, Supindham et al. [9] reported a 100 % HPV co-infection rate in the anal specimens of HIV-positive MSM in Thailand, with the majority being multiple HPV infections (mean 4.8 HPV types). The mean number of anal HPV types detected in HPV-positive MSM in this study was 4.5 types, which increased to 5.7 types among HIV-positive MSM ($p < 0.001$). The highest number of HPV types detected in a single anal sample was 15 HPV types in an HIV-positive participant co-infected with anal gonorrhoea and chlamydia. The mean number of HPV types in the oropharynx and urine was 1.7 and 1.4 types respectively, and the number of HPV types at these anatomical sites did not differ significantly according to HIV status. Multiple anal HPV infections are a cause for concern due to the strong association with anal intraepithelial neoplasia (AIN) and the development to high-grade AIN and anal cancer [29, 30].

Oro-pharyngeal HPV infections are much less common in adults than anogenital HPV infections [31]. King et al. [14] reported that the majority of HPV infections detected in the oral cavity of MSM in London were single HPV types. However, the incidence of HPV-related oro-pharyngeal cancers in the general population is increasing relative to other oral cancers associated with alcohol and tobacco use. A number of HR-HPV types have been implicated in carcinogenesis and tumour progression at different anatomical sites and are mainly due to the actions of their E6 and E7 viral oncogenes, which induce and maintain cellular transformation [32]. The majority of oro-pharyngeal squamous cell carcinomas (OPSCC) (+ – 90 % of cases) are associated with HPV-16 infection; however other HR-HPV types have also been identified in HPV-positive OPSCC and these types, although rare, constitute an important subset of oro-pharyngeal cancers which should not be ignored [33]. A few studies have reported associations between non-HPV-16 high-risk types and oro-pharyngeal cancer after controlling for or excluding HPV-16 infection [34–36]. A large US case–control study demonstrated that combined infections with HPV-16 and other HR-HPV types significantly increased the risk of head and neck squamous cell carcinoma [36]. Further studies are needed to determine whether oro-pharyngeal tumours containing non-HPV-16 high-risk types present less often with lymph node metastases and have better treatment outcomes [33, 37]. Davidson et al [38] reported a HPV prevalence of 5.6 % in oral rinse and gargle samples among male factory workers in Pretoria, South Africa, aged 17 - 64 years. Although oral sex was not common in this population, it was practised among men identified with HR-HPV infection [38]. Performing oral and oro-anal sex on men and women were not associated with oro-pharyngeal HPV infections in this study. However, HIV-positive MSM had significantly more oro-pharyngeal HPV infections (17.1 % in HIV-positive vs. 7.1 % in HIV-negative; $p = 0.029$), including LR-HPV infections (11.4 % in HIV-positive vs. 3.6 % in HIV-negative; $p = 0.032$). It is not clear if the increased oral HPV incidence in HIV-positive individuals is due to HIV-related immunosuppression or due to risky sexual practises [39]. In Italy, Parisi et al. [40] detected HPV in the oral specimens of approximately 20 % of HIV-infected MSM, which is lower than that reported by Blas et al. [41] (44.3 %) in Peru, but higher than the oro-pharyngeal HPV prevalence rates in HIV-positive MSM reported in this study. In our study, having any HPV infection or a LR-HPV infection in the oropharynx were the only oro-pharyngeal HPV groupings associated with being HIV-positive. No differences were observed between HIV-negative and HIV-positive MSM with regards to the prevalence of single HPV types, multiple HPV types, HR-HPV or HPV vaccine types detected in the oropharynx.

This study showed that MSM only had over three times more anal HPV infections and over 6 times more oro-pharyngeal HPV infections than MSMW. Anal HPV prevalence rates among MSM only were significantly higher for all HPV groupings, except for single HPV type prevalence. Having any oro-pharyngeal HPV infection or an oro-pharyngeal HR-HPV infection were the only oro-pharyngeal HPV groupings that showed significant differences between MSM only and MSMW. No significant differences were observed in the prevalence of HPV in urine between MSM only and MSMW. Compared to other male populations higher anal HPV prevalence rates are frequently reported for MSM only [19, 24, 42]. Limited information is available in the literature describing HPV prevalence rates in MSMW, especially anal HPV prevalence rates. Lu et al. [43] studied the sero-prevalence of quadrivalent HPV vaccine types (HPV-6,11,16,18) among men with different sexual practises in Brazil, Mexico and USA (The *HIM* study) and found MSMW to have lower HPV seroprevalence rates than MSM but higher than in MSW. Genital HPV prevalence analysis in the same *HIM* study cohort showed that MSMW had higher HPV prevalence rates on the penis and scrotum compared to MSM and MSW, which could be attributed to increased number of sex partners and increased frequency of insertive sex acts among MSMW. In our study, in comparison with the MSM only group, significantly fewer MSMW were HIV-positive, practised receptive anal intercourse with men whilst more MSMW practised insertive anal intercourse with men. These sexual practises could account for the absence of gonococcal and chlamydial co-infections detected in the anal canal of MSMW and the increased number of chlamydial co-infections detected in the urine of MSMW. MSMW were also less likely to be syphilis seropositive. Even though anal HPV infection among MSMW who practise receptive anal intercourse could be linked to these sexual practises, anal HPV transmission can also be attributed to other factors, similar to those found among HPV-infected MSW, such as transmission through skin contact, sharing sex toys or vertical transmission. Genital HPV genotypes have been detected on fingers and HPV transmission between ano-genital sites and hands have previously been reported among heterosexual couples [44]. These alternative modes of HPV transmission could explain the observation that 17.3 % of men who indicated no history of receptive anal intercourse had HPV detected in the anal canal.

This study had a number of limitations. Firstly, the relatively small sample size may have resulted in the misidentification of some predictors of HPV infection, especially in oro-pharyngeal and urine samples where the prevalence of HPV was low. Secondly, the liquid oral rinse sampling method has been shown to have a higher sensitivity than oro-pharyngeal swabs for the detection of HPV in the mouth and throat and therefore the use of oro-pharyngeal swabs in this study could have decreased the HPV detection rate in the oropharynx [13]. Thirdly, we were only able to test DNA extracts from urine as an indicator of urethral HPV infection. This was due to the sampling undertaken in the primary study; the true prevalence of penile HPV may have been higher than that reported here if penile samples had also been available for additional HPV testing. Fourthly, the participants attended one clinic in Cape Town and the findings of this study might not be generalized to the South African MSM population.

In keeping with South Africa's National Strategic Plan for HIV and AIDS, STIs and TB, scaling up services for most at risk populations (including MSM) to reduce HIV/STI burden should be prioritised. For HPV, these efforts include targeted behavioural interventions such as promotion of proper and consistent condom use, medical male circumcision to reduce the incidence, prevalence and persistence of HPV infections in MSM and HPV vaccination of boys. The South African government is currently providing free HPV vaccinations for 9–10 year old girls in all public schools in South Africa but it is unlikely that MSM would benefit from herd immunity due to female vaccination roll-out and it would be optimal to vaccinate boys directly. Randomised controlled trials have shown HPV vaccination to be highly efficacious in MSM with the potential to substantially reduce the burden of HPV-associated disease in this population [45]. More studies are needed to determine the natural history and burden of HPV-associated diseases in South African MSM in order to formulate effective HPV prevention strategies for the future.

Conclusions

A high prevalence of anal HPV infection was observed in this MSM population in Cape Town. All HPV groupings (any HPV, LR-HPV, HR-HPV, single type, multiple type, quadrivalent vaccine types) were more prevalent in the anal canal of HIV-positive MSM. Risk factors associated with any HPV, HR-HPV and multiple HPV types in the anal canal included having sex with men only, being HIV-positive and practising receptive anal intercourse. No risk factors were independently associated with oropharyngeal HPV infection or HPV detected in urine. Targeted interventions and HPV vaccination of boys should be considered to reduce the burden of HPV-related diseases among MSM in South Africa.

Abbreviations

AOR, adjusted odds ratio; CI, confidence interval; COR, crude odds ratio; HIV, human immunodeficiency virus; HPV, human papillomavirus; HR, high-risk; IQR, interquartile range; ISH, *in situ* hybridisation; ITCMH, Ivan Toms Centre for Men's Health; LA, linear Array; LR, low-risk; MSM, men-who-have-sex-with-men; MSMW, men-who-have-sex-with-men-and-women; MSW, men-who-have-sex-with-women; NICD, National Institute for Communicable Diseases; SD, standard deviation; SPM, sexual partner matrix; STI, sexually transmitted infection; TGW, transgender women

Acknowledgments

The authors would like to thank staff that collected specimens and questionnaire data at the Ivan Toms Centre for Men's Health in Woodstock, Cape Town and study participants for their cooperation in this study. Special thanks go to Dr Tendesayi Kufa-Chakezha for her assistance with statistical analysis and general comments related to the manuscript.

Funding

The sub study was funded by the Global Disease Detection (GDD) programme grant no. 1U19GH000622-01 while the main study received funding and support from PEPFAR/USAID and the Anova Health Institute NPC. The Anova Health Institute NPC is supported by the US President's Emergency Plan for AIDS Relief (PEPFAR) program via the US Agency for International Development, (USAID) under Cooperative Agreement No. AID-674-A-12-00015.

Authors' contributions

EEM worked on the conceptualization of the sub study, study design, ethics approval, laboratory testing, data analysis, interpretation of data and manuscript preparation; KR worked on study design, ethics approval, specimen and data collection, interpretation of data and manuscript preparation; TFC worked on data analysis and interpretation of data; HS and JM worked on the conceptualization of the original study and manuscript preparation; DAL worked on the conceptualization of the study, interpretation of data and manuscript preparation. All authors read and approved the final manuscript.

Competing interests

The authors declare that they have no competing interests.

Consent for publication

Not applicable.

Author details

[1]Centre for HIV and Sexually Transmitted Infections, National Institute for Communicable Diseases, National Health Laboratory Service, Johannesburg, South Africa. [2]Anova Health Institute, Johannesburg, South Africa. [3]Anova Health Institute, Cape Town, South Africa. [4]Department of Medicine, Division of Infectious Diseases and HIV Medicine, University of Cape Town, Cape Town, South Africa. [5]Division of Epidemiology and Biostatistics, School of Public Health, University of the Witwatersrand, Johannesburg, South Africa. [6]Division of Epidemiology & Biostatistics, School of Public & Family Medicine, University of Cape Town, Cape Town, South Africa. [7]Western Sydney Sexual Health Centre, Western Sydney Local Health District, Parramatta, Australia. [8]Marie Bashir Institute for Infectious Diseases and Biosecurity & Sydney Medical School-Westmead, University of Sydney, Sydney, Australia.

References

1. Giuliano AR, Tortolero-Luna G, Ferrer E, Burchell AN, de Sanjose S, Kjaer SK, Munoz N, Schiffman M, Bosch FX. Epidemiology of human papillomavirus infection in men, cancers other than cervical and benign conditions. Vaccine. 2008;26 Suppl 10:K17–28.
2. Rositch AF, Mao L, Hudgens MG, Moses S, Agot K, Backes DM, Nyagaya E, Snijders PJ, Meijer CJ, Bailey RC, et al. Risk of HIV acquisition among circumcised and uncircumcised young men with penile human papillomavirus infection. AIDS. 2014;28(5):745–52.
3. Mbulawa ZZ, Marais DJ, Johnson LF, Coetzee D, Williamson AL. Impact of human immunodeficiency virus on the natural history of human papillomavirus genital infection in South African men and women. J Infect Dis. 2012;206(1):15–27.

4. Shisana O, Rehle T, Simbayi LC, Zuma K, Jooste S, Zungu N, Labadarios D, Onoya D. South African National HIV Prevalence, Incidence and Behaviour Survey. Cape Town: HSRC Press; 2012. ISBN 978-0-7969-2456-8 2014.
5. Human Sciences Research Council. Three cities study: high levels of HIV infection found among men who have sex with men: The South African Marang Men's Project. 2014. http://www.hsrc.ac.za/en/media-briefs/hiv-aids-stis-and-tb/marang. Accessed 13 Aug 2015.
6. Baggaley RF, White RG, Boily MC. HIV transmission risk through anal intercourse: systematic review, meta-analysis and implications for HIV prevention. Int J Epidemiol. 2010;39(4):1048–63.
7. Machalek DA, Poynten M, Jin F, Fairley CK, Farnsworth A, Garland SM, Hillman RJ, Petoumenos K, Roberts J, Tabrizi SN, et al. Anal human papillomavirus infection and associated neoplastic lesions in men who have sex with men: a systematic review and meta-analysis. Lancet Oncol. 2012;13(5):487–500.
8. Mendez-Martinez R, Rivera-Martinez NE, Crabtree-Ramirez B, Sierra-Madero JG, Caro-Vega Y, Galvan SC, de Leon DC, Garcia-Carranca A. Multiple human papillomavirus infections are highly prevalent in the anal canal of human immunodeficiency virus-positive men who have sex with men. BMC Infect Dis. 2014;14:671.
9. Supindham T, Chariyalertsak S, Utaipat U, Miura T, Ruanpeng D, Chotirosniramit N, Kosashunhanan N, Sugandhavesa P, Saokhieo P, Songsupa R, et al. High Prevalence and Genotype Diversity of Anal HPV Infection among MSM in Northern Thailand. PLoS One. 2015;10(5):e0124499.
10. Wirtz AL, Zelaya CE, Peryshkina A, McGowan I, Cranston RD, Latkin C, Galai N, Mogilniy V, Dzhigun P, Kostetskaya I, et al. Anal human papillomavirus and HIV: A cross-sectional study among men who have sex with men in Moscow, Russia, 2012-2013. Euro Surveill. 2015;20(15):pii=21095.
11. Hu Y, Qian HZ, Sun J, Gao L, Yin L, Li X, Xiao D, Li D, Sun X, Ruan Y, et al. Anal human papillomavirus infection among HIV-infected and uninfected men who have sex with men in Beijing, China. J Acquir Immune Defic Syndr. 2013;64(1):103–14.
12. de Pokomandy A, Rouleau D, Ghattas G, Vezina S, Cote P, Macleod J, Allaire G, Franco EL, Coutlee F. Prevalence, clearance, and incidence of anal human papillomavirus infection in HIV-infected men: the HIPVIRG cohort study. J Infect Dis. 2009;199(7):965–73.
13. Read TR, Hocking JS, Vodstrcil LA, Tabrizi SN, McCullough MJ, Grulich AE; Garland SM, Bradshaw CS, Chen MY, Fairley CK. Oral human papillomavirus in men having sex with men: risk-factors and sampling. PLoS One. 2012; 7(11):e49324.
14. King EM, Gilson R, Beddows S, Soldan K, Panwar K, Young C, Jit M, Edmunds WJ, Sonnenberg P. Oral human papillomavirus (HPV) infection in men who have sex with men: prevalence and lack of anogenital concordance. Sex Transm Infect. 2015;91(4):284–6.
15. Shigehara K, Sasagawa T, Namiki M. Human papillomavirus infection and pathogenesis in urothelial cells: a mini-review. J Infect Chemother. 2014; 20(12):741–7.
16. SANAC. National Strategic Plan on HIV, STIs and TB: 2012-2016. Edited by SANAC. Pretoria: SANAC; 2012.
17. Rebe K, Lewis D, Myer L, de Swardt G, Struthers H, Kamkuemah M, McIntyre J. A Cross Sectional Analysis of Gonococcal and Chlamydial Infections among Men-Who-Have-Sex-with-Men in Cape Town, South Africa. PLoS One. 2015;10(9):e0138315.
18. South African Department of Health. First Line Comprehensive Management and Control of Sexually Transmitted Infections (STIs). Protocol for the management of a person with a sexually transmitted infection according to the essential drug list. 2003. Department of Health. http://www.nicd.ac.za/assets/files/STI%20Book%202008%20Edited(1).pdf. Accessed 07 June 2016.
19. Nyitray AG, da Silva RJ C, Baggio ML, Lu B, Smith D, Abrahamsen M, Papenfuss M, Villa LL, Lazcano-Ponce E, Giuliano AR. Age-specific prevalence of and risk factors for anal human papillomavirus (HPV) among men who have sex with women and men who have sex with men: the HPV in men (HIM) study. J Infect Dis. 2011;203(1):49–57.
20. Goldstone S, Palefsky JM, Giuliano AR, Moreira Jr ED, Aranda C, Jessen H, Hillman RJ, Ferris DG, Coutlee F, Liaw KL, et al. Prevalence of and risk factors for human papillomavirus (HPV) infection among HIV-seronegative men who have sex with men. J Infect Dis. 2011;203(1):66–74.
21. Quinn R, Salvatierra J, Solari V, Calderon M, Ton TG, Zunt JR. Human papillomavirus infection in men who have sex with men in Lima, Peru. AIDS Res Hum Retroviruses. 2012;28(12):1734–8.
22. Latini A, Dona MG, Ronchetti L, Giglio A, Moretto D, Colafigli M, Laquintana V, Frasca M, Zaccarelli M, Antinori A, et al. Prevalence of anal human papillomavirus infection and cytologic abnormalities among HIV-infected and HIV-uninfected men who have sex with men. J Int AIDS Soc. 2014;17(4 Suppl 3):19662.
23. Zou H, Tabrizi SN, Grulich AE, Garland SM, Hocking JS, Bradshaw CS, Morrow A, Prestage G, Cornall AM, Fairley CK, et al. Early acquisition of anogenital human papillomavirus among teenage men who have sex with men. J Infect Dis. 2014;209(5):642–51.
24. Colon-Lopez V, Ortiz AP, Del Toro-Mejias L, Clatts MC, Palefsky JM. Epidemiology of anal HPV infection in high-risk men attending a sexually transmitted infection clinic in Puerto Rico. PLoS One. 2014;9(1):e83209.
25. Silverberg MJ, Lau B, Justice AC, Engels E, Gill MJ, Goedert JJ, Kirk GD, D'Souza G, Bosch RJ, Brooks JT, et al. Risk of anal cancer in HIV-infected and HIV-uninfected individuals in North America. Clin Infect Dis. 2012;54(7):1026–34.
26. Gao L, Zhou F, Li X, Yang Y, Ruan Y, Jin Q. Anal HPV infection in HIV-positive men who have sex with men from China. PLoS One. 2010;5(12):e15256.
27. Torres M, Gonzalez C, del Romero J, Viciana P, Ocampo A, Rodriguez-Fortunez P, Masia M, Blanco JR, Portilla J, Rodriguez C, et al. Anal human papillomavirus genotype distribution in HIV-infected men who have sex with men by geographical origin, age, and cytological status in a Spanish cohort. J Clin Microbiol. 2013;51(11):3512–20.
28. Sahasrabuddhe VV, Castle PE, Follansbee S, Borgonovo S, Tokugawa D, Schwartz LM, Lorey TS, LaMere BJ, Gage JC, Fetterman B, et al. Human papillomavirus genotype attribution and estimation of preventable fraction of anal intraepithelial neoplasia cases among HIV-infected men who have sex with men. J Infect Dis. 2013;207(3):392–401.
29. Coutlee F, de Pokomandy A, Franco EL. Epidemiology, natural history and risk factors for anal intraepithelial neoplasia. Sex Health. 2012;9(6):547–55.
30. Sendagorta E, Herranz P, Guadalajara H, Zamora FX. [Early detection of anal intraepithelial neoplasia in high-risk patients]. Actas Dermosifiliogr. 2011; 102(10):757–65.
31. D'Souza G, Fakhry C, Sugar EA, Seaberg EC, Weber K, Minkoff HL, Anastos K, Palefsky JM, Gillison ML. Six-month natural history of oral versus cervical human papillomavirus infection. Int J Cancer. 2007;121(1):143–50.
32. Narisawa-Saito M, Kiyono T. Basic mechanisms of high-risk human papillomavirus-induced carcinogenesis: roles of E6 and E7 proteins. Cancer Sci. 2007;98(10):1505–11.
33. Walline HM, Komarck C, McHugh JB, Byrd SA, Spector ME, Hauff SJ, Graham MP, Bellile E, Moyer JS, Prince ME, et al. High-risk human papillomavirus detection in oropharyngeal, nasopharyngeal, and oral cavity cancers: comparison of multiple methods. JAMA Otolaryngol Head Neck Surg. 2013;139(12):1320–7.
34. Anantharaman D, Gheit T, Waterboer T, Abedi-Ardekani B, Carreira C, McKay-Chopin S, Gaborieau V, Marron M, Lagiou P, Ahrens W, et al. Human papillomavirus infections and upper aero-digestive tract cancers: the ARCAGE study. J Natl Cancer Inst. 2013;105(8):536–45.
35. Ribeiro KB, Levi JE, Pawlita M, Koifman S, Matos E, Eluf-Neto J, Wunsch-Filho V, Curado MP, Shangina O, Zaridze D, et al. Low human papillomavirus prevalence in head and neck cancer: results from two large case-control studies in high-incidence regions. Int J Epidemiol. 2011;40(2):489–502.
36. Michaud DS, Langevin SM, Eliot M, Nelson HH, Pawlita M, McClean MD, Kelsey KT. High-risk HPV types and head and neck cancer. Int J Cancer. 2014;135(7):1653–61.
37. Nichols AC, Dhaliwal SS, Palma DA, Basmaji J, Chapeskie C, Dowthwaite S, Franklin JH, Fung K, Kwan K, Wehrli B, et al. Does HPV type affect outcome in oropharyngeal cancer? J Otolaryngol Head Neck Surg. 2013;42:9.
38. Davidson CL, Richter KL, Van der Linde M, Coetsee J, Boy SC. Prevalence of oral and oropharyngeal human papillomavirus in a sample of South African men: a pilot study. S Afr Med J. 2014;104(5):358–61.
39. Mooij SH, Boot HJ, Speksnijder AG, Meijer CJ, King AJ, Verhagen DW, de Vries HJ, Quint WG, Molijn A, de Koning MN, et al. Six-month incidence and persistence of oral HPV infection in HIV-negative and HIV-infected men who have sex with men. PLoS One. 2014;9(6):e98955.
40. Parisi SG, Cruciani M, Scaggiante R, Boldrin C, Andreis S, Dal Bello F, Pagni S, Barelli A, Sattin A, Mengoli C, et al. Anal and oral human papillomavirus (HPV) infection in HIV-infected subjects in northern Italy: a longitudinal cohort study among men who have sex with men. BMC Infect Dis. 2011;11:150.
41. Blas MM, Brown B, Menacho L, Alva IE, Silva-Santisteban A, Carcamo C. HPV

Prevalence in Multiple Anatomical Sites among Men Who Have Sex with Men in Peru. PLoS One. 2015;10(10):e0139524.

42. Nyitray AG, da Silva RJ C, Baggio ML, Smith D, Abrahamsen M, Papenfuss M, Lin HY, Quiterio M, Salmeron J, Lazcano-Ponce E, et al. Six-month incidence, persistence, and factors associated with persistence of anal human papillomavirus in men: the HPV in men study. J Infect Dis. 2011;204(11):1711–22.
43. Lu B, Viscidi RP, Lee JH, Wu Y, Villa LL, Lazcano-Ponce E, da Silva RJ, Baggio ML, Quiterio M, Salmeron J, et al. Human papillomavirus (HPV) 6, 11, 16, and 18 seroprevalence is associated with sexual practice and age: results from the multinational HPV Infection in Men Study (HIM Study). Cancer Epidemiol Biomarkers Prev. 2011;20(5):990–1002.
44. Hernandez BY, Wilkens LR, Zhu X, Thompson P, McDuffie K, Shvetsov YB, Kamemoto LE, Killeen J, Ning L, Goodman MT. Transmission of human papillomavirus in heterosexual couples. Emerg Infect Dis. 2008;14(6):888–94.
45. Palefsky J, Giuliano A. Quadrivalent HPV vaccine efficacy in men having sex with men. Malmo: Paper presented at: International Papillomavirus Conference; May 2009; 2009.

3

Comparison of DNA testing strategies in monitoring human papillomavirus infection prevalence through simulation

Carol Y. Lin[1*] and Ling Li[2]

Abstract

Background: HPV DNA diagnostic tests for epidemiology monitoring (research purpose) or cervical cancer screening (clinical purpose) have often been considered separately. Women with positive Linear Array (LA) polymerase chain reaction (PCR) research test results typically are neither informed nor referred for colposcopy. Recently, a sequential testing by using Hybrid Capture 2 (HC2) HPV clinical test as a triage before genotype by LA has been adopted for monitoring HPV infections. Also, HC2 has been reported as a more feasible screening approach for cervical cancer in low-resource countries. Thus, knowing the performance of testing strategies incorporating HPV clinical test (i.e., HC2-only or using HC2 as a triage before genotype by LA) compared with LA-only testing in measuring HPV prevalence will be informative for public health practice.

Method: We conducted a Monte Carlo simulation study. Data were generated using mathematical algorithms. We designated the reported HPV infection prevalence in the U.S. and Latin America as the "true" underlying type-specific HPV prevalence. Analytical sensitivity of HC2 for detecting 14 high-risk (oncogenic) types was considered to be less than LA. Estimated-to-true prevalence ratios and percentage reductions were calculated.

Results: When the "true" HPV prevalence was designated as the reported prevalence in the U.S., with LA genotyping sensitivity and specificity of (0.95, 0.95), estimated-to-true prevalence ratios of 14 high-risk types were 2.132, 1.056, 0.958 for LA-only, HC2-only, and sequential testing, respectively. Estimated-to-true prevalence ratios of two vaccine-associated high-risk types were 2.359 and 1.063 for LA-only and sequential testing, respectively. When designated type-specific prevalence of HPV16 and 18 were reduced by 50 %, using either LA-only or sequential testing, prevalence estimates were reduced by 18 %.

Conclusion: Estimated-to-true HPV infection prevalence ratios using LA-only testing strategy are generally higher than using HC2-only or using HC2 as a triage before genotype by LA. HPV clinical testing can be incorporated to monitor HPV prevalence or vaccine effectiveness. Caution is needed when comparing apparent prevalence from different testing strategies.

Keywords: HPV prevalence, PCR, HPV clinical test, HPV vaccine effectiveness, Cervical cancer screening

* Correspondence: clin@cdc.gov
[1]Centers for Disease Control and Prevention, Atlanta, GA, USA
Full list of author information is available at the end of the article

Background

Cervical cancer is the third most common cancer among women and the second most frequent cause of cancer-related deaths, accounting for approximately 300,000 deaths annually worldwide [1]. More than 80 % of these cervical cancer related deaths occurs in low-resource countries [2]. Human papillomavirus (HPV) infections have been identified as a necessary cause of cervical cancer [3–5]. Screening and vaccination are the best strategies for reducing cervical cancer incidence. HPV-clinical DNA testing has been considered as a more cost- effective and feasible approach [3]. Since HPV vaccination was introduced in 2006, many developed countries also have initiated HPV immunization programs for adolescents [6–8]. While the high cost of HPV vaccination remains a barrier, HPV vaccine has been introduced in some developing countries successfully [9]. Because cervical cancer outcomes take years to observe, monitoring HPV infections has served as an early indication of vaccine effectiveness [7, 10–13]. In this study, we compare three HPV DNA testing strategies for monitoring HPV infection prevalence.

Molecular testing methods are available for detecting HPV infections for research or for clinical purposes. Polymerase chain reaction (PCR)-based DNA genotyping tests using target amplification technique can detect the existence of minute amounts of virus and have been considered as the "gold standard" for detecting infectious organisms [14, 15]. Linear Array (LA) genotyping assay is the commercialized version of PCR genotyping testing designed to standardize the PCR process for detecting existence of HPV DNA for research purposes. The LA genotyping assay is based on PCR amplification of a 450-bp sequence of the L1 region by using PGMY09/11 primer, hybridization of the amplified product to oligonucleotide probes, and their detection by colorimetric reaction [16]. LA can detect 37 HPV genotypes simultaneously. The test has been used in epidemiological and clinical research studies to detect HPV infections and is also the most widely used assay by HPV LabNet laboratories to monitor HPV infection prevalence for HPV vaccine effectiveness [17]. By comparison, commercially available Digene Hybrid Capture 2 (HC2) clinical-HPV assay uses the signal amplified hybridization microplate-based technique to detect HPV DNA presence. The HC2 clinical HPV test is an aggregate test that detects 13 high-risk (oncogenic) types (HPV16, 18, 31, 33, 35, 39, 45, 51, 52, 56, 58, 59, and 68), and because of cross-reactivity, it can also detect HPV66. HC2 is designed to detect high enough viral loads (i.e., clinically relevant viral loads), and it has been used as a co-test with the Papanicolaou smear test or a clinical test alone for screening women likely to develop or who have already developed cervical cancer. The HC2 assay has also been used as a reference test in studies evaluating newly developed clinical-HPV assays [18, 19].

PCR genotyping test has been used to monitor HPV infection prevalence and vaccine effectiveness for research purposes because of its high analytical sensitivity. Women with positive PCR genotyping test results typically are neither informed nor referred for colposcopy, and the PCR processing procedures can be complex and labor-intensive. Recently, a sequential testing strategy using HC2 as a triage and genotype only those HC2 positive specimens by LA PCR has been used to monitor HPV infections in China and England [20, 21]. Using PCR genotyping assays to monitor HPV infections is also not feasible in low-resource countries [22–24]. Alternatively, HC2 has been reported as a more feasible screening approach in low-resource countries [3, 23] because HC2 (particularly, *care*HPV, the developed countries version of HC2) does not require special facilities and is less labor-intensive than PCR-based methods [22, 25, 26]. Thus, knowing the performance of testing strategies incorporating HPV-clinical HC2, compared with using LA-only PCR testing, in measuring HPV infection prevalence will be informative for public health practice.

Since sensitivities and specificities of these testing strategies may not be easily obtained and the true HPV infection prevalence is normally not known, we use Monte Carlo simulation approach to compare different testing strategies. Simulation methods have been used for answering "what-if" questions. For example, IF the "true" prevalence level is "a" and IF the sensitivity/specificity of the test is "b"/"c", the simulation will provide information on what we expect to measure as the apparent prevalence (estimate) and thus the difference (bias) between the "true" and apparent prevalence (estimate). In this study, we use the reported HPV prevalence from the US and Latin America as the "true" HPV prevalence level. What we try to answer is, if the "true" prevalence is at the level as the reported prevalence in the US and Latin America and we use the test with sensitivity and specificity as specified, what is the apparent prevalence based on the testing strategy (i.e., LA-only, HC2-only, and sequential testing by using HC2 as a triage and genotyped by LA for HC2-positive specimens)? What is the ratio of the apparent prevalence to the "true" prevalence?

Methods

Simulation setup

The Monte Carlo simulation approach similar to Lin et al. [27, 28] was extended to incorporate various testing strategies. Analytical sensitivity is the probability of truly infected subjects with a positive test result; analytical specificity is the probability of truly uninfected subjects with a negative result. Mathematical algorithms with designated values of "true" underlying type-specific prevalence, genotyping assay analytical sensitivity and specificity, and correlations among HPV types were used to generate data." True" type-specific infectious statuses were determined on the basis of the designated type-specific prevalence. The genotyping test results were determined based on the basis of type-specific infection status and genotyping test performance (i.e., analytical sensitivity and specificity). Without loss of generalizability, the total number of subjects in each data set was set at 4,000, and correlations between HPV types were set at 0.06. For each simulated data set, there are "true" type-specific infectious status of 14 high-risk (oncogenic) types, the LA genotyping test results of 14 high-risk types and the HC2 result for each of the 4000 subject. Five hundred data sets were generated for each scenario. Mean and standard deviation of the "true" and apparent prevalence (estimates) of 500 data sets were calculated. Mathematical algorithms related to our simulation setup were given in the literature [27, 28].

To simulate scenarios on the basis of both high- and low-resource regions, the reported prevalence of the 14 high-risk HPV types for the United States and Latin America were designated as the known "true" underlying type-specific prevalence (Fig. 1) [29, 30]. HPV type-specific prevalence in Latin America was lower than in the United States, and the relative HPV infection prevalence was also different.

LA genotyping assay (type-specific) analytical sensitivity and specificity were initially set as (0.95, 0.95) to reflect the scenarios where specimens were carefully handled and PCR procedures were conducted adequately. Since various factors (i.e., precisely executing processing procedures, number and quality of virus genomes presented in the samples, etc.) could affect the performance of LA, LA genotyping assay analytical sensitivity and specificity were subsequently varied from (0.95, 0.95) to (0.95, 0.90), (0.95, 0.85), (0.90, 0.90), (0.90, 0.85), (0.85, 0.85), (0.80, 0.80). The idealistic scenario, LA genotyping assay analytical performance reached (1.00, 1.00), was also considered.

To obtain HC2 results, we based our study on the test results of 8,403 women participating in the U.S. NHANES (2003–2010) study with both LA and HC2 test conducted [9]. Forty-five percent of subjects with at least one LA-positive test among 14 high-risk HPV types also tested positive by HC2, and 93 % of subjects with all LA type-specific negative results also tested negative by HC2. This was equivalent to that the analytical sensitivity of HC2 in detecting any of the 14 high-risk HPV types was approximately 50 % lower than LA, but the analytical specificity was similar.

For each simulated data set, the data included the "true" type-specific infectious status of 14 high-risk types, the LA genotyping test results of 14 high-risk types and the HC2 result of the 4,000 subject. Using the simulated data, the "true" prevalence, estimated prevalence and estimated-to-"true" prevalence ratios from

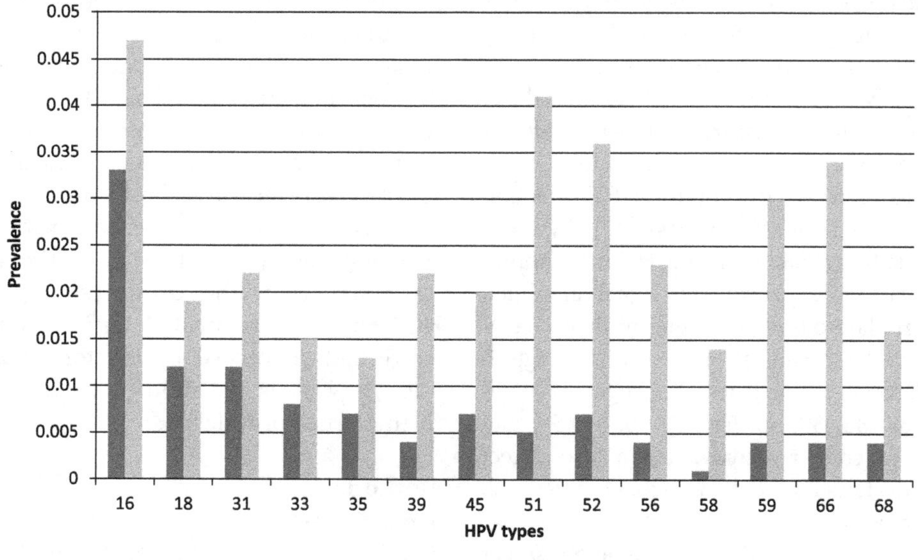

Fig. 1 The reported type-specific prevalence of the 14 high-risk (oncogenic) types of the United States and Latin America

Table 1 Designated and estimated prevalence of the 14 high-risk virus types by Linear Array (LA)-only, Hybrid Capture (HC2)-only, and sequential testing strategies in the United States and Latin America

Genotyping assay performance	Time	Designated composite prevalence (SD)	LA-only		HC2-only		Sequential test	
			Composite prevalence estimate (SD)	Estimate-to-true ratio	Composite prevalence estimate (SD)	Estimate-to-true ratio	Composite prevalence estimate (SD)	Estimate-to-true ratio
United States								
Sen = 1.00 Spe = 1.00	Baseline	0.287 (0.007)	0.287 (0.007)	1.000	0.180 (0.006)	0.628	0.129 (0.005)	0.446
	Reduced	0.265 (0.007)	0.265 (0.007)	1.000	0.172 (0.006)	0.657	0.124 (0.005)	0.468
	% Reduction	7.6	7.6		0.3		3.9	
Sen = 0.95 Spe = 0.95	Baseline	0.287 (0.007)	0.612 (0.008)	2.132	0.303 (0.007)	1.056	0.275 (0.007)	0.958
	Reduced	0.265 (0.007)	0.602 (0.008)	2.272	0.299 (0.007)	1.128	0.271 (0.007)	1.023
	% Reduction	7.6	1.6		1.3		1.5	
Sen = 0.95 Spe = 0.90	Baseline	0.287 (0.007)	0.792 (0.006)	2.760	0.371 (0.008)	1.293	0.356 (0.008)	1.240
	Reduced	0.265 (0.007)	0.787 (0.007)	2.970	0.369 (0.008)	1.392	0.354 (0.008)	1.340
	% Reduction	8.0	0.6		0.5		0.6	
Sen = 0.90 Spe = 0.90	Baseline	0.287 (0.007)	0.788 (0.006)	2.746	0.370 (0.007)	1.289	0.355 (0.007)	1.237
	Reduced	0.265 (0.007)	0.783 (0.007)	2.955	0.368 (0.007)	1.389	0.352 (0.002)	1.328
	% Reduction	7.7	0.6		0.5		0.8	
Sen = 0.90 Spe = 0.85	Baseline	0.287 (0.007)	0.887 (0.005)	3.091	0.407 (0.008)	1.418	0.399 (0.008)	1.390
	Reduced	0.265 (0.007)	0.885 (0.005)	3.340	0.405 (0.008)	1.528	0.397 (0.008)	1.498
	% Reduction	8.0	2.5		0.5		0.3	
Sen = 0.85 Spe = 0.85	Baseline	0.287 (0.007)	0.885 (0.005)	2.979	0.407 (0.007)	1.418	0.399 (0.007)	1.390
	Reduced	0.265 (0.007)	0.883 (0.005)	3.332	0.405 (0.007)	1.528	0.397 (0.007)	1.498
	% Reduction	8.0	2.2		0.5		0.3	
Sen = 0.80 Spe = 0.80	Baseline	0.286 (0.007)	0.939 (0.004)	3.283	0.426 (0.008)	1.489	0.422 (0.008)	1.475
	Reduced	0.265 (0.007)	0.938 (0.004)	3.540	0.424 (0.008)	1.600	0.421 (0.008)	1.589
	% Reduction	8.0	1.2		4.7		0.2	
Latin America								
Sen = 1.00 Spe = 1.00	Baseline	0.104 (0.005)	0.104 (0.005)	1.000	0.110 (0.005)	1.058	0.048 (0.003)	0.461
	Reduced	0.084 (0.004)	0.084 (0.004)	1.000	0.103 (0.005)	1.220	0.039 (0.003)	0.464
	% Reduction	19.2	19.2		6.3		18.7	
Sen = 0.95 Spe = 0.95	Baseline	0.104 (0.005)	0.527 (0.008)	5.067	0.270 (0.007)	2.596	0.237 (0.007)	2.279
	Reduced	0.084 (0.004)	0.518 (0.008)	6.167	0.267 (0.007)	3.179	0.233 (0.006)	2.774
	% Reduction	19.2	1.7		1.1		1.7	
Sen = 0.95 Spe = 0.90	Baseline	0.104 (0.005)	0.749 (0.007)	7.202	0.355 (0.007)	3.413	0.338 (0.007)	3.250
	Reduced	0.084 (0.005)	0.745 (0.007)	8.869	0.353 (0.007)	4.202	0.335 (0.007)	3.988
	% Reduction	19.2	0.5		0.6		0.8	
Sen = 0.90 Spe = 0.90	Baseline	0.104 (0.004)	0.748 (0.007)	7.192	0.354 (0.008)	3.404	0.337 (0.008)	3.240
	Reduced	0.084 (0.004)	0.743 (0.007)	8.845	0.353 (0.008)	4.202	0.335 (0.008)	3.988
	% Reduction	19.2	0.7		0.3		0.6	
Sen = 0.90 Spe = 0.85	Baseline	0.104 (0.005)	0.867 (0.006)	8.337	0.400 (0.008)	3.846	0.390 (0.008)	3.750
	Reduced	0.084 (0.004)	0.865 (0.005)	10.298	0.399 (0.008)	4.750	0.390 (0.008)	4.643
	% Reduction	19.2	0.3		0.2		0	
Sen = 0.85 Spe = 0.85	Baseline	0.104 (0.005)	0.866 (0.005)	8.327	0.399 (0.007)	3.837	0.389 (0.007)	3.740
	Reduced	0.084 (0.004)	0.864 (0.005)	10.286	0.398 (0.007)	4.738	0.388 (0.007)	4.619

Table 1 Designated and estimated prevalence of the 14 high-risk virus types by Linear Array (LA)-only, Hybrid Capture (HC2)-only, and sequential testing strategies in the United States and Latin America *(Continued)*

	% Reduction	19.2	0.2		0.2		0.2	
Sen = 0.80 Spe = 0.80	Baseline	0.104 (0.005)	0.930 (0.004)	8.942	0.424 (0.008)	4.077	0.419 (0.008)	4.029
	Reduced	0.084 (0.004)	0.929 (0.004)	11.060	0.423 (0.008)	5.036	0.418 (0.008)	4.976
	% Reduction	19.2	0.1		0.2		0.2	

Type-specific prevalence at baseline, in the United States: HPV16 = 0.047; HPV18 = 0.019; HPV31 = 0.022; HPV33 = 0.015; HPV35 = 0.013; HPV39 = 0.022; HPV45 = 0.020; HPV51 = 0.041; HPV52 = 0.036; HPV56 = 0.023; HPV58 = 0.014; HPV59 = 0.030; HPV66 = 0.034; and HPV68 = 0.016; in Latin America: HPV16 = 0.033; HPV18 = 0.012; HPV31 = 0.012; HPV33 = 0.008; HPV35 = 0.007; HPV39 = 0.004; HPV45 = 0.007; HPV51 = 0.005; HPV52 = 0.007; HPV56 = 0.004; HPV58 = 0.001; HPV59 = 0.004; HPV66 = 0.004; and HPV68 = 0.004

Reduced: HPV16 and HPV18 are reduced by 50 %

Abbreviations: *SD* standard deviation, *Sen* sensitivity, *Spe* specificity

various testing strategies based on the following definition were calculated.

"True" and estimated infection prevalence

Four outcome measures: 14 oncogenic high-risk types, 2 vaccine-associated high-risk types (HPV16 or HPV18 based on bivalent and quadrivalent HPV vaccine), type-specific HPV16, and type-specific HPV 18 were considered. HPV 16 and HPV 18 infections account for approximately 70 % of invasive cervical cancer globally [31, 32]. The "true" prevalence of each outcome measure was defined as the proportion of subjects having HPV infections. The "true" infection status of the four outcome measures were defined as follows: for each subject, the "true" positive infection status of the 14 high-risk types or the 2 vaccine-associated high-risk types was defined as having at least one of the 14 high-risk or the 2 vaccine-associated high-risk types, respectively. The "true" positive type-specific infection status of HPV16/HPV18 was defined as having type-specific infection of HPV16/HPV18.

Apparent prevalence (estimates) of each outcome measure was defined as a proportion of subjects with positive test results from different testing strategies. For the LA-only testing strategy, specimens taken from all subjects were genotyped by LA, therefore, the type-specific results of 14 HPV type were available. A positive LA test outcome of the 14 high-risk types and the 2 vaccine-associated high-risk types was defined as having at least one positive LA type-specific result of the 14 high-risk types and two positive vaccine-associated high-risk types, respectively. A positive test outcome of individual type-specific HPV16 or HPV18 was defined as having a positive HPV16 or HPV18 LA genotyping result, respectively.

For the HC2 clinical HPV testing-only strategy, specimens of all subjects were tested by HC2, therefore, HC2 results were available for all subjects. A positive HC2 test result was defined as subjects with at least one of the 14 high-risk HPV types. Since HC2 test result was an aggregate result, no type-specific result was available.

For the sequential testing strategy, specimens of all subjects were tested by HC2 first, and only those specimens with positive HC2 results were genotyped by LA. Therefore, for HC2 negative subjects, the LA type-specific results were not available. A positive sequential test outcome of the 14 high-risk types was defined as having both HC2-positive and at least one positive LA type-specific result of the 14 high-risk types. Similarly, a positive sequential test outcome of the two vaccine-associated high-risk types was defined as having a positive HC2 result and at least one positive LA type-specific result of two vaccine-associated high-risk types. A positive sequential test outcome of HPV16/HPV18 was defined as having positive HC2 and HPV16/HPV18 type-specific LA results.

The estimated-to-true prevalence ratio was calculated to examine how well prevalence estimates that were based on different testing strategies measured the designated "true" prevalence. A ratio >1 indicated the prevalence estimate overestimated the designated "true" prevalence. A ratio <1 indicated the prevalence estimate underestimated the designated "true" prevalence. To examine vaccine effectiveness, for demonstration purpose, the designated "true" type-specific prevalence of vaccine-associated high-risk types (i.e., HPV16 and HPV18) were reduced by 50 %. Percentage reductions of prevalence estimates of the 14 high-risk types, two vaccine-associated high-risk types, HPV16, and HPV18 that were based on different testing strategies were calculated.

Results

Apparent prevalence (estimates) of the 14 high-risk HPV types by various testing strategies are given in Table 1. In the idealistic scenario, when the analytic sensitivity and specificity of LA genotyping assay reach (1.00, 1.00), as expected, the LA-only testing strategy performs the best. When LA genotyping assay sensitivity and specificity are ≤0.95 and ≤0.95, respectively, prevalence estimates from all three testing strategies generally overestimat designated infection prevalence of the 14 high-

Table 2 Designated and estimated prevalence of two vaccine-associated high-risk types by Linear Array (LA)-only and sequential testing strategies in the United States and Latin America

Genotyping assay performance	Time	Designated composite prevalence (SD)	LA only		Sequential testing	
			Composite prevalence estimate (SD)	Estimate-to-true ratio	Composite prevalence estimate (SD)	Estimate-to-true ratio
United States						
Sen = 1.00 Spe = 1.00	Baseline	0.064 (0.004)	0.064 (0.004)	1.000	0.029 (0.003)	0.453
	Reduced	0.032 (0.003)	0.032 (0.003)	1.000	0.015 (0.002)	0.469
	% reduction	50	50		48	
Sen = 0.95 Spe = 0.95	Baseline	0.064 (0.004)	0.151 (0.006)	2.359	0.068 (0.004)	1.063
	Reduced	0.032 (0.003)	0.124 (0.005)	3.875	0.056 (0.004)	1.750
	% Reduction	50	17.9		17.6	
Sen = 0.95 Spe = 0.90	Baseline	0.064 (0.004)	0.287 (0.007)	4.484	0.107 (0.005)	1.672
	Reduced	0.032 (0.003)	0.213 (0.006)	6.656	0.096 (0.004)	3.000
	% Reduction	50	25.8		10.3	
Sen = 0.90 Spe = 0.90	Baseline	0.064 (0.004)	0.234 (0.007)	3.656	0.105 (0.005)	1.641
	Reduced	0.032 (0.003)	0.211 (0.006)	6.594	0.095 (0.005)	2.969
	% Reduction	0.50	9.8		9.5	
Sen = 0.90 Spe = 0.85	Baseline	0.064 (0.004)	0.314 (0.008)	4.906	0.142 (0.006)	2.219
	Reduced	0.032 (0.003)	0.294 (0.007)	9.188	0.132 (0.006)	4.125
	% Reduction	50	6.4		7.0	
Sen = 0.85 Spe = 0.85	Baseline	0.064 (0.004)	0.312 (0.007)	4.875	0.141 (0.005)	2.219
	Reduced	0.032 (0.003)	0.293 (0.008)	9.156	0.132 (0.005)	4.125
	% Reduction	50	42		7.0	
Sen = 0.80 Spe = 0.80	Baseline	0.064 (0.004)	0.385 (0.008)	6.016	0.173 (0.006)	2.703
	Reduced	0.032 (0.003)	0.371 (0.007)	11.594	0.167 (0.005)	5.219
	% Reduction	50	4.2		3.5	
Latin America						
Sen = 1.00 Spe = 1.00	Baseline	0.045 (0.003)	0.045 (0.003)	1.000	0.020 (0.002)	0.444
	Reduced	0.022 (0.002)	0.022 (0.002)	1.000	0.010 (0.002)	0.455
	% Reduction	51	5.1		5.0	
Sen = 0.95 Spe = 0.95	Baseline	0.045 (0.003)	0.135 (0.005)	3.000	0.060 (0.004)	1.333
	Reduced	0.022 (0.002)	0.116 (0.005)	5.273	0.052 (0.003)	2.364
	% Reduction	51	14.1		13.3	
Sen = 0.95 Spe = 0.90	Baseline	0.045 (0.003)	0.222 (0.007)	4.933	0.099 (0.005)	2.200
	Reduced	0.022 (0.002)	0.205 (0.006)	9.318	0.093 (0.005)	4.227
	% Reduction	51	7.6		6.1	
Sen = 0.90 Spe = 0.90	Baseline	0.045 (0.003)	0.219 (0.006)	4.867	0.099 (0.005)	2.200
	Reduced	0.022 (0.002)	0.204 (0.006)	8.870	0.092 (0.005)	4.000
	% Reduction	51	6.8		7.1	
Sen = 0.90 Spe = 0.85	Baseline	0.045 (0.003)	0.302 (0.007)	6.711	0.136 (0.005)	3.022
	Reduced	0.022 (0.002)	0.288 (0.007)	13.091	0.130 (0.005)	5.909
	% Reduction	51	4.6		4.4	
Sen = 0.85 Spe = 0.85	Baseline	0.045 (0.003)	0.300 (0.007)	6.667	0.135 (0.005)	3.000
	Reduced	0.022 (0.002)	0.288 (0.007)	13.091	0.129 (0.005)	5.864

Table 2 Designated and estimated prevalence of two vaccine-associated high-risk types by Linear Array (LA)-only and sequential testing strategies in the United States and Latin America *(Continued)*

	% Reduction	51	4.6		4.4	
Sen = 0.80 Spe = 0.80	Baseline	0.044 (0.003)	0.376 (0.007)	8.545	0.169 (0.006)	3.841
	Reduced	0.022 (0.002)	0.366 (0.007)	16.63	0.165 (0.006)	7.500
	% Reduction	50	2.7		2.4	

Type-specific prevalence at baseline, in the United States: HPV16 = 0.047 and HPV18 = 0.019; in Latin America: HPV16 = 0.033 and HPV18 = 0.012
Reduced: HPV16 and HPV18 are reduced by 50 %
Abbreviations: *SD* standard deviation, *Sen*, sensitivity, Spe, specificity

risk types. The prevalence estimate from the LA-only testing strategy is higher than the HC2-only or sequential testing strategies.

Estimated-to-true prevalence ratios are larger in the Latin America scenarios than in the U.S. scenarios because the designated "true" type-specific infections are lower in Latin America. When LA genotyping assay sensitivity and specificity are equal to (0.95,0.95) and the designated individual type-specific infection prevalence rates of HPV16 and HPV18 are reduced by 50 %, the designated "true" composite infection prevalence of 14 high-risk types is decreased by 7.6 % in the United States and 19.2 % in Latin America. The estimated reductions of 14 high-risk types from the LA-only, HC2-only, and sequential testing strategies are similar (1.6 %, 1.3 %, and 1.5 % for the United States and 1.7 %, 1.1 %, and 1.7 % for Latin America) and much lower than the designated "true" percentage reduction.

When LA genotyping assay sensitivity and specificity are ≤0.95 and ≤0.95, respectively, using either the LA-only or the sequential testing strategy overestimates the designated "true" prevalence of the two vaccine-associated high-risk types (Table 2). The prevalence estimates using the LA-only testing strategy are higher than using the sequential testing strategy. Similarly, compared with the U.S. scenarios, estimated-to-true prevalence ratios are higher when the "true" prevalence is designated as the reported prevalence in Latin America. When the designated "true" type-specific prevalence of HPV16 and HPV18 are reduced by 50 %, composite prevalence estimates calculated on the basis of either the LA-only or the sequential testing strategy underestimate the designated reduction.

Designated "true" and estimated type-specific prevalence for HPV16 are displayed in Table 3 and for HPV18 in Table 4. When LA genotyping sensitivity and specificity reach (1.00 1.00), LA-only performs best. The sequential testing strategy typically underestimates the designated underlying prevalence. When LA genotyping assay sensitivity and specificity are ≤0.95 and ≤0.95, respectively, the prevalence estimates from the LA-only testing strategy generally overestimate the designated "true" infection prevalence of HPV16 or HPV18. For HPV16, in certain scenarios, the prevalence estimates from sequential testing strategies underestimate the designated prevalence. Similarly, reducing the designated individual type-specific prevalence of HPV16 and HPV18 by 50 % when using either the LA-only or the sequential testing strategy underestimates the designated reduction.

Discussion

With >80 % of the cervical cancer-related deaths occurring in low-resource countries where women in most of these countries typically do not have access to effective screening or treatment before, successful introduction of using HPV-clinical test to screen cervical cancer is substantially beneficial in identifying women at risk of developing severe cervical cell abnormalities for cervical cancer prevention [3]. Availability of using HPV-clinical testing to screen cervical cancer in low-resource countries might allow public health officials to use the data to monitor HPV infection in ways not previously possible. Since HPV diagnostic testing strategies for epidemiological monitoring and cervical cancer screening have been considered separately, we have used a Monte Carlo simulation approach to investigate how well the apparent prevalence based on HC2-only and sequential testing strategies compared to LA-only measures the designated "true" prevalence. The results suggest that HPV clinical testing can be incorporated to monitor HPV prevalence or vaccine effectiveness and the apparent prevalence based on different testing strategies can be different.

Our simulation study is based on the assumption that analytical sensitivity of HC2 for detecting existence of the 14 high-risk HPV types is lower than LA-only but the analytical specificity is similar between the two. The HC2 clinical test is designed to detect high enough viral loads (i.e., clinically relevant viral loads). Analytical sensitivity of the LA is at the sub-picogram level of HPV DNA and analytical sensitivity of HC2 is at the picogram level [33–36]. Therefore, among infected subjects, the number of subjects who test LA positive is higher than the number of subjects who test HC2 positive. The magnitude of difference between analytical sensitivities of LA and HC2 depends on the distribution of the viral

Table 3 Designated and estimated prevalence of HPV16 by Linear Array (LA)-only and sequential testing strategies in the United States and Latin America

Genotyping assay performance	Time	Designated composite prevalence (SD)	LA only		Sequential testing	
			Composite prevalence estimate (SD)	Estimate-to-true ratio	Composite prevalence estimate (SD)	Estimate-to-true ratio
United States						
Sen = 1.00 Spe = 1.00	Baseline	0.047 (0.003)	0.047 (0.003)	1.000	0.009 (0.002)	0.191
	Reduced	0.023 (0.002)	0.023 (0.002)	1.000	0.004 (0.001)	0.173
	% Reduction	51.1	51.1		50	
Sen = 0.95 Spe = 0.95	Baseline	0.047 (0.003)	0.092 (0.004)	1.958	0.028 (0.003)	0.596
	Reduced	0.023 (0.002)	0.071 (0.004)	3.087	0.021 (0.002)	0.913
	% Reduction	51.1	22.8		0.7	
Sen = 0.95 Spe = 0.90	Baseline	0.047 (0.003)	0.140 (0.006)	2.979	0.052 (0.004)	1.106
	Reduced	0.023 (0.002)	0.120 (0.005)	5.217	0.044 (0.003)	1.913
	% Reduction	51.1	14.3		15.4	
Sen = 0.90 Spe = 0.90	Baseline	0.047 (0.003)	0.138 (0.005)	2.936	0.051 (0.003)	1.085
	Reduced	0.023 (0.002)	0.119 (0.005)	5.174	0.044 (0.003)	1.913
	% Reduction	51.1	13.8		13.7	
Sen = 0.90 Spe = 0.85	Baseline	0.047 (0.003)	0.185 (0.006)	3.936	0.075 (0.004)	1.596
	Reduced	0.023 (0.002)	0.167 (0.007)	7.261	0.068 (0.004)	2.957
	% Reduction	51.1	9.7		9.3	
Sen = 0.85 Spe = 0.85	Baseline	0.047 (0.003)	0.183 (0.006)	3.894	0.074 (0.004)	1.574
	Reduced	0.023 (0.002)	0.166 (0.006)	7.217	0.068 (0.004)	2.957
	% Reduction	51.1	9.3		8.1	
Sen = 0.80 Spe = 0.80	Baseline	0.047 (0.003)	0.228 (0.006)	4.851	0.097 (0.005)	2.064
	Reduced	0.024 (0.002)	0.214 (0.006)	8.917	0.091 (0.005)	3.792
	% Reduction	51.1	6.1		6.2	
Latin America						
Sen = 1.00 Spe = 1.00	Baseline	0.033 (0.003)	0.033 (0.003)	1.000	0.004 (0.001)	0.125
	Reduced	0.016 (0.002)	0.016 (0.002)	1.000	0.002 (0.001)	0.125
	% Reduction	51.5	51.5		50	
Sen = 0.95 Spe = 0.95	Baseline	0.033 (0.003)	0.080 (0.004)	2.424	0.022 (0.002)	0.667
	Reduced	0.016 (0.002)	0.065 (0.004)	4.063	0.017 (0.002)	1.063
	% Reduction	51.5	18.7		22.7	
Sen = 0.95 Spe = 0.90	Baseline	0.033 (0.003)	0.128 (0.005)	3.879	0.046 (0.003)	1.394
	Reduced	0.016 (0.002)	0.114 (0.005)	7.125	0.040 (0.003)	2.500
	% Reduction	51.5	10.9		13.0	
Sen = 0.90 Spe = 0.90	Baseline	0.033 (0.003)	0.126 (0.005)	3.818	0.045 (0.003)	1.364
	Reduced	0.016 (0.002)	0.113 (0.005)	7.063	0.040 (0.003)	2.500
	% Reduction	51.5	10.3		11.1	
Sen = 0.90 Spe = 0.85	Baseline	0.033 (0.003)	0.175 (0.006)	5.303	0.070 (0.004)	2.121
	Reduced	0.016 (0.002)	0.162 (0.006)	10.125	0.065 (0.004)	4.063
	% Reduction	51.5	7.4		7.1	
Sen = 0.85 Spe = 0.85	Baseline	0.033 (0.003)	0.173 (0.006)	5.242	0.069 (0.004)	2.091
	Reduced	0.016 (0.002)	0.161 (0.005)	10.062	0.064 (0.004)	4.000

Table 3 Designated and estimated prevalence of HPV16 by Linear Array (LA)-only and sequential testing strategies in the United States and Latin America *(Continued)*

	% Reduction	51.5	6.9		7.2	
Sen = 0.80 Spe = 0.80	Baseline	0.033 (0.003)	0.219 (0.006)	6.636	0.093 (0.005)	2.818
	Reduced	0.016 (0.002)	0.209 (0.006)	13.064	0.089 (0.004)	5.563
	% Reduction	51.5	4.5		4.3	

Type-specific prevalence at baseline, in the United States: HPV16 = 0.047; in Latin America: HPV16 = 0.033
Reduced: HPV16 is reduced by 50 %
Abbreviations: *SD* standard deviation, *Sen* sensitivity, *Spe* specificity

load of the infected subjects. When a large portion of the HPV infected subjects are with lower viral load (i.e., lower than the HC2 detection limit of 5,000 genomes), the analytical sensitivity of LA is much higher than HC2. When a smaller portion of the HPV infected subjects is with lower viral load, the analytical sensitivity of LA is closer to the analytical sensitivity of HC2. In our study, the association between HC2 and LA test results is based on samples from 8,403 women in the U.S. NHANES (2003 to 2010) studies for whom both LA and HC2 test results collected. It is equivalent to the scenario of analytical sensitivity of HC2 being approximately 50 % lower than LA, but specificity being similar. We further investigate the scenario, HC2 and LA results are more agreeable, which is based on the pap cohort Study [37]. Among 1,849 women, 83 % of LA test-positive subjects were tested positive by using HC2, and 84 % of LA test-negative subjects were also tested negative by using HC2. This is equivalent to analytical sensitivity of HC2 for detecting the 14 high-risk types is approximately 15 % lower than LA, but analytical specificity is similar. As expected, the conclusions are similar (simulation results not shown).

For demonstration purpose, the 50 % reduction of type 16 and 18 prevalence is chosen in this simulation study. The estimated vaccine effectiveness (reduction in prevalence) in the literature [9] is much lower than 50 % because of low coverage rate. Since the objective is to examine three testing strategies when infection prevalence is reduced, the 50 % reduction serves the purpose.

We consider type-specific infections to be correlated because the risk factors of getting infected by various virus types are similar and subjects with weaker immune system are more likely to get infected and stay infected. The correlations between HPV types in this simulation study were set to be 0.06 which was based on the average value of 91 pairwise correlations of the LA genotyping results of the 14 high-risk HPV types in the 2003–2006 National Health and Nutrition Examination Surveys (NHANES).

Discussion of using PCR genotyping assay to monitor HPV is given elsewhere [27]. Estimated-to-true prevalence ratios using the LA-only testing strategy are high. It is because we still get enough false-positives in a low-prevalence setting even when specificity is as high as 0.95, therefore, overestimate the "true" prevalence substantially. Taking a type-specific HPV infection as an example, this result can be easily seen from the following equation:

Apparent prevalence = sensitivity*true prevalence + (1-specificity) * (1- true prevalence).

The influence of the "true" prevalence level on the magnitude of overestimation can also be seen by comparing results from the US with those form the Latin America. The magnitude of over-estimation is more severe in Latin America. This is because the "true" type-specific infection prevalence is generally lower in Latin America.

The simulation results suggest that clinical-HC2 can be used as a triage before genotype to monitor HPV prevalence. Compared with LA-only testing strategy, that estimated-to-true prevalence ratios using the sequential testing strategy are closer to 1. In addition, the sequential testing strategy might be more compatible with cervical cancer screening programs. HC2 results for women aged ≥30 years can be used to screen for cervical cancer. In contrast, subjects with positive LA results are neither informed nor referred for colposcopy. Also, sequential testing strategy might reduce costs by greatly reducing the number of genotyping tests [38].

The simulation results also reveal that HC2-only can be used to monitor HPV prevalence of the 14 high-risk types, despite HC2 having lower analytical sensitivity than LA. The estimated-to-true prevalence ratios of the 14 high-risk HPV types from an HC2-only testing strategy are closer to 1 than the LA-only testing strategy. When the designated "true" underlying vaccine-associated high-risk types (HPV16 and HPV18) are reduced by 50 %, similar to using the LA-only testing strategy, prevalence estimates of the 14 high-risk types from HC2-only testing strategy also decline. Either using the LA-only or the HC2-only testing strategy underestimates the designated "true" reduction.

Other possible benefits exist to incorporating the HC2 clinical test for monitoring HPV infections. HC2

Table 4 Designated and estimated prevalence of HPV18 by Linear Assay (LA)-only and sequential testing strategies in the United States and Latin America

Genotyping assay performance	Time	Designated composite prevalence (SD)	LA only		Sequential testing	
			Composite prevalence estimate (SD)	Estimate-to-true ratio	Composite prevalence estimate (SD)	Estimate-to-true ratio
United States						
Sen = 1.00 Spe = 1.00	Baseline	0.019 (0.002)	0.019 (0.002)	1.000	0.003 (0.001)	0.158
	Reduced	0.009 (0.002)	0.009 (0.002)	1.000	0.002 (0.001)	0.222
	% Reduction	52	52		33	
Sen = 0.95 Spe = 0.95	Baseline	0.019 (0.002)	0.067 (0.004)	3.526	0.020 (0.002)	1.053
	Reduced	0.009 (0.002)	0.058 (0.004)	6.444	0.017 (0.002)	1.889
	% Reduction	52	13.4		15	
Sen = 0.95 Spe = 0.90	Baseline	0.019 (0.002)	0.116 (0.005)	6.105	0.043 (0.003)	2.263
	Reduced	0.009 (0.002)	0.108 (0.005)	12.000	0.040 (0.003)	4.444
	% Reduction	52	6.9		7	
Sen = 0.90 Spe = 0.90	Baseline	0.019 (0.002)	0.115 (0.005)	6.052	0.042 (0.003)	2.210
	Reduced	0.009 (0.002)	0.107 (0.005)	11.889	0.039 (0.003)	4.333
	% Reduction	52	7.0		7.1	
Sen = 0.90 Spe = 0.85	Baseline	0.019 (0.002)	0.164 (0.006)	8.632	0.066 (0.004)	3.474
	Reduced	0.009 (0.002)	0.157 (0.006)	17.444	0.064 (0.004)	7.111
	% Reduction	52	4.3		3.0	
Sen = 0.85 Spe = 0.85	Baseline	0.019 (0.002)	0.163 (0.006)	8.579	0.066 (0.004)	3.474
	Reduced	0.009 (0.002)	0.156 (0.006)	17.33	0.063 (0.004)	7.000
	% Reduction	52	4.3		4.5	
Sen = 0.80 Spe = 0.80	Baseline	0.019 (0.002)	0.211 (0.006)	11.105	0.090 (0.004)	4.737
	Reduced	0.009 (0.002)	0.206 (0.006)	22.889	0.088 (0.005)	9.778
	% Reduction	52	2.3		2.2	
Latin America						
Sen = 1.00 Spe = 1.00	Baseline	0.012 (0.002)	0.012 (0.002)	1.000	0.003 (0.001)	0.250
	Reduced	0.006 (0.002)	0.006 (0.002)	1.000	0.001 (0.001)	0.167
	% Reduction	50	50		50	
Sen = 0.95 Spe = 0.95	Baseline	0.012 (0.002)	0.061 (0.004)	5.083	0.016 (0.002)	1.333
	Reduced	0.006 (0.002)	0.056 (0.004)	9.333	0.015 (0.002)	2.500
	% Reduction	50	8.2		6.3	
Sen = 0.95 Spe = 0.90	Baseline	0.012 (0.002)	0.110 (0.005)	9.167	0.039 (0.003)	3.250
	Reduced	0.006 (0.001)	0.105 (0.005)	17.500	0.037 (0.003)	6.167
	% Reduction	50	4.5		5.1	
Sen = 0.90 Spe = 0.90	Baseline	0.012 (0.002)	0.109 (0.005)	9.083	0.039 (0.003)	3.250
	Reduced	0.006 (0.001)	0.105 (0.005)	17.500	0.037 (0.003)	6.167
	% Reduction	50	3.7		5.1	
Sen = 0.90 Spe = 0.85	Baseline	0.012 (0.002)	0.159 (0.006)	13.250	0.063 (0.004)	5.250
	Reduced	0.006 (0.001)	0.154 (0.006)	25.667	0.062 (0.004)	10.333
	% Reduction	50	3.1		1.6	
Sen = 0.85 Spe = 0.85	Baseline	0.012 (0.002)	0.158 (0.006)	13.167	0.063 (0.004)	5.250
	Reduced	0.006 (0.001)	0.154 (0.005)	25.667	0.061 (0.004)	10.166

Table 4 Designated and estimated prevalence of HPV18 by Linear Assay (LA)-only and sequential testing strategies in the United States and Latin America *(Continued)*

	% Reduction	50	3.1		3.1	
Sen = 0.80 Spe = 0.80	Baseline	0.012 (0.002)	0.207 (0.006)	17.250	0.087 (0.004)	7.250
	Reduced	0.006 (0.001)	0.204 (0.006)	34.000	0.086 (0.004)	14.333
	% Reduction	50	1.1		1.1	

Type-specific prevalence at baseline, in the US: HPV18 = 0.019; in Latin America: HPV18 = 0.012
Reduced: HPV18 is reduced by 50 %
Abbreviations: *SD* standard deviation, *Sen* sensitivity, *Spe* specificity

(particularly, careHPV, the developed countries version of HC2) procedures are less complex and less labor-intensive, therefore, less subject to human error. HC2 testing using the automation provided by a rapid capture system can achieve high-volume throughput [39]. Also, performance (sensitivities and specificities) of commercially manufactured HC2 has been reported to be highly reliable and reproducible in cervical cancer screening setting [22, 40]. High repeatability and consistent performance of HC2 testing allows public health professionals to compare HPV prevalence estimates of the 14 high-risk types across different geographic areas.

The simulations were conducted on the basis of an assumption that analytical sensitivity of LA-only testing is higher than sensitivity of HC2-only testing. When PCR procedures are performed incorrectly according to standard protocols, performance of LA might be worse than the performance of HC2, which was not considered in our study. Additionally, we did not consider the scenarios of cross-protection or type replacement attributable to vaccination in this simulation study because evidence of cross-protection and type replacement is inconclusive [41]. Conducting a cost-benefit analysis to compare LA-only testing strategy with HC2 as a triage before LA for monitoring HPV prevalence among specific age groups or within regions might be beneficial. Bias introduced because of study design (e.g., sampling strategy), confounders (e.g., demographic characteristics or sexual behaviors), or missing data are also beyond the scope of this paper. Future studies are needed to investigate the impact of those factors. Future study can also be extended to incorporate the newly approved Cobas HPV-clinical test and nine-valent HPV vaccine.

Conclusion

Estimated-to-true HPV infection prevalence ratios using LA-only testing strategy are generally higher than using HC2-only or using HC2 as a triage before genotype by LA. Clinical HPV test can be incorporated to monitor HPV infection prevalence. Data from screening through HPV-clinical test may be utilized for epidemiological monitoring. Caution is needed since the intervention effectiveness can be underestimated and the apparent prevalence from different testing strategies can be different.

Abbreviations

DNA: Deoxyribonucleic acid; HC2: Hybrid Capture 2; HPV: Human papillomavirus; LA: Linear Array; PCR: Polymerase chain reaction

Acknowledgment

The authors are grateful to Dr. Timothy Green for clarifying the simulation method in the introduction and Dr. Alula Hadgu for independently reproducing and verifying the simulation results. The authors also thank Drs. Timothy Green, Alula Hadgu, Joseph Gastwirth, Kyle Bernstein and Kim Miller for their constructive comments and/or support. The findings and conclusions in this report are those of the authors and do not necessarily represent the official position of the U.S. Centers for Disease Control and Prevention.

Funding

No funding was obtained for this study.

Authors' contributions

CL, LL participated in designing the study and drafting the manuscript. CL performed and executed the simulation. All authors read and approved the final manuscript.

Competing of interests

The authors declare that they have no competing interests.

Consent for publication

Not applicable.

Disclaimer

The findings and conclusions in this report are those of the authors and do not necessarily represent the official position of the Centers for Disease Control and Prevention.

Author details

[1]Centers for Disease Control and Prevention, Atlanta, GA, USA. [2]United Arab Emirates University, Al Ain, UAE.

References

1. Termrusnfrunglert W, Havanond P, Khemapech N, et al. Cost and effectiveness evaluation of prophylactic HPV vaccine in developing countries. Value Health. 2012;15(1 Suppl):S29–34.

2. Agosti JM, Goldie SJ. Introducing HPV vaccine in developing countries-key challenges and issues. N Engl J Med. 2007;356:1908–10.
3. Flores YN, Bishai DM, Lorincz A, et al. HPV testing for cervical cancer screening appears more cost-effective than Papanicolau cytology in Mexico. Cancer Cause Control. 2011;22:261–72.
4. Jit M, Demarteau N, Elbasha E, Ginsberg G, Kim J, Praditsitthikorn N, Sinanovic E, Hutubessy R. Human papillomavirus vaccine introduction in low-income and middle-income countries: guidance on the use of cost-effectiveness models. BMC Med. 2011;9:54.
5. Tsiodras S, Georgoulakis J, Chranioti A, Voulgaris Z, Psyrri A, Tsivilika A, Panayiotides J, Karakitsos P. Hybrid capture vs PCR screening of cervical human papilloma virus infections. Cytological and histological associations in 1270 women. BMC Cancer. 2010;10:53.
6. Kok I, Rosmalen J, Dillner J, Arbyn M, Sasieni P, Iftner T, Ballegooijen M. Primary screening for human papillomavirus compared with cytology screening for cervical cancer in European settings: cost effectiveness analysis based on a Dutch microsimulation model. BMJ. 2012;344:e670.
7. Tabrizi SN, Brotherton JM, Kaldor JM, Skinner SR Cummins E, Liu B, Bateson D, McNamee K, Garefalakis M, Garland SM. Fall in human papillomavirus prevalence following a national vaccination program. J Infectious Diseases. 2012;206(11):1645–51.
8. Markowitz LE, Tsu V, Deeks SL, Cubie H, Wang SA, Vcari AS, Brotherton JM. Human papillomavirus vaccine introduction –the first five years. Vaccine. 2012;55:F139–48.
9. Markowitz LE, Hariri S, Lin CY, Dunne EF, Steinau M, McQuillan G, Unger ER. Reduction in Human Papillomavirus (HPV) Prevalence Among Young Women Following HPV Vaccine Introduction in the United States, National Health and Nutrition Examination Surveys, 2003–2010. J Infectious Diseases. 2013;208(3):385–93.
10. Simard EP, Jemal A. Commentary: Infection-related cancers in low- and middle-income countries: challenges and opportunities. Int J Epidemiol. 2013;42(1):228–9.
11. Wong CA, Saraiya M, Hariri S, Echert L, Howlett R I, Markowitz L, Brotherton JMl, Sinka K, Martinez-Montazez OG, Kjaer SK, Dunne EF, Approaches to monitoring biological outcomes for HPV vaccination: challenges of early adopter countries. Vaccine. 2011;29(5):878–885.
12. Gaffga NH, Flagg EW, Weinstock HS, Shlay JC, Ghanem KG, Koutsky LA, Kerndt PR, Hsu KK, Unger ER, Datta SD. Monitoring HPV type-specific prevalence over time through clinic-based surveillance: A perspective on vaccine effectiveness. Vaccine. 2012;30:1959–64.
13. Kahn J, Brown D, Ding L, Widdice L, Shew M, Susan S, Bernstein D, Glynn M, Bernstein D. Vaccine-type human papillomavirus and evidence of herd protection after vaccine introduction. Pediatrics. 2012;130(2):e249–56.
14. Sandri MT, Lentati P, Benini E, Dell'Orto P, Zorzino L, Carozzi FM, Maisonneuve P, Passerini R, Salvatici M, Casadio C, Boveri S, Sideri M. Comparison of the Digene HC2 assay and the Roche AMPLICOR human Papillomavirus (HPV) Test for detection of high-risk HPV genotypes in cervical samples. J Clin Microbiol. 2006;44(6):2141–6.
15. Kulmala SM, Syrjanen S, Shabalova I, Petrovichev N, Kozachenko V, Podistov J, Ivanchenko O, Zakarenko S, Nerovjna R, Kljukina L. Branovskaja M, Grunberga V, Juschenko A, tosi P, Santopietro R, Syrjanen and NIS Cohort Study Group. Human Papillomavirus Testing with the Hybrid Capture 2 Assay and PCR as screening tools. J. Clin. Microbiol. 2004;42(6):2470–2475.
16. Sabol I, Salakova M, Smahelova J, Pawlita M, Schmitt M, Gasperov NM, Grce M, Tachezy R. Evaluation of Different techniques for identification of human papillomavirus types of low prevalence. J Clin Microbiol. 2008;46(5):1606.
17. Human Papillomavirus Laboratory Manual. Geneva, Switzerland: World Health Organization. http://whqlibdoc.who.int/hq/2010/WHO_IVB_10.12_eng.pdf. Accessed 2010.
18. Cuzick J, Clavel C, Petry KU, et al. Overview of the European and North American studies on HPV testing in primary cervical cancer screening. Int J Cancer. 2006;119:1095–101.
19. Park Y, Lee E, Choi J, Jeong S, Kim HS. Comparison of the Abbott Real Time High-Risk Human Papillomavirus (HPV), Roche Cobas HPV, and Hybrid Capture 2 assays to direct sequencing and genotyping of HPV DNA. J Clin Microbiol. 2012;50(7):2359–65.
20. Howell-Jones R, Silva N, Akpan M, Oakeshott P, Carder C, Coupland L, Sillis S, Mallinson H, Ellis V, Frodsham D, Robinson TI, Gill ON, Beddows S, Soldan K. Prevalence of human papillomavirus (HPV) infections in sexually active adolescents and young women in England, prior to widespread HPV immunization. Vaccine. 2012,30:3867–75.
21. Wu EQ, Liu B, Cui JF, Chen W, Wang JB, Lu L, Niyazi M, Zhao C, Ren SD, Li CQ, Gong XZ, Smith JS, Belinson JL, Liaw KL, Velicer C, Qiao YL. Prevalence of type-specific human papillomavirus and pap results in Chinese women: a multi-center, population-based cross-sectional study. Cancer Causes Control. 2013;24:795–803.
22. Villa LL, Denny L. Methods for detection of HPV infection and its clinical utility. Int J Gynecol Obstetrics. 2006;94:571–80.
23. Iftner T, Villa LL. Human Papillomavirus Technologies. J Natl Cancer Inst Monogr. 2003;31:80–8.
24. Zhao FH, Lin MJ, Chen F, Hu SY, Zhang R, Belinson JL, Sellors JW, Franceschi S, Qiao YL, Castle PE. Cervical Cancer Screening Group in China. Performance of high-risk human papillomavirus DNA testing as a primary screen for cervical cancer: a pooled analysis of individual patient data from 17 population-based studies from China. Lancet Oncol. 2010;11(12):1160–71.
25. Qiao YL, Sellors JW, Eder PS, Bao YP, Lim JM, Zhao FH, Weigl B, Zhang WH, Peck RB, Li L, Chen F, Pan QJ, Lorincz AT. A new HPV-DNA test for cervical-cancer screening in developing regions: a cross-sectional study of clinical accuracy in rural China. Lancet Oncol. 2008;9(10):929–36.
26. Jeronimo J, Bansil P, Lim J, Peck R, Paul P, Amador JJ, Mirembe F, Byamugisha J, Poli UR, Satyanarayana L, Asthana S, START-UP Study Group. A multicountry evaluation of careHPV testing, visual inspection with acetic acid, and papanicolaou testing for the detection of cervical cancer. Int J Gynecol Cancer. 2014;24(3):576–85.
27. Lin CY. Evaluation of using composite HPV genotyping assay results to monitor human papillomavirus infection burden through simulation. BMC Infect Dis. 2015;15:123.
28. Lin CY, Barnhart XH, Kosinski AS. The weighted generalized estimating equations approach for the evaluation of medical diagnostic test at subunit level. Biom J. 2006;5:758–71.
29. Hariri S, Unger E, Sternberg M, Dunne E, Swan D, Patel S, Markowitz L. Prevalence of genital human papillomavirus among females in the United States, the National Health and Nutrition Examination Survey, 2003–2006. J Infectious Disease. 2011;204(4):566–73.
30. Bruni L, Diaz M, Gastellsague X, Ferrer E, Bosch X, Sanjose S. Cervical human papillomavirus prevalence in 5 continents: meta-analysis of 1 million women with normal cytological findings. J Infectious Disease. 2010;202:1789–99.
31. Stoler MH, Wright T, Sharma A, Apple R, Gutekunst K, Wright T, et al. High-Risk Human Papillomavirus Testing in Women with ASC-US cytology. Am Soc Clin Path. 2011;135:468–75.
32. de Sanjose S, Quint WG, Alemany L, Geraets DT, Klaustermeier JE, Lloveras B, et al. Human papillomavirus genotype attribution in invasive cervical cancer: a retrospective cross-sectional worldwide study. Lancet Oncol. 2010;11:1048–56.
33. Molijin A, Kleter B, Quint W, Doorn LV. Molecular diagnosis of human papillomavirus (HPV) infections. J Clin Virol. 2005;32suppl1:s43–51.
34. Cope JU, Hildesheim A, Schiffman MH, Manos MM, Lorincz AT, Burk RD, et al. The viral origin of cervical cancer in Rabat, Morocco. Int J Cancer. 1998;75:546–55.
35. Smits HL, Bollen LJ, Tjong-A-Hung SP, Vonk J, van der Velden J, ten Kate FJ, et al. Intermethod variation in detection of human papillomavirus DNA in cervical smears. J Clin Microbiol. 1995;33:2631–6.
36. Snijders PJF, van den Brule AJC, Meijer CJLM. The clinical relevance of human papillomavirus testing: relationship between analytical and clinical sensitivity. J Pathology. 2003;201:1–6.
37. Gage JC, Sadorra M, LaMere BJ, Kail R, Aldrich C, Kinney W, Fetterman B, Lorey T, Schiffman M, Catles P, the PaP Cohort Study Group. Comparison of the cobas Human Papillomavirus (HPV) Test with the Hybrid Capture 2 and Linear Array HPV DNA Tests. J Clin Microbiol. 2012;50(1):61–5.
38. Meites E, Lin C, Unger E, Steinau M, Patel S, Markowitz L, Hariri S. Can clinical tests help monitor human papillomavirus vaccine impact?. International Journal of Cancer. 2013;1103–1106
39. Gravitte P, Schiffman M, Solomon D, Wheeler CM, Castle PE. A comparison of linear array and hybrid capture 2 for detection of carcinogenic human papillomavirus and cervical precancer in ASCUS-LSIL Triage study. Cancer Epidemiology Biomarkers Prevention. 2008;17:1248–54.
40. Carozzi FM, Mistro AD, Confortini M, Sani C, Puliti D, Trevisan R, Marco LD, Tos G, Girlando S, Paolo DP. Pellegrini, Schiboni ML, Crucitti P, Pierotti P, MD, Vignato A, Ronco G, Reproducibility of HPV DNA Testing by Hybrid Capture 2 in a Screening Setting: Intralaboratory and Interlaboratory Quality Control in Seven Laboratories Participating in the Same Clinical Trial. Am J Clin Pathol. 2005;124(5):716–21.
41. Pons-Salort M, Thiébaut A, Guillemot D, Favre M, Delarocque-Astagneau E. HPV genotype replacement: too early to tell". Lancet Infections. 2013;12(12):1012.

4

High-risk human papillomavirus infection and abnormal cervical cytology among Nepali and Bhutanese refugee women living in eastern Nepal

Madhav P. Bhatta[1*], Derek C. Johnson[2], Mingma Lama[3], Shilu Aryal[4], Pema Lhaki[3] and Sadeep Shrestha[5]

Abstract

Background: Cervical cancer is the leading cause of cancer morbidity and mortality among women in Nepal and Bhutan. Data on high-risk human papillomavirus (HR-HPV) infection and cervical abnormalities among Nepali and Bhutanese women are sparse. The objectives of this study were to assess and compare the prevalence of HR-HPV infection and cervical abnormalities among Nepali and Bhutanese women living in Jhapa District in eastern Nepal; and examine the risk factors for HR-HPV infection and cervical abnormalities in those women.

Methods: Study participants were recruited from a women's health camp organized by NFCC-International, a Nepal-based non-governmental organization, in 2014. Consenting participants were administered a demographic and health questionnaire and cervico-vaginal specimens collected. Both self-collected and clinician-collected cervico-vaginal specimens were tested for HR-HPV infection. Cytologic exam was performed on clinician-collected samples and cervical cytology results were categorized according to the Bethesda classification. A participant was classified as a Bhutanese if they were either born in Bhutan or currently lived in one of the United Nations administered Bhutanese refugee camps in Jhapa; otherwise, the participant was classified as a Nepali.

Results: Of the 647 study participants, 15.9% were Bhutanese women living in refugee camps and the overall age (± standard deviation) was 38.8 ± 8.2 years. The prevalence of HR-HPV infection was 8.9% and abnormal cervical cytology was 7.1% respectively, with no significant difference in HR-HPV positivity ($p = 0.399$) or abnormal cervical cytology ($p = 0.698$) between Nepali and Bhutanese women. Compared to women whose husbands had not migrated for employment, women whose husbands had migrated outside of the district had 3.30 times (95% Confidence Interval [CI]: 1.13–9.64) the odds of being HR-HPV positive and women whose husbands had migrated outside the country had 2.92 times (95% CI: 1.32–6.49) the odds of having abnormal cervical cytology.

Conclusions: HR-HPV positivity and abnormal cervical cytology were similar among Nepali and Bhutanese women. Husbands migrating for employment within or outside the country was a significant risk factor for high-risk HPV infection and cervical cytology, indicating the important role spousal behavior may play in HR-HPV acquisition and cervical abnormalities among these women.

Keywords: High-risk human papillomavirus, Abnormal cervical cytology, Nepal, Bhutanese refugee, Risk factors, Spousal migration

* Correspondence: mbhatta@kent.edu
[1]Department of Biostatistics, Environmental Health Sciences, and Epidemiology, College of Public Health Kent State University, PO Box 5190, Kent, OH 44242, USA
Full list of author information is available at the end of the article

Background

Cervical cancer is the leading cause of cancer morbidity and mortality among women in Nepal and Bhutan. The International Agency for Research on Cancer estimates of cervical cancer incidence and mortality in 2012 in Nepal were 22.4 and 18.4 per 100,000, and in Bhutan were 17.1 and 11.3 per 100,000 [1]. Cervical cancer is caused by an infection with a "high-risk" human papillomavirus (HR-HPV), which is sexually transmitted and is common among sexually active individuals [2]. Limited data on the prevalence of HR-HPV types in South Asian countries suggest a range of 8–18% in the general female population [3–6]. Specifically, in Nepal, our previous study among women from a rural far-western hilly region found an HR-HPV prevalence of 9.5% [3]. Another study among urban and semi-urban women in the south-central plains region of Nepal reported an HR-HPV prevalence of 8.6% [4]. To the best of our knowledge, there are currently no studies estimating the prevalence of HR-HPV and cervical cancer rates among women in eastern Nepal.

The Bhutanese population consists of three major ethnic groups: the Ngalops, the Lhotshampas, and the Scharchops. The Ngalops are the ethnic majority, and the Scharchops and the Lhotshampas are the two ethnic minority groups. The Lhotshampas are Bhutanese of Nepali origin, whose ancestors migrated to Bhutan, but they share cultural and linguistic similarities with Nepalis. A large proportion of the Lhotshampas in Bhutan fled the country in the early 1990s to escape ethnic and religious persecution and have been living as refugees in eastern Nepal. In the past 8 years, over 100,000 of these Lhotshampas Bhutanese refugees have been resettled in western countries, most notably in the United States [7]. Although over 100,000 have been resettled, about 20,000 still live in refugee camps and the shared socio-cultural similarities between these Bhutanese refugees and the Nepali population in eastern Nepal may indicate a similar risk of HPV and cervical cancer in the two groups. Currently there are no data on HR-HPV prevalence, cervical abnormality, or cervical cancer among Bhutanese refugee women living in Nepal or other countries. Similarly, data on HR-HPV prevalence and cervical abnormality among Bhutanese women in Bhutan are limited as well. A 2014 population-based survey conducted in women from the capital of Bhutan found an HR-HPV prevalence of 18% [6]. However, HPV and cervical cancer data among Bhutanese women in other parts of the country are lacking.

Both Nepali and Bhutanese populations have geographic and ethnic differences that may potentially influence the risk for HPV infections and cervical cancer in these populations. Despite the exodus of a significant proportion of Lhotshampas, or the Bhutanese of Nepali descent from the country, they still make up about a third of Bhutan's population. Understanding the epidemiology of HPV and cervical cancer abnormalities and the risk factors for cervical cancer in the Nepali and Bhutanese populations is important for prevention of cervical cancer. Thus, the objectives of this study were to assess and compare the prevalence of HR-HPV infection and cervical abnormalities among Nepali and Bhutanese women living in Jhapa District in eastern Nepal; and examine the risk factors for HR-HPV infection and cervical abnormalities among these women. The results of this study have relevance for the understanding of the epidemiology of HPV and cervical cancer among Nepali and Lhotshampa Bhutanese women living in Bhutan, Nepal, and western countries.

Methods

Study setting

This study was conducted in Damak Municipality in Jhapa District located in the Terai (lowland) region of eastern Nepal. From the early 1990s Jhapa has been the site of five of the seven United Nations administered refugee camps for Bhutanese refugees in Nepal [8]. The estimated population of the district in 2014 was 855,600. Jhapa is one of the most developed districts in Nepal with high levels of literacy, economic development, transportation infrastructure, and healthcare facilities [9, 10].

Participant recruitment and consent process

The study participants were recruited from a reproductive health camp organized by NFCC-International, a Nepal-based non-governmental organization, in 2014. Eligibility criteria for participation in the study included: being older than 18 years; able to provide informed consent; not menstruating; having a cervix; currently not being pregnant. Eligible women who were interested in participating in the study were read and explained the informed consent form, and a written informed consent was obtained before enrollment. Women who were not eligible or refused to participate in the study received the same health services as those participating in the study. Institutional review boards from Kent State University, the University of Alabama at Birmingham, and the Nepal Health Research Council approved the study.

Demographic and health risk questionnaire

The participants in the study were administered a demographic and health risk questionnaire that we developed and used in our previous studies in Nepal. The details of the development and the pilot testing of the questionnaire have been previously described [3, 11, 12]. The survey questionnaire included questions related to socioeconomic indicators, behavioral risk, reproductive health, and migration related factors. The questionnaire was administered by trained, native Nepali speaking research staff.

The demographic characteristics and behavioral risk profile assessed in the study included age, marital status, education, nationality, number of children, previously married or not, age at marriage, husband previously married or not, number of life-time sexual partners, age of sexual debut, current alcohol use, current tobacco smoking, and whether the husband had migrated for work inside Nepal to other districts or outside Nepal. Assessment and classification of nationality was based on answers to two questions: the country of birth or whether they lived in U.N. administered refugee camps in Nepal. A participant was considered a Bhutanese if they either indicated that they were born in Bhutan or currently lived in one of the refugee camps; otherwise, the participant was classified as a Nepali.

Biological specimens and laboratory analyses

Study protocols for biological sample collection and laboratory analyses have been described in detail previously [3]. During pelvic examinations trained auxiliary nurse midwives collected cervico-vaginal specimens using the APTIMA® Cervical Specimen Collection and Transport (CSCT) kit (Hologic/Gen-Probe, San Diego, CA). Cervico-vaginal samples were transported to the Hologic/Gen-Probe, Inc. laboratory in San Diego for HPV testing. Laboratory testing of HPV was first performed using a generic APTIMA® HR-HPV mRNA (APTIMA® HPV) probe (Hologic/Gen-Probe, San Diego, CA) to detect the presence of E6/E7 mRNA from at least one of 14 different types of HR-HPV (HPV 16, 18, 31, 33, 35, 39, 45, 51, 52, 56, 58, 59, 66, and 68). Samples with a positive HR-HPV test using the generic probe were then were retested with APTIMA® HPV16 18/45 Genotype Assay to detect the presence of HPV16 or HPV18/45 genotypes. Cervico-vaginal samples for cervical cytology were collected in ThinPrep® PreservCyt® medium (Hologic/Gen-Probe, San Diego, CA) and assessed for research purposes with results classified according to the Bethesda criteria. Women with abnormal cervical cytology were referred to local healthcare facilities for further evaluation, testing and clinical follow-up.

Outcomes and risk factors of interest

HR-HPV infection and abnormal cervical cytology were the two outcomes of interest assessed in this study. HR-HPV infection was defined as testing positive for at least one of the following HPV types: HPV 16, 18, 31, 33, 35, 39, 45, 51, 52, 56, 58, 59, 66, and 68. Cervical cytology was categorized as being either "Normal" or "Abnormal" based on the Bethesda classification system. "Normal" cervical cytology included those samples classified as benign cellular changes, results within normal limits (WNL), atypical squamous cells of undetermined significance (ASCUS), or actinomycosis. "Abnormal" cervical cytology included low-grade squamous intraepithelial lesion (LSIL), high-grade squamous intraepithelial lesion (HSIL), squamous cell carcinoma (SCC), atypical glandular cells of undetermined Significance (AGUS), or atypical squamous cells-cannot exclude high-grade (ASC-H).

Potential risk factors for HR-HPV infection and abnormal cervical cytology assessed in this study included: age (<45 [reproductive age] vs. ≥45 years); formal education (none vs. some); married more than once or 'previously married' (yes vs. no); husband married more than once or 'husband previously married' (yes vs. no); number of children (≤1, 2, 3 or ≥4); nationality (Nepali vs. Bhutanese); drink alcohol (yes vs. no); smoke any types of tobacco (yes vs. no); husband migrated for work (no, yes- migrated outside the district, or yes-migrated outside the country).

Statistical analyses

The cervico-vaginal samples were available for HR-HPV testing for 701 women and cervical cytology assessment for 688 women. A total of 679 women completed the survey questionnaires and provided information on nationality. Frequency distribution and proportions were computed for categorical variables and mean (± standard deviation) were computed for continuous variables to describe the demographic and risk behavioral profile for the overall as well as the sample stratified by nationality. Prevalence and 95% confidence interval (95% CI) for HR-HPV infection and cervical cytology were computed for overall and by nationality. The relationship between independent variables described above and the two main outcome variables (HR-HPV infection and abnormal cervical cytology) was assessed using univariable and multivariable logistic regression models. Crude and adjusted Odds Ratio (OR) and corresponding 95% CI and *p*-value are reported. The multivariable logistic regression models included the following independent variables: nationality; age; formal education; and husband migrated for work. SAS version 9.3 (SAS Institute, Cary, NC) was used to perform all statistical analyses.

Results

Demographic characteristics and risk behavioral profile

Of the 679 women who completed the survey questionnaires, 574 (84.1%) were Nepali and 105 (15.9%) were Bhutanese. Table 1 provides the demographic and risk factor profile of the participants in the study. The mean age of the sample was 38.8 (±8.2) years, with Nepali women being significantly older than Bhutanese women [39.5 (±8.1) vs. 35.0 (±7.8) years; p <0.001]. All the women, except one, were currently married, widowed or divorced, with a mean age at marriage of 19.2 (±4.0) years. Nepali women were significantly more likely to report being currently married compared to Bhutanese women (98.3 vs. 92.8%; $p = 0.001$). They also reported an

Table 1 Demographic Characteristics and Risk Behavioral Profile of Samples of Nepali and Bhutanese Women Living in Eastern Nepal

Characteristics	n (%)			
	Overall*	Nepali	Bhutanese	
	679 (100.0)	574 (84.1)	105 (15.9)	p- value
Age, years				<0.0001
19–30	24 (3.5)	6 (1.1)	18 (17.4)	
30–34	226 (33.3)	187 (32.6)	39 (37.1)	
35–39	122 (18.0)	104 (18.1)	18 (17.1)	
40–44	115 (16.9)	98 (17.1)	17 (16.2)	
45–69	192 (28.3)	179 (31.2)	13 (12.4)	
Formal education				
None	219 (32.3)	179 (32.2)	40 (38.1)	0.1640
Some	460 (67.5)	395 (68.8)	65 (61.9)	
Marital Status				
Currently married	630 (97.5)	540 (98.4)	90 (92.8)	0.0011
Other†	16 (2.5)	9 (1.6)	7 (7.2)	
Previously married				<0.0001
Yes	14 (2.2)	6 (1.1)	8 (8.1)	
No	634 (97.8)	543 (98.9)	91 (91.9)	
Husband previously married				0.8481
Yes	69 (10.6)	59 (10.7)	10 (10.1)	
No	579 (89.4)	490 (89.3)	89 (89.9)	
Number of children				<0.0001
≤ 1	138 (21.0)	98 (17.6)	40 (40.4)	
2	259 (39.4)	240 (43.0)	19 (19.2)	
3	160 (24.4)	140 (25.1)	20 (20.2)	
≥ 4	100 (15.2)	80 (14.4)	20 (20.2)	
Drink alcohol				0.0010
Yes	55 (8.7)	38 (7.1)	17 (17.4)	
No	576 (91.3)	495 (92.9)	81 (82.7)	
Smoke				0.0326
Yes	60 (9.4)	45 (8.3)	15 (15.2)	
No	579 (90.6)	495 (91.7)	84 (84.8)	
Husband migrated for work				0.0432
No	398 (74.5)	328 (72.6)	70 (85.3)	
Outside the district	24 (4.5)	21 (4.6)	3 (3.7)	
Outside the country	112 (21.0)	103 (22.8)	9 (11.0)	

*Not all values may add to 679 due to missing data; Number of missing values for: Age = 0 (0%); Formal education = 0 (0%); Marital status = 33 (4.9%); Previously married = 31 (4.6%); Husband previously married = 31 (4.6%); Number of children = 22 (3.2%); Drink alcohol = 48 (7.1%); Smoke = 40 (5.9%); and Husband migrated for work = 145 (21.5%)
†Includes single ($n = 1$), divorced/separated ($n = 6$), or widowed ($n = 9$) women

older age at marriage than Bhutanese women [19.2 (±4.0) vs. 18.0 (±3.9) years; $p = 0.003$]. Bhutanese women were significantly more likely to report being married more than once (or previously married) (8.1 vs. 1.1%; $p < 0.001$). About 11% of the women reported that their husband had been previously married. The mean number of children reported was 2.4 (±1.3). About 29% of the women reported no formal education. There was no significant difference between Nepali and Bhutanese women in regards to husband being previously married, or the level of formal education.

The mean number of life-time sexual partner reported was 1.0, with no significant difference between two groups. The mean age at first sexual debut was 19.3 (±4.1) years with Bhutanese women [18.2 (±4.1) years] reporting a younger age than Nepali women [19.6 (±4.0) years]; a difference that coincided with the difference in the mean age of marriage. About 9% of the women reported drinking alcohol and currently smoking. Bhutanese women were significantly more likely to report drinking alcohol (17.4 vs. 7.1%; $p = 0.001$) and current smoking (15.1 vs. 8.0%; $p = 0.033$) than Nepali women. Over a quarter of the women reported that their husbands had migrated for work, with 21% reporting migration outside the country. Nepali women were almost two-times more likely to reported spousal migration for employment than Bhutanese women (27.4 vs. 14.7%; $p = 0.04$).

High-risk HPV infection and cervical cytology

In the 713 cervico-vaginal samples available for HR-HPV testing, the prevalence of HR-HPV positivity was 8.4% (95% CI: 6.4–10.5%). When including only the participants who answered the nationality questions ($n = 641$), the prevalence of HR-positivity was 8.9% (95% CI: 6.7–11.1%) with no significance difference in HR-HPV prevalence between Nepali and Bhutanese women ($p = 0.399$). Among HR-HPV positive women, 41.7% were positive for HPV 16, 18 or 45 with no significant difference between the two groups ($p = 0.850$). Among HR-HPV positive women, abnormal cervical cytology was 33.3% compared to 5.0% among HR-HPV negative women ($p < 0.001$).

The prevalence of abnormal cervical cytology in the 640 satisfactory samples (out of 688 total samples) was 7.3% (95% CI: 5.3–9.4%). When including only women with the information on nationality ($n = 576$), the prevalence of abnormal cervical cytology was 7.1% with no significance difference between Nepali and Bhutanese women ($p = 0.698$). There was also no significant difference in cervical cytology results among women with and without the nationality information (results not shown). HR-HPV positivity was strongly associated with abnormal cervical cytology [OR = 9.6; 95% CI: 4.9–14.9]. Table 2 provides details on HR-HPV positivity and cervical cytology data among Nepali and Bhutanese women.

Table 3 presents results of the univariable analyses of the risk factors for HR-HPV positivity and abnormal cervical cytology. In the multivariable analysis, women whose husbands had migrated outside of the districts were 3.30 times

(95% CI: 1.13–9.64) as likely to be HR-HPV positive compared to women whose husbands had not migrated for employment (Table 4). Similarly, in the multivariable analysis, women who husbands had migrated outside the country for work had 2.92 times the odds of having abnormal cervical cytology (95% CI: 1.32–6.49) compared to women whose husband had not (Table 4).

Discussion

This study, conducted among a community-based sample of Nepali and Bhutanese women living in the eastern Terai region of Nepal, found an HR-HPV prevalence of 8.9%. The observed prevalence of HR-HPV in this study is similar to our previous observation of a 9.6% HR-HPV prevalence in a sample of women from the far-western hilly region of Nepal [3]. Similar prevalence (9.9%) of HR-HPV has been observed in the neighboring Indian state of Uttar Pradesh [13]. The previously mentioned 2014 study from Bhutan reported an overall HPV prevalence of 26%, and HR-HPV prevalence of 18%, in a sample of general population women from the capital city of Thimpu [6]. Any HPV positivity prevalence among the Lhotsampas (Bhutanese of Nepali descent) was reported at 19.8%. While the study did not report HR-HPV separately for the Lhotsampa women, assuming the ratio of HR-HPV positivity to any HPV positivity in this group is similar to the general population in Bhutan, the expected prevalence of HR-HPV among the Lhotsampa women is likely to be around 14%. Among Bhutanese women in our sample, the prevalence of HR-HPV was 11%. However, the small sample size of Bhutanese women in our study and the fact that most of them were originally from the rural south of Bhutan make the comparison of HR-HPV prevalence between our sample of Lhotsampa Bhutanese women with those from the capital of Bhutan problematic. In any case, our study adds to the growing body of literature on the population level data on the HR-HPV distribution among Nepali and Bhutanese women in particular, and South-Asian women in general, which is critical for estimating the cervical cancer risk and targeted intervention efforts locally, and globally among South Asian diaspora.

Table 2 High-risk Human Papillomavirus (HPV) Infection and Abnormal Cervical Cytology in Samples of Nepali and Bhutanese Women Living in Eastern Nepal

	n (%)			
	Overall	Nepali	Bhutanese	p- value
High-risk HPV infection (n = 641)				0.3993
No	584 (91.1)	496 (91.5)	88 (88.9)	
Yes	57 (8.9)	46 (8.5)	11 (11.1)	
Cervical cytology† (n = 576)				0.6982
Normal	535 (92.9)	458 (92.7)	77 (93.9)	
Abnormal	41 (7.1)	36 (7.3)	5 (6.1)	
Cytology results in detail				0.5387
Normal				
WNL	473 (82.1)	406 (82.4)	66 (80.5)	
ASCUS	62 (10.8)	51 (10.3)	11 (13.4)	
Abnormal				
ASC-H	7 (1.2)	5 (1.0)	2 (2.4)	
AGUS	10 (1.7)	10 (2.0)	C (0.0)	
LSIL	20 (3.5)	18 (3.6)	2 (2.4)	
HSIL	4 (0.7)	3 (0.6)	1 (1.2)	

†Cervical cytology classification: "Normal" includes: benign cellular changes, *WNL* results Within Normal Limits, *ASCUS* Atypical Squamous Cells of Undetermined Significance, or actinomycosis; "Abnormal" includes: *ASC-H* Atypical Squamous Cells- cannot exclude High-grade, *LSIL* Low-grade Squamous Intraepithelial Lesion, *HSIL* High-grade Squamous Intraepithelial Lesion, *AGUS* Atypical Glandular Cells of Undetermined Significance; and Squamous Cell Carcinoma (none in this sample)

In addition to the HPV vaccine, primary prevention efforts for HPV infection and cervical cancer focus on the reduction of sexual exposure to HPV through behavioral interventions for the woman and her sexual partner. In our study, we found that almost all the women had one life-time sexual partner—the husband—and the age of sexual debut coincided with the age of marriage. These results on the number of life-time sexual partners, and the age of sexual debut and marriage for Nepali women are consistent with other population-based data [14]. So, for most Nepali women, the husband's sexual behavior is a key determinant of her risk of HPV acquisition and, thus, the cervical cancer. This observation is supported by our findings that the employment-related migration of the husband within and outside Nepal is associated with an increased risk of HR-HPV infection and cervical abnormalities. We found that women who reported that their husband had migrated outside the district of their residence for employment purposes were almost five times as likely to have an HR-HPV infection compared to women whose husband had no history of employment-related migration. Similarly, women who reported their husband had migrated outside the country for employment were almost three times as likely to have abnormal cervical cytology compared to women with a husband without a history of employment-related migration. These observation have tremendous implications for the primary prevention measures for HPV infection and cervical cancer in Nepal.

Previous studies have shown that men who are engaged in professions that require travel or have migrated for employment have been found to be at a higher-risk of STIs including migrant workers from Nepal to India and other countries [15–17]. Men, when away from their wives or partners for an extended period of time, are likely to engage in high-risk sexual behaviors, including multiple sexual partners and sex without condoms, with other high-risk sexual partners including commercial sex workers. This puts a married woman in Nepal, who may

Table 3 Univariable Analyses of Risk Factors for High-risk Human Papillomavirus (HPV) Infection and Abnormal Cervical Cytology in a Sample of Nepali and Bhutanese Women Living in Eastern Nepal

Risk Factor	High-risk HPV					Cervical Cytology†				
	n (%)					n (%)				
	Total	Positive	Negative	OR (95% CI)§	p- value	Total	Abnormal	Normal	OR (95% CI)§	p- value
Nationality										
Nepali	542 (84.6)	46 (8.5)	496 (91.5)	1.00		494 (14.2)	36 (7.3)	458 (92.7)	1.00	
Bhutanese	99 (15.4)	11 (11.1)	88 (88.9)	1.35 (0.67–2.70)	0.4000	82 (85.8)	5 (6.1)	77 (93.9)	0.83 (0.31–2.17)	0.6984
Total	641 (100.0)	57 (8.9)	584 (91.1)			576 (100.0)	41 (7.1)	535 (92.9)		
Age, years										
45–69	175 (27.4)	9 (5.1)	166 (94.9)	1.00		151 (26.3)	10 (6.6)	141 (93.4)	1.00	
19–44	464 (72.6)	48 (10.3)	416 (89.7)	2.13 (1.02–4.44)	0.0438	423 (73.7)	31 (7.3)	392 (92.7)	1.12 (0.53–2.33)	0.7725
Total	639 (100.0)	57 (8.9)	582 (91.1)			574 (100.0)	41 (7.1)	533 (92.9)		
Formal education										
None	185 (28.9)	15 (8.1)	170 (91.9)	1.00		162 (28.1)	9 (5.6)	153 (94.4)	1.00	
Some	456 (71.1)	42 (9.2)	414 (90.8)	1.15 (0.62–2.13)	0.6570	414 (71.9)	32 (7.7)	382 (92.3)	1.42 (0.66–3.05)	0.3642
Total	641 (100.0)	57 (8.9)	584 (91.1)			576 (100.0)	41 (7.1)	535 (92.9)		
Current marital Status										
Other*	15 (2.5)	0 (0.0)	15 (100.0)			13 (0.0)	0 (0.0)	13 (100.0)		
Married	595 (97.5)	54 (9.1)	541 (88.7)	**		535 (100.0)	41 (7.7)	494 (92.3)	**	
Total	610 (100.0)	54 (9.1)	556 (90.9)			548 (100.0)	41 (7.5)	507 (92.5)		
Previously married										
No	603 (97.7)	54 (9.0)	549 (91.0)			540 (97.6)	39 (7.2)	501 (92.8)		
Yes	14 (2.3)	1 (7.1)	13 (92.9)	***		13 (2.4)	1 (7.7)	12 (92.3)	***	
Total	617 (100.0)	55 (8.9)	562 (91.1)			553 (100.0)	40 (7.2)	513 (92.8)		
Husband previously married										
No	550 (89.1)	49 (8.9)	501 (91.1)	1.00		490 (88.9)	36 (7.3)	454 (92.7)	1.00	
Yes	67 (10.9)	6 (9.0)	61 (91.0)	1.01 (0.41–2.45)	0.9900	61 (11.1)	4 (6.6)	57 (93.4)	1.13 (0.39–3.29)	0.8228
Total	617 (100.0)	55 (8.9)	562 (91.1)			551 (100.0)	40 (7.3)	511 (92.7)		
Number of children										
≤ 1	130 (20.9)	13 (10.0)	117 (90.0)	1.00		119 (21.2)	14 (11.8)	105 (88.2)	1.00	-
2	242 (38.8)	22 (9.1)	220 (90.9)	0.90 (0.44–1.85)	0.7746	219 (39.1)	13 (5.9)	206 (94.1)	0.47 (0.22–1.04)	0.0637
3	154 (24.7)	11 (7.1)	143 (92.9)	0.69 (0.30–1.60)	0.3907	137 (24.5)	8 (5.8)	129 (94.2)	0.47 (0.19–1.15)	0.0977
≥ 4	97 (15.6)	9 (9.3)	88 (90.7)	0.92 (0.38–2.25)	0.8557	85 (15.2)	6 (7.1)	79 (92.9)	0.57 (0.21–1.55)	0.2700
Total	623 (100.0)	55 (8.8)	568 (91.2)			560 (100.0)	41 (7.3)	519 (92.7)		
Drink alcohol										
No	573 (91.4)	49 (8.6)	524 (91.4)	1.00	-	515 (91.5)	34 (6.6)	481 (93.4)	1.00	
Yes	54 (8.6)	6 (11.1)	48 (88.9	1.34 (0.55–3.28)	0.5258	48 (8.5)	6 (12.5)	42 (87.5)	2.02 (0.80–5.09)	0.1353
Total	627 (100.0)	55 (8.8)	572 (91.2)			563 (100.0)	40 (7.6)	523 (92.4)		
Currently smoke										
No	550 (90.8)	50 (9.1)	500 (90.7)			517 (90.8)	38 (7.4)	479 (92.7)		
Yes	56 (9.2)	2 (3.6)	54 (96.4)	***		47 (9.2)	3 (6.4)	44 (93.6)	***	
Total	606 (100.0)	52 (8.6)	554 (91.4)			564 (100.0)	41 (7.3)	523 (92.7)		
Husband migrated for work										
No	393 (74.6)	30 (7.6)	363 (92.4)	1.00		354 (74.2)	17 (4.8)	337 (95.2)	1.00	

Table 3 Univariable Analyses of Risk Factors for High-risk Human Papillomavirus (HPV) Infection and Abnormal Cervical Cytology in a Sample of Nepali and Bhutanese Women Living in Eastern Nepal *(Continued)*

Outside the district	23 (4.4)	5 (21.7)	18 (78.3)	3.36 (1.17–9.69)	0.0248	19 (4.0)	1 (5.3)	18 (87.5)	***	
Outside the country	111 (21.0)	10 (9.0)	101 (91.0)	1.20 (0.57–2.53)	0.6363	104 (21.8)	13 (12.5)	91 (94.7)	2.83 (1.33–6.05)	0.0073
Total	527 (100.0)	45 (8.5)	582 (91.5)			477 (100.0)	31 (6.5)	446 (93.5)		

[†]Cervical cytology classification: "Normal" includes: benign cellular changes, *WNL* results Within Normal Limits, *ASCUS* Atypical Squamous Cells of Undetermined Significance, or actinomycosis; "Abnormal" includes: *ASC-H* Atypical Squamous Cells- cannot exclude High-grade, *LSIL* Low-grade Squamous Intraepithelial Lesion, *HSIL* High-grade Squamous Intraepithelial Lesion, *AGUS* Atypical Glandular Cells of Undetermined Significance; and Squamous Cell Carcinoma (none in this sample)
[§]OR (95% CI) = Odds Ratio (95% Confidence Interval)
*Other included single, divorced/separated, and widowed women
**OR undefined
***Too few data to estimate an OR

only have one life-time sexual partner, at a heightened risk for HPV and cervical cancer. With over 2 million Nepalis (7% of the total population), primarily men [18], engaged in migrant work within and outside of the country annually, a significant proportion of the women in Nepal are at an increased risk of STI infections, including HPV infection, and cervical cancer. Thus, the behavioral interventions for reducing HPV infection and cervical cancer in Nepal should target husbands and partners as they are likely the primary source of infection for the majority of the women.

We observed that over 7% of the women in the study had abnormal cervical cytology. These women were referred to the regional hospital for further testing, diagnosis, and follow-up treatment and care. Early detection using the cytology smears or non-cytology based screening methods, diagnosis, and treatment, when necessary, of these cytologic abnormalities has been the cornerstone of the cervical cancer prevention over the last several decades globally. The visual inspection with acetic acid (VIA) method is the official protocol of the government for cervical screening in Nepal. However, only a very small proportion of Nepali women get this cervical cancer screening annually. A recent nation-wide survey of women reported that only 13% of women were aware of a cervical cancer screening test and only 5% had ever undergone a cervical cancer screening test [19]. Lack of screening, diagnosis, and treatment for women with abnormal cervical cytology continues to pose a significant barrier for cervical cancer prevention among Nepali women. Along with primary prevention through HPV vaccination and decreasing sexual exposure to HPV infection, the provision of

Table 4 Multivariable Analyses of Risk Factors for High-risk Human Papillomavirus (HPV) Infection and Abnormal Cervical Cytology in a Sample of Nepali and Bhutanese Women Living in Eastern Nepal

Risk Factor	High-risk HPV (n = 527)		Abnormal Cervical Cytology[†] (n = 476)	
	aOR (95% CI)[§]	*p*- value	aOR (95% CI)[§]	*p*- value
Nationality				
Nepali	1.00	-	1.00	-
Bhutanese	1.31 (0.59–2.92)	0.5046	1.05 (0.34–3.19)	0.9368
Age, years				
45–69	1.00	-	1.00	-
19–44	2.06 (0.84–5.04)	0.1141	0.92 (0.35–2.44)	0.8665
Formal education				
None	1.00	-	1.00	-
Some	0.72 (0.35–1.49)	0.3780	0.93 (0.37–2.30)	0.8662
Husband migrated for work				
No	1.00	-	1.00	-
Outside the district	3.30 (1.13–9.64)	0.0294	1.13 (0.14–9.00)	0.9112
Outside the country	1.14 (0.53–2.48)	0.7346	2.92 (1.32–6.49)	0.0084

[†]Cervical cytology classification: "Normal" includes: benign cellular changes, *WNL* results Within Normal Limits, *ASCUS* Atypical Squamous Cells of Undetermined Significance, or actinomycosis; "Abnormal" includes: *ASC-H* Atypical Squamous Cells- cannot exclude High-grade, *LSIL* Low-grade Squamous Intraepithelial Lesion, *HSIL* High-grade Squamous Intraepithelial Lesion, *AGUS* Atypical Glandular Cells of Undetermined Significance; and Squamous Cell Carcinoma (none in this sample)
[§]aOR (95% CI) = adjusted odds ratio (95% Confidence Interval); multivariable models included all the variables listed for each outcome

screening with follow-up diagnosis and treatment is vital, if Nepal is to reduce cervical cancer morbidity and mortality.

To the best of our knowledge, this is the first study that has assessed the prevalence of HR-HPV infection and cervical abnormalities among Bhutanese women living in Nepal or western countries. There are about 20,000 Bhutanese refugees still living in Nepal and about 100,000 have been resettled in western countries, most notably in the United States [6]. The findings of the study have implications in cervical cancer prevention among Bhutanese women in Bhutan, Nepal, and western countries. A small study (n = 42) conducted among resettled Bhutanese women in the United States found that only 22.2% report ever hearing of a Pap test and 13.9% report ever having one [20]. Moreover, this study also reported that only one in three women perceived themselves to be susceptible to cervical cancer. The results of the current study show that Bhutanese women are at risk of HR-HPV infection and cervical cancer. This highlight the need for increasing awareness in this population regarding cervical cancer as a potential health risk, its cause and the available primary and secondary prevention modalities as first steps towards cervical cancer prevention efforts.

The study results should be interpreted in the context of the strengths and limitations of the study. The sample for the study was recruited from a health camp as a convenience sample. Thus, the Nepali women in the study may not be a representative sample of all the Nepali women living in Jhapa district. Similarly, the Bhutanese women in the study may not a representative sample of the Bhutanese refugee women in the camps. Moreover, the majority of Bhutanese refugees in Nepal have been resettled in western countries, thus, those still remaining in Nepal and participating in the study may suffer from selection bias. However, as the first study among this group to assess HR-HPV infection and cervical abnormalities, the results provide important preliminary information on the cervical cancer risk in this population. As a cross-sectional study, we measured the prevalence of HR-HPV infection, not the life-time exposure or persistence of HPV, which are better predictors of cervical precancerous lesions. However, HPV prevalence data is still a useful proxy for assessing cervical cancer risk, when longitudinal data are not available. Also, our study used an mRNA based test to detect the presence of HR-HPV, a test that detects the expression of genes related to E6/E7. Most population-based studies of HPV prevalence have relied on DNA-based techniques to detect the presence of the HR-HPV virus genome. Thus, the prevalence observed in our study may not be directly comparable to studies using DNA-based techniques.

Conclusions

The prevalence of HR-HPV and abnormal cervical cytology among Nepali and Bhutanese women in eastern Nepal were similar to the prevalence observed in our previous study conducted in far-western Nepal [3]. While the sexual risk behaviors reported by the women indicated them as being a low-risk for HPV infection, husband's migration outside the district or the country was a significant risk factor for high-risk HPV infection and cervical cytology. Employment-related migration is a surrogate for high-risk sexual behavior among men. These findings highlight the important role husband's sexual behavior plays in HPV infection and cervical cancer risk among Nepali and Nepali women. Since the HPV vaccine is not widely available and used in Nepal yet, and millions of women are too old to be vaccinated, an important prevention effort for cervical cancer needs to focus on reducing high-risk sexual behaviors among men. The low level of knowledge regarding cervical cancer cause and prevention methods observed among Nepali and Bhutanese-Nepali women [12, 20] highlight the need for health education to increase the knowledge and awareness of the risk factors for HPV infection and cervical cancer risk.

Abbreviations

HPV: Human papillomavirus; HR: High-risk; UN: United Nations; US: United States

Acknowledgements

We thank the study participants, without whose participation we would not have been able to conduct the study. We also thank the staff at NFCC-International who organized the health camp and helped with the sample collection. We would like to acknowledge the assistance of the Nepal Ministry of Health Family Health Division with the logistics of the health camp and data collection.We would like to thank Bellamy Cla Hawkins, Suzanne Newton, and Stephanie E. Tison for their assistance with data entry and data cleaning

Funding

The study was supported in part by the pilot fund from College of Public Health, Kent State University and the Department of Epidemiology, School of Public Health, University of Alabama at Birmingham and Derek Johnson was supported by a National Institutes of Health Cancer Prevention and Control Training Grant (R25CA47888). Hologic/GenProbe Inc. (San Diego) donated reagents and kits and provided testing of HPV and liquid cytology. The funders had no role in the study design, data collection and analysis, decision to publish, or preparation of the manuscript.

Authors' contributions

MPB, DCJ, and SS conceptualized the study. MB conducted the data analysis, interpreted resulted and lead in the writing of the manuscript. ML, SA, and PL performed the fieldwork and data collection. DCJ performed the data management. SS contributed to interpretation of the results and the manuscript writing. All authors read and approved the final manuscript.

Competing interests

The authors declare that they have no competing interests.

Consent for publication

Not applicable.

Author details
[1]Department of Biostatistics, Environmental Health Sciences, and Epidemiology, College of Public Health Kent State University, PO Box 5190, Kent, OH 44242, USA. [2]Department of Public Health & Community Medicine, Tufts University School of Medicine, Boston, MA, USA. [3]NFCC, International, Kathmandu, Nepal. [4]Family Health Division, Nepal Ministry of Health, Kathmandu, Nepal. [5]Department of Epidemiology, School of Public Health, University of Alabama at Birmingham, Birmingham, AL, USA.

References

1. IARC. Cancer Today. Population fact sheet: South-Central Asia. Available at: http://gco.iarc.fr/today/fact-sheets-populations?population=921&sex=2#collapse4. Accessed 1 Sep 2016.
2. Crosbie EJ, Einstein MH, Franceschi F, Kitchener HC. Human papillomavirus and cervical cancer. Lancet. 2013;382(9895):889–99.
3. Johnson D, Bhatta MP, Smith JS, Kempf MC, Broker TR, Vermund SH, et al. Assessment of high-risk human papillomavirus infections using clinician- and self-collected cervical sampling methods in rural women from Far Western Nepal. PLoS One. 2014;9(6):e101255.
4. Sherpa AT, Clifford GM, Vaccarella S, Shrestha S, Nygård M, Karki BS, et al. Human papillomavirus infection in women with and without cervical cancer in Nepal. Cancer Causes Control. 2010;21:323–30.
5. Bhatla N, Lal N, Bao YP, Ng T, Qiao YL. A meta-analysis of human papillomavirus type-distribution in women from South Asia: implications for vaccination. Vaccine. 2008;26:2811–7.
6. Tshomo U, Franceschi S, Dorji D, Baussano I, Tenet V, Snijders PJ, Meijer CJ, Bleeker MC, Gheit T, Tommasino M, Clifford GM. Human papillomavirus infection in Bhutan at the moment of implementation of a national HPV vaccination programme. BMC Infect Dis. 2014;14:408.
7. UNHCR. Resettlement of Bhutanese refugees surpasses 100,000 mark. 19 November 2015. www.unhcr.org/en-us/news/latest/2015/11/564dded46/resettlement-bhutanese-refugees-surpasses-100000-mark.html. Accessed 1 Sep 2016.
8. UNCHR. Global Focus—Nepal. http://reporting.unhcr.org/node/10316#_ga=1.137969456.1299581115.1472585269. Accessed 1 Sep 2016.
9. Central Bureau of Statistics. Government of Nepal National Planning Commission. Population Atlas of Nepal, 214. http://cbs.gov.np/sectoral_statistics/population/populationmonographnepa_2014. Accessed 1 Sept 2016.
10. Government of Nepal National Planning Commission. Nepal Human Development Report 2014. http://www.npc.gov.np/images/category/NHDR_Report_20141.pdf. Accessed 1 Sept 2016.
11. Jonson D, Lhaki P, Bhatta MP, Smith JS, Kempf MC, Smith JS, et al. Spousal migration and human papillomavirus infection among women in rural western Nepal. Int Health. 2016;8(4):261–8.
12. Johnson D, Bhatta MP, Gurung S, Aryal S, Lhaki P, Shrestha S. Knowledge and awareness of human papillomavirus (HPV), cervical cancer and HPV vaccine among women in two distinct Nepali communities. Asian Pac J Cancer Prev. 2014;15(19):8287–93.
13. Srivastava S, Gupta S, Roy JK. High prevalence of oncogenic HPV-16 in cervical smears of asymptomatic women of eastern Uttar Pradesh, India: a population-based study. J Biosci. 2012;37:63–72.
14. Ministry of Health and Population (MOHP) [Nepal], New ERA, and ICF International Inc. 2012. Nepal Demographic and Health Survey 2011. Kathmandu, Nepal: Ministry of Health and Population, New ERA, andICF International, Calverton, Maryland. http://dhsprogram.com/pubs/pdf/FR257/FR257%5B13April2012%5D.pdf. Accessed 1 Sep 2016
15. Bam K, Thapa R, Newman MS, Bhatt LP, Bhatta SK. Sexual behavior and condom use among seasonal Dalit migrant laborers to India from Far West, Nepal: a qualitative study. PLoS One. 2013;8(9):e74903.
16. Poudel KC, Okumura J, Sherchand JB, Jimba M, Murakami I, Wakai S. Mumbai disease in far western Nepal: HIV infection and syphilis among male migrant-returnees and non-migrants. Trop Med Int Health. 2003; 8(10):933–9.
17. Poudel KC, Jimba M, Okumura J, Joshi AB, Wakai S. Migrants' risky sexual behaviours in India and at home in far western Nepal. Trop Med Int Health. 2004;9(8):897–903.
18. Ministry of Labour and Employment [Nepal]. Labour migration for employment–A status report for Nepal: 2013/2014 . Kathmandu, Nepal, 2014. http://www.ilo.org/kathmandu/whatwedo/publications/WCMS_312137/lang–en/index.htm. Accessed 1 Sep 2016
19. Ranjit A, Gupta S, Shrestha R, Kushner AL, Nwomeh BC, Groen RS. Awareness and prevalence of cervical cancer screening among women in Nepal. International J Gynecol Obstet. 2016;134(1):37–40.
20. Haworth RJ, Margalit R, Ross C, Nepal T, Soliman AS. Knowledge, attitudes, and practices for cervical cancer screening among the Bhutanese refugee community in Omaha, Nebraska. J Community Health. 2014;39(5):872–8.

5

Human papillomavirus infection in Rwanda at the moment of implementation of a national HPV vaccination programme

Fidele Ngabo[1,2], Silvia Franceschi[3], Iacopo Baussano[3], M. Chantal Umulisa[1], Peter J. F. Snijders[4], Anne M. Uyterlinde[4], Fulvio Lazzarato[3,5], Vanessa Tenet[3], Maurice Gatera[1], Agnes Binagwaho[1,6,7] and Gary M. Clifford[3*]

Abstract

Background: Cervical cancer is the most common female cancer in Rwanda that, in 2011, became the first African country to implement a national vaccination programme against human papillomavirus (HPV).

Methods: To provide a robust baseline for future evaluations of vaccine effectiveness, cervical cell specimens were obtained from 2508 women aged 18–69 years from the general population in Kigali, Rwanda, during 2013/14. 20 % of women were HIV-positive. Samples were used for liquid-based cytology and HPV testing (44 types) with GP5+/6+ PCR.

Results: HPV prevalence was 34 %, being highest (54 %) in women ≤19 years and decreasing to 20 % at age ≥50. Prevalence of high risk (HR) HPV and cytological abnormalities was 22 and 11 % respectively (including 2 % with high-grade squamous intraepithelial lesions, HSIL) decreasing with age. Age-standardised prevalence of HR HPV was 22 % (or 19 % among HIV-negative women), and HPV16 was the most common type. Prevalence of HPV and cytological abnormalities were significantly higher in HIV-positive than HIV-negative women, and the difference increased with age. Other significant risk factors for HPV positivity in multivariate analyses were high lifetime number of sexual partners, receiving cash for sex, and being a farmer. 40 % of women with HSIL were infected with HPV16/18 and there was no significant difference between HIV-positive and HIV-negative women.

Conclusions: This study confirms Rwanda to be a setting of high prevalence of HPV and cervical disease that is worsened by HIV. These data will serve as a robust baseline for future evaluations of HPV vaccine programme effectiveness.

Keywords: Human papillomavirus, Human immunodeficiency virus, Prevalence, Cervical cancer, Rwanda

Background

Cervical cancer represents by far the most common cancer among females in Rwanda, and has a high age-standardised incidence rate of approximately 42 cases per 100,000 women per year [1] that is typical of many sub-Saharan African countries. In response to this high burden, Rwanda became the first African country to initiate a national vaccination programme against human papillomavirus (HPV), the necessary cause of cervical cancer. In 2011, over 92,000 girls in primary school grade six (approximately 12 years old) were vaccinated with quadrivalent (HPV16/18/6/11) HPV vaccine. The three-dose vaccination coverage was estimated at 93 % in the target population [2]. During 2012 and 2013, a catch-up vaccination targeted girls also in secondary school grade three (approximately 15 years old) whereas from 2014, vaccination has reverted to targeting primary school grade six only.

However, the impact of HPV vaccination on cervical cancer will likely not be observed for 20 years at least, so earlier evidence of vaccine programme effectiveness is important to encourage planners in Rwanda and other African countries to sustain their programmes. To this end, the Rwandan Ministry of Health, in collaboration with the International Agency for Research on Cancer

* Correspondence: clifford@iarc.fr
[3]International Agency for Research on Cancer, 150 cours Albert Thomas, 69372 Lyon Cedex 08, France
Full list of author information is available at the enc of the article

(IARC), initiated a series of studies to evaluate the early impact of HPV vaccination on HPV prevalence.

A pre-vaccination study of the prevalence of, and risk factors for, HPV infection, was initiated in 2011 according to the standard protocol of the IARC HPV prevalence surveys [3]. Cervicovaginal samples were collected from women aged 18–69 years living in the capital, Kigali, with a particular effort to oversample women ≤25 years of age in whom the impact of vaccination on HPV prevalence should be seen the earliest. The influence of HIV positivity, which is known to be an important determinant of HPV prevalence and may affect the future effectiveness of HPV vaccination, was also evaluated.

Methods

Population

Between July 2013 and May 2014, a survey was conducted by the Ministry of Health of Rwanda in collaboration with the IARC, Lyon, France. The study aim was to enrol 2500 women from the general population using an age-stratified approach, namely 1000 women aged below 25 years old, 500 women aged 25 to 29 years old, 200 women in each 5-year age group between 30–34 and 45–49 years, and 200 women aged ≥50 years. All mentally and physically competent women were eligible for the study, regardless of their marital status, with exception of those who were known to be pregnant.

All participants were residents of Nyarugenge District, Kigali and were recruited in two ways: 1) A population-based invitation of women aged 18–69 years residing in pre-defined areas of Nyarugenge District was made through community workers and community meetings. Women were invited to attend the Reproductive Health Department of the district hospital (Muhima). Participation rates are difficult to estimate due to the uncertainty on the number of women who had been reached by the information campaign. 2) An additional opportunistic approach was used to recruit women aged ≤29 years who were spontaneously attending Muhima hospital or eight other health centers in the Nyarugenge District (Muhima, Butamwa, Rugarama, Mwendo, Corum, Gitega, Kabusunzu, Biryogo). Principal reasons for consultation were family planning, childhood vaccination, post-natal care services and HIV-related services. Study procedures were undertaken in the centre where the woman was consulting and very few refusals were recorded.

Following signature of an informed consent form, a structured risk questionnaire was administered to all study participants, and data transferred electronically to IARC via a specifically designed on-line webpage/application.

A cytobrush (Cervex-Brush, Rovers Medical Devices B.V., The Netherlands) was used for the collection of exfoliated cervical cells from the endocervix and ectocervix for all women. The brush containing cellular material was placed in a vial containing PreservCyt medium (Cytyc, Boxbourough, MA, USA) and stored at +4C until shipment.

Women aged ≥30 years old also underwent screening by visual inspection with acetic acid (VIA). Women with visible abnormalities of the cervix, and/or who were positive for high risk (HR) HPV infection (for which results became available at a later date, see below) were to be recalled for a second VIA and treatment according to national protocols (including cryotherapy, thermo coagulation or loop electrosurgical excision of the cervix transition zone). Biopsies were to be taken from all HPV-positive women, either VIA-directed to a visible lesion or randomly from 12 o'clock of the transformation zone in the absence of a visible lesion, prior to any treatment. Histological confirmation of cervical tissue was performed at the Department of Pathology at the Kigali Teaching University Hospital. Histology results are the subject of ongoing quality control and, apart from invasive cervical cancer, are not reported here. Among women ≤29 years, no VIA was performed, nor were HR HPV-positive women recalled for follow-up.

HPV testing and liquid based cytology (LBC)

HPV testing was performed on exfoliated cervical cells in the Department of Pathology at the VU University Medical Center, Amsterdam. DNA was extracted from the PreservCyt sample using magnetic beads (Macherey-Nagel) on a robotic system (Hamilton Robotics) according to the manufacturer's instructions. Beta-Globin PCR analysis was conducted first to confirm the presence of human DNA in all specimens [4]. The presence of HPV DNA was determined by conducting a general primer GP5+/6+ – mediated PCR, which permits the detection of a broad spectrum of genital HPV types [5]. HPV positivity was assessed by hybridization of PCR products in an enzyme immunoassay with two oligoprobe cocktails that, together, detect 44 mucosal HPV types. Subsequent HPV genotyping was conducted by reverse-line blot hybridization of GP5+/6+ PCR products [6]. HPV types considered HR types for this analysis were HPV16, 18, 31, 33, 35, 39, 45, 51, 52, 56, 58, 59, and 68 [7]; possible HR types HPV26, 30, 34, 53, 66, 67, 69, 70, 73, 82, and 85; low-risk (LR) types HPV6, 11, 32, 40, 42, 43, 44, 54, 55, 57, 61, 64, 71, 72, 81, 83, 84, 86, 89, and 90.

Liquid-based cytology slides were prepared using a Thin Prep 3000 processor (Cytyc-Hologic), and were read at the Department of Pathology at the Vrije University Medical Center, Amsterdam, The Netherlands. Cytological diagnoses were reported according to CISOE-A standards [8] and were translated into

Bethesda 2001 terminology system as 1) normal, 2) atypical squamous cells of undetermined significance; atypical squamous cells cannot exclude high-grade lesion; atypical glandular cells of undetermined significance; low-grade squamous intraepithelial lesions (ASCUS/ASC-H/AGUS/LSIL), 3) high-grade squamous intraepithelial lesions (HSIL), or 4) invasive cancer.

Statistical analyses

Age-standardised HPV prevalence was computed using the world standardised population to allow comparisons of HPV prevalence with other IARC HPV surveys [9]. Adjusted prevalence ratios (PR) for HPV positivity and corresponding 95 % confidence intervals (CI) were computed using two binomial regression models with a log link, the first adjusted for age group (<24; 25–34, 35–44 and ≥45 years) only, and a second model that adjusted additionally for lifetime sexual partners (1, 2 or ≥3) and HIV status (positive, negative, unknown). Risk trends were assessed by considering categories as continuous variables. Effect modification of HIV status on the association between HPV16/18 positivity and cytology was tested using the log-likelihood ratio test.

Results

General female population

Of 2511 participants providing cervical cell samples, 2508 had valid HPV results and were included in the following analyses, including 1233 and 1275 recruited at Muhima Hospital and health centres, respectively. Ninety nine percent of women reported no HPV vaccination and 98 % no history of previous cervical cancer screening. Among the 2391 women with a valid result on LBC, 255 (11 %) had an abnormal cytological diagnosis, including 210 (9 %) with ASCUS/ASC-H/AGUS/LSIL and 45 (2 %) with HSIL.

Overall HPV prevalence was 34 %, being 29 % among women with normal cytology (Table 1). The prevalence of HPV was 73 and 96 % in ASCUS/ASC-H/AGUS/LSIL and HSIL, respectively. In total, 480 (19 %) women had single-type and 377 (15 %) had multiple-type infections. Crude and age-standardised prevalence of HR HPV types was 22 %. Prevalence of possible HR HPV and LR HPV was 10 and 15 % respectively. HPV16 was the most common HPV type in women with normal cytology (4 %), ASCUS/ASC-H/AGUS/LSIL (11 %), and HSIL (29 %). HPV52 and HPV35 were the next most common HR types in women with normal cytology and ASCUS/ASC-H/AGUS/LSIL, compared to HPV18 and HPV58 in HSIL. Four invasive cervical cancers were found in the study population (2 HPV16, 1 HPV33, 1 HPV negative), and two additional invasive cervical cancers among participants without a valid sample for HPV and cytology.

Figure 1 shows the age-specific prevalence of HPV and cytological abnormalities, with HPV-positive women classified hierarchically into (1) HPV16 and/or 18, (2) other HR types and (3) LR types only. Overall HPV prevalence was highest (54 %) among women ≤19 years, and decreased with age, down to 20 % among women aged ≥50 years. Prevalence of cytological abnormalities showed no clear trend by age group.

A total of 490 (20 %) study participants self-reported to be HIV-positive, and 1414 (56 %) to be HIV-negative. An additional 604 (24 %) who reported not to know their HIV-status are hereafter considered as HIV-negative, based on similar risk factor profiles and sensitivity analyses after the exclusion of women with unknown HIV status. Eighty-four percent of HIV-positive women were receiving combined anti-retroviral therapy (cART) (data not shown). Of note, HIV-positive women represented 11 % of the study population below age 25 but 34 % in those age 45 or older.

Table 2 shows the relationship between HPV positivity and selected women's characteristics. In the age-adjusted model, variables significantly associated with HPV positivity were age group, occupation, tobacco use, marital status, number of lifetime sexual partners, history of receiving cash for sex, the presence of anogenital warts, HIV positivity, number of pregnancies and contraceptive use in the last year. Additional adjustment for the two strongest risk factors, lifetime number of sexual partners and HIV, attenuated most PRs for HPV positivity, and the remaining significant associations included age group (PR for ≥45 vs ≤24 years = 0.45; 95 % CI: 0.37–0.55), marital status (PR for single versus married = 1.16; 95 % CI: 1.02–1.30), being a farmer (PR for farmers versus housewives = 0.78; 95 % CI: 0.66–0.92), number of lifetime sexual partners (PR for ≥3 vs 1 = 1.53; 95 % CI: 1.33–1.77), HIV positivity (PR = 1.54; 95 % CI: 1.36–1.75), number of pregnancies (PR for ≥4 vs 1 = 0.78; 95 % CI: 0.63–0.97), and use of contraceptive methods in the last year (PR for any = 0.82; 95 % CI: 0.74–0.91). Among contraceptive methods, condom did not reach statistical significance in multi-variate analysis. No significant associations with HPV positivity were seen for body mass index (5 % underweight, 7 % obese), age at menarche (median = 14 years), age at first sexual intercourse (median = 18 years), nor difference in age with partner at first sexual intercourse (median = 5 years younger) (data not shown).

In addition to total HPV prevalence, HR HPV prevalence was also significantly higher among HIV-positive (32 %) than in HIV-negative (20 %) women. Figure 2 shows prevalence of HR HPV infection, and of cytological abnormalities among HR HPV-positive women,

Table 1 Prevalence of human papillomavirus (HPV) types by cytological findings and overall, among 2508 women. Rwanda, 2013–2014

HPV type	Normal (*N* = 2136)		ASCUS/ASC-H/LSIL (*n* = 210)		HSIL (*n* = 45)		Total (*n* = 2508) [a]	
	N	%	N	%	N	%	N	%
Negative	1510	70.7	56	26.7	2	4.4	1651	65.8
Positive	626	29.3	154	73.3	43	95.6	857	34.2
Multiple	250	11.7	85	40.5	23	51.1	377	15.0
High-risk								
16	88	4.1	23	11.0	13	28.9	131	5.2
18	31	1.5	13	6.2	6	13.3	52	2.1
31	35	1.6	12	5.7	4	8.9	54	2.2
33	29	1.4	4	1.9	3	6.7	36	1.4
35	48	2.2	20	9.5	4	8.9	75	3.0
39	22	1.0	10	4.8	2	4.4	37	1.5
45	36	1.7	12	5.7	4	8.9	55	2.2
51	29	1.4	14	6.7	2	4.4	47	1.9
52	50	2.3	20	9.5	3	6.7	76	3.0
56	38	1.8	13	6.2	4	8.9	59	2.4
58	38	1.8	17	8.1	9	20.0	68	2.7
59	28	1.3	6	2.9	0	0.0	36	1.4
68	11	0.5	2	1.0	2	4.4	16	0.6
Any	378	17.7	113	53.8	40	88.9	557	22.2
Possibly high-risk								
26	9	0.4	4	1.9	3	6.7	16	0.6
30	11	0.5	6	2.9	1	2.2	18	0.7
34	0	0.0	1	0.5	0	0.0	1	0.0
53	13	0.6	11	5.2	2	4.4	26	1.0
66	39	1.8	18	8.6	1	2.2	63	2.5
67	53	2.5	8	3.8	5	11.1	68	2.7
69	11	0.5	5	2.4	0	0.0	17	0.7
70	30	1.4	8	3.8	0	0.0	38	1.5
73	13	0.6	2	1.0	1	2.2	19	0.8
82	11	0.5	6	2.9	0	0.0	18	0.7
85	4	0.2	1	0.5	1	2.2	6	0.2
Any	167	7.8	60	28.6	10	22.2	248	9.9
Low risk								
6	28	1.3	10	4.8	0	0.0	40	1.6
11	15	0.7	4	1.9	0	0.0	20	0.8
Any	282	13.2	59	28.1	10	22.2	368	14.7

[a]Including 117 women with missing/inadequate cytology

stratified by age group and HIV positivity. PRs for HR HPV prevalence by HIV-positivity increased with increasing age from 1.6 (95 % CI: 1.3–2.0) in women below age 25 up to 4.0 (95 % CI: 2.3–7.0) in women aged 45 or older (Fig. 2). The percentage of HR HPV-positive that had cytological abnormalities was significantly higher in HIV-positive than HIV-negative women below age 25 (PR = 1.7, 95 % CI: 1.2–2.6) but similar in older age groups.

The proportion of women who were positive for HPV16/18 is shown in Table 3, by cytological diagnosis and HIV status. Overall, the proportion of HPV16/18-positive women increased from 5.5 % in normal cytology up to 40 % in HSIL with no statistically significant

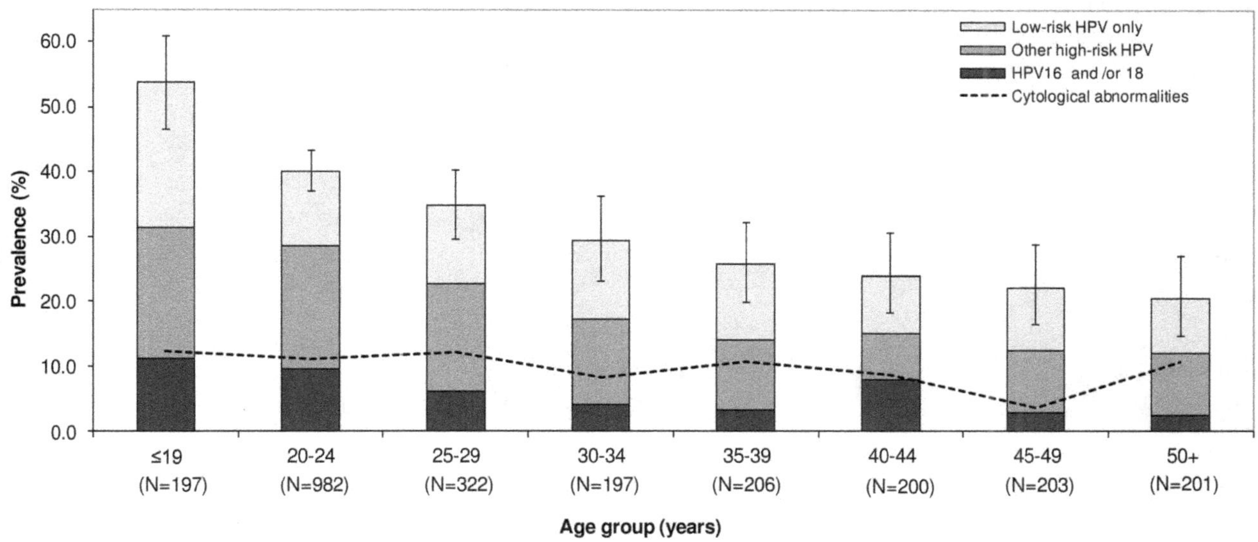

Fig. 1 Age-specific prevalence of human papillomavirus (HPV) DNA and of cytological abnormalities among 2508 women. Rwanda, 2013–2014

heterogeneity by HIV status (p for heterogeneity = 0.33) (Table 3).

Of 976 women that underwent VIA, only 5 % were classified as positive and only one of the 22 HSILs detected in this group of women was VIA-positive (data not shown).

Discussion

We describe the epidemiology of HPV infection in the adult female population of Rwanda soon after the country successfully embarked upon a national programme of HPV vaccination. Data represent that of an almost entirely vaccine- and screening-naive population and disclose a high prevalence of HPV infection (34 %), particularly among women ≤19 years (54 %). Findings can be robustly compared with other IARC HPV surveys that were conducted according to a similar protocol. In this respect, the age-standardised HR HPV prevalence of 22 % in Rwanda (or 19 % in HIV-negative women) ranks below that of Guinea (31 %) [10] and Mongolia (25 %) [11], is similar to the prevalence detected in Nigeria (18 %) [12] and Vanuatu (19 %) [13], but remains more elevated than that found in many other areas known to be at high-risk for cervical cancer, including that in India (12 %) [14] and Colombia (10 %) [15]. The high prevalence of HSIL and cervical cancer in the study population is consistent with recent estimates of high cervical cancer incidence in Rwanda [1].

HPV16 was by far the most frequently detected type in Rwanda, increasing from 4 % of normal cytology up to 29 % of HSIL. This agrees with a meta-analysis in which the proportion of HPV16-positive HSIL in Africa was 30 %, and lower than in other world regions [16]. Vaccine types HPV16 and/or 18 accounting for 42 % of HSIL, and a relatively high importance of HPV35 and HPV58 in Rwanda are also consistent with previous African studies [16]. The importance of HPV16 and 18 increased with the severity of cytological lesions similarly in HIV-negative and HIV-positive, and we did not observe any statistically significant under-representation of HPV16/18 in HIV-positive HSIL, as has been suggested by meta-analyses [17].

HIV infection was associated with higher prevalence of HPV, confirming previous findings from Rwanda [18–20]; sub-Saharan Africa [21–25] and elsewhere [17]. This association persisted after adjustment for lifetime number of sexual partners, confirming an independent effect of HIV-infection beyond that of confounding by sexual behaviour. Indeed, lower CD4+ cell counts (a specific measure of HIV-related immunosuppression) are known to be negatively associated with the prevalence [26–29], persistence [30], and cumulative incidence [31] of HPV infection.

In agreement with our present findings, some studies in sub-Saharan African populations have reported declining HPV prevalence with age [21, 32–34], whereas others have showed HPV prevalence remaining equally high [10, 12, 35–37], or even increasing [38] in middle and old age. Even if it declined, HR HPV prevalence remained 10–15 % in women age 35 or older in Rwanda, suggesting that a large proportion of women might test positive for HPV-based screening and require diagnostic follow-up and treatment. This problem particularly applies to HIV-positive women, among whom HR HPV prevalence decreased less with age than among HIV-negative women.

Risk factors, other than HIV and age group, associated with cervical HPV infection were mostly proxies of sexual behaviour, as identified in previous HPV prevalence

Table 2 Prevalence ratios (PR) for human papillomavirus (HPV) positivity and corresponding 95 % confidence intervals (CIs) according to selected characteristics among 2508 women. Rwanda, 2013–2014

Characteristic	N women [a]	HPV-positive (%)	Adjusted [b] PR	95 % CI	Adjusted [c] PR	95 % CI
Age-group (years)						
≤ 24	1179	500 (42.4)	1	-	1	-
25–34	519	170 (32.8)	0.77	0.67–0.89	0.71	0.62–0.82
35–44	406	101 (24.9)	0.59	0.49–0.70	0.52	0.44–0.63
≥ 45	404	86 (21.3)	0.50	0.41–0.61	0.45	0.37–0.55
Chi²(1) for trend			*p <0.001*		*p <0.001*	
Education (Years)						
Non-literate 0–5	325	122 (37.5)	1	-	1	-
Literate 0–5	640	226 (35.3)	0.86	0.73–1.03	0.97	0.82–1.14
Literate 6–10	1123	383 (34.1)	0.88	0.75–1.03	1.00	0.86–1.17
Literate ≥11	420	126 (30.0)	0.85	0.70–1.04	0.99	0.82–1.20
Chi²(1) for trend			*p =0.199*		*p =0.849*	
Occupation						
Housewife	964	366 (38.0)	1	-	1	-
Shopkeeper/salesman	391	154 (39.4)	1.13	0.98–1.31	1.03	0.90–1.18
Manual worker	400	132 (33.0)	0.90	0.77–1.06	0.92	0.79–1.08
Teacher/health worker/Student/Clerical staff	188	56 (29.8)	0.93	0.73–1.17	0.92	0.73–1.15
Farmer	532	134 (25.2)	0.72	0.61–0.85	0.78	0.66–0.92
Tobacco use						
Never	2276	766 (33.7)	1	-	1	-
Ever	230	91 (39.6)	1.45	1.23–1.71	1.13	0.96–1.32
Marital status						
Married or cohabiting	1734	533 (30.7)	1	-	1	-
Single	444	212 (47.8)	1.35	1.20–1.53	1.16	1.02–1.30
Separated/widowed	330	112 (33.9)	1.38	1.17–1.63	1.16	0.98–1.37
Lifetime sexual partners[d]						
1	1131	294 (26.0)	1	-	1	-
2	701	263 (37.5)	1.45	1.26–1.65	1.37	1.20–1.56
3	281	128 (45.6)	} 1.84[e]	1.62–2.10	1.53[e]	1.33–1.77
≥ 4	248	116 (46.8)				
Chi²(1) for trend			*p <0.001*		*p <0.001*	
Sexual activity in the last year						
Yes	2189	766 (35.0)	1	-	1	-
No	299	84 (28.1)	1.07	0.87–1.30	0.93	0.77–1.14
History of receiving cash for sex[d]						
Never	2333	769 (33.0)	1	-	1	-
Ever	154	85 (55.2)	1.59	1.37–1.84	1.14	0.98–1.33
Evidence of anogenital warts						
No	2395	814 (34.0)	1	-	1	-
Yes	113	43 (38.1)	1.35	1.07–1.72	1.09	0.88–1.35
HIV status						
Negative	1414	450 (31.8)	1	-	1	-
Unknown	604	166 (27.5)	1.01	0.87–1.18	1.02	0.87–1.18

Table 2 Prevalence ratios (PR) for human papillomavirus (HPV) positivity and corresponding 95 % confidence intervals (CIs) according to selected characteristics among 2508 women. Rwanda, 2013–2014 *(Continued)*

Positive	490	241 (49.2)	1.84	1.65–2.06	1.54	1.36–1.75
Number of pregnancies						
Nulliparous	237	101 (42.6)	1.15	0.97–1.36	0.99	0.85–1.15
1	804	327 (40.7)	1	-	1	-
2-3	840	285 (33.9)	0.94	0.83–1.08	0.85	0.75–0.97
≥4	616	141 (22.9)	0.85	0.67–1.06	0.78	0.63–0.97
$Chi^2(1)$ for trend			*p =0.010*		*p =0.006*	
Contraceptive use in the last year						
No	1146	422 (36.8)	1	-	1	-
Yes	1359	432 (31.8)	0.80	0.72–0.89	0.82	0.74–0.91
Hormonal	1005	339 (33.7)	0.82	0.73–0.92	0.84	0.75–0.96
Intra Uterine Device	185	54 (29.2)	0.79	0.62–1.00	0.79	0.62–1.00
Condom	72	25 (34.7)	0.92	0.67–1.27	0.86	0.64–1.16
Other/two or more of above	97	14 (14.4)	0.48	0.29–0.78	0.45	0.26–0.78

[a]Some figures do not add up to the total due to missing values
[b]Adjusted for age as appropriate
[c]Adjusted for age, HIV status and lifetime sexual partners as appropriate
[d]three virgins excluded
[e]PR ratio is calculated for "three lifetime sexual partners or more"

surveys. Lifetime number of sexual partners, being single, and history of receiving cash for sex (albeit rarely reported), were positively associated with HPV prevalence in multivariate analyses. Multiparity and recent use of contraceptives were also significantly and negatively associated with HPV positivity. Lower prevalence in farmers than other occupational groups suggest the possibility of an urban–rural gradient in the frequency of the infection. Residual confounding by sexual behaviour on the association with occupation, multiparity, and contraceptive use is difficult to rule out [39, 40].

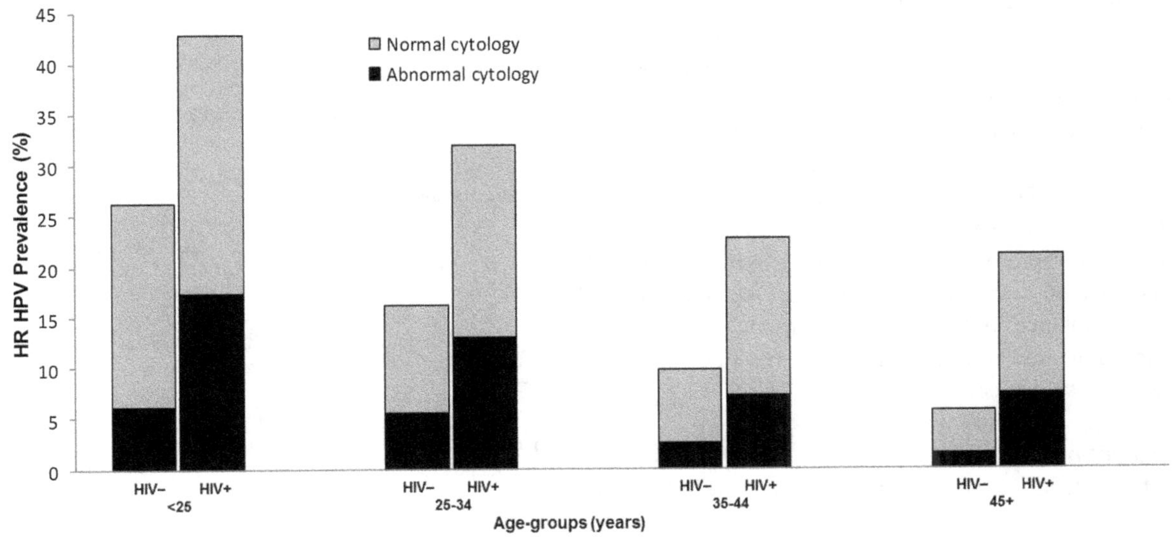

	HIV-	HIV+	PR (95% CI)	HIV-	HIV+	PR (95% CI)	HIV-	HIV+	PR (95% CI)	HIV-	HIV+	PR (95% CI)
Total	1053	126		419	100		279	127		267	137	
HR HPV+	286	56	1.6 (1.3-2.0)	72	35	2.0 (1.5-2.9)	28	31	2.4 (1.5-3.9)	16	33	4.0 (2.3-7.0)
Cyto+ among HRHPV+	22.7%	39.3%	p=0.009	31.9%	37.1%	p=0.593	25.0%	29.0%	p=0.728	25.0%	30.3%	p=0.700

Fig. 2 Age-specific prevalence of HR HPV infection, and of cytological abnormalities among HR HPV-positive women, stratified by HIV status among 2508 women. Rwanda, 2013–2014

Table 3 Positivity for human papillomavirus (HPV)16/18 among 2508 women, according to cytological findings and HIV status. Rwanda, 2013–2014

Cytology	HIV negative		HIV positive		Total	
	N	HPV16/18-pos n (%)	N	HPV16/18-pos n (%)	N	HPV16/18-pos n (%)
Normal	1749	91 (5.2)	387	26 (6.7)	2136	117 (5.5)
ASCUS/ASC-H/LSIL	146	26 (17.8)	64	8 (12.5)	210	34 (16.2)
HSIL	27	11 (40.7)	18	7 (38.9)	45	18 (40.0)
	p-value for heterogeneity by HIV status[a] = 0.33					

[a]log-likelihood ratio test (see methods)

Although only 2 % of study participants reported a prior Pap smear, the current study coincided with the initiation of screening and treatment programmes based on VIA, and/or testing for HPV DNA with careHPV (QIAGEN, Hilden, Germany) with use of VIA to triage HPV-positives for treatment [41]. A potential warning about the performance of VIA in this setting comes from the finding that, despite very high HR HPV prevalence, VIA detected abnormalities in only 5 % of women in this high-risk population, and missed the vast majority of HSIL. This mirrors findings from other IARC HPV surveys [10, 42].

This study has strengths and weaknesses. Strengths include the relatively large number of women, especially young women, and the use of high-quality HPV testing and liquid-based cytology. HPV infection is asymptomatic and self-selection of women by level of HPV risk is unlikely to have occurred. The large number of HIV-positive women in our study will allow the opportunity to estimate HPV vaccine effectiveness in this high-risk group separately but also raises the question of whether our study population is representative of the general female population in Kigali, and Rwanda as a whole. HIV-positive women are over-represented in our survey in comparison to the general population [43]. In particular, HIV-positive women (in the vast majority under cART treatment) were clearly more willing to accept screening invitations, or to be spontaneously seeking medical care, than HIV-negative women and represented approximately one third of study women age 35 or older. Had overall age-standardised HR HPV prevalence been estimated among HIV-negative women only, however, findings would have not been very different: 19 % instead of 22 %.

Conclusions

The findings of this study confirm Rwanda to be a setting of high prevalence of HPV and cervical disease that is worsened by HIV co-infection. These data will serve as a robust baseline for evaluations of HPV vaccine programme effectiveness in future cohorts of vaccinated girls.

Ethics approval and consent to participate

The present study had the approval of the Health Research Committee and Rwanda National Ethical

Consent for publication

Not applicable.

Abbreviations

ASCUS/ASC-H/AGUS/LSIL: atypical squamous cells of undetermined significance, atypical squamous cells cannot exclude high-grade lesion or atypical glandular cells of undetermined significance, low-grade squamous intraepithelial lesions; cART: combined anti-retroviral therapy; CI: confidence interval; HPV: human papillomavirus; HR: high-risk; HSIL: high-grade squamous intraepithelial lesions; IARC: International Agency for Research on Cancer; LR: low-risk; PR: prevalence ratio; VIA: visual inspection with acetic acid.

Competing interests

P.J.F. Snijders has Honoraria from Speakers Bureau from Roche, Gen-Probe, Qiagen, Abbott and Seegene and has a minority stake in Self-screen. No competing interests were disclosed by the other authors.

Authors' contributions

GC and SF conceived the study protocol. FN, MG and AG were involved in the development of the study methodology and infrastructure in Rwanda. MCU supervised the study protocol and data entry in Rwanda. IB, FL and VT were responsible for designing the electronic supports for data acquisition and/or statistical analyses. PS and AU were responsible for HPV testing and cytological reading, respectively. GC wrote the first draft of the manuscript. All authors were involved in the interpretation of the analyses and gave input to the final manuscript. All authors read and approved the final manuscript.

Acknowledgements

We would like to thank Marcelline Mahirwe and Evodie Mudaheranwa, the staff of Muhima Hospital, the staff in the health centres of Muhima, Butamwa, Rugarama, Mwendo, Corum, Gitega, Kabusunzu and Biryogo for their contribution to the field work in Rwanda. We also acknowledge the help of Dr Venerand Bigirimana, Pathologist at Kigali University Hospital for histological confirmation of biopsies, and Veronique Chabanis and Susan Gamon at IARC for administrative assistance.

Funding

The support for this project came from the Rwandan Ministry of Health, the International Agency for Research on Cancer and grants from the Bill & Melinda Gates Foundation, USA (grant numbers 35537 and OPP1053353). The Bill & Melinda Gates Foundation did not have any role in the writing process of this manuscript.

Author details

[1]Ministry of Health of Rwanda, Kigali, Rwanda. [2]Université Libre de Bruxelles, Ecole de Santé Publique, Brussels, Belgium. [3]International Agency for Research on Cancer, 150 cours Albert Thomas, 69372 Lyon Cedex 08, France. [4]Department of Pathology, VU University Medical Center, De Boelelaan 1117,

1081 HV Amsterdam, The Netherlands. [5]Unit of Cancer Epidemiology, Department of Medical Sciences, University of Turin, Turin, Italy. [6]Harvard Medical School, Boston, MA, USA. [7]Geisel School of Medicine, Dartmouth, Hanover, USA.

References

1. Ferlay J, Soerjomataram I, Ervik M, Dikshit R, Eser S, Mathers C, Rebelo M, Parkin DM, Forman D, and Bray F. GLOBOCAN 2012 v1.0, Cancer Incidence and Mortality Worldwide: IARC CancerBase No. 11 [Internet]. Lyon, France: International Agency for Research on Cancer; http://globocan.iarc.fr. Accessed 20 June 15.
2. Binagwaho A, Wagner CM, Gatera M, Karema C, Nutt CT, Ngabo F. Achieving high coverage in Rwanda's national human papillomavirus vaccination programme. Bull World Health Organ. 2012;90:623–8.
3. Clifford GM, Gallus S, Herrero R, Munoz N, Snijders PJ, Vaccarella S, Anh PT, Ferreccio C, Hieu NT, Matos E, Molano M, Rajkumar R, Ronco G, de Sanjosé S, Shin HR, Sukvirach S, Thomas JO, Tunsakul S, Meijer CJ, Franceschi S, and the IARC HPV Prevalence Surveys Study Group. Worldwide distribution of human papillomavirus types in cytologically normal women in the International Agency for Research on Cancer HPV prevalence surveys: a pooled analysis. Lancet. 2005;366:991–8.
4. Roda Husman AM, Snijders PJ, Stel HV, van den Brule AJ, Meijer CJ, Walboomers JM. Processing of long-stored archival cervical smears for human papillomavirus detection by the polymerase chain reaction. Br J Cancer. 1995;72:412–7.
5. Jacobs MV, Walboomers JM, Snijders PJ, Voorhorst FJ, Verheijen RH, Fransen-Daalmeijer N, Meijer CJ. Distribution of 37 mucosotropic HPV types in women with cytologically normal cervical smears: the age-related patterns for high-risk and low-risk types. Int J Cancer. 2000;87:221–7.
6. van den Brule AJ, Pol R, Fransen-Daalmeijer N, Schouls LM, Meijer CJ, Snijders PJ. GP5+/6+ PCR followed by reverse line blot analysis enables rapid and high-throughput identification of human papillomavirus genotypes. J Clin Microbiol. 2002;40:779–87.
7. IARC. Human papillomaviruses. IARC Monogr Eval Carcinog Risks Hum. 2007; 90:1–636. http://monographs.iarc.fr/ENG/Monographs/vol90/index.php. Accessed 20 June 15.
8. Bulk S, van Kemenade FJ, Rozendaal L, Meijer CJ. The Dutch CISOE-A framework for cytology reporting increases efficacy of screening upon standardisation since 1996. J Clin Pathol. 2004;57:388–93.
9. Crosbie EJ, Einstein MH, Franceschi S, Kitchener HC. Human papillomavirus and cervical cancer. Lancet. 2013;382:889–99.
10. Keita N, Clifford GM, Koulibaly M, Douno K, Kabba I, Haba M, Sylla BS, van Kemenade FJ, Snijders PJ, Meijer CJ, Franceschi S. HPV infection in women with and without cervical cancer in Conakry, Guinea. Br J Cancer. 2009;101:202–8.
11. Dondog B, Clifford GM, Vaccarella S, Waterboer T, Unurjargal D, Avirmed D, Enkhtuya S, Kommoss F, Wentzensen N, Snijders PJ, Meijer CJ, Franceschi S, Pawlita M. Human papillomavirus infection in Ulaanbaatar, Mongolia: a population-based study. Cancer Epidemiol Biomarkers Prev. 2008;17:1731–8.
12. Thomas JO, Herrero R, Omigbodun AA, Ojemakinde K, Ajayi IO, Fawole A, Oladepo O, Smith JS, Arslan A, Munoz N, Snijders PJ, Meijer CJ, Franceschi S. Prevalence of papillomavirus infection in women in Ibadan, Nigeria: a population-based study. Br J Cancer. 2004;90:638–45.
13. Aruhuri B, Tarivonda L, Tenet V, Sinha R, Snijders PJ, Clifford G, Pang J, McAdam M, Meijer CJ, Frazer IH, Franceschi S. Prevalence of cervical Human Papillomavirus (HPV) infection in Vanuatu. Cancer Prev Res (Phila). 2012;5:746–53.
14. Franceschi S, Rajkumar R, Snijders PJF, Arslan A. Mahé C, Plummer M, Sankaranarayanan R, Cherian J, Meijer CJLM, Weiderpass E. Papillomavirus infection in rural women in southern India. Br J Cancer. 2005;92:601–6.
15. Molano M, Posso H, Weiderpass E, van den Brule AJ, Ronderos M, Franceschi S, Meijer CJ, Arslan A, Munoz N, and the HPV Study Group. Prevalence and determinants of HPV infection among Colombian women with normal cytology. Br J Cancer. 2002;87:324–33.
16. Guan P, Howell-Jones R, Li N, Bruni L, de Sanjosé S, Franceschi S, Clifford GM. Human papillomavirus types in 115,789 HPV-positive women: a meta-analysis from cervical infection to cancer. Int J Cancer. 2012;131:2349–59.
17. Clifford GM, Goncalves MA, Franceschi S, for the HPV and HIV Study Group. Human papillomavirus types among women infected with HIV: a meta-analysis. AIDS. 2006;20:2337–44.
18. Sinayobye J, Sklar M, Hoover DR, Shi Q, Dusingize JC, Cohen M, Mutimura E, Asiimwe-Kateera B, Castle PE, Strickler H, Anastos K. Prevalence and risk factors for High-Risk Human Papillomavirus (hrHPV) infection among HIV-infected and Uninfected Rwandan women: implications for hrHPV-based screening in Rwanda. Infect Agent Cancer. 2014;9:40.
19. Singh DK, Anastos K, Hoover DR, Burk RD, Shi Q, Ngendahayo L, Mutimura E, Cajigas A, Bigirimani V, Cai X, Rwamwejo J, Vuolo M, Cohen M, Castle PE. Human papillomavirus infection and cervical cytology in HIV-infected and HIV-uninfected Rwandan women. J Infect Dis. 2009;199:1851–61.
20. Veldhuijzen NJ, Braunstein SL, Vyankandondera J, Ingabire C, Ntirushwa J, Kestelyn E, Tuijn C, Wit FW, Umutoni A, Uwineza M, Crucitti T, van de Wijgert JH. The epidemiology of human papillomavirus infection in HIV-positive and HIV-negative high-risk women in Kigali, Rwanda. BMC Infect Dis. 2011;11:333.
21. Womack SD, Chirenje ZM, Gaffikin L, Blumenthal PD, McGrath JA, Chipato T, Ngwalle S, Munjoma M, Shah KV. HPV-based cervical cancer screening in a population at high risk for HIV infection. Int J Cancer. 2000;85:206–10.
22. Safaeian M, Kiddugavu M, Gravitt PE, Gange SJ, Ssekasanvu J, Murokora D, Sklar M, Serwadda D, Wawer MJ, Shah KV, Gray R. Determinants of incidence and clearance of high-risk human papillomavirus infections in rural Rakai, Uganda. Cancer Epidemiol Biomarkers Prev. 2008;17:1300–7.
23. Akarolo-Anthony SN, Al-Mujtaba M, Famooto AO, Dareng EO, Olaniyan OB, Offiong R, Wheeler CM, Adebamowo CA. HIV associated high-risk HPV infection among Nigerian women. BMC Infect Dis. 2013;13:521.
24. Hanisch RA, Sow PS, Toure M, Dem A, Dembele B, Toure P, Winer RL, Hughes JP, Gottlieb GS, Feng Q, Kiviat NB, Hawes SE. Influence of HIV-1 and/or HIV-2 infection and CD4 count on cervical HPV DNA detection in women from Senegal, West Africa. J Clin Virol. 2013;58:696–702.
25. Dartell M, Rasch V, Munk C, Kahesa C, Mwaiselage J, Iftner T, Kjaer SK. Risk factors for high-risk human papillomavirus detection among HIV-negative and HIV-positive women from Tanzania. Sex Transm Dis. 2013;40:737–43.
26. Chaturvedi AK, Dumestre J, Gaffga AM, Mire KM, Clark RA, Braly PS, Dunlap K, Beckel TE, Hammons AF, Kissinger PJ, Hagensee ME. Prevalence of human papillomavirus genotypes in women from three clinical settings. J Med Virol. 2005;75:105–13.
27. Strickler HD, Palefsky JM, Shah KV, Anastos K, Klein RS, Minkoff H, Duerr A, Massad LS, Celentano DD, Hall C, Fazzari M, Cu-Uvin S, Bacon M, Schuman P, Levine AM, Durante AJ, Gange S, Melnick S, Burk RD. Human papillomavirus type 16 and immune status in human immunodeficiency virus-seropositive women. J Natl Cancer Inst. 2003;95:1062–71.
28. Strickler HD, Burk RD, Fazzari M, Anastos K, Minkoff H, Massad LS, Hall C, Bacon M, Levine AM, Watts DH, Silverberg MJ, Xue X, Schlecht NF, Melnick S, Palefsky JM. Natural history and possible reactivation of human papillomavirus in human immunodeficiency virus-positive women. J Natl Cancer Inst. 2005;97:577–86.
29. Harris TG, Burk RD, Palefsky JM, Massad LS, Bang JY, Anastos K, Minkoff H, Hall CB, Bacon MC, Levine AM, Watts DH, Silverberg MJ, Xue X, Melnick SL, Strickler HD. Incidence of cervical squamous intraepithelial lesions associated with HIV serostatus, CD4 cell counts, and human papillomavirus test results. JAMA. 2005;293:1471–6.
30. Rowhani-Rahbar A, Hawes SE, Sow PS, Toure P, Feng Q, Dem A, Dembele B, Critchlow CW, N'Doye I, Kiviat NB. The impact of HIV status and type on the clearance of human papillomavirus infection among Senegalese women. J Infect Dis. 2007;196:887–94.
31. Massad LS, Xie X, Burk R, Keller MJ, Minkoff H, D'Souza G, Watts DH, Palefsky J, Young M, Levine AM, Cohen M, Strickler HD. Long-term cumulative detection of human papillomavirus among HIV seropositive women. AIDS. 2014;28:2601–8.
32. Serwadda D, Wawer MJ, Shah KV, Sewankambo NK, Daniel R, Li C, Lorincz A, Meehan MP, Wabwire-Mangen F, Gray RH. Use of a hybrid capture assay of self-collected vaginal swabs in rural Uganda for detection of human papillomavirus. J Infect Dis. 1999;180:1316–9.
33. Castellsagué X, Menendez C, Loscertales MP, Kornegay JR, dos Santos F, Gomez-Olive FX, Lloveras B, Abarca N, Vaz N, Barreto A, Bosch FX, Alonso P. Human papillomavirus genotypes in rural Mozambique. Lancet. 2001;358:1429–30.
34. de Vuyst H, Steyaert S, Van Renterghem L, Claeys P, Muchiri L, Sitati S, Vansteelandt S, Quint W, Kleter B, Van Marck E, Temmerman M. Distribution

of human papillomavirus in a family planning population in Nairobi, Kenya. Sex Transm Dis. 2003;30:137–42.

35. Gage JC, Ajenifuja KO, Wentzensen NA, Adepiti AC, Eklund C, Reilly M, Hutchinson M, Wacholder S, Harford J, Soliman AS, Burk RD, Schiffman M. The age-specific prevalence of human papillomavirus and risk of cytologic abnormalities in rural Nigeria: Implications for screen-and-treat strategies. Int J Cancer. 2012;130:2111–7.
36. Kuhn L, Denny L, Pollack A, Lorincz A, Richart RM, Wright TC. Human papillomavirus DNA testing for cervical cancer screening in low-resource settings. J Natl Cancer Inst. 2000;92:818–25.
37. Wall SR, Scherf CF, Morison L, Hart KW, West B, Ekpo G, Fiander AN, Man S, Gelder CM, Walraven G, Borysiewicz LK. Cervical human papillomavirus infection and squamous intraepithelial lesions in rural Gambia, West Africa: viral sequence analysis and epidemiology. Br J Cancer. 2005;93:1068–76.
38. Xi LF, Toure P, Critchlow CW, Hawes SE, Dembele B, Sow PS, Kiviat NB. Prevalence of specific types of human papillomavirus and cervical squamous intraepithelial lesions in consecutive, previously unscreened, West-African women over 35 years of age. Int J Cancer. 2003;103:803–9.
39. Vaccarella S, Herrero R, Dai M, Snijders PJ, Meijer CJ, Thomas JO, Hoang Anh PT, Ferreccio C, Matos E, Posso H, de SS, Shin HR, Sukvirach S, Lazcano-Ponce E, Ronco G, Rajkumar R, Qiao YL, Munoz N, Franceschi S. Reproductive factors, oral contraceptive use, and human papillomavirus infection: pooled analysis of the IARC HPV prevalence surveys. Cancer Epidemiol Biomarkers Prev. 2006;15:2148–53.
40. Vaccarella S, Franceschi S, Herrero R, Munoz N, Snijders PJF, Clifford GM, Smith JS, Lazcano-Ponce E, Sukvirach S, Shin HR, de Sanjose S, Molano M, Matos E, Ferreccio C, Anh PTH, Thomas JO, Meijer CJLM, and the IARC HPV Prevalence Surveys Study Group. Sexual behavior, condom use and HPV: pooled analysis of the International Agency for Research on Cancer HPV Prevalence Surveys. Cancer Epidemiol Biomarkers Prev. 2006;15:326–33.
41. Binagwaho A, Ngabo F, Wagner CM, Mugeni C, Gatera M, Nutt CT, Nsanzimana S. Integration of comprehensive women's health programmes into health systems: cervical cancer prevention, care and control in Rwanda. Bull World Health Organ. 2013;91:697–703.
42. Li N, Shi JF, Franceschi S, Zhang WH, Dai M, Liu B, Zhang YZ, Li LK, Wu RF, De VH, Plummer M, Qiao YL, Clifford G. Different cervical cancer screening approaches in a Chinese multicentre study. Br J Cancer. 2009;100:532–7.
43. Rwanda Biomedical Center. Rwanda Global AIDS Response Progress Report 2014. Rwanda, Kigali: Republic of Rwanda, Ministry of Health; http://www.unaids.org/sites/default/files/country/documents/RWA_narrative_report_2014.pdf. Accessed 20 May 15

6

HPV prevalence and type distribution in Cypriot women with cervical cytological abnormalities

George Krashias[*†], Dana Koptides[†] and Christina Christodoulou

Abstract

Background: Human papillomavirus (HPV) is the most common sexually transmitted agent, and it can cause cervical lesions and cancer in females. Currently, information regarding the prevalence of HPV in Cyprus is lacking. The aim of this study was to evaluate the HPV type-specific prevalence in 596 women, aged 19–65 years, with cytological abnormalities. Additionally, in a subset of 348 women for whom cytology results of the Pap test were available, the association between HPV infection and cervical disease was investigated.

Methods: HPV detection and typing was carried out using PCR and restriction fragment length polymorphism analysis, respectively.

Results: Overall, the HPV prevalence was 72.8%, and it was shown to be age dependent, with a decreasing prevalence until the age of 45 years ($p = 0.0018$, χ^2). Two hundred and fifty-eight women (59.4%) were infected with high-risk HPV, 151 (34.8%) with low-risk HPV, and 25 (5.8%) with HPV types of unknown risk. The most common high-risk HPV type was HPV16 (17.7%), followed by HPV31 (12.9%), HPV58 (7.1%), HPV68 (4.6%), HPV18 (4.1%), and HPV56 (3.7%). Among the women for whom cytology results were available, 268 (77%) were HPV positive, with a sample distribution as follows: 188 (74%) had atypical squamous cells of undetermined significance (ASCUS), 61 (85.9%) had low-grade squamous intraepithelial lesion (L-SIL), and 19 (82.6%) had high-grade squamous intraepithelial lesion (H-SIL). HPV16 was the most common type among women affected by L-SIL (19.7%) and H-SIL (15.8%), with HPV31 being the most common type in women affected by ASCUS (16.5%).

Conclusions: The present study provides the first epidemiological data related to HPV prevalence and type distribution in Cypriot women with cytological abnormalities.

Keywords: Human papillomavirus (HPV), Prevalence, Typing, Age distribution, Cytology, Cyprus

Background

Human papillomavirus (HPV) is the most common sexually transmitted pathogen in both men and women. Accumulating epidemiological evidence supports a strong association between HPV and genital warts as well as cancer of the cervix, vulva, vagina, anus, and penis [1–3]. Cervical cancer is the second most common cancer in women worldwide [3, 4]. It is estimated that approximately 500,000 new cases of cervical cancer are diagnosed each year, with a 56% mortality rate in the developing world [3, 4].

Currently, over 100 different HPV types have been described, and they can be further subdivided into low-risk and high-risk types according to their oncogenic potential [5]. According to the International Agency for Research on Cancer (IARC) Monograph (2012), there are 13 high-risk HPV (HR-HPV) types, including HPV16, 18, 31, 33, 35, 39, 45, 51, 52, 56, 58, 59, and 68 [3, 6, 7]. HPV16 and 18 have been associated with 70% of cervical cancer cases [6, 8, 9], with other HR-HPV types being responsible for 20% of cervical cancers globally [6, 8, 9]. Low-risk HPV (LR-HPV) types include HPV6, 11, 42, 43, and 44, which

* Correspondence: georgek@cing.ac.cy
[†]Equal contributors
Department of Molecular Virology, The Cyprus Institute of Neurology and Genetics, 6 International Airport Avenue, 2370 Nicosia, Cyprus

are known to be associated with hyperplastic lesions such as genital warts [5].

The oncogenic potential of particular HPV types highlights the importance of the detection and typing of different HPV isolates. The results of HPV testing have significant prognostic and therapeutic implications, providing clinicians with valuable information for deciding the most appropriate course of action for each individual patient [10]. In addition, data regarding HPV type-specific distribution can provide a valuable tool in the quest for the implementation of vaccination programmes against cervical cancer. Currently, there are three prophylactic HPV vaccines available (Gardasil, Gardasil 9, and Cervarix) that are approved for use in many countries around the world [11–13]. All three vaccines provide protection against infection with HR-HPV16 and HR-HPV18. Gardasil also includes prevention against LR-HPV6 and LR-HPV11, whereas the recently approved Gardasil 9 expands protection further by adding five additional HR-HPV types (31, 33, 45, 52, and 58) [11–13]. Until recently, Cyprus was one of the very few EU countries yet to introduce a national HPV immunization programme. In January 2016, the Health Ministry introduced an HPV vaccination programme for all 12-year-old girls.

The government of Cyprus has not yet established any form of a national health system, and thus, cervical screening in the country is performed on an ad hoc basis and can be conducted in public or private hospitals or clinics [14]. To the best of our knowledge, epidemiological studies in Cyprus regarding the distribution of HPV types in the general population or in women with cytological abnormalities are still lacking. This study aimed to provide data regarding HPV prevalence and type distribution in Cypriot women with cervical cytological abnormalities. Importantly, the data presented here could provide a valuable baseline for assessing the impact of the newly introduced vaccination programme in the future.

Methods

Study population

The data for the present study were gathered between October 2012 and May 2015 from the results of diagnostic HPV testing of samples from women with abnormal Pap tests that were referred by experienced gynaecologists. The study included cervicovaginal wash samples from 596 women [mean age 37.3 years, standard deviation (SD) 11.9 years, range 19–65 years] attending private or governmental gynaecological outpatient clinics in Cyprus. The samples were tested for HPV at the Molecular Virology department of the Cyprus Institute of Neurology and Genetics. Cytology results were available only for a subgroup of 348 women. Based on the Bethesda system classification [15] cervical cytological samples were classified as follows: atypical squamous cells of undetermined significance (ASCUS), low-grade squamous intraepithelial lesion (L-SIL) or high-grade squamous intraepithelial lesion (H-SIL). Age class distribution among the participating women is reported in Table 1.

Extraction of DNA and detection of HPV infection by PCR

Cervicovaginal wash samples were collected by washing the cervical and vaginal wall with 10 mL of normal saline and then immediately shipped at 4 °C to the Molecular Virology department, where DNA extraction was performed the same day. Each vial was vortexed for 15 s before use. Starting material (400 μL) was then used for DNA extraction using the iPrep PureLink Virus Kit (Life Technologies, Carlsbad, CA, USA), according to manufacturer's instructions. The resulting DNA was immediately processed for the detection and typing of HPV DNA.

A PCR assay using the MY09/MY11 L1 consensus primer set was performed as previously described [16]. Specifically, the test uses the primers MY09 (reverse: 5′ CGT CCM ARR GGA WAC TGA TC 3′) and MY11 (forward: 5′ GCM CAG GGW CAT AAY AAT GG 3′) to amplify approximately a 450 bp fragment within the L1 open reading frame in the HPV genome [16]. To provide a control for sampling and cell adequacy, extraction, and amplification, an additional primer pair targeting human beta globin was used as previously described [17]. The HPV PCR test was performed in a 60 μL reaction containing 6 μL of the isolated DNA, 1× PCR buffer, 4.5 mM $MgCl_2$, 0.2 mM dNTPs, 0.5 μM of forward and reverse primers each, and 2.5 U of AmpliTaq Gold DNA polymerase (Roche Molecular Systems Inc., USA). The amplification reactions were performed using an MJR PTN-200 PCR machine (MJ Research Inc., Watertown, MA, USA) with the following conditions: initial denaturation for 10 min at 95 °C, followed by 40 cycles of 15 s at 95 °C, 20 s at 55 °C, 30 s at 72 °C, and finally at 72 °C for 5 min. The resulting PCR products were evaluated by electrophoresis on a 1.8% agarose gel stained with ethidium bromide.

HPV genotyping by restriction fragment length polymorphism (RFLP) analysis

Typing of HPV-DNA-positive samples was performed by restriction digestion of PCR products. Each restriction reaction was performed separately in a final volume of 20 μL using 5–7 μL of crude MY09/11 PCR product, 2 μL of 10× recommended restriction buffer, and 5–10 U of the following restriction endonucleases: EcoRI, BamHI, HinfI, DraI, PstI (all from New England BioLabs, Ipswich, MA, USA), according to the manufacturer's

Table 1 Results of HPV detection by age and cytology

	Outcomes of HPV detection and typing, *N*/% (95% C.I)					
	HPV-	HPV+	HR-HPV+	LR-HPV+	UR-HPV+	Total (%)
Total[a]	162/27.2% (23.8–30.9)	434/72.8% (69.1–76.2)	258/59.4% (54.8–64)	151/34.8% (30.5–39.4)	25/5.8% (3.9–8.4)	596 (100%)
Age[a] (years)						
≤ 25	15/15.3% (9.4–23.8)	83/84.7% (76.2–90.6)	52/62.6% (51.9–72.3)	31/37.4% (27.7–48.1)	0 (0%) (<0.01–7.2)	98 (100%)
26–35	48/23.1% (17.9–29.3)	160/76.9% (70.7–82.2)	98/61.3% (53.5–68.5)	54/33.7% (26.9–41.4)	8/5% (2.4–9.7)	208 (100%)
36–45	49/36.6% (28.9–45)	85/63.4% (55–71.1)	48/56.5% (45.9–66.5)	28/32.9% (23.9–43.5)	9/10.6% (5.5–19.1)	134 (100%)
≥ 46	50/32.1% (25.2--39.7)	106/67.9% (60.3–74.8)	60/56.6% (47.1–65.7)	38/35.8% (27.4–45.3)	8/7.6% (3.7–14.4)	156 (100%)
Cytology[b]						
ASCUS	66/26% (21–31.7)	188/74% (68.3–79)	117/62.2% (55.1–68.9)	62/33% (26.7–40)	9/4.8% (2.4–9)	254 (100%)
L-SIL	10/14.1% (7.6–24.2)	61/85.9% (75.8–92.4)	37/60.7% (48.1–72)	22/36.1% (25.2–48.6)	2/3.2% (0.3–11.9)	71 (100%)
H-SIL	4/17.4% (6.4–37.7)	19/82.6% (62.3–93.6)	11/57.9% (36.2–76.9)	7/36.8% (19.1–59.1)	1/5.3% (<0.01–26.5)	23 (100%)

[a]HPV detection and typing in 596 women
[b]HPV detection and typing in 348 women for which cytology results were available

instructions. Reactions were incubated at 37 °C for 1 h. Digested products were electrophoretically separated on 2% agarose gels supplemented with ethidium bromide in parallel with a 100 bp DNA ladder (New England BioLabs, Ipswich, MA). In cases where the HPV types were unidentifiable due to the similarity of restriction profile, or a mixture of HPV types was detected, a second round of restriction digestion of PCR products was performed using the above protocol with the following restriction endonucleases: AccI, HaeIII, HincII, HindIII, SpeI, and SspI (all from New England BioLabs, Ipswich, MA), according to the manufacturer's instructions.

Following the RFLP analysis, individual HPV genotypes were classified into HR, LR, and unknown risk (UR). Classification of HR-HPV genotypes followed the IARC Monograph (2012) [7] and included HPV genotypes 16, 18, 31, 33, 35, 39, 45, 51, 52, 56, 58, 59, and 68. The LR group included HPV genotypes 6, 11, 42, 44, 53, 54, 55, 61, 66, 70, 73, 81, 82, and 89. The UR group included HPV genotypes 34, 62, 67, 83, 84, 85, 90, 91, and 118.

Statistical analysis

Overall HPV prevalence was initially determined in all 596 samples included in the study, followed by analysis to determine type-specific distribution in those samples with HPV-positive status. These results were also analysed in the context of the different age groups. The association between HPV infection and individual genotypes with the three different groups of cytology result (ASCUS, L-SIL, H-SIL) was assessed in 348 samples for which cytology results were available.

The GraphPad Prism software version 5 (GraphPad, San Diego, CA, USA) was used for statistical analysis. Fisher's exact test was used to compare proportions where appropriate. Trends in proportion were tested using the chi-square test (χ^2). Proportions were computed with the corresponding 95% confidence intervals (95% CI) according to the modified Wald method [18]. All statistical tests were two-sided, and all P values of <0.05 were considered statistically significant.

Ethical approval

This study was exempted from ethical approval by the Cyprus National Bioethics Committee (Reference no: EEBK/21.1.02.01.05). Ethical approval and informed consent was not required because all the data utilized for the present study were generated following diagnostic HPV tests of cervicovaginal wash samples that were referred to the department of Molecular Virology by experienced gynaecologists as part of a diagnostic procedure in women with an abnormal Pap test.

Results

HPV prevalence and age distribution

Of the 596 women tested, 434 women (72.8%) were positive for at least one HPV type; the prevalence among age groups is listed in Table 1. Overall, the HPV prevalence was age dependent, with a decreasing prevalence until the age of 45 years (p = 0.0018, χ^2). The highest prevalence of HPV was detected in women ≤25 years (84.7%), followed by women aged 26–35 years (76.9%), and women ≥46 years (67.9%), and the lowest prevalence of HPV infection (63.4%) was found in women between 36 and 45 years (Table 1).

HPV genotype distribution

The 434 samples identified to be positive for HPV DNA were further analysed to identify the infecting HPV genotype. In total, 36 HPV types were identified and stratified according to their oncogenic potential into the following three categories: 13 HR-HPV types (HPV16, 18, 31, 33, 35, 39, 45, 51, 52, 56, 58, 59, and 68), 14 LR-HPV types (HPV6, 11, 42, 44, 53, 54, 55, 61, 66, 70, 73, 81, 82, and 89), and 9 types for which the risk is still unknown (UR-HPV) (HPV34, 62, 67, 83, 84, 85, 90, 91, and 118). The prevalences of HR-HPV, LR-HPV, and UR-HPV are listed in Table 1. In general, regardless of patient age, the HR-HPV types were the most frequent (59.4% of the overall HPV prevalence), with the highest prevalence (62.6%) in women ≤25 years. Although not age dependent ($p > 0.05$, χ^2), the prevalence of HR-HPV types declined marginally as age increased up to the group of women ≥46 years of age (26–35: 61.3%; 36–45: 56.5%; ≥46: 56.6%). In contrast, the prevalence of UR-HPV appeared to be age dependent ($p = 0.0232$, χ^2), with an increasing prevalence with increasing age up to the 36–45 age group (10.6%). No significant association could be established between the LR-HPV group and any of the age groups. The prevalence of LR-HPV types ranged from 37.4% in the youngest age group, to 33.7%, 32.9% and 35.8% in the age groups 26–35, 36–45, and ≥46 respectively (Table 1).

Detailed analysis of the prevalence of individual HPV genotypes in the whole cohort of samples revealed that HR-HPV16 was the most common type detected (17.7%), followed by HR-HPV31 (12.9%) (Fig. 1). The remaining HR-HPV types detected in order of decreasing prevalence were HPV58 (7.1%), HPV68 (4.6%), HPV18 (4.1%), HPV56 (3.7%), HPV51 (3.5%), HPV45 (2.5%), HPV33 (2.3%), HPV39 (1.8%), HPV35 (1.6%), HPV52 (1.4%), and HPV59 (1.2%) (Fig. 1). Overall, the frequencies of infections with HPV types of LR and UR were lower than the occurrence of HR-HPV infections, with the most common LR- and UR-HPV types being HPV53 (11.3%) and HPV84 (2.5%) respectively (Fig. 1).

Multiple infections

Co-infection with two or more HPV types was observed in 99 of the 434 HPV-positive samples (22.8%). Dual infections accounted for 18.7% of all positive samples, with three and four viruses detected in 3.9% and 0.2% of positive samples, respectively. Table 2 summarizes the prevalence of each HPV type in single vs. multiple infections. Overall, HPV16 was the most common genotype detected in multiple infections (5.8%), followed by HPV31 (4.8%), HPV53 (4.6%), HPV6 and HPV58 (2.8%), and HPV66 (2.1%). HPV types that were not present in conjunction with other viruses included HPV67, HPV85, HPV90, and HPV118, which were each present in only 1 or 2 samples.

Prevalence of HPV types stratified by the cervical cytological result

In the subgroup of 348 women for whom a cytology result was available, 254 (73%) were affected by ASCUS, 71 (20.4%) by L-SIL and 23 (6.6%) by H-SIL (Table 1). HPV DNA was detected in 268 out of 348 of these samples (77%). Among women with a cytology result of ASCUS, L-SIL and H-SIL, 74%, 85.9% and 82.6% were infected with HPV, respectively (Table 1).

The prevalence of HR-HPV, LR-HPV and UR-HPV types among HPV-positive samples diagnosed with ASCUS, L-SIL and H-SIL is also listed in Table 1. Irrespective of cytology results, HR-HPV genotypes were detected with the highest prevalence in all three cytology classes (ASCUS: 62.2%, L-SIL: 60.7%, H-SIL: 57.9%). The second most prevalent HPV genotypes that were detected belonged to the LR-HPV group, with their prevalence ranging from 33% in the ASCUS group to 36.1% in the L-SIL group and 36.8% in the H-SIL group. No significant

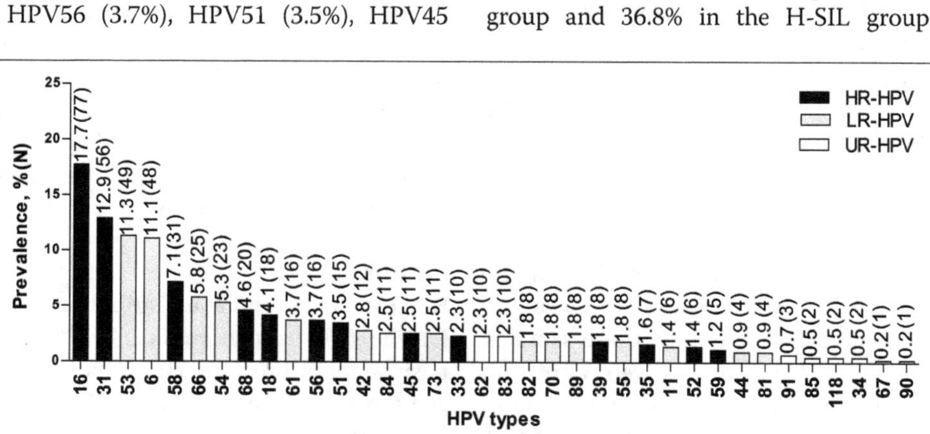

Fig. 1 Overall HPV type-specific distribution in decreasing order of prevalence among HPV-positive women ($N = 434$)

Table 2 Distribution of infections in 434 HPV-positive women, by HPV genotypes detected by PCR-RFLP

Genotypes	Infections	
	Single, *N* (%)	Multiple, *N* (%)
HR-HPV		
HPV16	52 (12%)	25 (5.8%)
HPV18	11 (2.5%)	7 (1.6%)
HPV31	35 (8.1%)	21 (4.8%)
HPV33	4 (0.9%)	6 (1.4%)
HPV35	5 (1.2%)	2 (0.5%)
HPV39	5 (1.2%)	3 (0.7%)
HPV45	6 (1.4%)	5 (1.2%)
HPV51	10 (2.3%)	5 (1.2%)
HPV52	1 (0.2%)	5 (1.2%)
HPV56	8 (1.8%)	8 (1.8%)
HPV58	19 (4.4%)	12 (2.8%)
HPV59	3 (0.7%)	2 (0.5%)
HPV68	14 (3.2%)	6 (1.4%)
LR-HPV		
HPV6	36 (8.3%)	12 (2.8%)
HPV11	3 (0.7%)	3 (0.7%)
HPV42	11 (2.5%)	1 (0.2%)
HPV44	2 (0.5%)	2 (0.5%)
HPV53	29 (6.7%)	20 (4.6%)
HPV54	17 (3.9%)	6 (1.4%)
HPV55	4 (0.9%)	4 (0.9%)
HPV61	10 (2.3%)	6 (1.4%)
HPV66	16 (3.7%)	9 (2.1%)
HPV70	6 (1.4%)	2 (0.5%)
HPV73	4 (0.9%)	7 (1.6%)
HPV81	3 (0.7%)	1 (0.2%)
HPV82	5 (1.2%)	3 (0.7%)
HPV89	6 (1.4)	2 (0.5%)
UR-HPV		
HPV34	1 (0.2%)	1 (0.2%)
HPV62	5 (1.2%)	5 (1.2%)
HPV67	1 (0.2%)	0 (0%)
HPV83	5 (1.2%)	5 (1.2%)
HPV84	6 (1.4%)	5 (1.2%)
HPV85	2 (0.5%)	0 (0.0%)
HPV90	1 (0.2%)	0 (0.0%)
HPV91	2 (0.5%)	1 (0.2%)
HPV118	2 (0.5%)	0 (0.0%)

association could be established between the different classes of cytological abnormalities and any of the HR-HPV, LR-HPV, and UR-HPV type groups ($p > 0.05$, χ^2).

Detailed analysis of the prevalence of individual HPV genotypes in the three different classes of cytological abnormalities revealed that the most prevalent HPV types were: HPV31 in 31 out of 188 HPV-positive women affected by ASCUS (16.5%), HPV16 in 12 out of 61 HPV-positive women affected by L-SIL (19.7%) and HPV16 in 3 out of 19 HPV-positive women affected by H-SIL (15.8%). The distribution and proportion of the HPV genotypes in different classes of cytological abnormalities are presented in Table 3.

Discussion

The analysis presented here is a study of the rate of HPV detection and type distribution in samples of women living in Cyprus that were referred because of an abnormal Pap test. To the best of our knowledge, this work is the first of its kind in this population.

Overall, the prevalence of HPV in the entire group (n = 596) was 72.8% (434 of 596). This result is consistent with previous studies of similar nature conducted in other European countries that reported HPV prevalence ranging from 35.3% to 88.9% among women with cytological abnormalities [19–27]. The results for each of these studies together with the methods used for analysis are listed in Table 4. The high HPV prevalence in our study group could be partly attributed to the fact that the referred samples were selected for molecular investigation by experienced specialists based on cytological abnormalities and therefore were more likely to have detectable HPV DNA as a result of a current HPV infection. Variations between studies most likely reflect differences in the population studied with respect to risk factors for exposure to HPV and methods used for analysis as well as triage for HPV testing by gynaecologists.

HPV prevalence stratified by age revealed an age-dependent association, in agreement with data reported in other European countries [21, 28, 29], reflecting a higher risk in young sexually active women that tend to have multiple partners [30].

In the present study, a spectrum of 36 genotypes were identified, with HR-HPV types being more frequently detected than LR-HPV types. Thirteen HR-HPV genotypes were detected in the sample cohort and accounted for 59.4% of HPV-positive samples, in accordance with other studies carried out in similar populations [19, 21, 27, 31]. Overall, the most prevalent genotype was HPV16, present in 17.7% of the specimens, followed by HR-HPV31, LR-HPV53, and LR-HPV6. These findings paralleled those of other studies, in which HPV16 and HPV31 were the predominant genotypes detected in women of European origin with cervical cytological

Table 3 Distribution and proportion of HPV genotypes in ASCUS, L-SIL, and H-SIL cytological lesions

Genotypes	Cytology result, *N* (%) ASCUS (*N* = 188)	L-SIL (*N* = 61)	H-SIL (*N* = 19)	Total[a] (%)
HR-HPV				
HPV16	26 (13.8%)	12 (19.7%)	3 (15.8%)	41 (15.3%)
HPV18	8 (4.3%)	2 (3.3%)	1 (5.3%)	11 (4.1%)
HPV31	31 (16.5%)	7 (11.5%)	2 (10.5%)	40 (14.9%)
HPV33	4 (2.1%)	2 (3.3%)	0 (0%)	6 (2.2%)
HPV35	3 (1.6%)	1 (1.6%)	0 (0%)	4 (1.5%)
HPV39	5 (2.7%)	2 (3.3%)	0 (0%)	7 (2.6%)
HPV45	5 (2.7%)	1 (1.6%)	2 (10.5%)	8 (3%)
HPV51	11 (5.9%)	1 (1.6%)	1 (5.3%)	13 (4.9%)
HPV52	0 (0%)	2 (3.3%)	2 (10.5%)	4 (1.5%)
HPV56	3 (1.6%)	6 (9.8%)	0 (0%)	9 (3.4%)
HPV58	18 (9.6%)	2 (3.3%)	0 (0%)	20 (7.5%)
HPV59	3 (1.6%)	1 (1.6%)	0 (0%)	4 (1.5%)
HPV68	8 (4.3%)	5 (8.2%)	1 (5.3%)	14 (5.2%)
LR-HPV				
HPV6	15 (8%)	7 (11.5%)	2 (10.5%)	24 (9%)
HPV11	2 (1.1%)	1 (1.6%)	0 (0%)	3 (1.1%)
HPV42	9 (4.8%)	1 (1.6%)	0 (0%)	10 (3.7%)
HPV44	1 (0.5%)	1 (1.6%)	1 (5.3%)	3 (1.1%)
HPV53	21 (11.2%)	5 (8.2%)	1 (5.3%)	27 (10.1%)
HPV54	6 (3.2%)	1 (1.6%)	2 (10.5%)	9 (3.4%)
HPV55	4 (2.1%)	0 (0%)	1 (5.3%)	5 (1.9%)
HPV61	11 (5.9%)	3 (4.9%)	0 (0%)	14 (5.2%)
HPV66	8 (4.3%)	7 (11.5%)	0 (0%)	15 (5.6%)
HPV70	2 (1.1%)	1 (1.6%)	0 (0%)	3 (1.1%)
HPV73	2 (1.1%)	3 (4.9%)	0 (0%)	5 (1.9%)
HPV81	3 (1.6%)	0 (0%)	0 (0%)	3 (1.1%)
HPV82	6 (3.2%)	0 (0%)	0 (0%)	6 (2.2%)
HPV89	4 (2.1%)	1 (1.6%)	1 (5.3%)	6 (2.2%)
UR-HPV				
HPV34	0 (0%)	1 (1.6%)	0 (0%)	1 (0.4%)
HPV62	1 (0.5%)	3 (4.9%)	0 (0%)	4 (1.5%)
HPV83	5 (2.7%)	0 (0%)	1 (5.3%)	6 (2.2%)
HPV84	5 (2.7%)	1 (1.6%)	2 (10.5%)	8 (3%)
HPV90	0 (0%)	1 (1.6%)	0 (0%)	1 (0.4%)
HPV91	1 (0.5%)	0 (0%)	0 (0%)	1 (0.4%)

[a]Overall prevalence of individual HPV types in 268 HPV-positive women with available cytology result

abnormalities [19, 27, 31–33]. HPV16 together with HPV18 are known to be responsible for approximately 70% of the cervical cancer cases worldwide [6, 8, 9]. The prevalence of HPV18 has been reported in other studies, ranging between 1.8% and 16.3% [20, 21, 23, 27]. In agreement with the aforementioned studies, the prevalence of HPV18 in the present study was 4.1%.

Our study showed that at least 22.8% of women were infected with two or more HPV genotypes, in accordance with other studies reporting a prevalence of multiple infections in 11% to 50% of cases [21, 23, 34]. The clinical significance of co-infection with multiple HPV genotypes remains uncertain, with some reports showing that the clearance rate in immunocompetent women is not

Table 4 Summary of European studies regarding the prevalence of HPV in women with cytological abnormalities

Authors (Year)	Citation	*N* (Country)	Method of Analysis	HPV+ (%)
Bonde et al. (2014)	[7]	5068 (Denmark)	CLART	88.9%
Capra et al. (2008)	[19]	970 (Italy)	Nested PCR/sequencing INNO-LiPA	37.7%
Delgado et al. (2012)	[20]	106 (Spain)	Linear Array	69.8%
Meloni et al. (2014)	[21]	650 (Italy)	INNO-LiPA	52.6%
Monsonego et al. (2008)	[22]	575 (France)	Linear Array Hybrid Capture II	88.1%
Panotopoulou et al. (2007)	[23]	997 (Greece)	PCR/sequencing	75.1%
Rassu et al. (2005)	[24]	1335 (Italy)	PCR-RFLP	35.3%
Simanaviciene et al. (2015)	[25]	547 (Lithuania)	PCR	67.6%
Spinillo et al. (2009)	[26]	1218 (Italy)	INNO-LiPA	69.9%
Yapijakis et al. (2008)	[27]	263 (Greece)	PCR-RFLP	81.7%

dependent on the number of genotypes involved in the infection [35]. Additionally, it is still not clear whether co-infection with multiple HPV genotypes increases the risk of progression to cancer [36, 37].

An increasing trend in the overall prevalence of HPV infection was observed in parallel with an increase in the degree of cervical cytological abnormalities (ASCUS: 74%, L-SIL: 85.9%, H-SIL: 82.6%). In agreement with our results showing HPV positivity in 82.6% of H-SIL cases, a meta-analysis conducted using data from 423 studies revealed an overall HPV prevalence in 84% and 85% of H-SIL cases in Europe and globally, respectively [38]. The prevalence of HR-HPV genotypes has been reported to increase with the grade of cytological lesions in some [28, 31, 39] but not all published studies [20, 21, 40]. In the present work, such an association was not observed, probably due to the low number of HPV-positive L-SIL and H-SIL cases that were included for analysis. An alternative explanation might be the lack of histological results as verification for the cytology results. As previously reported, almost 40% of women with an ASCUS diagnosis could be histologically confirmed as high-grade cervical neoplasia [41]. Nevertheless, HR-HPV types were more frequently detected than LR-HPV types in all three classes of precancerous lesions (ASCUS: 62.2% vs 33%, L-SIL: 60.7% vs 36.1%, H-SIL: 57.9% vs 36.8%), highlighting the need for more frequent follow-up examinations in women who are HR-HPV-positive.

Among individual HPV types, HPV16 was the most frequently identified type in both the L-SIL (19.7%) and the H-SIL (15.8%) group, confirming that HPV16 is the most frequent HPV type associated with high-grade lesions, as was previously reported [32, 33]. The current literature suggests that HPV16 and HPV18 are more likely to progress to cervical cancer than L-SIL and H-SIL with other HPV genotypes [32, 33]. Therefore, it could be of potential benefit to the patient if HPV16- and/or HPV18-infected SIL cases are separated from those infected with other HR-HPV types for closer monitoring and surveillance. Regarding the prevalence of HPV18 in the present study, this HPV type was detected at a low prevalence in all three classes of cytological abnormalities, with the highest prevalence detected in the H-SIL group (5.3%) followed by the ASCUS group (4.3%) and the L-SIL group (3.3%). A meta-analysis carried out with data from 55 studies of women showing a prevalence of HPV18 in L-SIL and H-SIL cases of 8.6% and 7% respectively [32, 33]. However, the results obtained for HPV18 should be interpreted cautiously because, as previously indicated, the number of L-SIL and H-SIL cases available for analysis in the present study was small. Nonetheless, it is interesting to note that the short time of progression to invasive cancer as a result of infection by HR-HPV types such as HPV18, with or without transition through the pre-invasive cases, might be an additional contributor to the low prevalence of HPV18 in L-SIL and H-SIL cases in our study.

Only few studies have addressed the prevalence of HPV in women with abnormal cytology in the geographical region in Eastern Mediterranean and Middle East. In Turkey, three studies showed an overall HPV prevalence ranging from 13.7% to 52% in women with abnormal cytology [42–44], with HR-HPV types detected in 27% and 20% of L-SIL and H-SIL cases [42]. In contrast, other studies in the surrounding region reported higher HPV prevalence rates in women with abnormal cytology, such as 84% in Jordan [45] and 100% in Egypt [46]. In the Jordanian study, HR-HPV prevalence was 72.2% and 78.6% of L-SIL and H-SIL cases, respectively [45]. In agreement with our results, HPV16 was the most common genotype detected in the above studies [42–46]. In terms of overall HPV positivity (72.8%) and HR-HPV prevalence in L-SIL (60.7%) and H-SIL (57.9%) cases, our results are discordant with the above studies. These discrepancies might be attributed to the differences in study populations and designs as well as due to the different methodologies used for sample analysis.

The current results should be evaluated in the context of the strengths and limitations of the study. A major strength of this study is the fact that it provides the first estimates of the prevalence of HPV and its type-specific distribution among women from Cyprus diagnosed with cytological abnormalities by Pap test. The presented study, however, is not without limitations. First, the results relied on samples referred to our laboratory for diagnostic purposes as convenience samples. Thus, these data cannot be considered nationally representative because the Cypriot women included in the study may not be a representative sample of all the Cypriot women living in the country. Another potential limitation is the extent of missing cytological data (41.6%) that required implementation of an amputation scheme during assessment of overall HPV prevalence and type-specific distribution in the groups with different cytological abnormalities. However, our analyses suggest that there was no selection bias when assessing HPV prevalence in only those samples for which cytology results were available, as overall HPV positivity in samples with cytology results as presented in the study (n = 348) (77%, 95% CI: 72.3–81.1) is very similar to HPV positivity of all analysed samples (n = 596) (72.8%, 95% CI: 69.1–76.2). In a similar manner, type-specific distribution in HPV-positive samples with available cytology results is comparable to type-specific distribution observed in all samples with HPV-positive status (Table 3 and Fig. 1). The present study analysed samples using an established PCR-RFLP methodology that was optimized and validated in our laboratory. Although an unassuming method of a seemingly bygone era, PCR-RFLP is a robust approach for detection and genotyping of HPV and shows excellent discriminatory power to differentiate the HPV in HR or LR groups and to identify single or multiple infections [47]. Current literature suggests additional HPV assays that are commercially available for HPV testing including Hybrid Capture 2, Linear Array, INNO-LiPa, CLART, PapilloCheck, Abbott real-time PCR, and COBAS 4800 HPV test [47]. From a screening perspective, it might therefore be interesting to show the robustness of our methodology compared to the above commercially available assays in future studies.

Beginning in January 2016, the Health Ministry of the Cyprus government has introduced an HPV vaccination programme for all 12-year-old girls. The use of genotyping assays could prove pivotal for monitoring the effect of this HPV vaccination programme. The results of the present study could also provide a baseline reference for a later comparison of HPV prevalence among vaccinated women. Additionally, the data on type-specific HPV distribution presented herein can provide a reference point for evaluating the efficacy of available vaccines in conferring cross-protection against non-vaccine types, monitoring at the same time undesirable phenomena such as HPV type replacement.

Conclusions

In conclusion, this study presents the first investigation into the prevalence of HPV infection and HPV genotype distribution in Cypriot women with abnormal cytological tests. Whether the presented results may reflect the HPV prevalence and genotype distribution in the general population remains to be seen in additional population-based epidemiological studies. Nevertheless, the high prevalence of HPV16 and HPV6 detected in the present study highlights the potential benefits of the introduction of a national HPV immunization programme. Furthermore, as seen in the present study, the circulation of HPV genotypes other than those targeted by the available HPV vaccines [11, 12] highlights the necessity of sustaining such screening programmes in the near future. Otherwise, it is possible that the available vaccines could cause a genotype redistribution with an increase in the number of women infected with HPV types other than those targeted by vaccines.

Abbreviations

ASCUS: atypical squamous cells of undetermined significance; HPV: human papillomavirus; HR: high-risk; H-SIL: high-grade squamous intraepithelial lesion; LR: low-risk; L-SIL: low-grade squamous intraepithelial lesion; RFLP: restriction fragment length polymorphism; UR: unknown risk

Acknowledgements

The authors are grateful to the Cyprus Institute of Neurology and Genetics and the members of the Molecular Virology departments for their assistance with this study.

Funding

This work was supported by the Cyprus Institute of Neurology and Genetics through grants provided for research purposes.

Authors' contributions

DK and CC conceived the study protocol. DK and GK were responsible for HPV testing, HPV typing, analysis and interpretation of the data, literature research, data collection, and statistical analyses. GK wrote the first draft of the manuscript. All authors gave input into the final manuscript. All authors read and approved the final manuscript.

Competing interests

The authors declare that they have no competing interests.

Consent for publication

Not applicable.

Ethics approval and consent to participate

The study was exempted from ethical approval by the Cyprus National Bioethics Committee (Reference no: EEBK/21.1.02.01.05). Ethical approval and signing of an informed consent form was not required because all the data utilized for the present study were generated following diagnostic HPV tests of cervicovaginal wash samples that were referred to the department of Molecular Virology by experienced gynaecologists, as part of an investigative procedure in women with an abnormal Pap test.

References

1. Bosch FX, Manos MM, Munoz N, Sherman M, Jansen AM, Peto J, Schiffman MH, Moreno V, Kurman R, Shah KV. Prevalence of human papillomavirus in cervical cancer: a worldwide perspective. International biological study on cervical cancer (IBSCC) study group. J Natl Cancer Inst. 1995;87:796–802.
2. Bosch FX, Lorincz A, Munoz N, Meijer CJ, Shah KV. The causal relation between human papillomavirus and cervical cancer. J Clin Pathol. 2002;55:244–65.
3. Munoz N, Bosch FX, de Sanjose S, Herrero R, Castellsague X, Shah KV, Snijders PJ, Meijer CJ. Epidemiologic classification of human papillomavirus types associated with cervical cancer. N Engl J Med. 2003;348:518–27.
4. Jemal A, Bray F, Center MM, Ferlay J, Ward E, Forman D. Global cancer statistics. CA Cancer J Clin. 2011;61:69–90.
5. Baseman JG, Koutsky LA. The epidemiology of human papillomavirus infections. J Clin Virol. 2005;32(Suppl 1):S16–24.
6. de Sanjose S, Quint WG, Alemany L, Geraets DT, Klaustermeier JE, Lloveras B, Tous S, Felix A, Bravo LE, Shin HR, Vallejos CS, de Ruiz PA, Lima MA, Guimera N, Clavero O, Alejo M, Llombart-Bosch A, Cheng-Yang C, Tatti SA, Kasamatsu E, Iljazovic E, Odida M, Prado R, Seoud M, Grce M, Usubutun A, Jain A, Suarez GA, Lombardi LE, Banjo A, Menendez C, Domingo EJ, Velasco J, Nessa A, Chichareon SC, Qiao YL, Lerma E, Garland SM, Sasagawa T, Ferrera A, Hammouda D, Mariani L, Pelayo A, Steiner I, Oliva E, Meijer CJ, Al-Jassar WF, Cruz E, Wright TC, Puras A, Llave CL, Tzardi M, Agorastos T, Garcia-Barriola V, Clavel C, Ordi J, Andujar M, Castellsague X, Sanchez GI, Nowakowski AM, Bornstein J, Munoz N, Bosch FX. Human papillomavirus genotype attribution in invasive cervical cancer: a retrospective cross-sectional worldwide study. Lancet Oncol. 2010;11:1048–1056.
7. Bonde J, Rebolj M, Ejegod DM, Preisler S, Lynge E, Rygaard C. HPV prevalence and genotype distribution in a population-based split-sample study of well-screened women using CLART HPV2 human papillomavirus genotype microarray system. BMC Infect Dis. 2014;14:413.
8. Walboomers JM, Jacobs MV, Manos MM, Bosch FX, Kummer JA, Shah KV, Snijders PJ, Peto J, Meijer CJ, Munoz N. Human papillomavirus is a necessary cause of invasive cervical cancer worldwide. J Pathol. 1999;189:12–9.
9. Lombard I, Vincent-Salomon A, Validire P, Zafrani B, de la Rochefordiere A, Clough K, Favre M, Pouillart P, Sastre-Garau X. Human papillomavirus genotype as a major determinant of the course of cervical cancer. J Clin Oncol. 1998;16:2613–9.
10. Rosales R, Rosales C. Immune therapy for human papillomaviruses-related cancers. World J Clin Oncol. 2014;5:1002–19.
11. Villa LL, Costa RL, Petta CA, Andrade RP, Paavonen J, Iversen OE, Olsson SE, Hoye J, Steinwall M, Riis-Johannessen G, Andersson-Ellstrom A, Elfgren K, Krogh G, Lehtinen M, Malm C, Tamms GM, Giacoletti K, Lupinacci L, Railkar R, Taddeo FJ, Bryan J, Esser MT, Sings HL, Saah AJ, Barr E. High sustained efficacy of a prophylactic quadrivalent human papillomavirus types 6/11/16/18 L1 virus-like particle vaccine through 5 years of follow-up. Br J Cancer. 2006;95:1459–66.
12. Harper DM, Franco EL, Wheeler CM, Moscicki AB. Romanowski B, Roteli-Martins CM, Jenkins D, Schuind A, Costa Clemens SA, Dubin G. Sustained efficacy up to 4.5 years of a bivalent L1 virus-like particle vaccine against human papillomavirus types 16 and 18: follow-up from a randomised control trial. Lancet. 2006;367:1247–1255.
13. Kirby T. FDA approves new upgraded Gardasil 9. Lancet Oncol. 2015;16:e56.
14. Papapetrou I, Charalambous G, Sissouras A, Jelastopulu E. Cervical cancer screening in the municipality of Nicosia. Cyprus-Coverage and association with socioeconomic determinants Austin Journal of Public Health and Epidemiology. 2016;3:1032.
15. Henry MR. The Bethesda system 2001: an update of new terminology for gynecologic cytology. Clin Lab Med. 2003;23:585–603.
16. Manos MM, Y. T, Wright DK, Lewis AJ, Broker TR, Wolinsky SM. The use of polymerase chain reaction amplification for the detection of genital human papillomaviruses. Cancer Cells 1989;7:209–214.
17. Saiki RK, Gelfand DH, Stoffel S, Scharf SJ, Higuchi R, Horn GT, Mullis KB, Erlich HA. Primer-directed enzymatic amplification of DNA with a thermostable DNA polymerase. Science. 1988;239:487–91.
18. Agresti A, Coull B. Aproximate is better than "exact" for interval estimation of binomial proportions. Am Stat. 1998;52:119–26.
19. Capra G, Giovannelli L, Bellavia C, Migliore MC, Caleca MP, Perino A, Ammatuna P. HPV genotype prevalence in cytologically abnormal cervical samples from women living in south Italy. Virus Res. 2008;133:195–200.
20. Delgado D, Marin JM, de Diego J, Guerra S, Gonzalez B, Barrios JL, Canut A. Human papillomavirus (HPV) genotype distribution in women with abnormal cervical cytology in the Basque Country. Spain Enferm Infecc Microbiol Clin. 2012;30:230–5.
21. Meloni A, Pilia R, Campagna M, Usai A, Masia G, Caredda V, Coppola RC. Prevalence and molecular epidemiology of human papillomavirus infection in italian women with cervical cytological abnormalities. J Public Health Res. 2014;3:157.
22. Monsonego J, Pollini G, Evrard MJ, Sednaoui P, Monfort L, Zerat L, Syrjanen K. Detection of human papillomavirus genotypes among high-risk women: a comparison of hybrid capture and linear array tests. Sex Transm Dis. 2008;35:521–7.
23. Panotopoulou E, Tserkezoglou A, Kouvousi M, Tsiaousi I, Chatzieleftheriou G, Daskalopoulou D, Magiakos G. Prevalence of human papillomavirus types 6, 11, 16, 18, 31, and 33 in a cohort of Greek women. J Med Virol. 2007;79: 1898–905.
24. Rassu M, Bertoloni G, Mengoli C, Peron A, Benedetti P, Palu G. HPV genotype prevalence in cervical specimens with abnormal cytology: a report from north-east Italy. Scand J Infect Dis. 2005;37:476–81.
25. Simanaviciene V, Gudleviciene Z, Popendikyte V, Dekaminaviciute D, Stumbryte A, Rubinaite V, Zvirbliene A. Studies on the prevalence of oncogenic HPV types among Lithuanian women with cervical pathology. J Med Virol. 2015;87:461–71.
26. Spinillo A, Dal Bello B, Gardella B, Roccio M, Dacco MD, Silini EM. Multiple human papillomavirus infection and high grade cervical intraepithelial neoplasia among women with cytological diagnosis of atypical squamous cells of undetermined significance or low grade squamous intraepithelial lesions. Gynecol Oncol. 2009;113:115–9.
27. Yapijakis C, Adamopoulou M, Antonopoulos G, Koufaliotis N, Vairaktaris E. Prevalence of HPV types in a cohort of Greeks with clinical indication of infection. Anticancer Res. 2008;28:2233–7.
28. Argyri E, Papaspyridakos S, Tsimplaki E, Michala L, Myriokefalitaki E, Papassideri I, Daskalopoulou D, Tsiaoussi I, Magiakos G, Panotopoulou E. A cross sectional study of HPV type prevalence according to age and cytology. BMC Infect Dis. 2013;13:53.
29. Kjaer SK, Breugelmans G, Munk C, Junge J, Watson M, Iftner T. Population-based prevalence, type- and age-specific distribution of HPV in women before introduction of an HPV-vaccination program in Denmark. Int J Cancer. 2008;123:1864–70.
30. Ethier KA, Kershaw T, Niccolai L, Lewis JB, Ickovics JR. Adolescent women underestimate their susceptibility to sexually transmitted infections. Sex Transm Infect. 2003;79:408–11.
31. Pista A, Oliveira A, Verdasca N, Ribeiro F. Single and multiple human papillomavirus infections in cervical abnormalities in Portuguese women. Clin Microbiol Infect. 2011;17:941–6.
32. Clifford GM, Rana RK, Franceschi S, Smith JS, Gough G, Pimenta JM. Human papillomavirus genotype distribution in low-grade cervical lesions: comparison by geographic region and with cervical cancer. Cancer Epidemiol Biomark Prev. 2005;14:1157–64.
33. Clifford GM, Smith JS, Aguado T, Franceschi S. Comparison of HPV type distribution in high-grade cervical lesions and cervical cancer: a meta-analysis. Br J Cancer. 2003;89:101–5.
34. Gargiulo F, De Francesco MA, Schreiber C, Ciravolo G, Salinaro F, Valloncini B, Manca N. Prevalence and distribution of single and multiple HPV infections in cytologically abnormal cervical samples from Italian women. Virus Res. 2007;125:176–82.
35. Molano M, Van den Brule A, Plummer M, Weiderpass E, Posso H, Arslan A, Meijer CJ, Munoz N, Franceschi S. Determinants of clearance of human papillomavirus infections in Colombian women with normal cytology: a population-based, 5-year follow-up study. Am J Epidemiol. 2003;158:486–94.
36. Agarossi A, Ferrazzi E, Parazzini F, Perno CF, Ghisoni L. Prevalence and type distribution of high-risk human papillomavirus infection in women undergoing voluntary cervical cancer screening in Italy. J Med Virol. 2009;81:529–35.
37. Broccolo F, Chiari S, Piana A, Castiglia P, Dell'Anna T, Garcia-Parra R, Maneo A, Villa A, Leone EB, Perego P, Maida A, Mangioni C, Cocuzza CE. Prevalence and viral load of oncogenic human papillomavirus types associated with cervical carcinoma in a population of North Italy. J Med Virol. 2009;81:278–87.
38. Guan P, Howell-Jones R, Li N, Bruni L, de Sanjose S, Franceschi S, Clifford GM. Human papillomavirus types in 115,789 HPV-positive women: a meta-analysis from cervical infection to cancer. Int J Cancer. 2012;131:2349–59.
39. Dickson EL, Vogel RI, Geller MA, Downs LS Jr. Cervical cytology and multiple type HPV infection: a study of 8182 women ages 31-65. Gynecol Oncol. 2014;133:405–8.
40. Moga MA, Irimie M, Oanta A, Pascu A, Burtea V. Type-specific prevalence of

human papillomavirus by cervical cytology among women in Brasov. Romania Asian Pac J Cancer Prev. 2014;15:6887–92.
41. Kinney WK, Manos MM, Hurley LB, Ransley JE. Where's the high-grade cervical neoplasia? The importance of minimally abnormal Papanicolaou diagnoses. Obstet Gynecol. 1998;91:973–6.
42. Dursun P, Ayhan A, Mutlu L, Caglar M, Haberal A, Gungor T, Ozat M, Ozgu E, Onan A, Taskiran C, Guner H, Yetimalar H, Kasap B, Yuce K, Salman MC, Sayal B, Dogan S, Harma M, Basaran M, Aydogmus H, Ergun Y, Sehirali S, Gultekin E, Kose S, Yildirim Y, Yenen M, Dede M, Alanbay I, Karaca R, Metindir J, Keskin L, Ustuner I, Avsar F, Yuksel H, Kirdar S. HPV types in Turkey: multicenter hospital based evaluation of 6388 patients in Turkish gynecologic oncology group centers. Turk Patoloji Derg. 2013;29:210–216.
43. Dursun P, Senger SS, Arslan H, Kuscu E, Ayhan A. Human papillomavirus (HPV) prevalence and types among Turkish women at a gynecology outpatient unit. BMC Infect Dis. 2009;9:191.
44. Ozalp SS, Us T, Arslan E, Oge T, Kasifoglu N. HPV DNA and pap smear test results in cases with and without cervical pathology. J Turk Ger Gynecol Assoc. 2012;13:8–14.
45. Obeidat B, Matalka I, Mohtaseb A, Jaradat S, Hayajneh W, Khasawneh R, Haddad H, Obeidat F. Prevalence and distribution of high-risk human papillomavirus genotypes in cervical carcinoma, low-grade, and high-grade squamous intraepithelial lesions in Jordanian women. Eur J Gynaecol Oncol. 2013;34:257–60.
46. Youssef MA, Abdelsalam L, Harfoush RA, Talaat IM, Elkattan E, Mohey A, Abdella RM, Farhan MS, Foad HA, Elsayed AM, Elkinaa NA, Ghaith D, Rashed ME, Ghafar MA, Khamis Y, Hosni AN. Prevalence of human papilloma virus (HPV) and its genotypes in cervical specimens of Egyptian women by linear array HPV genotyping test. Infect Agent Cancer. 2016;11:6.
47. Abreu AL, Souza RP, Gimenes F, Consolaro ME. A review of methods for detect human papillomavirus infection. Virol J. 2012;9:262.

7

Quality assurance of human papillomavirus (HPV) testing in the implementation of HPV primary screening in Norway: an inter-laboratory reproducibility study

Birgit Engesæter[1], Bianca van Diermen Hidle[2], Mona Hansen[3], Pia Moltu[2], Kjersti Mangseth Staby[4], Siri Borchgrevink-Persen[5], Olav K. Vintermyr[4,6], Stefan Lönnberg[1], Mari Nygård[1], Emiel A. M. Janssen[2,7], Philip E. Castle[8] and Irene Kraus Christiansen[3*]

Abstract

Background: Human papillomavirus (HPV) testing as primary screening for cervical cancer is currently being implemented in Norway in a randomized controlled fashion, involving three laboratories. As part of the quality assurance programme of the implementation, an evaluation of the inter-laboratory reproducibility of the HPV test was initiated, to ensure satisfactory HPV test reliability in all three laboratories.

Methods: The HPV test used is the cobas 4800 HPV Test, detecting 14 high-risk types with individual HPV genotype results for HPV16 and HPV18. In addition to the three laboratories involved in the implementation, the Norwegian HPV reference laboratory was included as a fourth comparative laboratory. A stratified sample of 500 cervical liquid based cytology (LBC) samples was used in the evaluation, with an aim towards a high-risk HPV positivity of ~25%. Samples were collected at one laboratory, anonymized, aliquoted, and distributed to the other laboratories.

Results: Comparison of the test results of all four laboratories revealed a 95.6% agreement, an 86.3% positive agreement and a kappa value of 0.94 (95% CI 0.92–0.97). For negative cytology specimens, there was a 95.8% overall agreement, a 67.4% positive agreement, and a kappa value of 0.88 (95% CI 0.80–0.93). For abnormal cytology specimens, there was a 95.8% overall agreement, a 95.5% positive agreement, and a kappa value of 0.86 (95% CI 0.71–0.97).

Conclusions: The study showed a high inter-laboratory reproducibility of HPV testing, implying satisfactory user performance and reliability in the laboratories involved in the implementation project. This is important knowledge and we recommend similar studies always to be performed prior to the introduction of new screening routines.

Keywords: Human papillomavirus, HPV, Cervical cancer screening, HPV primary screening, HPV testing, Quality assurance, Cobas 4800 HPV Test, Inter-laboratory reproducibility

* Correspondence: irene.kraus.christiansen@ahus.no
[3]Department of Microbiology and Infection Control, Akershus University Hospital, Lørenskog, Norway
Full list of author information is available at the end of the article

Background

Identification of the association between high-risk human papillomavirus (HR-HPV) and cervical carcinogenesis has led to revolutionary advances in cervical cancer screening, including sensitive, molecular HPV tests that improve early detection of cervical precancerous lesions. In Norway, HPV testing was introduced in triage of women diagnosed with ASC-US (atypical squamous cells of undetermined significance) and LSIL (low-grade squamous intraepithelial lesions) in 2005. Based on randomized clinical trials of HR-HPV detection conducted in Europe, as well as recommendations by the European guidelines for quality assurance in cervical cancer screening [1–3], HPV testing in primary screening has been introduced in several European countries during the last few years. The more sensitive and objective HPV test is proposed to increase health benefit and reduce the harms associated with screening. In addition, the objectivity of the test implies better reproducibility compared to cytology [4]. Still, primary HPV-based screening has been and is controversial, related to the low clinical specificity of HPV DNA tests. HPV DNA testing will identify several infections never leading to dysplasia or cancer, especially in younger age-groups. Of this reason, HPV primary screening is commonly introduced for women above the age of 30. Also, low specificity of HPV DNA testing is partly compensated for by cytological triage of HPV positive women (http://www.kreftregisteret.no/hpv-algoritme).

In 2015, gradual implementation of primary HPV screening in the Norwegian cervical cancer screening programme was initiated. Women in the age group 34–69 years resident in four (of a total of 19) counties in Norway, are randomized to HPV testing or cytology according to their date of birth. The HPV analyses are performed by three laboratories located at Stavanger University Hospital, Stavanger, Haukeland University Hospital, Bergen and St. Olavs Hospital, Trondheim University Hospital, Trondheim. After competitive bidding, the cobas 4800 HPV Test (Roche Diagnostics) was selected for the implementation. In 2014, the cobas HPV Test was U.S. Food and Drug-approved for use in primary cervical cancer screening for women 25 year and older.

In addition to good clinical performance, reproducibility of laboratory results is fundamental for safe screening. To confirm satisfactory HPV test reproducibility and user performance within the screening programme, an evaluation of inter-laboratory reproducibility between the three service laboratories involved in the implementation was performed. The Norwegian HPV reference laboratory (Akershus University Hospital, Lørenskog), with cobas 4800 HPV Test accreditation since 2011, contributed as a fourth evaluator. Two of the three service laboratories had no previous experience with the test, and a shared laboratory handbook containing necessary standard operating procedures (SOPs) for HPV testing was prepared to ensure standardized methods. The inter-laboratory evaluation of HPV testing reported here was considered part of the quality assurance programme of the implementation of HPV primary screening in Norway, aiming to confirm satisfactory user performance and reliability in each of the three laboratories.

Methods

Clinical material and study design

Residual material of cervical liquid based cytology (LBC) samples (in PreservCyt medium, Hologic, Bedford, MA, USA) taken as part of the cervical cancer screening programme in Norway, was used. The samples were collected at Stavanger University Hospital, Department of Pathology, in the time period December 16th 2014 to May 21st 2015. All ages were included (comprising ages 16–81 years).

Two-sided Z test (kappa statistic) for agreement between two rates was used for sample size determination [5]. Power calculation showed that a sample size of 480 subjects achieved 86% power to detect a true Kappa value of 0.80 in a test of H0: Kappa = 0.69 vs. H1: Kappa <> 0.69. The power calculation was based on a significance level of 0.05. A total of 500 samples were collected with a composition aiming to provide an approximate prevalence of high-risk HPV of 25%. In order to reach that goal, 100 samples were selected based on the cytological results, either high-risk HPV DNA positive ASC-US or LSIL samples; or HSIL (high-grade squamous intraepithelial lesion) or ASC-H (atypical squamous cells, cannot rule out HSIL), assumed to be HPV positive. In addition, 400 consecutive samples without regard to their cytological results were included.

For ethical reasons, all samples were anonymized before HPV analysis. Cytological diagnoses were recorded prior to anonymization, important for the final evaluation of the results. For HSIL and ASC-H samples, a high concordance is essential. For NILM (negative for intra-epithelial lesions or malignancy) samples, with a generally lower viral load expected, a certain degree of discordance is expected due to the stochasticity of the PCR process. Due to anonymization of the samples, review of cytological diagnoses and/or comparison to histological results was not feasible.

One sample was excluded from the analyses due to empty sample tube upon arrival at one laboratory. Hence, the presented data are based on results from 499 samples.

Considering all 499 samples, 24% presented samples with cellular changes (ASC-US 7%, LSIL 7%, ASC-H 2% and HSIL 8%), while 5% was unsatisfactory for cytological evaluation. The sample distribution according to cytological result is given in Table 1.

HPV determination

The cobas 4800 HPV Test is a fully automated, qualitative multiplex assay, including full sample preparation (cobas x 480) and HPV detection (cobas z 480 Analyser) based on real-time polymerase chain reaction (PCR) technology. The method detects 14 high-risk types, including individual HPV genotype results for HPV16 and HPV18. The other 12 types are reported concurrently by a pooled result (HR-HPV). Beta-globin is used as an internal quality control for each sample. The system is provided with an advanced result algorithm for the calculation of distinct HPV positive, HPV negative or invalid (negative beta-globin) results and the ability to review reaction curves manually is not routinely available for users. In addition, of various indicated reasons, the sample may come up as "failed", with the most common explanations being clots or insufficient sample volume.

Results are reported through four channels specific for HPV16, HPV18, HR-HPV, or beta-globin, respectively. Each channel has a distinct cut-off value, based on cycle threshold (Ct) values to distinguish a clinically positive from a negative sample. The cut-off values are 40.5, 40.0, 40.0 and 40.0 for the four channels HPV16, HPV18, HR-HPV and beta-globlin, respectively [6]. Sets of positive controls (one for each channel; HPV16, HPV18 and HPV39) and negative controls are included for each set-up. The 960 sample kit was used by all laboratories.

Preparation and distribution of clinical material

Cytology was interpreted according to the Bethesda system as unsatisfactory, NILM, ASC-US, LSIL, ASC-H and HSIL. After registration of cytological diagnosis, the samples were anonymized and given a study identification number. The samples were stored within the validated storage parameters ascribed by the manufacturer, which says a maximum of 6 months at 2–30 °C. Each LBC sample was vigorously mixed by using a vortex machine and aliquoted to four Sarstedt tubes (1.25 ml to each tube allowing two runs with the cobas HPV Test). The first set of aliquots was analysed by lab A, the second by lab B, the third by lab C and the fourth by lab D (The Norwegian HPV reference laboratory).

Performance at the individual laboratory

Each laboratory (A, B, C and D) tested one set of aliquots blinded for all information except for the study identification number. The samples were run within the same defined period of two weeks. Samples were scanned directly onto the instrument and a work-list ("work order") was created. The analysis was performed according to the shared SOPs (www.kreftregisteret.no/laboratoriemappe). Samples obtaining "failed" results in the first analysis were rerun once. If persistent, the sample was reported as failed, and a flag explaining the reason for not being analyzed was attached. Remaining sample material after analysis was discarded. Results (raw data) of the testing from each lab were exported to Excel (Microsoft Office) and sent to the Cancer Registry of Norway for analysis and interpretation.

Statistical analyses

The inter-laboratory reproducibility was assessed by comparison of the test results using percentage agreement, positive percentage agreement and Fleiss' kappa statistics. Differences in test results were compared pairwise between the laboratories using McNemar test. Stata version 14.1 (Stata Corporation, College Station) was used for the analyses.

Results

HPV test results showed a mean HPV positivity rate of 28.9% for the four laboratories, varying from 28.3 to 29.3% (Table 2). Table 2 shows the frequency of HPV negative, HPV positive and failed samples for the laboratories, stratified on the cytological categories NILM, ASC-US, LSIL, ASC-H/HSIL and unsatisfactory.

Agreement between the laboratories was calculated by overall percentage agreement, positive percentage agreement and Fleiss' kappa. Comparison of the results from all four laboratories revealed 95.6% overall agreement, 86.3% positive agreement and a kappa value of 0.94 (95% CI 0.92–0.97) (Table 2). A pairwise comparison (not adjusted for multiple comparisons) did not reveal a significant difference between the results from the four laboratories ($p > 0.05$). Reproducibility between the laboratories was not dependent on cytological

Table 1 Distribution of cytological diagnoses among the 499 samples

	NILM $N = 355$	ASC-US $N = 36$	LSIL $N = 33$	ASC-H $N = 11$	HSIL $N = 38$	Unsatisfactory $N = 27$
100 selected samples	0	28[a]	28[a]	11	33	0
399 consecutive samples	354	8	5	0	5	27

[a]HPV positive samples

NILM negative for intraepithelial lesion or malignancy, *ASC-US* atypical squamous cells of undetermined significance, *LSIL* low-grade squamous intraepithelial lesion, *ASC-H* atypical squamous cells, cannot exclude a high-grade lesion, *HSIL* high-grade squamous intraepithelial lesion

Table 2 Frequencies of HPV negative, HPV positive and failed samples considering all 499 samples, stratified on cytological categories

	All (*n* = 499)			NILM (*n* = 354)			ASC-US (*n* = 36)			LSIL (*n* = 33)			ASC-H/HSIL (*n* = 49)			Unsatisfactory (*n* = 27)			ASC-US or more severe (*n* = 118)		
	#pos (%)	#neg (%)	#failed (%)	#pos (%)	#neg (%)	#failed (%)	#pos (%)	#neg (%)	#failed (%)	#pos (%)	#neg (%)	#failed (%)	#pos (%)	#neg (%)	#failed (%)	#pos (%)	#neg (%)	#failed (%)	#pos (%)	#neg (%)	#failed (%)
Lab A	145 (29.1)	350 (70.1)	4 (0.8)	34 (9.6)	317 (89.6)	3 (0.8)	32 (88.9)	4 (11.1)	0 (0.0)	33 (100.0)	0 (0.0)	0 (0.0)	44 (89.8)	5 (10.2)	0 (0.0)	2 (7.4)	24 (88.9)	1 (3.7)	109 (92.4)	9 (7.6)	0 (0.0)
Lab B	145 (29.1)	346 (69.3)	8 (1.6)	34 (9.6)	314 (88.7)	6 (1.7)	33 (91.7)	3 (8.3)	0 (0.0)	31 (93.9)	0 (0.0)	2 (6.1)	44 (89.8)	5 (10.2)	0 (0.0)	2 (11.1)	24 (88.9)	0 (0.0)	108 (91.5)	8 (6.8)	2 (1.7)
Lab C	141 (28.3)	355 (71.1)	3 (0.6)	32 (9.0)	321 (90.7)	1 (0.3)	31 (86.1)	4 (11.1)	1 (2.8)	32 (96.8)	0 (0.0)	1 (3.0)	44 (89.8)	5 (10.2)	0 (0.0)	2 (7.4)	25 (92.6)	0 (0.0)	107 (90.7)	9 (7.6)	2 (1.7)
Lab D	146 (29.3)	353 (70.7)	0 (0.0)	35 (9.9)	319 (90.1)	0 (0.0)	32 (88.9)	4 (11.1)	0 (0.0)	33 (100.0)	0 (0.0)	0 (0.0)	44 (89.8)	5 (10.2)	0 (0.0)	2 (7.4)	25 (92.6)	0 (0.0)	109 (92.4)	9 (7.6)	0 (0.0)
% Overall Agreement	95.6 (93.8–97.2)			95.8 (93.5–97.7)			94.4 (86.1–100.0)			90.9 (78.8–100.0)			100.0 (100.0–100.0)			92.6 (81.5–100.0)			95.8 (92.4–99.2)		
% Positive Agreement	90.8 (85.9–94.9)			79.4 (65.1–91.5)			93.9 (84.8–100.0)			90.9 (78.8–100.0)			100.0 (100.0–100.0)			66.7 (0.0–100.0)			95.5 (91.4–99.1)		
Kappa	0.94 (0.92–0.97)			0.88 (0.80–0.93)			0.86 (0.52–1.00)			n/a			1.0			0.78 (−0.03–1.00)			0.86 (0.71–0.97)		

Agreement statistics with 95% confidence intervals between the laboratories are shown

NILM negative for intraepithelial lesion or malignancy, *ASC-US* atypical squamous cells of undetermined significance, *LSIL* low-grade squamous intraepithelial lesion, *ASC-H* atypical squamous cells, cannot exclude a high-grade lesion, *HSIL* high-grade squamous intraepithelial lesion

interpretation. Notably, a 100% agreement was obtained for the samples with the most severe cytological interpretation (ASC-H and HSIL) (Table 2). The lowest inter-laboratory agreement was observed among results from women with unsatisfactory cytology ($n = 27$) with the overall percent agreement of 92.6 and a kappa value of 0.78.

Of the 499 samples, 22 samples showed discordant results (Table 3). For 19 samples, one of the four laboratories showed discordancy compared to the three other laboratories. For two samples, two and two laboratories had the same results. Only one sample showed three different results (HPV positive, HPV negative and failed). Two categories of discordant results were observed; 1) Discordancy in terms of a failed sample for at least one laboratory ($n = 12$), and 2) Discordancy in terms of HPV positive vs HPV negative results ($n = 10$). Comparison of the test results from all four laboratories, excluding the failed samples, showed 98.2% overall agreement, 93.9% positive agreement and a kappa value of 0.98 (95% CI 0.96–0.99). The four involved laboratories reported in total 15 failed samples. In a clinical setting, these women would be recalled to take a new cell sample from the cervix. Almost all of these samples (14/15) came up with the flag X3 "Clot was detected; Sample was not processed".

Table 3 Samples with discordant HPV test results (HPV positive, HPV negative, failed) between the four laboratories

Cytological finding	Lab A	Lab B	Lab C	Lab D	
Unsatisfactory	failed	negative	negative	negative	*
NILM	failed	negative	negative	negative	*
NILM	failed	negative	failed	negative	*
NILM	negative	failed	negative	negative	*
NILM	negative	failed	negative	negative	*
NILM	negative	failed	negative	negative	*
NILM	negative	failed	negative	negative	*
NILM	negative	failed	negative	negative	*
ASCUS	positive	positive	failed	positive	*
LSIL	positive	failed	positive	positive	*
LSIL	positive	failed	positive	positive	*
LSIL	positive	positive	failed	positive	*
Unsatisfactory	negative	positive	negative	negative	**
NILM	failed	failed	negative	positive	**
NILM	positive	negative	negative	negative	**
NILM	positive	positive	negative	negative	**
NILM	positive	positive	positive	negative	**
NILM	negative	positive	negative	negative	**
NILM	negative	positive	negative	positive	**
NILM	negative	negative	negative	positive	**
NILM	negative	negative	negative	positive	**
ASCUS	negative	positive	negative	negative	**

*Samples for which at least one laboratory reported a failed result, and the women would be recalled to take a new call sample from the cervix

** True discordant samples; would lead to different clinical follow-up procedures

NILM negative for intraepithelial lesion or malignancy, *ASC-US* atypical squamous cells of undetermined significance, *LSIL* low-grade squamous intraepithelial lesion

For the 10 true discordant samples, different follow-up procedures would be recommended; seven of the samples had NILM cytology, two ASC-US, three LSIL and one unsatisfactory, emphasizing that none had severe cytological abnormalities (ASC-H or HSIL). The Ct-values of the discordant samples (Additional file 1: Table S1) were generally above 38.4 (with two exceptions), and hence close to the clinical Ct cut-off values. The Ct-values of beta-globin were for all samples between 25.5 and 28, indicating sufficient quality of the input DNA.

The cobas HPV Test detects HPV16, HPV18 and 12 additional high-risk types in a pooled analysis. In total, nine samples showed discordant genotype results (Additional file 2: Table S2). No samples showed complete discordance, i.e., there was always partial concordance between the genotypes. Concordance after including genotype information, showed 93.8% overall agreement, 78.7% positive agreement and a kappa value of 0.93 (95% CI 0.91–0.96) (Table 3). Calculation was also performed stratifying multiple infections according to oncogenic potential of the HPV types present; HPV16>HPV18>HR-HPV. The results showed 94.4% overall agreement, 82.5% positive agreement and kappa value of 0.94 (95% CI 0.91–0.96) (Table 4).

Discussion

Safe implementation of primary HPV testing in cervical screening programmes is dependent on reliable test results to maximize the benefits of HPV testing. Currently, implementation of primary HPV screening is on-going in Norway, involving women resident in four counties (and three laboratories). The screening interval for women with a negative HPV test is 5 years, compared to 3 years with cytology, and endeavors to minimize false negative results is particularly important. An evaluation of the inter-laboratory reproducibility of the HPV testing was initiated as part of the quality assurance programme. In addition to the three laboratories involved in the implementation, the Norwegian HPV reference laboratory contributed as a fourth comparing laboratory. For yearly quality control, the laboratories are attending the Quality Control for Molecular Diagnostics (QCMD) HPV DNA external quality assessment (EQA) programme.

In general, the HPV testing showed high reproducibility between the four sites. Both overall, and after stratification according to cytological diagnoses and HPV

Table 4 Agreement of HPV test results between the four laboratories including HPV genotype information

Test results compared	Overall percentage agreement	Positive percentage agreement	k value (95% CI)	Number of samples
Multiple genotypes taken into consideration	93.8	78.7	0.93 (0.91–0.96)	499
Highest risk genotype taken into consideration	94.4	82.5	0.94 (0.91–0.96)	499

Calculations were performed both with and without taking multiple infections into consideration. For calculation not considering multiple infections, HPV type category with highest oncogenic potential was the deciding factor; HPV16>HPV18>HR-HPV

genotypes, high agreement between the laboratories was observed, with kappa values above 0.85. The overall agreement including all samples was 95.6% (95% CI 93.8–97.4%) and the kappa value was 0.95. These results are well above the recommended lower confidence bound of 87% overall agreement and kappa value of at least 0.5, suggested by "Guidelines for HPV test DNA requirement for primary cervical cancer screening" authored by Meijer et al. [7].

Detection of HPV is dependent on the number of viral DNA copies present in the sample. A negative test result does not guarantee absence of HPV DNA in the sample, just that the level is below a defined threshold value based on the clinical characteristics of the test [8]. In this evaluation, ten samples showed positive vs negative discordant results, which according to the current screening algorithm would result in different follow-up of the women (http://www.kreftregisteret.no/hpv-algoritme). For the discordant results, samples with HPV positive outcomes had high Ct-values (>38.4) with two exceptions, implying low levels of viral DNA. The discrepancy in test results (HPV negative vs HPV positive) may be associated with the inherent stochasticity of the PCR process, i.e., whether the Ct-value will be below or above the clinical Ct-threshold value for samples with low viral load, may be related to coincidence. Accordingly, discordant results may also be explained by intra-laboratory variability.

All samples with a severe cytological diagnosis (ASC-H or HSIL) had concordant results. This is regarded as a significant finding due to the importance in identifying these women when HPV testing is introduced as a primary screening test. High-grade lesions generally have higher viral loads, possibly also explaining the higher concordance rate among these samples. It is noteworthy however, that four HSIL samples had an HPV negative test result in all four laboratories. Based on the close relation between HSIL and HPV infection, false positive cytology results or false negative HPV results are likely explanations. HPV testing, although sensitive, may not capture all cases of disease and hence, these may be true false negative cases. Due to the anonymisation of samples, recalling of the cytology results and/or comparison with histological data was, however, not feasible. In the end, given the aim of this study, the concordance in test results between the laboratories was considered a central finding.

According to the algorithm for primary HPV screening in Norway, HPV genotypes are not reported and all HPV-positive women have a cytological reflex evaluation. Still, categorizing the genotypes based on the cobas HPV Test results, may be of interest as it has been suggested that HPV16 and/or HPV18 positive women should have a more aggressive follow-up regime compared to women positive for the HR-HPV category [9]. In the present data, discordant results related to genotypes were observed for nine samples. Discordance in terms of HPV16/18 versus HR-HPV, is seen for four samples. Discrepancy in genotype results may be related to the multiplex PCR process where targets in the reaction compete with each other for resources.

The cobas 4800 instrument automatically "approves" the results based on algorithmic criteria in the software. Accordingly, samples may fail to provide a result. Failed samples are often explained by insufficient material, too much material or cellular aggregates, or may be a result of insufficient mixing of the samples before loading on the instrument. Failed samples were rerun, and upon a second fail reported as failed in the study report. This is a common procedure also in routine screening, where the women are recalled for a new sample after two failed analyses. For 11 of the 13 samples reported as "failed" (Table 3), the failure was only reported from one laboratory, suggesting the failure being related to technical issues in the laboratory rather than to the quality of the sample. Samples should before loading always be visually inspected, evaluating the need for additional mixing or even removal of cellular aggregates. For primary screening, this is however not always feasible due to high quantity of samples and use of the instrument cobas p 480 for automated sample handling. A suggested procedure would be to evaluate samples prior to reloading after a failed result.

Along with the implementation of primary HPV testing, proper directions for quality assessment is paramount. In Norway, several initiatives are on-going. Centralization of HPV testing and cytology reading is in process to ensure a sound environment with high molecular biology competence for HPV testing and with sufficient amount of cytology samples to satisfy "the European guidelines for quality assurance in cervical cancer screening" of 15,000 samples per year for each analyzing laboratory [3]. Laboratories performing HPV testing should have, and maintain, accreditation to ISO15189 standard. Among others, this involves that each laboratory should have SOPs describing all steps from sample arrival to report. In addition, internal quality assurance (ICA) should ensure that systematic method verification is performed and approved upon the implementation of a new HPV test, documenting for example internal reproducibility of the assay. Also, the introduction of kit independent controls should be considered, which is important not only as an independent control for each run, but also for the verification of analytical stability over time. As a necessary supplement to ICA, all laboratories should regularly participate to international EQA programmes in order to evaluate and document adequate performance, as the QCMD HPV DNA programme. There is, however, a prominent need for additional panels specifically designed for HPV-based screening, evaluating performance based on clinical cut-off values in the test. Importantly, such a proficiency screening panel is planned by the WHO HPV LabNet-programme [10], which would constitute an important contribution to quality assurance of HPV-based cervical cancer screening. Awaiting such a panel, Norway will, in addition to participation in the QCMD programme, continue with circulation of samples between laboratories every second year as part of the continuous quality assurance of the screening programme. Essentially, we support the message given by Carozzi and collegues [11], emphasizing the need for international efforts in order to establish quality guidelines in line with the change to HPV-based screening in several countries.

Study constraints

For ethical reasons, all samples were anonymized before HPV-analysis and consequently, comparison to histological results was not feasible. This would have been valuable in order to better explain the HPV negative HSIL samples observed. In the implementation pilot, only the cobas HPV Test is used and cell samples are collected in PreservCyt media. Lacking assessment of reproducibility between several HPV tests and transport media entails a limitation to the generality of this evaluation, but fulfil the requirement for the Norwegian implementation.

Conclusions

Transition from HPV testing as a secondary screening test to primary HPV testing requires a significant reorganization of laboratory activities. Laboratory staff needs good information and training to be able to contribute at a high professional level. The assessment of the inter-laboratory reproducibility of the HPV testing is an important contribution to the quality assurance. Overall, the results in this study show a high inter-laboratory reproducibility of the HPV testing with the cobas HPV Test, certifying satisfactory laboratory performance in each of the three laboratories involved in the implementation of HPV primary screening in Norway. This is important knowledge and we recommend similar studies always to be performed prior to the introduction of new screening routines.

Additional files

Additional file 1: Table S1. Ct-values for HPV and beta-globin detection in samples with discordant results. The Ct-values of the discordant samples were generally above 38.4 (with two exceptions), and hence close to the clinical Ct cut-off values. The Ct-values of beta-globin were for all samples between 25.5 and 28, indicating sufficient quality of the input DNA.

Additional file 2: Table S2. Discordant genotype results among HPV positive samples. Nine samples showed discordant genotype results. No samples showed complete discordance, i.e., there was always partial concordance between the genotypes.

Abbreviations

ASC-H: Atypical squamous cells, cannot rule out HSIL; ASC-US: Atypical squamous cells of undetermined significance; EQA: External quality assessment; HPV: Human papillomavirus; HR-HPV: High-risk human papillomavirus; HSIL: High-grade squamous intraepithelial lesions; IQA: Internal quality assurance; LBC: Liquid based cytology; LSIL: Low-grade squamous intraepithelial lesions; NILM: Negative for intra-epithelial lesions or malignancy; QCMD: Quality control for molecular diagnostics; SOP: Standard operating procedure

Acknowledgements

We thank Linda Vos at The Cancer Registry of Norway for statistical support.

Funding

This research received no specific grant from any funding agency in the public, commercial, or not-for-profit sectors.

Authors' contributions

BE made substantial contributions to statistical analysis, interpretation of data and writing of the manuscript. BDH contributed to design of the study, was responsible for the collection, aliquotation and distribution of clinical samples and has revised the manuscript for important intellectual content. MH made substantial contributions to acquisition and interpretation of data and has revised the manuscript for important intellectual content. PM, KMS and SBP made substantial contributions to laboratory analysis and acquisition of data, and have revised the manuscript for important intellectual content. OKV, SL and MN made contributions to conception and design of the study and have revised the manuscript for important intellectual content. EAMJ contributed to design, collection of samples and ethical approval of the study, and has revised the manuscript for important intellectual content. PEC made substantial contribution to conception and design of the study and statistical analysis, and has revised the manuscript for important intellectual content. IKC made substantial contributions to conception and design, interpretation of data and writing of the manuscript. All authors have given final approval of the version to be published.

Competing interests

PEC reports personal fees from Roche, outside the submitted work. No conflicts of interest were disclosed by the other authors.

Consent for publication

Not applicable.

Author details

[1]Cancer Registry of Norway, Oslo, Norway. [2]Department of Pathology, Stavanger University Hospital, Stavanger, Norway. [3]Department of Microbiology and Infection Control, Akershus University Hospital, Lørenskog, Norway. [4]Department of Pathology, Haukeland University Hospital, Bergen, Norway. [5]Department of Pathology and Medical Genetics, St. Olavs Hospital, Trondheim University Hospital, Trondheim, Norway. [6]The Gade Laboratory for Pathology, Department of Clinical Medicine (K1), University of Bergen, Bergen, Norway. [7]Department of Mathematics and Natural Sciences, University of Stavanger, Stavanger, Norway. [8]Albert Einstein College of Medicine, Bronx, NY, USA.

References

1. Arbyn M, Ronco G, Anttila A, Meijer CJ, Poljak M, Ogilvie G, Koliopoulos G, Naucler P, Sankaranarayanan R, Peto J. Evidence regarding human papillomavirus testing in secondary prevention of cervical cancer. Vaccine. 2012;30 Suppl 5:F88–99.
2. Ronco G, Giorgi-Rossi P, Carozzi F, Confortini M, Dalla Palma P, Del Mistro A, Ghiringhello B, Girlando S, Gillio-Tos A, De Marco L, et al. Efficacy of human papillomavirus testing for the detection of invasive cervical cancers and cervical intraepithelial neoplasia: a randomised controlled trial. Lancet Oncol. 2010;11(3):249–57.
3. Anttila A, Arbyn M, De Vuyst H, Dillner J, Dillner L, Franceschi S, Patnik J, Ronco G, Segnan N, Suinio E, et al. European guidelines for quality assurance in cervical cancer screening. Supplements. 2nd ed. Luxembourg: Publication Office of the European Union; 2015.
4. Stoler MH, Schiffman M, Atypical Squamous Cells of Undetermined Significance-Low-grade Squamous Intraepithelial Lesion Triage Study G. Interobserver reproducibility of cervical cytologic and histologic interpretations: realistic estimates from the ASCUS-LSIL Triage Study. JAMA. 2001;285(11):1500–5.
5. Flack VF, Lachenbruch PA, Schouten HJA. Sample size determinations for the two rater kappa statistic. Psychometrika. 1988;53(3):321–5.
6. Wright TC Jr, Stoler MH, Behrens CM, Apple R, Derion T, Wright TL. The ATHENA human papillomavirus study: design, methods, and baseline results. Am J Obstet Gynecol. 2012;206(1):46 e41-46 e11
7. Meijer CJ, Berkhof J, Castle PE, Hesselink AT, Franco EL, Ronco G, Arbyn M, Bosch FX, Cuzick J, Dillner J, et al. Guidelines for human papillomavirus DNA test requirements for primary cervical cancer screening in women 30 years and older. Int J Cancer. 2009;124(3):516–20.
8. Rao A, Young S, Erlich H, Boyle S, Krevolin M, Sun R, Apple R, Behrens C. Development and characterization of the cobas human papillomavirus test. J Clin Microbiol. 2013;51(5):1478–84.
9. Schiffman M, Boyle S, Raine-Bennett T, Katki HA, Gage JC, Wentzensen N, Kornegay JR, Apple R, Aldrich C, Erlich HA, et al. The role of human papillomavirus genotyping in cervical cancer screening: a large-scale evaluation of the cobas HPV test. Cancer Epidemiol Biomarkers Prev. 2015; 24(9):1304–10.
10. Eklund C, Forslund O, Wallin KL, Dillner J. Global improvement in genotyping of human papillomavirus DNA: the 2011 HPV LabNet International Proficiency Study. J Clin Microbiol. 2014;52(2):449–59.
11. Carozzi FM, Del Mistro A, Cuschieri K, Frayle H, Sani C, Burroni E. HPV testing for primary cervical screening: laboratory issues and evolving requirements for robust quality assurance. J Clin Virol. 2016;76 Suppl 1:S22–8.

8

Independent prognostic role of human papillomavirus genotype in cervical cancer

Dong Hang[1], Meiqun Jia[1], Hongxia Ma[1], Jing Zhou[1], Xiaoshuang Feng[2], Zhangyan Lyu[2], Jian Yin[2], Hong Cui[2], Yin Yin[1], Guangfu Jin[1], Zhibin Hu[1,3], Hongbing Shen[1,3], Kai Zhang[4*], Ni Li[2*] and Min Dai[2*]

Abstract

Background: Although the correlation of HPV genotype with cervical precursor lesions and invasive cancer has been confirmed, the role of HPV genotype in cervical cancer prognosis is less conclusive. This study aims to systematically investigate the independent prognostic role of HPV genotype in cervical cancer.

Methods: A total of 306 eligible patients provided cervical cell specimens for HPV genotyping before therapy and had a median follow-up time of 54 months after diagnosis. Survival times were measured from the date of diagnosis to the date of cervical cancer-related death (overall survival, OS) and from the date of diagnosis to the date of recurrence or metastasis (disease free survival, DFS). Log-rank tests and Cox proportional hazard models were performed to evaluate the association between HPV genotype and survival times.

Results: A total of 12 types of high-risk HPV were detected and the leading ten types belong to two species: alpha-9 and alpha-7. HPV16 and 18 were the two most common types, with the prevalence of 60.8% and 8.8%, respectively. In the univariate analysis, HPV16-positive cases were associated with better OS ($P = 0.037$) and HPV16-related species alpha-9 predicted better OS and DFS (both $P < 0.01$). After adjusting for age, FIGO stage, and therapy, HPV16 showed a hazard ratio (HR) of 0.36 (95% CI: 0.18, 0.74; $P = 0.005$) for OS, and alpha-9 resulted in a HR of 0.17 (95% CI: 0.08, 0.37; $P < 0.001$) for OS and 0.32 (95% CI: 0.17, 0.59; $P < 0.001$) for DFS.

Conclusions: HPV genotype poses differential prognoses for cervical cancer patients. The presence of HPV16 and its related species alpha-9 indicates an improved survival.

Keywords: Cervical cancer, Prognosis, Human papillomavirus, Genotype

Background

Cervical cancer is the fourth most common malignancy in females worldwide, with an estimated 527,600 new cases and 265,700 deaths per year [1]. The etiological relationship has been well established between human papillomavirus (HPV) and cervical cancer. Recently, more than 170 HPV genotypes have been identified and classified according to their L1 open reading frame [2]. When HPVs have 60–70% genomic nucleotide similarity, they are clustered into the same species. Two HPV species, alpha-7 (HPV18, 39, 45, 59, 68, and 70) and alpha-9 (HPV16, 31, 33, 35, 52, 58, and 67), are responsible for over 80% of all cervical cancer cases [3].

Although there has been much evidence on the role of HPV genotype in cervical precursor lesions and invasive cancer, it remains unclear whether they affect prognosis of cervical cancer. Furthermore, existing results on the relationship of HPV genotype with survival are heterogeneous. For example, early evidence showed that HPV16 positivity predicted poor prognosis and was associated with histological features of prognostic significance such as squamous cell carcinomas, pelvic node metastases, and lymphatic space invasion [4]. But some studies reported that HPV18 positivity, rather than HPV16, is a poor prognostic factor [5, 6]. Histologic type of adenocarcinomas, pelvic lymph node metastasis, and deeper stromal invasion was more common in HPV18-caused

* Correspondence:
kai87968@sina.com; nli@cicams.ac.cn; daimin2002@hotmail.com
[4]Department of Cancer Prevention, National Cancer Centre/Cancer Hospital, Chinese Academy of Medical Sciences and Peking Union Medical College, Beijing 100021, China
[2]Program Office for Cancer Screening in Urban China, National Cancer Centre/Cancer Hospital, Chinese Academy of Medical Sciences and Peking Union Medical College, Beijing 100021, China

cervical cancer [6]. In addition, HPV31-related and HPV58-related types were found to be associated with better survival outcome [7, 8]. However, no prognostic value of HPV type was reported by the other studies [9, 10]. The inconsistency may be attributed to the significant differences in sample size, length of follow-up, assay methods, and adjustment for known prognostic factors.

To better understand the role of HPV genotype in prognosis of patients with cervical cancer, we assessed the association of HPV genotype with overall survival (OS, the time between the date of diagnosis and the date of cervical cancer-related death) and disease free survival (DFS, the time between the date of diagnosis and the date of recurrence, distant metastasis, or the last follow-up) among 306 cases of cervical cancer from China.

Methods

Patients

Cervical cancer patients were consecutively recruited from Cancer Hospital, Chinese Academy of Medical Sciences from 2010 to 2012. We included patients who had a first diagnosis of histologically confirmed invasive cervical cancer, and the sampling of cervical exfoliated cells for HPV genotyping were taken by a gynecologist before therapy. Patients were excluded for the following criteria: a history of hysterectomy or conization, recurrent cervical cancer, other preexisting malignancies, and those with less than two months of survival after completing therapy. Patient's age, FIGO stage, tumor histology, and pathologic variables were retrieved from medical records. This study was approved by the ethics committees of National Cancer Centre/Cancer Hospital, Chinese Academy of Medical Sciences, and all patients provided informed written consent before study enrollment.

HPV genotyping

Genomic DNA was extracted from cervical cell specimens manually by using QIAamp DNA Mini Kit, according to the manufacture's protocol (Qiagen, Valencia, CA, USA). The quality of extracted DNA was assessed by PCR with a set of primers for the housekeeping gene β-actin (forward primer, 5′-GAAATCGTGCGTGACATTAA-3′; reverse primer 5′-AAGGAAGGCTGGAAGA.

GTG-3′). All β-actin positive specimens were tested for HPV DNA by following the manufacturer's protocol of a HPV GenoArray Test Kit (HybriBio, Beijing, China), which is a Chinese FDA-approved assay for HPV genotyping. A total of 21 HPV types could be detected simultaneously, including 13 high-risk (HR) types (HPV16, 18, 31, 33, 35, 39, 45, 51, 52, 56, 58, 59, and 68), two intermediate-risk types (HPV53 and 66), and six low-risk HPV types (HPV6, 11, 42, 43, 44, and 81).

Treatment and follow up

Treatment information was retrieved from medical records and was summarized and grouped as follows: surgery alone (radical hysterectomy and pelvic lymphadenectomy); surgery plus adjunctive chemotherapy (CT), radiotherapy (RT) or chemoradiotherapy (CRT); concurrent chemoradiotherapy (CCRT); CT or RT only. Each patient was followed up every 3 months in the first year and every 6 months in the next years by personal or family contacts, until June 2016. Hospital medical records were obtained in order to confirm the reported events. Only validated events were included in analysis. Overall survival (OS) was defined as the time between the date of diagnosis and the date of cervical cancer-related death or the last follow-up. Disease-free survival (DFS) was measured from the date of diagnosis to the date of recurrence, distant metastasis, or the last follow-up.

Statistical analysis

The data were analyzed by using the Stata version 11.0 (Stata Corporation, Texas, USA). To assess the potential of HPV type as a prognostic biomarker for cervical cancer patients with no matter single or multiple infections, all cases were included for HPV16 and 18 survival analysis. Multiple infections with only alpha-9 types were included for alpha-9 survival analysis. Survival curves were generated using the Kaplan-Meier method, and comparisons were performed using the log–rank test. Multivariate analyses of the factors associated with OS and DFS were done using Cox proportional hazard regression model. In the stratified analysis, the chi-square test-based Q-statistic was applied to test the heterogeneity between subgroups defined by age, FIGO stage, and treatment. All P values presented were two-sided and were assumed significant as $P < 0.05$.

Results

Patient characteristics

The demographic and clinical characteristics of cervical cancer patients are summarized in Table 1. This study included 306 women with a median age of 48 years (range: 26–71 years). The most common histological type was squamous cell carcinoma (96.7%) and the others were adenocarcinoma (AC) and adeno-squamous carcinoma (ASC). Most of patients were diagnosed with FIGO stage I-II (81.0%). Seventy-eight patients (25.5%) received surgery, and 21 (6.9%) surgery plus CT/RT/CRT, 160 (52.3%) CCRT, 47 (15.4%) CT or RT only.

HPV genotypes

A total of 12 types of high-risk HPV were detected in this study (Table 2). The top three types were HPV16 (60.8%), 18 (8.8%), and 52 (5.9%). In the leading ten types, five (HPV16, 52, 33, 31, 58) were alpha-9 and the

Table 1 Characteristics of cervical cancer patients

Characteristics	Patients (N = 306)	
	No.	%
Age, years		
Median	48	
Range	26–71	
< 40	45	14.71
40–50	133	43.46
> 50	128	41.83
Histologic type[a]		
SCC	296	96.73
AC/ASC	10	3.26
FIGO stage		
I	105	34.31
II	143	46.73
III	52	16.99
IV	6	1.96
Differentiation		
Poor	87	28.43
Moderate	126	41.18
Well	11	3.59
Unclassified	82	26.80
Treatment[b]		
Surgery	78	25.49
Surgery plus CT/RT/CRT	21	6.86
CCRT	160	52.29
CT or RT only	47	15.36

[a]*SCC* squamous cell carcinoma, *AC* adenocarcinoma, *ASC* adeno-squamous carcinoma
[b]*CT* chemotherapy, *RT* radiotherapy, *CRT* chemoradiotherapy, *CCRT* concurrent chemoradiotherapy

others (HPV18, 39, 59, 68, 45) were alpha-7. Of 306 patients, 268 (87.6%) harbored single-type and 38 (12.4%) contained multiple-type infections. As shown in Additional file 1: Table S1, HPV16 (81.6%, 31/38) and 52 (42.1%, 16/38) were the predominant types that made up the multiple infections.

Survival analysis

The mean number of follow-up was 5 for each patient and the median time for these follow ups was 54 (range, 3–75) months. A total of 58 patients (19.0%) had experienced treatment failure, including 27 recurrences and 38 distant metastases (7 patients had both). In addition, 34 deaths (11.1%) were attributed to cervical cancer. The 5-year OS rate for the entire cohort was 87.1% (95% CI: 82.1–90.8%), and the corresponding DFS rate was 78.3% (95% CI: 72.5–83.1%).

In univariate analysis (Table 3), FIGO stage IV was significantly associated with poorer OS (P < 0.001) and DFS (P < 0.001), while primary surgical treatment was associated with a better OS (P = 0.004) and DFS (P = 0.019). Of note, patients infected with HPV16 had a better OS than those with any other types (P = 0.037) (Fig. 1a). HPV16-related species alpha-9 also posed a better OS (P < 0.001) and DFS (P = 0.005), compared to alpha-7 (Fig. 1b and c). No significant association with prognosis was found for HR-HPV multiple infections, HPV18 and the other types.

In multivariate models with adjustment for patients' age, FIGO stage, and treatment, HPV16 was independently associated with better OS (HR = 0.36, 95% CI: 0.18, 0.74; P = 0.005) (Table 3). Infection with the five alpha-9 types was independently associated with better OS (HR = 0.17, 95% CI: 0.08–0.37; P < 0.001) and DFS (HR = 0.32, 95% CI: 0.17–0.59; P < 0.001). Further analysis suggested that HPV52/33/31/58 group had more favorable OS (HR = 0.12, 95% CI: 0.02–0.57; P = 0.008) and DFS (HR = 0.21, 95% CI: 0.06, 0.77; P = 0.018) (Additional file 1: Table S2). Given the limitation of statistical power, we did not find meaningful results when analyzing these four types individually.

To better understand the effect of HPV genotype on cervical cancer survival, stratified analyses based on age, FIGO stage, and treatment were performed. Although the protective effects of HPV16 and alpha-9 were more evident among those with FIGO stage III/IV and those receiving primary RT and/or CT, no significant difference was detected between subgroups (homogeneity test P > 0.05 for all) (Additional file 1: Table S3).

Discussion

Despite recent progress in multimodal treatments, the clinical outcome of cervical cancer remains unfavorable. TNM or FIGO classification based on cervical pathology has insufficient predictive ability, because significant differences in survival are often observed for the same stage. Thus, it is highly necessary to explore additional biomarkers for the identification of a more effective therapeutic strategy against cervical cancer. In this study, we investigated prognostic value of HPV genotype for patients with cervical cancer. A total of 12 HR types were identified and HPV16 positivity was independently associated with lower risk of cervical cancer death than the group of the other 11 HR types. In addition, alpha-9 species including five HR types (16, 52, 33, 31, and 58) was a predictor of better survival compared with alpha-7 species group including the other five HR types (18, 39, 59, 68, and 45).

Substantial differences in risk for high-grade cervical intraepithelial neoplasia (CIN) and cervical cancer have been revealed between HR HPV types, in which HPV16 and HPV18 confer the highest risk [11, 12] However, the relationship between HPV genotype and cervical cancer

Table 2 Distribution of HR-HPV types in cervical cancer patients

HR-HPV type[a]		Species	SCC[b] (*N* = 296)	AC/ASC[c] (*N* = 10)	Total (%)
Single infection					268 (87.58)
	16	alpha-9	184	2	186 (60.78)
	18	alpha-7	24	3	27 (8.82)
	52	alpha-9	17	1	18 (5.88)
	39	alpha-7	8	0	8 (2.61)
	33	alpha-9	6	0	6 (1.96)
	31	alpha-9	5	0	5 (1.63)
	58	alpha-9	4	1	5 (1.63)
	59	alpha-7	4	0	4 (1.31)
	68	alpha-7	4	0	4 (1.31)
	45	alpha-7	3	0	3 (0.98)
	51	alpha-5	1	0	1 (0.33)
	56	alpha-10	1	0	1 (0.33)
Multiple infection			35	3	38 (12.42)
Alpha-7 only			43	3	46 (15.03)
Alpha-9 only			237	4	241 (78.76)

[a]*HR-HPV* high risk human papillomavirus
[b]*SCC* squamous cell carcinoma.
[c]*AC* adenocarcinoma, *ASC* adeno-squamous carcinoma

prognosis has been controversial. Plich et al. identified HPV16 infection as a poor prognostic factor in 204 patients treated by primary radical hysterectomy and pelvic lymphadenectomy [4]. Conversely, another study showed that HPV16 positivity was significantly associated with improved prognosis in the whole series of cervical AC/ASC and also in subgroup receiving primary RT/CCRT [13]. In our study, the results supported the hypothesis that HPV16 has a favorable impact on the prognosis of cervical cancer. Further, we demonstrated that HPV16-related alpha-9 species significantly lowers the risk of cervical cancer-related death and recurrence/metastasis than the alpha-7 species, which was consistent with a previous study in patients undergoing primary radiotherapy [14]. Moreover, although several studies found that HPV18 positivity was associated with poorer prognosis of patients receiving primary surgery [5, 15, 16], other studies [17, 18] and ours failed to support the relationship. Given the much lower prevalence of HPV18 in cervical cancer than HPV16, independent studies with large sample size are needed to assess the impact of HPV18 on patients' prognosis. In addition, because the HPV genotyping kit used in this study does not cover HPV67 and 70, which are high-risk types for cervical cancer, the impact of HPV67 and 70 on prognosis remains to be determined.

The underlying mechanisms that result in the tumors caused by HPV16 and the alpha-9 species being less aggressive are still undetermined. Interestingly, HPV status has been recognized as a strong and independent factor for favorable survival of patients with oropharyngeal cancer (OPC) [19, 20]. According to a systematic review, HPV prevalence was 35.6% (95% CI: 32.6–38.7%) in OPC specimens, and HPV16 accounted for a larger majority of HPV-positive OPC (86.7%; 95% CI, 82.6–90.1%) [21]. A better response to chemotherapy and radiation was observed for HPV-positive OPC [22–24]. In a worldwide survey of HPV genotype in cervix cancer, 61% of tumors were positive for HPV16 and 83% were positive for the alpha-9 species [3], similar to the data in our study. In vitro studies have revealed significant differences in biological behaviors between HPV types. For example, HPV16 is associated with a higher level of tumor apoptosis than HPV18, affording one possible explanation for more radiosensitive cervical cancer with HPV16 [25]. In addition, HR-HPV E6 proteins could interact with cellular PDZ domain-containing proteins to promote cell immortalization, invasion, and epithelial-to-mesenchymal transition (EMT) characteristics [26, 27]. There are significant differences in the interactions of HPV16 and HPV18 E6 with the PDZ domain-containing proteins, because a critical difference exists in the amino acid residue at the PDZ-binding motifs of the two E6 proteins [28]. This difference exists not only between HPV16 and HPV18, but also between the alpha-9 and alpha-7 species. Whether the variation in the PDZ domain-binding capacities determines the observed differential therapeutic response is worth additional exploration.

Table 3 Univariate and multivariate analyses of prognostic factors for cervical cancer patients

Variable	Overall survival					Disease free survival				
	3-Year Rate (95% CI)	5-Year Rate (95% CI)	P^e	Adjusted HR (95% CI)[f]	P^b	3-Year Rate (95% CI)	5-Year Rate (95% CI)	P^e	Adjusted HR (95% CI)[f]	P^f
Age, years										
< 40	93.18 (80.33, 97.75)	93.18 (80.33, 97.75)	0.634	1.00		86.43 (72.24, 93.67)	78.58 (62.60, 88.34)	0.956	1.00	
40–50	91.20 (84.67, 95.03)	85.39 (76.26, 91.21)		1.74 (0.49, 6.20)	0.390	83.84 (76.07, 89.26)	78.48 (68.81, 85.46)		0.72 (0.32, 1.60)	0.417
> 50	91.75 (85.20, 95.47)	86.99 (79.22, 92.00)		1.09 (0.30, 4.04)	0.893	87.78 (80.55, 92.45)	78.01 (68.46, 84.99)		0.56 (0.25, 1.30)	0.177
Histologic type[a]										
SCC	91.77 (87.87, 94.46)	87.07 (81.97, 90.81)	0.943			85.79 (81.13, 89.37)	77.96 (71.96, 82.82)	0.478		
AC/ASC	87.50 (38.70, 98.14)	87.50 (38.70, 98.14)				87.50 (38.70, 98.14)	87.50 (38.70, 98.14)			
FIGO stage[b]										
I	95.82 (89.23, 98.41)	94.73 (87.79, 97.77)	**<0.001**	1.00		93.83 (86.78, 97.18)	86.60 (75.90, 92.76)	**<0.001**	1.00	
II	95.68 (90.63, 98.04)	88.83 (79.72, 94.00)		0.98 (0.27, 3.50)	0.970	89.86 (83.48, 93.87)	84.14 (76.10, 89.65)		1.20 (0.43, 3.36)	0.735
III	74.66 (59.67, 84.76)	70.20 (54.87, 81.17)		3.40 (0.92, 12.52)	0.066	66.66 (51.44, 78.08)	53.52 (37.74, 66.96)		4.54 (1.53, 13.42)	**0.006**
IV	60.00 (12.57, 88.18)	40.00 (5.20, 75.28)		9.91 (1.87, 52.39)	0.007	16.67 (0.77, 51.68)	16.67 (0.77, 51.68)		13.21 (3.24, 53.82)	**<0.001**
Differentiation										
Poor	90.36 (81.64, 95.07)	86.83 (76.49,92.82)	0.383			83.23 (73.31, 89.71)	68.83 (55.26, 79.03)	0.068		
Moderate	90.68 (83.80, 94.73)	88.08 (80.70,92.77)				88.27 (80.98, 92.88)	82.83 (73.70, 89.02)			
Well	90.91 (50.81, 98.67)	72.73 (37.08,90.28)				63.64 (29.69, 84.52)	63.64 (29.69, 84.52)			
Unclassified										
Treatment[§]										
Surgery	100	98.53 (90.02, 99.79)	**0.004**	1.00		96.05 (88.24, 98.71)	84.25 (66.36, 93.09)	**0.019**	1.00	
Surgery plus CT/RT/CRT	100	93.75 (63.23, 99.10)		3.98 (0.25, 64.19)	0.331	95.00 (69.47, 99.28)	95.00 (69.47, 99.28)		0.43 (0.52, 3.56)	0.433
CCRT	90.02 (83.99, 93.87)	82.55 (74.02, 88.49)		8.26 (0.87, 78.75	0.066	83.34 (76.34, 88.43)	73.83 (65.27, 80.60)		1.44 (0.44, 4.74)	0.545
CR or RT	79.55 (64.38, 88.79)	79.55 (64.38, 88.79)		13.91 (1.59, 121.54)	0.017	73.37 (57.89, 83.91)	73.37 (57.89, 83.91)		1.92 (0.63, 5.88)	0.253
HPV16										
Negative	83.09 (73.10, 89.63)	81.77 (71.57, 88.60)	**0.037**	1.00		82.89 (72.81, 89.50)	75.71 (64.69, 83.71)	0.342		
Positive	95.17 (91.21, 97.37)	88.93 (82.31, 93.17)		**0.36 (0.18, 0.74)**	**0.005**	87.07 (81.70, 90.95)	79.03 (71.40, 84.84)			
HPV18										
Negative	91.87 (87.80, 94.62)	87.58 (82.23, 91.40)	0.404			86.49 (81.69, 90.11)	78.76 (72.58, 83.71)	0.69		
Positive	90.04 (72.14, 96.69)	83.12 (64.02, 92.62)				80.85 (62.18, 90.93)	74.63 (52.38, 87.60)			

Table 3 Univariate and multivariate analyses of prognostic factors for cervical cancer patients *(Continued)*

HR-HPV species[d]										
Alpha-7	74.38 (58.47, 84.93)	71.81 (55.65, 82.94)	**<0.001**	1.00		76.32 (60.41, 86.51)	62.96 (45.04, 76.47)	**0.005**	1.00	
Alpha-9	94.34 (90.44, 96.67)	90.42 (84.82, 94.02)		**0.17 (0.08, 0.37)**	**<0.001**	87.89 (82.93, 91.47)	80.88 (74.33, 85.92)		**0.32 (0.17, 0.59)**	**<0.001**
HR-HPV pattern										
Single	90.90 (86.61, 93.86)	87.04 (81.66, 90.94)	0.939			85.47 (80.51, 89.25)	77.41 (71.06, 82.53)	0.389		
Multiple	97.30 (82.32, 99.61)	87.77 (70.52, 95.24)				88.83 (72.85, 95.67)	85.54 (68.53, 93.75)			

[a]SCC, squamous cell carcinoma; AC, adenocarcinoma; ASC, adeno-squamous carcinoma
[b]FIGO, International Federation of Gynecology and Obstetrics
[c]CT, chemotherapy; RT, radiotherapy; CRT, chemoradiotherapy; CCRT, concurrent chemoradiotherapy
[d]HR-HPV, high risk human papillomavirus
[e]Calculated by using the log-rank test. Bold values indicate $P < 0.05$
[f]Adjusted for age, FIGO stage, and treatment in the Cox regression models

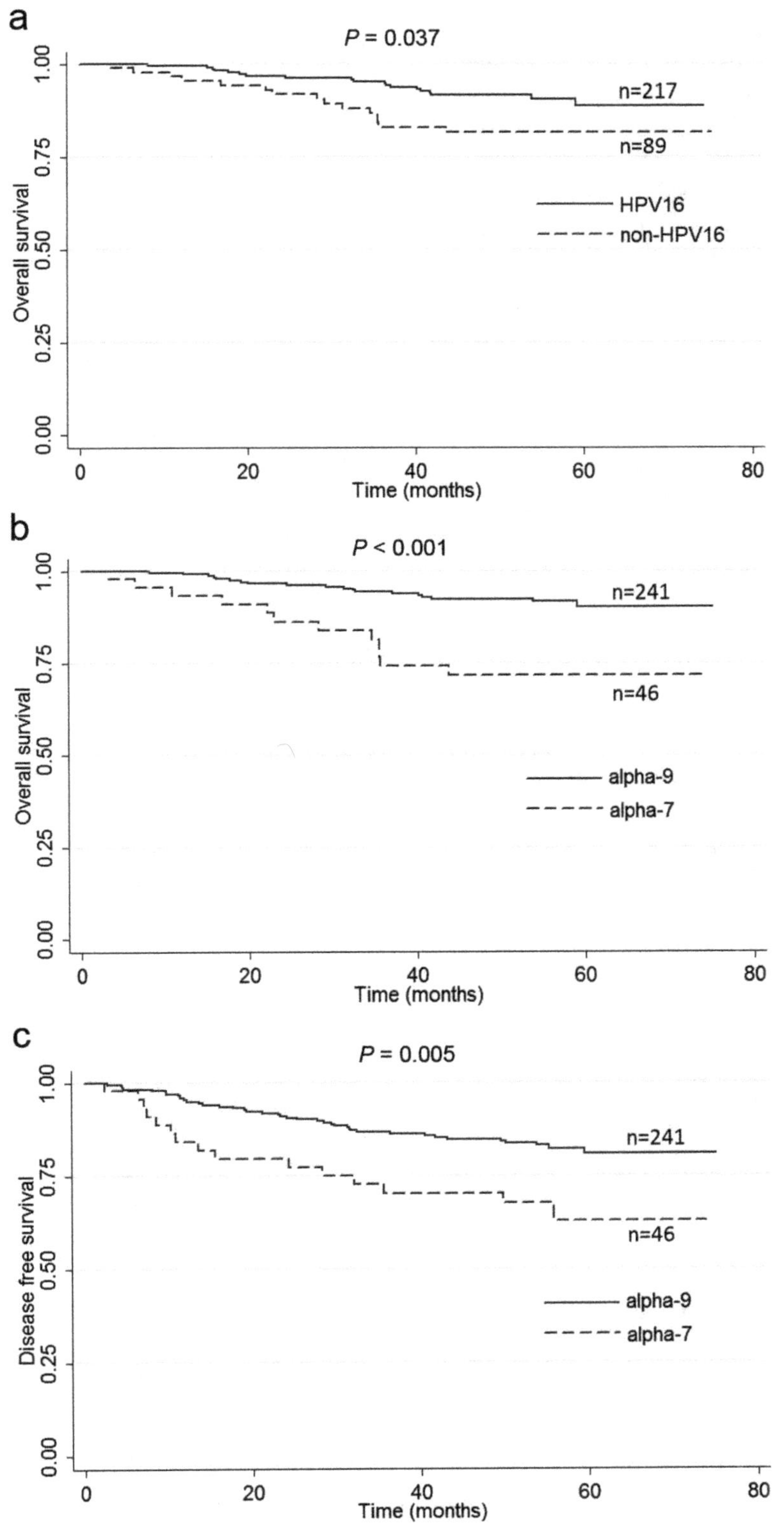

Fig. 1 The role of HPV genotype in cervical cancer prognosis. **a** Kaplan-Meier overall survival (OS) curves for HPV16 and non-HPV16 types; (**b**) Kaplan-Meier OS curves for the alpha-7 and alpha-9 species; (**c**) Kaplan-Meier disease free survival (DFS) curves for the alpha-7 and alpha-9 species

Conclusions

Our results demonstrated the independent prognostic value of HPV genotype in cervical cancer. HPV genotyping could potentially help to stratify cervical cancer patients for more effective therapeutic regimens. Patients with alpha-9-caused cervical cancer may receive less aggressive therapy to reduce side effects, while those with alpha-7 positivity may require more aggressive treatment and closer monitoring. Identifying the mechanisms by which the alpha-7 species leads to a poorer prognosis could help to improve the outcome of cervical cancer patients.

Abbreviations

AC: Adenocarcinoma; ASC: Adeno-squamous carcinoma; CCRT: Concurrent chemoradiotherapy; CRT: Chemoradiotherapy; CT: Chemotherapy; DFS: Disease free survival; EMT: Epithelial-to-mesenchymal transition; HPV: Human papillomavirus; HR: Hazard ratio; OPC: Oropharyngeal cancer; OS: Overall survival; RT: Radiotherapy

Acknowledgements

Not applicable.

Funding

This study was supported by the National Natural Science Fund from the National Natural Science Foundation of China (81,502,873, 81,373,079 and 81,673,265), Research Special Fund for Public Welfare Industry of Health (201402003), Natural Science Foundation of Jiangsu Province for Youth (BK20150997), PUMC Youth Fund (3,332,016,131 and 33,320,140,168), Natural Science Foundation of the Higher Education Institutions of Jiangsu Province (15KJB330001), Priority Academic Program for the Development of Jiangsu Higher Education Institutions (Public Health and Preventive Medicine), and Beijing Nova Program (xx2012067).

Authors' contributions

DH performed statistical analyses and drafted the initial manuscript. MJ, JZ, and XF did the experiments. HM checked statistical results. ZL, JY, HC, and YY collected the clinical data and cervical exfoliated cell samples. GJ, ZH, and HS supervised the follow-up and revised the manuscript critically. KZ, NL, and MD obtained financial support and were responsible for study design and interpretation of results. All authors read and approved the final manuscript.

Competing interests

The authors declare that they have no competing interests.

Consent for publication

Not applicable.

Author details

[1]Department of Epidemiology and Biostatistics, School of Public Health, Nanjing Medical University, Nanjing 211166, China. [2]Program Office for Cancer Screening in Urban China, National Cancer Centre/Cancer Hospital, Chinese Academy of Medical Sciences and Peking Union Medical College, Beijing 100021, China. [3]State Key Laboratory of Reproductive Medicine, Nanjing Medical University, Nanjing 211166, China. [4]Department of Cancer Prevention, National Cancer Centre/Cancer Hospital, Chinese Academy of Medical Sciences and Peking Union Medical College, Beijing 100021, China.

References

1. Torre LA, Bray F, Siegel RL, Ferlay J, Lortet-Tieulent J, Jemal A. Global cancer statistics, 2012. CA Cancer J Clin. 2015;65(2):87–108.
2. de Villiers EM. Cross-roads in the classification of papillomaviruses. Virology. 2013;445(1–2):2–10.
3. de Sanjose S, Quint WG, Alemany L, Geraets DT, Klaustermeier JE, Lloveras B, et al. Human papillomavirus genotype attribution in invasive cervical cancer: a retrospective cross-sectional worldwide study. Lancet Oncol. 2010;11(11):1048–56.
4. Pilch H, Gunzel S, Schaffer U, Tanner B, Brockerhoff P, Maeurer M, et al. The presence of HPV DNA in cervical cancer: correlation with clinico-pathologic parameters and prognostic significance: 10 years experience at the Department of Obstetrics and Gynecology of the Mainz University. International journal of gynecological cancer : official journal of the International Gynecological Cancer Society. 2001;11(1):39–48.
5. Lai CH, Chang CJ, Huang HJ, Hsueh S, Chao A, Yang JE, et al. Role of human papillomavirus genotype in prognosis of early-stage cervical cancer undergoing primary surgery. J Clin Oncol. 2007;25(24):3628–34.
6. Im SS, Wilczynski SP, Burger RA, Monk BJ. Early stage cervical cancers containing human papillomavirus type 18 DNA have more nodal metastasis and deeper stromal invasion. Clinical cancer research : an official journal of the American Association for Cancer Research. 2003;9(11):4145–50.
7. Huang LW, Chao SL, Hwang JL. Human papillomavirus-31-related types predict better survival in cervical carcinoma. Cancer. 2004;100(2):327–34.
8. Lai HC, Sun CA, Yu MH, Chen HJ, Liu HS, Chu TY. Favorable clinical outcome of cervical cancers infected with human papilloma virus type 58 and related types. Int J Cancer. 1999;84(6):553–7.
9. Fule T, Csapo Z, Mathe M, Tatrai P, Laszlo V, Papp Z, et al. Prognostic significance of high-risk HPV status in advanced cervical cancers and pelvic lymph nodes. Gynecol Oncol. 2006;100(3):570–8.
10. Zampronha Rde A, Freitas-Junior R, Murta EF, Michelin MA, Barbaresco AA, Adad SJ, et al. Human papillomavirus types 16 and 18 and the prognosis of patients with stage I cervical cancer. Clinics (Sao Paulo). 2013;68(6):809–14.
11. Song X, Sturgis EM, Huang Z, Li X, Li C, Wei Q, et al. Potentially functional variants of p14ARF are associated with HPV-positive oropharyngeal cancer patients and survival after definitive chemoradiotherapy. Carcinogenesis. 2014;35(1):62–8.
12. Schuler S, Ponnath M, Engel J, Ortmann O. Ovarian epithelial tumors and reproductive factors: a systematic review. Arch Gynecol Obstet. 2013;287(6):1187–204.
13. Lai CH, Chou HH, Chang CJ, Wang CC, Hsueh S, Huang YT, et al. Clinical implications of human papillomavirus genotype in cervical adeno-adenosquamous carcinoma. Eur J Cancer. 2013;49(3):633–41.
14. Hang DR, Islam SE, Sharma KH, Kuo SW, Zhang CZ, Wang JJ. Annealing effects on the optical and morphological properties of ZnO nanorods on AZO substrate by using aqueous solution method at low temperature. Nanoscale Res Lett. 2014;9(1):632.
15. Yang SH, Kong SK, Lee SH, Lim SY, Park CY. Human papillomavirus 18 as a poor prognostic factor in stage I-IIA cervical cancer following primary surgical treatment. Obstet Gynecol Sci. 2014;57(6):492–500.
16. Kang WD, Kim CH, Cho MK, Kim JW, Cho HY, Kim YH, et al. HPV-18 is a poor prognostic factor, unlike the HPV viral load, in patients with stage IB-IIA cervical cancer undergoing radical hysterectomy. Gynecol Oncol. 2011;121(3):546–50.
17. Tong SY, Lee YS, Park JS, Namkoong SE. Human papillomavirus genotype as a prognostic factor in carcinoma of the uterine cervix. Int J Gynecol Cancer. 2007;17(6):1307–13.
18. Cuschieri K, Brewster DH, Graham C, Nicoll S, Williams AR, Murray GI, et al. Influence of HPV type on prognosis in patients diagnosed with invasive cervical cancer. Int J Cancer. 2014;135(11):2721–6.
19. Gillison ML, Alemany L, Snijders PJ, Chaturvedi A, Steinberg BM, Schwartz S, et al. Human papillomavirus and diseases of the upper airway: head and neck cancer and respiratory papillomatosis. Vaccine. 2012;30(Suppl 5):F34–54.
20. Ang KK, Harris J, Wheeler R, Weber R, Rosenthal DI, Nguyen-Tan PF, et al. Human papillomavirus and survival of patients with oropharyngeal cancer. N Engl J Med. 2010;363(1):24–35.
21. Kreimer AR, Clifford GM, Boyle P, Franceschi S. Human papillomavirus types in head and neck squamous cell carcinomas worldwide: a systematic review. Cancer Epidemiol Biomark Prev. 2005;14(2):467–75.
22. Fakhry C, Westra WH, Li S, Cmelak A, Ridge JA, Pinto H, et al. Improved survival of patients with human papillomavirus-positive head and neck

squamous cell carcinoma in a prospective clinical trial. J Natl Cancer Inst. 2008;100(4):261–9.

23. Worden FP, Kumar B, Lee JS, Wolf GT, Cordell KG, Taylor JM, et al. Chemoselection as a strategy for organ preservation in advanced oropharynx cancer: response and survival positively associated with HPV16 copy number. J Clin Oncol. 2008;26(19):3138–46.
24. Lassen P, Eriksen JG, Hamilton-Dutoit S, Tramm T, Alsner J, Overgaard J. Effect of HPV-associated p16INK4A expression on response to radiotherapy and survival in squamous cell carcinoma of the head and neck. J Clin Oncol. 2009;27(12):1992–8.
25. Arends MJ, Wyllie AH, Bird CC. Human papillomavirus type 18 is associated with less apoptosis in fibroblast tumours than human papillomavirus type 16. Br J Cancer. 1995;72(3):646–9.
26. Spanos WC, Hoover A, Harris GF, Wu S, Strand GL, Anderson ME, et al. The PDZ binding motif of human papillomavirus type 16 E6 induces PTPN13 loss, which allows anchorage-independent growth and synergizes with ras for invasive growth. J Virol. 2008;82(5):2493–500.
27. Watson RA, Thomas M, Banks L, Roberts S. Activity of the human papillomavirus E6 PDZ-binding motif correlates with an enhanced morphological transformation of immortalized human keratinocytes. J Cell Sci. 2003;116(Pt 24):4925–34.
28. Thomas M, Massimi P, Navarro C, Borg JP, Banks L. The hScrib/Dlg apico-basal control complex is differentially targeted by HPV-16 and HPV-18 E6 proteins. Oncogene. 2005;24(41):6222–30.

9

Population-based prevalence of cervical infection with human papillomavirus genotypes 16 and 18 and other high risk types in Tlaxcala, Mexico

Samantha E. Rudolph[1,2], Attila Lorincz[3], Cosette M. Wheeler[4], Patti Gravitt[4], Eduardo Lazcano-Ponce[5], Leticia Torres-Ibarra[5*], Leith León-Maldonado[6], Paula Ramírez[2,5], Berenice Rivera[2,5], Rubí Hernández[5], Eduardo L. Franco[7], Jack Cuzick[3], Pablo Méndez-Hernández[8,9], Jorge Salmerón[2] and FRIDA Study Group

Abstract

Background: Cervical cancer remains an important cause of cancer mortality for Mexican women. HPV 16/18 typing may help to improve cervical cancer screening. Here we present the prevalence of high-risk human papillomavirus (hrHPV) including HPV16 and HPV18 from the FRIDA (Forwarding Research for Improved Detection and Access) population.

Methods: Beginning in 2013, we recruited 30,829 women aged 30–64 in Tlaxcala, Mexico. Cervical samples were collected and tested for 14 hrHPV genotypes (16, 18, 31, 33, 35, 39, 45, 51, 52, 56, 58, 59, 66, and 68). We used logistic regression to estimate odds ratios with 95 % confidence intervals for hrHPV infections according to putative risk factors.

Results: Prevalence of infection with any of the 14 hrHPV types was 11.0 %. The age-specific prevalence of all hrHPV formed a U-shaped curve with a higher prevalence for women aged 30–39 and 50–64 than women aged 40–49. Across all age groups, 2.0 % of women were positive for HPV16 and/or HPV18 (HPV16/18), respectively. HPV16/18 prevalence also showed a U-shaped curve with increased prevalence estimates for women aged both 30–39 and 60–64. Both prevalence curves had a significant quadratic age coefficient. Infections with hrHPV were positively associated with an increased number of lifetime sexual partners, a history of sexually transmitted disease, being unmarried, use of hormonal contraception, having a history of smoking and reported condom use in the multivariate model.

Conclusions: The FRIDA population has a bimodal distribution of both hrHPV and HPV16/18 positivity with higher prevalences at ages 30–39 and 60–64. These findings will help to evaluate triage algorithms based on HPV genotyping.

Keywords: Human papillomavirus DNA testing, HPV16/18, Prevalence, Risk factors, Mexico

Abbreviations: CI, Confidence intervals; CIN, Cervical intraepithelial neoplasia; FRIDA, Forwarding research for improved detection and access; HPV, Human papillomavirus; hrHPV, high-risk human papillomavirus; IUD, Intrauterine device; ORs, Odds ratios; STIs, Sexually transmitted infections

* Correspondence: leticia.torres@insp.mx
[5]Centro de Investigación en Salud Poblacional, Instituto Nacional de Salud Pública, Avenida Universidad 655, Colonia Sta. María Ahuacatitlán, 62100 Cuernavaca, Morelos, Mexico
Full list of author information is available at the end of the article

Background

Cervical cancer is the second most fatal cancer for women in Mexico [1]. Chronic infection with high-risk human papillomavirus (hrHPV), one of the world's most prevalent sexually transmitted infections (STIs), is a necessary cause of cervical cancer [2]. Over 100 types of HPV have been established. Among these, 15 HPV types are classified as carcinogenic or high risk (16, 18, 31, 33, 35, 39, 45, 51, 52, 56, 58, 59, 68, 73, and 82) [3]. From the point of view of cervical pathology, however, two types—HPV16 and 18—account for the vast majority of cervical cancer cases. Worldwide, HPV16 alone accounts for almost 60 % of cases, and HPV18 accounts for another 10 % of cases [4].

Because many countries in the developing world including Mexico do not have reliable cancer registries, it is difficult to ascertain the incidence of disease. Without incidence rates, resource allocation cannot fully reflect the differing needs of the various health districts. The prevalence of hrHPV, particularly HPV16 and HPV18, can be used as a valuable predictor of cervical cancer incidence [5].

Wise resource allocation will become more important as the cervical cancer prevention landscape in Mexico shifts. In 2008, Mexico began using hrHPV testing instead of cervical cytology for primary screening in the public sector, and then in 2012, Mexico introduced a universal HPV vaccination program for all girls in the 5th grade of elementary school [6]. The impact of the vaccine, however, will not be seen for at least a generation, and therefore, research groups in Mexico and throughout the developing world are seeking to establish their cervical cancer screening program. At the current time, Mexican health services cannot support a screening program in which all hrHPV positive women are sent for further diagnostic work-up [7]. Indeed only a small percentage of hrHPV positive women will actually ever develop high grade cervical intraepithelial neoplasia (CIN) [8].

To avoid overburdening the local services, researchers are now working to identify a reliable triage testing strategy for hrHPV positive women. While cytology seems to be an obvious triage option given the existing infrastructure, we are also trying alternatives because of the difficulty of maintaining high-quality cytology in Mexico [9]. One potentially important option for the triage of hrHPV positive women would be to identify those positive for HPV16 and HPV18 for further evaluation and diagnostic confirmation. Results of the Roche ATHENA trial in the US demonstrate the strong promise of HPV16/18 based triage strategies to increase diagnostic efficiency without sacrificing sensitivity of disease detection [10]. Indeed Roche has recently received FDA approval for its test to triage HPV16/18 positive women for diagnostic follow-up. The feasibility of a similar screening strategy in Mexico will rest on the prevalence of HPV16 and HPV18 and the positive predictive value of these types for high grade CIN.

The prevalence of HPV16 and HPV18 within the general population has not been well described in Mexico. The last population-based study to report on the prevalence of HPV16 and HPV18 in Mexico was published over a decade ago in 2001 [11]. More recent studies have only looked at small convenience samples [12–14]. The present study is part of a larger study, FRIDA (Forwarding Research for Improved Detection and Access), a population-based demonstration project designed to evaluate the performance and cost-effectiveness of triage alternatives for cervical cancer screening in Tlaxcala, Mexico. While a number of small studies have reported on the type-specific prevalence of HPV16 and HPV18 in Mexico [11–18], the present study is the largest to do so with population-based representation.

Methods

Study population

We studied specimens and data from the FRIDA study, an on-going population-based demonstration project that began in Tlaxcala, Mexico in August 2013. Women 30 to 64 years of age living within our target health district in Tlaxcala, Mexico are being recruited directly by healthcare personnel within preventive, family planning and gynecological health services during routine visits. This target health district includes approximately 100 health care facilities. The complete FRIDA cohort is projected to include more than 80% of the target population of over 100,000 women aged 30 to 64 years. Although the Tlaxcala cervical cancer screening program continuously invites women for screening at regular time intervals, women are generally tested opportunistically, with screening usually being initiated by the woman herself. This preliminary analysis includes results from the first 31,629 women enrolled in the demonstration project who came to the the clinic health care settings. Women then were invited at the clinic into the study. Women who were pregnant or had had a hysterectomy were excluded, leaving a total of 30,829 women in the present analysis (Fig. 1).

The study proposal was reviewed and approved by the research and ethics committees of the Instituto Nacional de Salud Pública (INSP) (1094), Comisión Federal para la Protección Contra Riesgos Sanitarios (CAS/OR/01/CAS/123300410C0044-3578/2012) and Secretaría de Salud del Estado de Tlaxcala (SS. DECI-OI-13/12). The purpose and procedures of the study were explained to all participants and informed verbal consent was obtained.

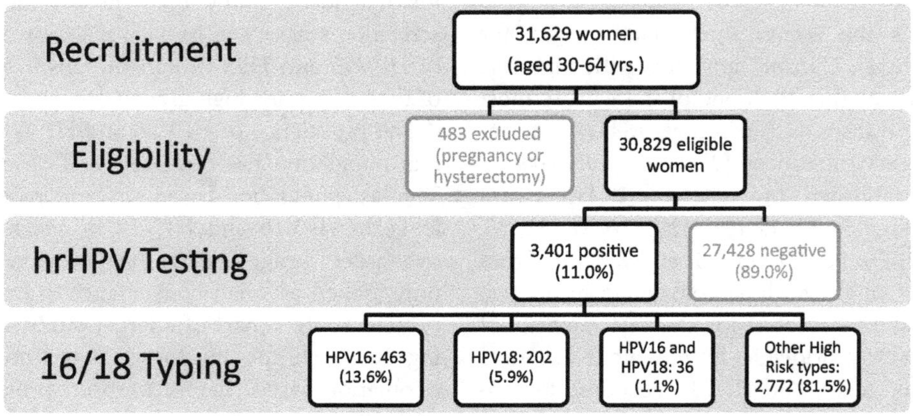

Fig. 1 Flow Chart of hrHPV Screening of the FRIDA Study Population. Women 30 to 64 years of age living within our target health district were invited by healthcare personnel. This study reports the results from the first 31,629 women who volunteered to participate in the Tlaxcala cervical cancer screening program. Four-hundred and eighty-three women were excluded, leaving 30,829 who had hrHPV results available, in the current analysis. Of those 30,829 women, 3,401 women were positive for hrHPV. Among those 3,401 women, 13.6 % were positive for HPV16, 5.9 % for HPV18 and 1.1 % for both HPV16 and HPV18 coinfection. These three categories indicate positivity independent of the presence of other hrHPV types. The last category of other high risk HPV types include women who tested positive for other hrHPV types (31, 33, 35, 39, 45, 51, 52, 56, 58, 59, 66, and 68), but neither HPV16 nor HPV18

Procedures

Health care personnel conducted face-to-face interviews of FRIDA study participants using pre-printed pen and paper surveys designed to elicit details of sexual behavior, history of STIs, parity, gynecologic and reproductive health histories, and other probable risk factors for cervical cancer.

Participants were then given a pelvic exam during which a cervical sample was collected using a Cervex-Brush® (Rovers®). This cervical sample was placed in a ThinPrep® vial (Hologic, Inc., Bedford, MA) and then 0.4 mL tested for hrHPV using Roche's cobas® 4800 system. This assay uses a PCR-based in-vitro test for the simultaneous detection of 14 hrHPV types (16, 18, 31, 33, 35, 39, 45, 51, 52, 56, 58, 59, 66, and 68) in liquid based cervical samples. The system detects HPV16 and HPV18 individually, and the remaining 12 hrHPV genotypes as a pool [19]. The testing was carried out at the HPV laboratory at the INSP in Cuernavaca, Mexico according to manufacturer's instructions (Roche Diagnostics).

Statistical analysis

Descriptive statistics were used to characterize the variables. Age, age of sexual debut, parity, and number of sexual partners were recorded as continuous, numeric variables, and then analyzed as categorical variables. Marital status, use of contraception (hormonal, IUD, condoms), history of previous STIs, and smoking history were both collected and analyzed as categorical variables. In the analysis, participants classified as hrHPV positive tested positive for any of the 14 hrHPV types including HPV16 and HPV18. Among these positives, participants were then classified as positive for HPV16 regardless of whether or not they also tested positive for another hrHPV type. Participants classified as positive for HPV18 were treated in the same way. The designation "HPV16/18" refers to participants who tested positive for either HPV16, HPV18, or both, regardless of other hrHPV types. The designation "HPV16/18 only" means these participants tested positive for HPV16 and/or HPV18, but no other hrHPV types. The "non-16/18 hrHPV only" group refers to women who tested positive for other hrHPV types (31, 33, 35, 39, 45, 51, 52, 56, 58, 59, 66, and 68), but neither HPV16 nor HPV18. The "HPV16/18 and other hrHPV types" group tested positive for HPV16 and/or HPV18 as well as another hrHPV type.

All pooled hrHPV, HPV16/18 only, non-16/18 hrHPV only, and HPV16/18 and other hrHPV type prevalence were estimated by age along with associated binomial 95 % confidence intervals (CI). Looking at the prevalence graphs by age categories, we decided to use a quadratic model for log odds as a function of age. Assuming that the quadratic models are approximately correct, the coefficient on age^2 is a rough measure of the steepness of the parabola. A formal test for differences in steepness of curves for different hrHPV categories was constructed by using the coefficient estimates and their standard errors. Because the sample sizes are large, a normal approximation was used.

We furthermore used logistic regression to compute odds ratios (ORs) with 95 % CIs to identify independent risk factors for hrHPV infections. ORs were adjusted for age to account for differences in age-group prevalence and for comparability with other population reports. Variables associated with hrHPV infections were adjusted for other covariates using multiple logistic regression analysis. Data analysis was conducted using STATA version 12.0 (StataCorp). A two-sided significance level of 0.05 was chosen to indicate statistical significance.

Results

Characteristics of the population

Nearly 97% of women who volunteered to participate in the Tlaxcala cervical cancer screening program met the inclusion study criteria. Approximately 31 % of the target population is included in this analysis. The distribution of ages screened does not perfectly reflect the target population. A higher proportion of women aged 30 to 49 were screened than older groups in the population. Approximately 3.4 % of women aged 60 to 64 were screened. The mean age of the study population was 41.8 years (data not shown).

Approximately 90 % of participants were married, and nearly two-thirds of participants were 18 or older when they initiated sexual activity. The majority of participants have been pregnant and almost 50 % report 3 or more live births. The vast majority of the study participants reported one lifetime sexual partner (71 %). A history of oral contraceptive use was reported by about 21 % of women and a little more than one-third (33 %) were using an IUD. Most women (83 %) reported not using a condom at all in the last 12 months. Histories of previous sexually transmitted infections were rare (3 %), and about 3 % of women reported ever having smoked (Table 1). Approximately 5.0 % self-reported a history of abnormal cervical cytology (data not shown) and 24.9 % of those women received treatment.

High risk HPV prevalence and risk profile

The estimated overall prevalence of hrHPV in this population was 11.0 % (95 % CI 10.7–11.4). High risk HPV DNA was detected in 13.7 % (95 % CI 12.9–14.5) of women aged 30 to 34 and in 11.3 % (95 % CI 10.6–12.1) of women aged 35 to 39. The prevalence estimates declined to 9.4 % (95 % CI 8.7–10.2), 8.8 % (95 % CI 7.9–9.6), and 10.2 % (95 % CI 9.2–11.4) for women aged 40–44, 45–49, and 50–54, respectively. High risk HPV detection then increased again to 11.4 % (95 % CI 10.1–12.9) and 11.3 % (95 % CI 9.5–13.4) for women aged 55 to 59 and 60 to 64, respectively (Table 1 and Fig. 2). In the multivariate model, women aged 30 to 39 were at higher risk of hrHPV infection than women aged 45 to 49, the reference group. The prevalence of hrHPV infections for the oldest age group, women aged 55 to 64, was also significantly different than the reference group, showing a clear U-shaped curve. The coefficients on age^2 were significant.

In addition to age related risks, being unmarried, having a history of oral contraceptive use, having a history of smoking, condom use, having more than one lifetime sexual partner, having two or more sexual partners in the last year, and a history of another STI were also found to be positively associated with hrHPV infections in the multivariate model ($p < 0.05$). This model adjusted for marital status, age at initiation of sexual intercourse, number of lifetime sexual partners, number of sexual partners in the last 12 months, history of hormonal contraception, condom use in the last 12 months, a history of a previous STI, and tobacco use. Age of sexual initiation was, significant only in the age adjusted model (Table 1).

Prevalence of hrHPV Infections by Type in the total screened population

Among all age groups, 9.0 % tested positive for non-16/18 hrHPV only. The distribution by age group showed a U-shaped curve with increased prevalence estimates for women in their 30s and as well as for women over the age of 50 (Table 2 and Fig. 3). The coefficients on age^2 were significant (Table 3).

Among all age groups, 1.5 and 0.7 % were positive at least for HPV16 and HPV18, respectively. By age group, the prevalence of HPV16/18 was highest for the youngest women in the population at 2.9 % (95 % CI 2.5–3.3) for ages 30–34 and 2.3 % (95 % CI 2.0–2.7) for ages 35–39. Prevalence estimates then declined to 1.8 % (95 % CI 1.5–2.1), 1.3 % (95 % CI 1.0–1.6), 1.4 % (95 % CI 1.0–1.8), and 1.5 % (95 % CI 1.1–2.2) for ages 40–44, 45–49, 50–54, and 55–59 (Table 2 and Fig. 2). Estimates then surge for women aged 60 to 64 to 2.2 % (95 % CI 1.5–3.3) (Table 2 and Fig. 2). The prevalence of HPV16 and HPV18 coinfection but neither hrHPV types was rare (0.08 %) (data not shown). The distribution by age group for women who only had HPV16/18 infections showed a marked U-shaped curve with an initial increase for women in their 30s, a decreased prevalence for women in their 40s and 50s, and a second increase in prevalence for women in their 60s (Table 2 and Fig. 3). Like the other prevalence curves, the coefficients on age^2 for HPV16/18 only infections is highly significant (Table 3).

Finally, the prevalence of coinfections with HPV16/18 and another hrHPV type was 0.7 %. The prevalence by age showed a similar U-shaped curve with increased estimates for the younger and older women in the population (Table 2 and Fig. 3). Again, this curve had a significant quadratic trend (Table 3). Overall, there was no significant difference between the quadratic terms for HPV16/18 and the non-16/18 hrHPV only curve. Furthermore, when the quadratic terms for HPV16/18 only and non-16/18 hrHPV only were compared, there was no significant difference ($p < 0.05$) (Table 3).

Table 1 Associations between hrHPV and Reproductive Health and Behavior Variables

	n (% of Total pop. screened)	hrHPV n	Prevalence hrHPV (95 % CI)	Age Adjusted OR (95 % CI)[a]	Multivariate Adjusted OR (95 % CI)[b]
Age (years)					
30–34	7,083 (23.0)	971	13.7 (12.9–14.5)	**1.65 (1.46–1.87)**	**1.61 (1.42–1.83)**
35-39	7,131 (23.1)	809	11.3 (10.6–12.1)	**1.33 (1.17-1.51)**	**1.31 (1.15–1.49)**
40–44	6,176 (20.0)	582	9.4 (8.7–10.2)	1.08 (0.95–1.24)	1.09 (0.95–1.25)
45–49	4,402 (14.3)	386	8.8 (7.9–9.6)	1 (ref)	1 (ref)
50–54	2,969 (9.6)	304	10.2 (9.2–11.4)	1.19 (1.01–1.39)	1.19 (1.01–1.40)
55–59	2,015 (6.5)	230	11.4 (10.1–12.9)	**1.34 (1.28–1.59)**	**1.32 (1.11–1.58)**
60–64	1,053 (3.4)	119	11.3 (9.5–13.4)	**1.33 (1.07–1.65)**	**1.34 (1.07–1.68)**
Total	30,829	3401	11.0 (10.7–11.4)		
Marital Status					
Unmarried	3, 362 (10.9)	600	17.9 (16.6–19.2)	**1.96 (1.78–2.16)**	**1.65 (1.48–1.83)**
Married/Civil Union	27,467 (89.1)	2,801	10.2 (9.8–10.6)	1 (ref)	1 (ref)
Age of Sexual Debut					
≤17	11,221 (36.4)	1,333	11.9 (11.3–12.5)	**1.13 (1.05–1.20)**	1.04 (0.97–1.13)
≥18	19,591 (63.6)	2,067	10.6 (10.1–11.0)	1 (ref)	1 (ref)
Number of Lifetime Sexual Partners[c]					
1 partner	21,832 (70.8)	1,950	8.9 (8.6–9.3)	1 (ref)	1 (ref)
2 partners	5,910 (19.2)	879	14.9 (14.0–15.8)	**1.77 (1.62–1.93)**	**1.61 (1.47–1.76)**
≥3 partners	2,940 (9.5)	556	18.9 (17.5–20.4)	**2.34 (2.11–2.59)**	**1.96 (1.75–2.19)**
Number of Sexual Partners in the Last 12 Months[c]					
0 partners	5,724 (18.6)	686	12.0 (11.2–12.9)	1 (ref)	1 (ref)
1 partner	24,792 (78.2)	2,659	10.7 (10.3–11.1)	0.87 (0.79–0.95)	0.96 (0.87–1.05)
≥2 partners	111 (0.4)	32	28.8 (21.2–37.9)	**2.9 (1.90–4.41)**	**1.75 (1.13–2.70)**
Parity					
0	7,091 (23.1)	785	11.1 (10.4–11.8)	1 (ref)	
1 or 2	8,511 (27.6)	967	11.4 (10.7–12.1)	1.04 (0.94–1.15)	
3 or more	15,049 (48.8)	1,631	10.8 (10.4–11.3)	1.05 (0.96–1.16)	
History of Hormonal Contraception					
Yes	6,417 (20.8)	790	12.3 (11.5–13.1)	**1.17 (1.07–1.27)**	1.10 (1.01–1.20)
No	24,154 (78.1)	2,587	10.7 (10.3–11.1)	1 (ref)	1 (ref)
Current IUD Use					
Yes	10,170 (33.0)	1,164	11.5 (10.8–12.1)	1.05 (0.98–1.14)	
No	19,887 (64.5)	2,153	10.8 (10.4–11.3)	1 (ref)	
Condom Use in the last 12 months					
Never	25,557 (82.9)	2,682	10.5 (10.1–10.9)	1 (ref)	1 (ref)
Almost always	2,777 (9.0)	373	13.4 (12.2–14.8)	**1.27 (1.13–1.43)**	1.15 (1.01–1.29)
Always	1,716 (5.6)	253	14.7 (13.1–16.5)	**1.42 (1.23–1.63)**	**1.26 (1.09–1.46)**
History of a Previous STI					
Yes	979 (3.2)	182	18.6 (16.3–21.1)	**1.91 (1.62–2.25)**	**1.54 (1.30–1.84)**
No	29,424 (95.4)	3,161	10.7 (10.4–11.1)	1 (ref)	1 (ref)
Tobacco Use					
Never	29,238 (94.8)	3,160	10.8 (10.5–11.2)	1 (ref)	1 (ref)
Ever	964 (3.1)	175	18.2 (15.8–20.7)	**1.77 (1.49–2.10)**	**1.23 (1.03–1.47)**

Abbreviations: *STI* sexually transmitted infections, *OR* odds ratio, *CI* confidence interval
[a]Odds ratios for all the variables with the exception of age itself are adjusted for age. Age was included in the model as a categorical variable (30–34, 35–39, 40–44, 45–49, 50–54, 55–59, 60–64); [b]Association test was adjusted for age, marital status, age of sexual debut, number of lifetime sexual partners, number of sexual partners in the last 12 months, history of hormonal contraception, condom use in the last 12 months, history of a previous STI, and tobacco use; [c]Women who reported zero lifetime sexual partners were excluded
Statistically significant *p* values ≤ 0.05 of the OR's are marked in bold font

Discussion

Our population-wide investigation provides a better representation of exposure to infection than a clinic-based population with abnormal cytology in whom HPV16 and HPV18 would be over-represented. The present study is not only the largest in Latin America and most current population based study to date, but is also the first to use Roche's cobas® 4800 system for hrHPV analysis. Roche's cobas® 4800 system has been shown to be a highly sensitive and specific test for the detection of hrHPV as well as HPV16 and HPV18 [20].

There has only been one other previous large population based study conducted in Mexico to report hrHPV type specific prevalence estimates. Although this previous study used a different design and methodology, the age distribution of hrHPV from this study shows a similar U-shaped curve with a first peak for the youngest women and a second peak for the oldest age group [11]. A similar U-shaped curve was found in both the Guanacaste cohort in Costa Rica [21] and a population of Colombian women [22]. Outside of Latin America, a meta-analysis of worldwide epidemiologic data also found this same U-shaped curve for developing nations throughout the world including Africa and Southeast Asia [23].

While the second peak of HPV infections for women up to ages 30 to 39 has been seen in diverse populations throughout the world [23, 24], in Central and South America this peak appears to be more prominent. Epidemiologic data suggests that this first peak of infection can be correlated with sexual initiation in younger women when they are exposed to HPV for the first time and their adaptive immune response has yet to develop [8].

The second peak of infections for women ages 60 to 64 in the FRIDA population is again only seen mirrored in populations throughout the developing world. In North America and throughout most of Europe, the prevalence of HPV infection declines consistently after the initial peak associated with sexual debut [23]. The reasons for this second peak of hrHPV DNA detection are unknown. Current theories suggest that this second peak may be the result of immune depression leading to reactivation of previous quiescent infections [25, 26], the

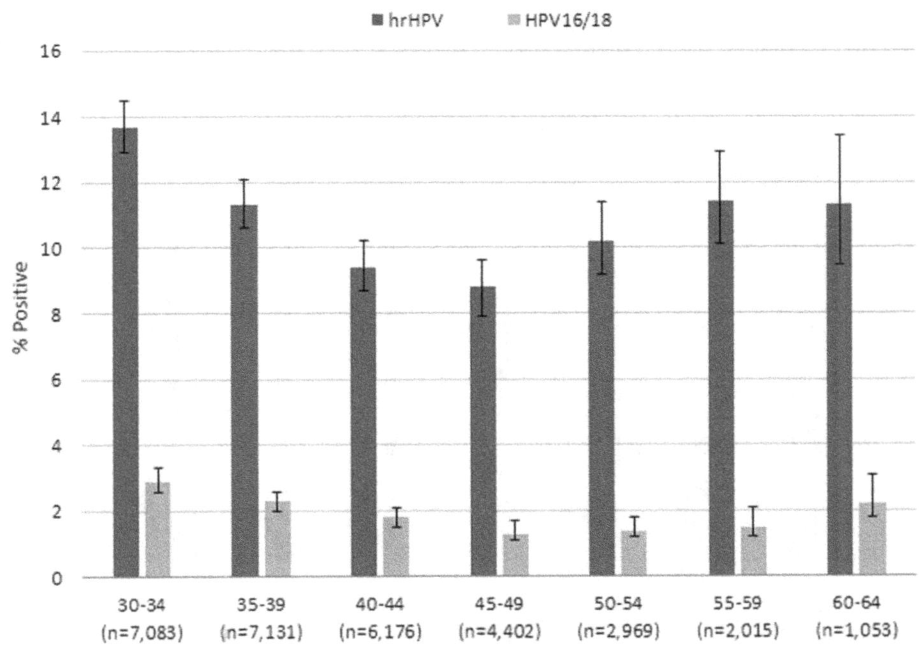

Fig. 2 Age Specific Prevalence of hrHPV and HPV16/18 with 95 % CI. The overall prevalence of hrHPV was 11.0 % in this population. Two percent of women overall were positive for HPV16 and/or HPV18 (HPV16/18). The prevalence of hrHPV overall and HPV16/18 by age group both show a bimodal distribution with an increased prevalence for the youngest women in the population aged 30–39 and a second bump of positivity for the oldest women aged 60 and above

Table 2 Type Specific Prevalence of hrHPV by Age

Age (years)	Total pop.	HPV16/18[a]	Non-16/18 hrHPV only	HPV16/18 only	HPV16/18 and Non-16/18 hrHPV
		% (95 % CI)	% (95 % CI)	% (95 % CI)	% (95 % CI)
30–34	7,083	2.9 (2.5–3.3)	10.8 (10.1–11.5)	1.8 (1.5–2.2)	1.1 (0.9–1.4)
35–39	7,131	2.3 (2.C–2.7)	9.1 (8.4–9.7)	1.5 (1.2–1.8)	0.8 (0.6–1.1)
40–44	6,176	1.8 (1.5–2.1)	7.7 (7.0–8.3)	1.3 (1.0–1.6)	0.5 (0.3–0.7)
45–49	4,402	1.3 (1.C–1.6)	7.5 (6.8–8.3)	0.8 (0.6–1.2)	0.4 (0.3–0.7)
50–54	2,969	1.4 (1.C–1.8)	8.9 (7.9–10.0)	0.6 (0.4–1.0)	0.7 (0.5–1.1)
55–59	2,015	1.5 (1.1–2.2)	9.9 (8.6–11.3)	0.9 (0.6–1.5)	0.6 (0.3–1.0)
60–64	1053	2.2 (1.5–3.3)	9.1 (7.5–11.0)	1.1 (0.7–2.0)	1.0 (0.6–1.9)
Total	30,829	2.0 (1.9–2.2)	9.0 (8.7–9.3)	1.3 (1.2–1.4)	0.7 (0.6–0.8)

Abbreviations: *CI* confidence interval

[a]HPV16/18 refers to women who are positive for HPV16 and/or 18 regardless of other hrHPV types for which they may or may not test positiv

acquisition of new hrHPV infections through changes in sexual behavior on the part of the women themselves and/or their partners, or a cohort effect [25, 27–29]. Another theory suggests that differences in screening programs may also play a role in the presence of this second peak. In countries with effective screening programs, the removal of precancerous lesions is believed to have an antigen-presenting effect to the immune system that may help protect against future HPV infections [30]. Based on this theory, in countries where screening programs do not identify and treat these precancerous lesions, women cannot benefit from this added immunologic boost.

For the FRIDA population, the U-shaped prevalence curve was also seen for HPV16/18 infections. This same pattern is seen in the Guanacaste cohort in Costa Rica [21] and in the previous Mexican study for HPV16, but not for HPV18 [11]. Overall, point estimates of HPV16/18 prevalence appear higher in other study populations throughout Latin America [9, 21, 23, 31], but due to different study designs, it is difficult to draw conclusions concerning the comparative burden of infections.

In addition to the differences seen among age groups, multiple sexual partners was found to be a risk factor for hrHPV infection. Other studies have found a similar association between an increased number of sexual

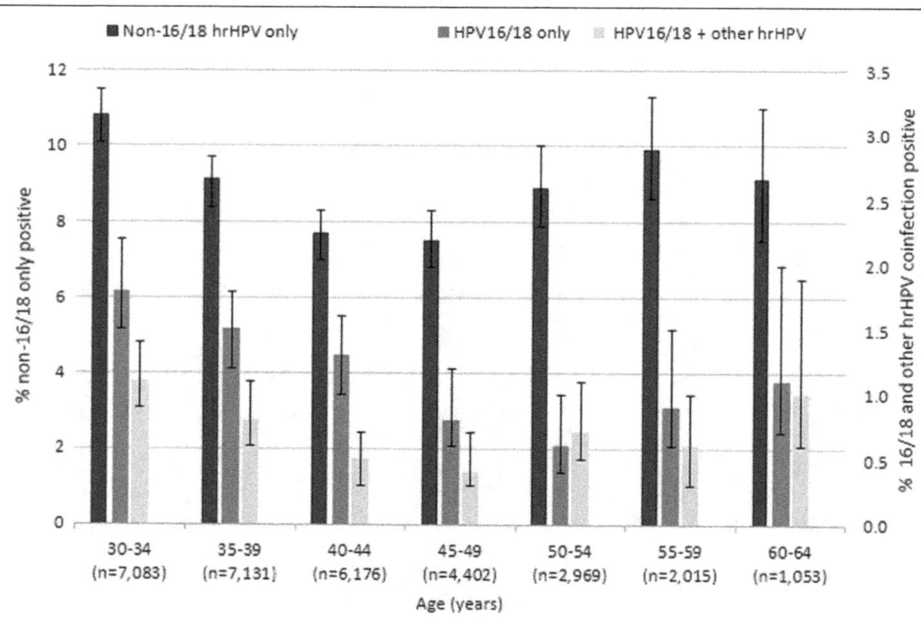

Fig. 3 Age Specific Prevalence of hrHPV Types with 95 % CI. The cobas® 4800 system delivers hrHPV results in three categories: HPV16, HPV18, and other hrHPV. Based on these results, we divided the population into three mutually exclusive categories: (1) women positive for only other hrHPV (non-16/18 hrHPV only), (2) women positive for HPV16 and/or HPV18 (HPV16/18), and (3) women positive for HPV16 and/18 as well as another hrHPV (HPV16/18 + other hrHPV). The prevalence of these three categories by age group shows a similar bimodal distribution with increased prevalence values for the youngest and oldest women in the population

Table 3 Quadratic Model for Log Odds of hrHPV and hrHPV by Type

	Coef. on age^2 (SD)	Coef. on age (SD)	Model *p* value	Two-tailed P values for Differences in Coefficient on Age^2
Any hrHPV	0.00178 (0.000299)	−0.1702 (0.0204)	<0.001	
HPV16/18[a]	0.00228 (0.000520)	−0.2302 (0.0458)	<0.001	0.206[b]
Non-16/18 hrHPV only	0.00155 (0.000250)	−0.1449 (0.0223)	<0.001	
HPV16/18 only	0.00147 (0.000681)	−0.1628 (0.0594)	0.031	1.098[c]
HPV16/18 and other hrHPV	0.00342 (0.000805)	−0.3246 (0.0717)	<0.001	

Abbreviation: *SD* standard deviation

[a]HPV16/18 refers to women who are positive for HPV16 and/or 18 regardless of other hrHPV types for which they may or may not test positive; [b]comparison non-16/18 hrHPV only vs HPV16/18; [c] comparison non-16/18 hrHPV only vs HPV16/18 only

partners and risk of hrHPV infection [26, 32, 33]. In contrast, age at first intercourse was not found to be an independent risk factor for hrHPV in this population, similar to other studies. However, we also acknowledge that there are previous studies reporting that the age of sexual debut is an independent risk factor by itself [34]. It should be noted that a particularity of FRIDA population was a younger age of sexual debut was highly correlated with having more than one lifetime sexual partner ($p < 0.001$) (data not shown).

This preliminary analysis only contains 30 % of the target population. With a larger population, our study will be better powered to describe HPV16/18 determinants. We furthermore acknowledge the possibility of social desirability bias with the sensitive, self-reported data, such a bias may have led to underestimation of certain risk factors. We attempted to limit such bias by providing a private space for the recruitment interviews.

In the absence of cervical screening or cancer registries in Mexico at the national, regional or state levels, these prevalence data can help to better inform resource allocation decisions. Sharma et al. developed a model whereby hrHPV prevalence data can be used to estimate cervical cancer risk [5]. While Sharma et al.'s models have been developed to predict cervical cancer incidence in developed countries, more data is needed in developing countries such as Mexico to refine these models so they can be better applied in the developing world [5]. Such a reliable model to determine cervical cancer risk would be a very valuable tool in Mexico and through the developing world. Nonetheless, it is important to note that the generalizability of the findings may be limited both within Mexico and outside of Mexico.

Beyond predicting cervical cancer risk, the prevalence data from this study can serve a number of additional uses from a policy perspective. First the prevalence information can be useful for evaluating the impact of HPV vaccination over the long term. While a number of surrogate endpoints of vaccine impact may be used, HPV type-specific prevalence data has become the standard early indicator of choice [35, 36], and thus these prevalence data may also be used as baseline to monitor vaccine effectiveness.

This prevalence information will furthermore be useful for policymakers trying to determine the best triage practices in Mexico. In 2013, our study group was able to show that primary screening for hrHPV is effective, but a secondary follow-up or triage test is needed to determine which women should be sent to colposcopy [7]. We attempted to send all hrHPV positive women to colposcopy, but found it was not only inefficient, but also overburdened the local health services. In this previous pilot, we sent nearly 11 % of women for colposcopy services. If we had triaged women based on HPV16/18, we would have only sent 2 % of women and still detected more than 70 % of disease [4]. Furthermore, some analyses suggest that the best alternative may be a combination of triage alternatives to offer high joint specificity to detect CIN2 or more, including other triage tests such as cytology, p16 or DNA methylation or at least evidence of 6 to 12 months of persistent hrHPV infection before referral [37]. A triage algorithm using HPV16/18 testing has been validated in the US [10], but needs to be further explored in Mexico. This prevalence data will help policymakers to determine whether or not the current infrastructure in Mexico can support the triage of HPV16 and HPV18 positive women. Further study is still needed to determine the performance and cost-effectiveness of HPV16 and HPV18 detection as an additional triage alternative for hrHPV positive women, and what additional testing may be required to ensure a more effective and safe cervical cancer screening program in Mexico.

The main strength of our study is our large, population-based approach. This is the first study in Mexico of this size to assess the prevalence of HPV16/18. This epidemiologic data will contribute to the creation of a more reliable strategy of cervical cancer prevention in Mexico.

Conclusion

This sub-analysis of the FRIDA study demonstrates the population level prevalence pattern of hrHPV and HPV16/18 by age in Mexico. Both hrHPV and HPV16/18 positivity have a bimodal distribution by age with higher prevalences at ages 30–39 and 60–64. Infections with hrHPV were also found to be positively associated with an increased number of lifetime sexual partners, a history of STIs, being unmarried, use of hormonal contraception, and reported condom use. Our results set the stage for an improved cervical cancer screening strategy in Mexico. While primary screening for hrHPV has already been instituted in Mexico, this prevalence data suggests the feasibility of HPV typing as an additional screening parameter nationwide.

Acknowledgments

Drs. Heidi Bauer, Karen Sokal-Gutierrez, and Maureen Lahiff helped to review the manuscript, and Dr. Lahiff and Dr. Ndola Prata further provided biostatistical support. The authors would also like to recognize the FRIDA study population for their generous participation as well as the Tlaxcala FRIDA field team for collecting the data and supervising field procedures.

*FRIDA Study Group: Samantha E. Rudolph, Attila Lorincz, Cosette Wheeler, Patti Gravitt, Eduardo Lazcano, Leticia Torres-Ibarra, Leith León, Paula Ramírez, Berenice Rivera, Eduardo L. Franco, Jack Cuzick, Pablo Méndez, Jorge Salmerón, Mauricio Hernández, Thomas C. Wright, Anna Barbara Moscicki, Yvonne Flores, Mark H. Stoler, Enrique Carmona, Kathleen M. Schmeler, David Bishai, Pilar Hernández, Daniel Alvarez, Elizabeth Barrios, Rubi Hernández, Indira Mendiola, and Vicente González.

Funding

This study was supported by the National Institute of Public Health of Mexico, the Coordinación de Investigación en Salud del Instituto Mexicano del Seguro Social, the Secretaría de Salud Tlaxcala, the Instituto Nacional de las Mujeres, and the Consejo Nacional de Ciencia y Tecnología [FOSISS 2013 202468]. Additional support has been provided by Roche Diagnostics, BD Diagnostics, DICIPA and Arbor Vita Corporation. The study sponsors did not played a role in designing the study, collecting, analyzing or interpreting the data, writing the report, or submitting this paper for publication. UC Berkeley Center for Global Public Health, Schoeneman Grant, Joint Medical Program Thesis Grant, and Cancer Research UK (C569/A10404).

Authors' contributions

SR, AL, CW, PG, ELP, LTI, EF, JC and JS were responsible for the study design and had full access to all the data in the study and take responsibility for the integrity of the data and the accuracy of the data analysis. JS, BR, PMH, LLM, LTI site investigators, contributed to study implementation and study coordination. BR, PR, LLM, LTI, RH and JS were responsible for the data collection and study supervision. SR, AL, CW, PG, LTI, ELP, JC and JS were responsible of drafting the manuscript and contributed to data interpretation. SR, RH and JC performed and reviewed the statistical analyses. All authors contributed ideas to the manuscript, provided critical revision of content, and approved the final version.

Competing interests

JS has received funding for research projects from Qiagen, GSK, Merck, Roche, Beckton Dickinson, Gen-Probe, DICIPA and Arbor Vita. ATL is a consultant for EVE Medical. CMW has received funding through the University of New Mexico for HPV vaccine studies (Merck and GSK) and reagents and equipment for HPV genotyping (Roche Molecular Systems).

Consent for publication

Not applicable.

Author details

[1]UC Berkeley-UCSF Joint Medical Program, Berkeley, CA, USA. [2]Unidad de Investigación Epidemiológica y en Servicios de Salud, Instituto Mexicano del Seguro Social, Cuernavaca, Morelos, México. [3]Wolfson Institute of Preventive Medicine, Barts and The London School of Medicine, Queen Mary University of London, London, UK. [4]Department of Pathology, University of New Mexico School of Medicine, Albuquerque, NM, USA. [5]Centro de Investigación en Salud Poblacional, Instituto Nacional de Salud Pública, Avenida Universidad 655, Colonia Sta. María Ahuacatitlán, 62100 Cuernavaca, Morelos, Mexico. [6]CONACYT, Centro de Investigación en Salud Poblacional, Instituto Nacional de Salud Pública, Cuernavaca, Morelos, México, USA. [7]Division of Cancer Epidemiology, McGill University, Montreal, Canada. [8]Departamento de Enseñanza, Capacitación e Investigación, Secretaría de Salud de Tlaxcala, Tlaxcala, Tlaxcala, Mexico. [9]Facultad de Ciencias de la Salud, Universidad Autónoma de Tlaxcala, Tlaxcala, Tlaxcala, Mexico.

References

1. Bruni L, Barrionuevo-Rosas L, Albero G, Aldea M, Serrano B, Valencia S, Brotons M, Mena M, Cosano R, Muñoz J, Bosch FX, de Sanjosé S, Castellsagué X. ICO Information Centre on HPV and Cancer (HPV Information Centre). Human Papillomavirus and Related Diseases in Mexico. Summary Report 2016-02-26. http://www.hpvcentre.net/statistics/reports/MEX.pdf. [Accesed 22 Aug 2016].
2. Walboomers JMM, Jacobs MV, Manos MM, Bosch FX, Kummer JA, Shah KV, Snijders PJF, Peto J, Meijer CJLM, Muñoz N. Human Papillomavirus is a necessary cause of invasive cervical cancer worldwide. J Pathol. 1999;189:12–9.
3. Muñoz N, Mendez F, Posso H, Molano M, van de Brule AJC, Ronderos M, Meijer CJLM, Muñoz A. Incidence, duration, and determinants of cervical human papillomavirus infection in a cohort of Colombian women with normal cytological results. J Infect Dis. 2004;190:2077–87.
4. de Sanjose S, Quint WG, Alemany L, Geraets DT, Klaustermeier JE, Lloveras B, Tous S, Felix A, Bravo LE, Shin H-R, Vallejos CS, de Ruiz PA, Lima MA, Guimera N, Clavero O, Alejo M, Llombart-Bosch A, Cheng-Yang C, Tatti SA, Kasamatsu E, Iljazovic E, Odida M, Prado R, Seoud M, Grce M, Usubutun A, Jain A, Suarez GA, Lombardi LE, Banjo A, et al. Human papillomavirus genotype attribution in invasive cervical cancer: a retrospective cross-sectional worldwide study. Lancet Oncol. 2010;11:1048–56.
5. Sharma M, Bruni L, Diaz M, Castellsagué X, de Sanjosé S, Bosch FX, Kim JJ. Using HPV prevalence to predict cervical cancer incidence. Int J Cancer. 2012;132:1895–900.
6. Kably-Ambe A, Ruiz-Moreno JA, Lazcano-Ponce E, Vargas-Hernandez VM, Aguado-Perez RA, Alonso-de Ruiz P. Consenso para la prevención del cáncer cervicouterino en México. Ginecol Obstet Mex. 2011;79:785–7.
7. Lazcano-Ponce E, Lorincz AT, Torres L, JJorge S, Cruz A, Rojas R, Hernandez P, Hernandez M. Specimen self-collection and HPV DNA screening in a pilot study of 100,242 women. Int J Cancer. 2013;135:109–16.
8. Moscicki A-B, Shiboski S, Broering J, Powell K, Clayton L, Jay N, Darragh TM, Brescia R, Kanowitz S, Miller SB, Stone J, Hanson E. The natural history of human papillomavirus infection as measured by repeated DNA testing in adolescent and young women. J Pediatr. 1998;132:277–84.
9. Lazcano-Ponce E, Lorincz AT, JJorge S, Fernández I, Cruz A, Hernandez P, Mejia I, Hernández-Ávila M. A pilot study of HPV DNA and cytology testing in 50,159 women in the routine Mexican Social Security Program. Cancer Causes Control. 2010;21:1693–700.
10. Cox JT, Castle PE, Behrens CM, Sharma A, Wright TC, Cuzick J, Group AHS. Comparison of cervical cancer screening strategies incorporating different combinations of cytology, HPV testing, and genotyping for HPV 16/18: results from the ATHENA HPV study. Ame J Obstet Gynecol. 2013;208:184.e1–184.e11.
11. Lazcano-Ponce E, Herrero R, Muñoz N, Cruz A, Shar KV, Alonso P, Hernandez P, JJorge S, Hernandez M. Epidemiology of HPV infection among Mexican women with normal cervical cytology. Int J Cancer. 2001;91:412–20.
12. Orozco-Colin A, Carrillo-García A, Méndez-Tenorio A, Ponce-de-León S, Mohar A, Maldonado-Rodríguez R, Guerra-Arias R, Flores-Gil O, Sotelo-Regil R, Lizano M. Geographical variation in human papillomavirus prevalence in Mexican women with normal cytology. Int J Infect Dis. 2010;14:e1082–7.
13. Velázquez-Márquez N, Paredes-Tello MA, Pérez-Terrón H, Santos-López G, Reyes-Leyva J, Vallejo-Ruiz V. Prevalence of human papillomavirus genotypes in women from a rural region of Puebla, Mexico. Int J Infect Dis. 2009;13:690–5.
14. Sánchez-Anguiano L, Alvarado-Esquivel C, Reyes-Romero M, Carrera-Rodríguez M. Human papillomavirus infection in women seeking cervical Papanicolaou cytology of Durango, Mexico: prevalence and genotypes. BMC Infect Dis. 2006;6:27.

15. Illades-Aguiar B, Cortés-Malagón E-M, Antonio-Véjar V, Zamudio-López N, Alarcón-Romero LDC, Fernández-Tilapa G, Hernández-Sotelo D, Terán-Porcayo M-A, Flores-Alfaro E, Leyva-Vázquez M-A. Cervical carcinoma in southern Mexico: human papillomavirus and cofactors. Cancer Detect Prev. 2009;32:300–7.
16. Illades-Aguiar B, del Carmen Alarcón-Romero L, Antonio-Véjar V, Zamudio-López N, Sales-Linares N, Flores-Alfaro E, Fernández-Tilapa G, Vences-Velázquez A, Muñoz-Valle JF, Leyva-Vázquez M-A. Prevalence and distribution of human papillomavirus types in cervical cancer, squamous intraepithelial lesions, and with no intraepithelial lesions in women from Southern Mexico. Gynecol Oncol. 2010;117:291–6.
17. Peralta-Rodriguez R, Romero-Morelos P, Villegas-Ruiz V, Mendoza-Rodriguez M, Taniguchi-Ponciano K, Gonzalez-Yebra B, Marrero-Rodriguez D, Salcedo M. Prevalence of human papillomavirus in the cervical epithelium of Mexican women: meta-analysis. Infect Agents Cancer. 2012;7:1–1.
18. Torroella-Kouri M, Morsberger S, Carrillo A, Mohar A, Meneses A, Ibarra M, Daniel RW, Ghaffari AM, Solorza G, Shah KV. HPV prevalence among Mexican women with neoplastic and normal cervixes. Gynecol Oncol. 1998;70:115–20.
19. Snijders PJF, Heideman DAM, Meijer CJLM. Methods for HPV detection in exfoliated cell and tissue specimens. APMIS. 2010;118:520–8.
20. Park Y, Lee E, Choi J, Jeong S, Kim HS. Comparison of the Abbott RealTime high-risk human papillomavirus (HPV), roche cobas HPV, and hybrid capture 2 assays to direct sequencing and genotyping of HPV DNA. J Clin Microbiol. 2012;50:2359–65.
21. Herrero R, Castle PE, Schiffman M, Bratti C, Hildesheim A, Morales J, Alfaro M, Sherman ME, Wacholder S, Chen S, Rodriguez AC, Burk RD. Epidemiologic profile of type-specific human papillomavirus infection and cervical neoplasia in Guanacaste, costa rica. J Infect Dis. 2005;191:1796–807.
22. Molano M, Posso H, Weiderpass E, van den Brule AJC, Ronderos M, Franceschi S, Meijer CJLM, Arslan A, Munoz N. Prevalence and determinants of HPV infection among Colombian women with normal cytology. Br J Cancer. 2002;87:324–33.
23. Bruni L, Diaz M, Castellsagué X, Ferrer E, Bosch FX, de Sanjose S. Cervical human papillomavirus prevalence in 5 continents: MetahAnalysis of 1 million women with normal cytological findings. J Infect Dis. 2010;202:1789–99.
24. Franceschi S, Herrero R, Clifford GM, Snijders PJF, Arslan A, Anh PTH, Bosch FX, Ferreccio C, Hieu NT, Lazcano-Ponce E, Matos E, Molano M, Qiao Y-L, Rajkumar R, Ronco G, de Sanjose S, Shin H-R, Sukvirach S, Thomas JO, Meijer CJLM, Muñoz N, the IARC HPV Prevalence Surveys Study Group. Variations in the age-specific curves of human papillomavirus prevalence in women worldwide. Int J Cancer. 2006;119:2677–84.
25. Gravitt PE. Evidence and impact of human papillomavirus latency. Open Virol J. 2012;6:198–203.
26. Rositch AF, Burke AE, Viscidi RP, Silver MI, Chang K, Gravitt PE. Contributions of recent and past sexual partnerships on incident human papillomavirus detection: acquisition and reactivation in older women. Cancer Res. 2012;72:6183–90.
27. Bosch FX, Burchell AN, Schiffman M, Giuliano AR, de Sanjose S, Bruni L, Tortolero-Luna G, Kjaer SK, Muñoz N. Epidemiology and natural history of human papillomavirus infections and type-specific implications in cervical neoplasia. Vaccine. 2008;26:K1–K16.
28. Trottier H, Ferreira S, Thomann P, Costa MC, Sobrinho JS, Prado JCM, Rohan TE, Villa LL, Franco EL. Human papillomavirus infection and reinfection in adult women: the role of sexual activity and natural immunity. Cancer Res. 2010;70:8569–77.
29. Gravitt PE, Rositch AF, Silver MI, Marks MA, Chang K, Burke AE, Viscidi RP. A cohort effect of the sexual revolution May Be masking an increase in human papillomavirus detection at menopause in the United States. J Infect Dis. 2013;207:272–80.
30. Passmore J-AS, Morroni C, Shapiro S, Williamson A-L, Hoffman M. Papanicolaou smears and cervical inflammatory cytokine responses. J Inflamm. 2007;4:8.
31. Matos E, Loria D, Amestoy GM, Herrera L, Prince MA, Moreno J, Krunfly C, van den Brule AJC, Meijer CJLM, Muñoz N, Herrero R. Prevalence of human papillomavirus infection among women in Concordia. Argentina: Sex Transm Dis. 2003;30:593–9.
32. Bahmanyar ER, Paavonen J, Naud P, JJorge S, Chow S-N, Apter D, Kitchener H, Castellsagué X, Teixeira JC, Skinner SR, Jaisamrarn U, Limson GA, Garland SM, Szarewski A, Romanowski B, Aoki F, Schwarz TF, Poppe WAJ, De Carvalho NS, Harper DM, Bosch FX, Raillard A, Descamps D, Struyf F, Lehtinen M, Dubin G. Group FTHPS: prevalence and risk factors for cervical HPV infection and abnormalities in young adult women at enrolment in the multinational PATRICIA trial. Gynecol Oncol. 2012;127:440–50.
33. Roura E, Iftner T, Vidart JA, Kjaer SK, Bosch FX, Muñoz N, Palacios S, Rodriguez MSM, Morillo C, Serradell L, Torcel-Pagnon L, Cortes J, Castellsagué X. Predictors of human papillomavirus infection in women undergoing routine cervical cancer screening in Spain: the CLEOPATRE study. BMC Infect Dis. 2012;12:1–13.
34. Kahn JA, Rosenthal SL, Succop PA, Ho GYF, Burk RD. Mediators of the association between Age of first sexual intercourse and subsequent human papillomavirus infection. Pediatrics. 2002;109:e5.
35. Wheeler CM, Hunt WC, Cuzick J, Langsfeld E, Pearse A, Montoya GD, Robertson M, Shearman CA, Castle PE. For the New Mexico HPV Pap registry steering committee: a population-based study of human papillomavirus genotype prevalence in the United States: baseline measures prior to mass human papillomavirus vaccination. Int J Cancer. 2012;132:198–207.
36. Chang Y, Brewer NT, Rinas AC, Schmitt K, Smith JS. Evaluating the impact of human papillomavirus vaccines. Vaccine. 2009;27:4355–62.
37. Beal CM, Salmerón J, Flores YN, Torres L, Granados-García V, Dugan E, Lazcano-Ponce E. Cost analysis of different cervical cancer screening strategies in Mexico. Salud Publica Mex. 2014;56:492–501.

10

Reproductive and genital health and risk of cervical human papillomavirus infection: results from the Ludwig-McGill cohort study

Eileen Shaw[1,2], Agnihotram V. Ramanakumar[1], Mariam El-Zein[1], Flavia R. Silva[1], Lenice Galan[3,4], Maria L. Baggio[3,4], Luisa L. Villa[3,4], Eduardo L. Franco[1,2*] and for the Ludwig-McGill Cohort Study

Abstract

Background: There are inconsistencies in the literature on reproductive and genital health determinants of human papillomavirus (HPV) infection, the primary cause of cervical cancer. We examined these factors in the Ludwig-McGill Cohort Study, a longitudinal, repeated-measurements investigation on the natural history of HPV infection.

Methods: We analyzed a cohort subset of 1867 women with one complete year of follow-up. We calculated odds ratios (OR) and 95 % confidence intervals (CI) for reproductive and genital health characteristics from questionnaire and laboratory data in relation to 1-year period prevalence of HPV infection. Two outcomes were measured; the first based on phylogenetic grouping of HPV types based on tissue tropism and oncogenicity (Alphapapillomavirus Subgenus 1: species 1, 8, 10 and 13; Subgenus 2: species 5, 6, 7, 9, 11; Subgenus 3: species 3, 4 and 14) and the second based on transient or persistent HPV infections.

Results: Lifetime (Subgenus 3 OR = 2.00, CI: 1.23–3.24) and current (Subgenus 3 OR = 2.00, CI: 1.15–3.47) condom use and use of contraceptive injections (Subgenus 1 OR = 1.96, CI: 1.22–3.16, Subgenus 2 OR = 1.34, CI: 1.00–1.79) were associated with increased risk of HPV infection. Intrauterine device use was protective (Subgenus 1 OR = 0.48, CI: 0.30–0.75, Subgenus 2 OR = 0.78, CI: 0.62–0.98). These factors were not associated with persistence of HPV infection. Tampon use, previous gynecologic infections and cervical inflammation were associated with an overall increased risk of HPV infection.

Conclusions: Cervical HPV infection was associated with reproductive and genital health factors. Further studies are necessary to confirm the low to moderate associations observed.

Keywords: Human papillomavirus, HPV, Cervical cancer, Reproductive health, Genital hygiene, Determinants

Background

Cervical cancer is the fourth most common cancer in women worldwide [1]. Despite recent advances in human papillomavirus (HPV) vaccines and screening programs, cervical cancer remains a large global health burden. HPV is a necessary cause of cervical cancer, but it is not sufficient. Therefore, identification of risk factors of HPV infection and cervical cancer may inform preventive strategies. Outside of sexual behavior characteristics and parity [2–4], there is a lack of consensus in the literature on determinants of HPV infection, particularly with respect to reproductive and genital health.

Condom use has been inconsistently associated with a decreased risk of HPV infection [5, 6]. Use of oral contraceptives (OCs) is associated with cervical carcinogenesis [7, 8], while use of intrauterine devices (IUDs) [9] and tubal sterilization [10] seems protective. However, evidence of a relationship between these factors and risk of HPV infection remains equivocal as there have been

* Correspondence: eduardo.franco@mcgill.ca
[1]Division of Cancer Epidemiology, Department of Oncology, McGill University, Montreal, Canada
[2]Department of Epidemiology, Biostatistics and Occupational Health, McGill University, 546 Pine Avenue West, Montreal, QC H2W 1S6, Canada

very few studies done in this field [10, 11]. An elevated risk of HPV infection is associated with other infections such as *Chlamydia trachomatis* [12, 13], human immunodeficiency virus (HIV) [14, 15], and bacterial vaginosis (BV) [16]. Despite these trends, inconsistencies remain concerning the magnitude and direction of effects, with a paucity of information on other factors.

This study focuses on the role of reproductive and genital health on cervical HPV infections using data from a large longitudinal study conducted to investigate the natural history of HPV infection.

Methods

Study design and participants

The design and methods of the Ludwig-McGill Cohort Study have been previously described [17]. The study enrolled women from São Paulo, Brazil, a high-risk area for cervical cancer. Briefly, women were recruited from a maternal and child health program for low-income families between 1993 and 1997. Eligible women must have: 1) been 18–60 years old 2) been permanent residents of São Paulo 3) had no intention of becoming pregnant over the next year 4) had an intact uterus without referral for hysterectomy 5) had no treatment for cervical disease within 6 months previous to enrolment and 6) reported no use of vaginal medication in the 2 days prior to enrolment. Signed, informed consent for participation in the study was obtained from all women. Follow-up of women occurred every 4 months in the first year and twice per year afterwards. The study was approved by the institutional review boards and ethical committees of McGill University, University of Toronto, the Ludwig Institute for Cancer Research and the Maternidade Escola Vila Nova Cachoeirinha clinic.

Data collection and procedures

Questionnaires were administered by one of two study nurses (MLB, LG) at each of the four visits in the first year and once per year afterwards. Baseline questionnaires collected detailed information on sexual and reproductive histories, and behavioural characteristics including smoking and hygiene habits. Cervical specimens were taken at each visit for conventional Pap cytology and molecular HPV testing. Ectocervical and endocervical cells were collected using an Accelon biosampler (Medscand Inc., Hollywood, FL). Pap smears were read and graded at the Jewish General Hospital (Montreal, Canada).

Presence of HPV DNA was detected using polymerase chain reaction to amplify a highly conserved segment of the L1 viral gene using PGMY consensus primers [18, 19]. Typing of the amplified product was performed by hybridization with individual oligonucleotide probes, and by restriction fragment-length polymorphism analysis to identify 40 different mucosal HPV types. We grouped types according to Alphapapillomavirus species clusters that exhibit comparable tissue tropism and biological behavior concerning cancer risk [20–23]. Subgenus 1 included HPV types 6, 11, 32, 40, 42, 44 and 54, from species α1, α8, α10 and α13. Subgenus 2 included HPV types 16, 18, 26, 31, 33, 34, 35, 39, 45, 51, 52, 53, 56, 58, 59, 66, 67, 68, 69, 70, 73 and 82, from species α5, α6, α7, α9 and α11. Subgenus 3 included HPV types 57, 61, 62, 71, 72, 81, 83, 84 and 89, from species α3, α4 and α14. Subgenus 1 and Subgenus 3 HPV types are part of subgenera whose members are not carcinogenic, whereas types in Subgenus 2 are mostly carcinogenic. Types in all three subgenus groups exhibit strong genital tropism but types from Subgenus 3 are mostly commensal agents that infect the vagina but produce no clinically identifiable lesions [20–23].

Exposure measurements and study outcomes

Aside from questions with predetermined answer choices, responses to open-ended questions were grouped into categorical variables, including comments disclosed to the administering nurses, but not explicitly asked (Additional file 1: Table S1). Some exposures were classified as "former", indicating lifetime use and "current", indicating use between the first and second visit as use between visits remained relatively constant over the first year of follow-up. We also grouped qualitative cytology results, which included reports on inflammation and bacterial or fungal infections into categories relating to cervical health conditions.

We used two HPV outcome variables. First, we considered 1-year period prevalence for infections from the above three phylogenetically-defined subgenus groups by taking into account HPV types detected cumulatively over the first four visits in the first year (enrolment and months 4, 8 and 12). Second, we categorized HPV infections into mutually exclusive transient or persistent infections in the first year. Transient HPV infections were those involving one positive HPV test result followed by two subsequent negative results. Persistent infections were two or more positive HPV test results of the same HPV group, with no more than one negative result between two positive test results. HPV test results that did not fall into these definitions were excluded.

Statistical analysis

We estimated odds ratios (ORs) and 95 % confidence intervals (CIs) for HPV outcomes using logistic regression models, adjusting for *a priori* (baseline age and lifetime number of sexual partners) and empirical confounders. The latter, identified using a 5 % change-in-estimate strategy, included race, marital status, education, age at first intercourse, age at menarche, number of pregnancies, smoking, alcohol drinking and years since last Pap smear.

For the analysis of 1-year period prevalence, we compared women with a specific group infection (Subgenus 1 = 108, Subgenus 2 = 495, Subgenus 3 = 131) to a floating control group of those who did not have that group infection. We called this the non-restricted analysis. Since concurrent and cumulative multiple-type infections were common in the cohort, we conducted separate analyses restricted to women who only harboured infections with HPV types from a single phylogenetic group (Subgenus 1 = 41, Subgenus 2 = 377, Subgenus 3 = 57). A fixed control group that included only HPV-negative women ($n = 1267$) was used in these restricted analyses. The restricted analyses, while compromising on precision, were intended to increase the validity of observed associations and were thus used to confirm associations seen in the non-restricted estimates. Adjusted ORs were calculated using the non-restricted crude estimate. All data were analyzed using Stata 12.0 (StataCorp, College Station, TX, USA).

Results

Of the 3589 eligible women, 2528 participants were enrolled in the Ludwig-McGill cohort study (Fig. 1), with an average follow-up time of 7 years. This analysis was restricted to 1867 women who had completed all four visits within the first year, representing 76 % of those enrolled in the study. Of these, 1267 women were HPV-negative and 600 women tested positive for any HPV infection on at least one of the four visits. Due to multiple infections in some women, there were a total of 734 type-specific HPV infections. For the second outcome indicator, there were 262 transient HPV infections, 282 persistent infections and 56 women were excluded from this analysis. At baseline, the mean age of participants was 32.9 (±8.7) years, and the mean number of lifetime sexual partners and pregnancies were 3.9 and 3.5,

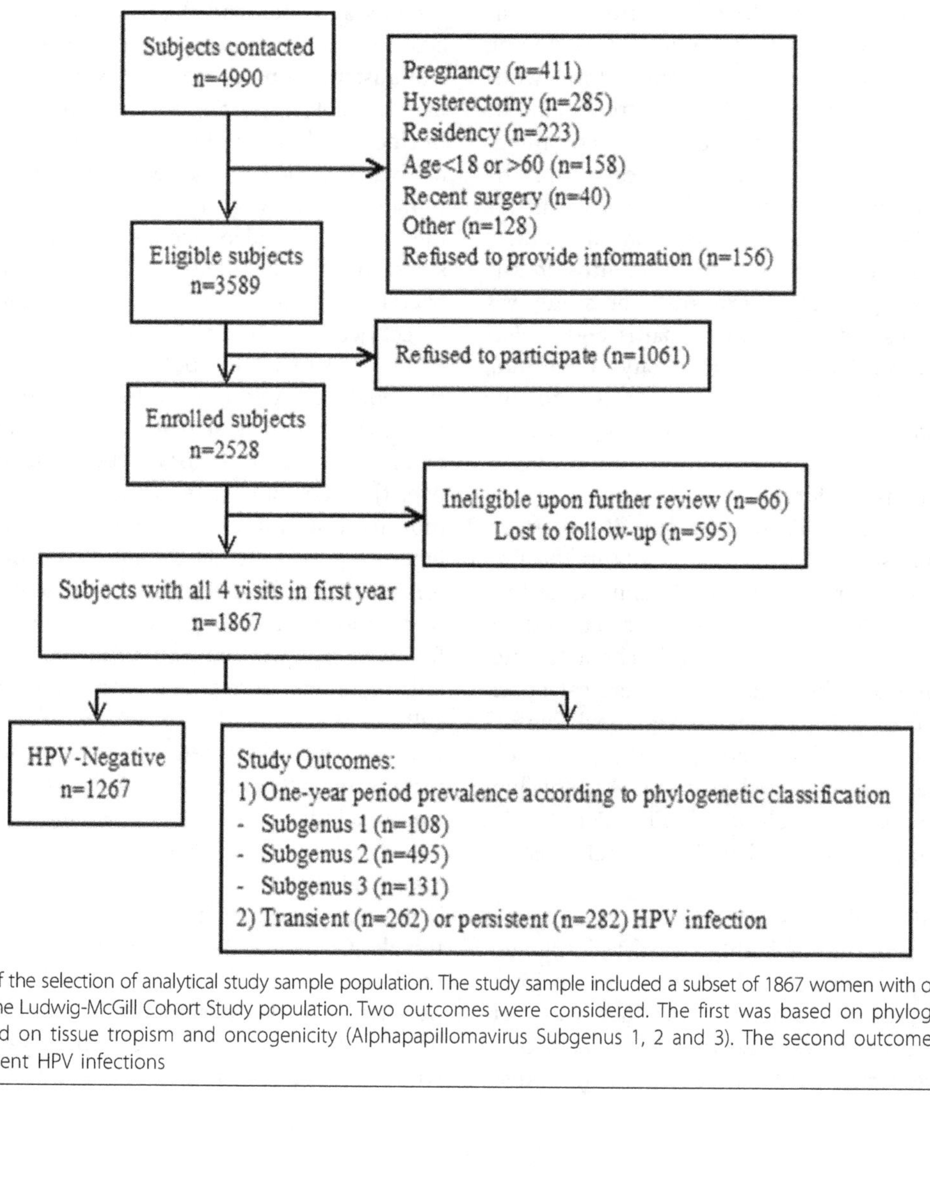

Fig. 1 Flow chart of the selection of analytical study sample population. The study sample included a subset of 1867 women with one complete year of follow-up from the Ludwig-McGill Cohort Study population. Two outcomes were considered. The first was based on phylogenetic grouping of HPV types based on tissue tropism and oncogenicity (Alphapapillomavirus Subgenus 1, 2 and 3). The second outcome was based on transient or persistent HPV infections

respectively. Only 19 % of women had completed high school or further education. Characteristics of this study population according to outcome variables are described in Additional file 1: Table S2.

Table 1 presents associations for reproductive and genital health factors with the first outcome of phylogenetic grouping of HPV types (Additional file 1: Table S3 refers to the restricted subsets). Results from the restricted crude analyses tended to reflect those of the non-restricted crude and adjusted analyses apart from the expected loss in precision in the restricted estimates. Table 2 presents these associations for the second outcome of transient and persistent infections.

Contraceptive methods

Both former (OR = 2.00, 95 % CI: 1.23–3.24) and current (OR = 2.00, 95 % CI: 1.15–3.47) condom use was significantly associated with an increased prevalence of Subgenus 3 HPV infections. Current condom use was also significantly associated with transient HPV infections (OR = 1.47, 95 % CI: 1.00–2.16). OC use was not significantly associated with any HPV outcome analyzed. Use of IUDs was protective across all HPV outcomes with significant effects in Subgenus 1 (OR = 0.48, 95 % CI: 0.30–0.75), Subgenus 2 (OR = 0.78, 95 % CI: 0.62–0.98) and transient (OR = 0.65, 95 % CI: 0.48–0.87) infections. Tubal sterilization had a predominantly protective, although insignificant, effect across all outcomes. Of the open-ended responses, use of contraceptive injections increased the prevalence of all HPV outcomes, with Subgenus 1 (OR = 1.96, 95 % CI: 1.22–3.16), Subgenus 2 (OR = 1.34, 95 % CI: 1.00–1.79) and transient (OR = 1.58, 95 % CI: 1.10–2.26) HPV infections being statistically significant. Natural and external products were not significantly associated with any HPV outcome, although there were not enough observations to calculate Subgenus 1 ORs.

Vaginal hygiene

Menstrual cloth use had a protective effect for Subgenus 2, transient and persistent HPV infections with a significant effect on Subgenus 1 infections (OR = 0.54, 95 % CI: 0.32–0.91). Conversely, all point estimates for hygienic tampon use were above the null with Subgenus 2 infections approaching borderline significance and transient infections being statistically significant (OR = 1.48, 95 % CI: 1.00–2.20). Frequent douching was not associated with most HPV outcomes, although there was a significantly protective effect on Subgenus 3 infections (OR = 0.11, 95 % CI: 0.02–0.81). There was also no effect of the types of douching products used, with the exception of "unknown" products and Subgenus 3 HPV infections (OR = 2.92, 95 % CI: 1.20–7.12). Lastly, genital discomfort, recent discomfort and reported pain/bleeding were not associated with any HPV infection outcome.

Gynecologic products

In general, no significant associations or trends were observed with the use of gynecologic products and some categories lacked observations. Of note, both former (OR = 2.09, 95 % CI: 1.10–3.98) and current (OR = 2.50, 95 % CI: 1.23–5.08) antibiotic use were associated with persistent HPV infections, while current antibiotic use (OR = 5.95, 95 % CI: 1.14–30.97) and former antifungal use (OR = 5.14, 95 % CI: 1.17–22.52) were significantly associated with Subgenus 1 infections. No significant trends were observed with the use of homemade gynecologic products, other than use of "unknown" homemade products and Subgenus 3 infections (OR = 5.33, 95 % CI: 1.80–15.85) and persistent HPV infections (OR = 3.20, 95 % CI: 1.00–10.24). Due to low numbers of women using these products, the CIs were very wide, indicating low precision in the estimates.

Vaginal health

From information volunteered by the participant and not explicitly asked in questionnaires, there were no significant associations between cervical ectropion and any HPV infection outcome. A self-report of gynecologic surgery was associated with an increased prevalence of Subgenus 1 HPV infections (OR = 2.05, 95 % CI: 1.11–3.79). Information on previous gynecologic infections or treatments volunteered by the participant was also associated with a significant increase in prevalence of Subgenus 1 HPV infections (OR = 1.73, 95 % CI: 1.13–2.65) with no association with other HPV outcomes. When previous history of gynecologic infections was explicitly asked, there were no significant associations between non-HPV-related infections and any HPV infection outcome. There was, however, a significant increase between previous HPV-related infections and Subgenus 1 (OR = 3.87, 95 % CI: 2.09–7.14), Subgenus 2 (OR = 2.02, 95 % CI: 1.27–3.19), transient (OR = 3.23, 95 % CI: 1.91–5.47) and persistent (OR = 2.46, 95 % CI: 1.40–4.31) HPV infections. Using qualitative notes from the cytology reports, there were no significant associations with bacterial or fungal infections and any HPV infection. General inflammation was positively associated with Subgenus 1 (OR = 2.10, 95 % CI: 1.37–3.22), Subgenus 2 (OR = 1.53, 95 % CI: 1.21–1.94), transient (OR = 1.73, 95 % CI: 1.27–2.35) and persistent (OR = 1.62, 95 % CI: 1.20–2.19) HPV infections.

Discussion

This study provides novel insights on reproductive health and vaginal hygiene factors in HPV infection. While some of these factors seemed to be associated

Table 1 Associations between reproductive health and vaginal hygiene factors and the 1-year period prevalence of HPV infection by phylogenetic group in the Ludwig-McGill cohort study

Variable	Subgenus 1[a] ($n = 108$)		Subgenus 2[a] ($n = 495$)		Subgenus 3[a] ($n = 131$)	
	OR[b]	95 % CI	OR[b]	95 % CI	OR[b]	95 % CI
Reproductive Health Factors						
Condom Use						
Former vs. Never	1.28	0.79, 2.07	0.90	0.71, 1.15	2.00	1.23, 3.24
Current vs. Never	1.43	0.83, 2.48	1.09	0.82, 1.45	2.00	1.15, 3.47
Oral Contraceptives						
< 6 years vs. Never	1.25	0.66, 1.38	0.98	0.71, 1.35	1.40	0.83, 2.37
6+ years vs. Never	1.23	0.60, 2.53	1.00	0.70, 1.43	0.62	0.32, 1.19
Intrauterine Device						
Yes vs. No	0.48	0.30, 0.75	0.78	0.62, 0.98	0.73	0.49, 1.08
Tubal Sterilization						
Yes vs. No	1.24	0.65, 1.36	0.84	0.59, 1.21	0.65	0.33, 1.30
Contraceptive Injection						
Yes vs. No	1.96	1.22, 3.16	1.34	1.00, 1.79	1.34	0.83, 2.17
Natural Products						
Yes vs. No	-	-	0.37	0.13, 1.05	0.74	0.17, 3.20
Vaginal Products						
Yes vs. No	-	-	0.82	0.37, 1.81	0.32	0.04, 2.40
Genital Health and Hygiene Factors						
Menstrual Cloth						
Yes vs. No	0.54	0.32, 0.91	0.93	0.74, 1.18	1.02	0.68, 1.53
Hygienic Tampon						
Yes vs. No	1.49	0.87, 2.54	1.33	0.98, 1.81	1.30	0.79, 2.14
Douching						
Frequent vs. Infrequent	1.20	0.53, 2.69	1.29	0.83, 2.00	0.11	0.02, 0.81
Douching Products						
Natural vs. None	0.96	0.60, 1.54	0.92	0.72, 1.17	0.90	0.57, 1.41
Medical vs. None	1.09	0.23, 5.15	0.97	0.46, 2.06	2.75	0.98, 7.73
Unknown vs. None	1.18	0.27, 5.22	0.51	0.21, 1.21	2.92	1.20, 7.12
Genital Discomfort						
Yes vs. No	0.96	0.64, 1.45	0.96	0.78, 1.20	0.89	0.60, 1.31
Recent Discomfort						
Yes vs. No	0.99	0.65, 1.50	1.11	0.89, 1.38	1.22	0.84, 1.75
Pain or Bleeding						
Yes vs. No	2.83	0.59, 13.51	1.14	0.34, 3.75	0.91	0.12, 7.00
Gynecologic Products						
Antibiotic						
Former vs. Never	3.86	0.86, 17.34	0.83	0.51, 1.33	1.43	0.52, 3.97
Current vs. Never	5.95	1.14, 30.97	0.97	0.53, 1.79	1.84	0.56, 6.02
Antifungal						
Former vs. Never	5.14	1.17, 22.52	1.10	0.70, 1.75	1.85	0.68, 5.02
Current vs. Never	1.64	0.22, 12.24	1.06	0.56, 2.02	1.74	0.49, 6.11

Table 1 Associations between reproductive health and vaginal hygiene factors and the 1-year period prevalence of HPV infection by phylogenetic group in the Ludwig-McGill cohort study *(Continued)*

Abrasion						
Former vs. Never	-	-	1.68	0.40, 7.72	-	-
Current vs. Never	-	-	1.10	0.08, 16.23	-	-
External Products						
Former vs. Never	0.75	0.20, 2.84	-	-	-	-
Current vs. Never	1.36	0.48, 3.89	-	-	-	-
Unknown Products						
Former vs. Never	2.82	0.64, 12.42	0.96	0.62, 1.49	2.21	0.81, 6.01
Current vs. Never	3.44	0.63, 18.68	1.10	0.60, 2.03	2.82	0.83, 9.53
Home-made Products						
Natural vs. None	1.22	0.78, 1.92	0.91	0.72, 1.15	0.98	0.66, 1.47
Medical vs. None	0.80	0.27, 2.40	1.26	0.77, 2.04	0.76	0.29, 2.02
Unknown vs. None	2.75	0.53, 14.15	1.33	0.45, 3.91	5.33	1.80, 15.82
Vaginal Health Characteristics						
Cervical Ectropion						
Yes vs. No	0.37	0.05, 2.77	0.89	0.42, 1.91	0.74	0.17, 3.10
Gynecologic Surgery						
Yes vs. No	2.05	1.11, 3.79	0.90	0.60, 1.37	0.89	0.42, 1.89
Gynecologic Treatment/Infection						
Yes vs. No	1.73	1.13, 2.65	1.17	0.92, 1.50	1.26	0.83, 1.89
Previous Gynecologic Infection						
HPV vs. None	3.87	2.09, 7.14	2.02	1.27, 3.19	1.21	0.54, 2.71
Non-HPV vs. None	1.33	0.81, 2.19	1.03	0.78, 1.34	1.27	0.82, 1.97
Cytology Observations						
Bacterial Infection						
Yes vs. No	1.28	0.63, 2.63	1.30	0.88, 1.91	1.31	0.68, 2.52
Fungal Infection						
Yes vs. No	1.25	0.61, 2.54	1.29	0.88, 1.87	1.48	0.83, 2.66
General Inflammation						
Yes vs. No	2.10	1.37, 3.22	1.53	1.21, 1.94	1.12	0.74, 1.69

[a] Subgenus 1 (HPVs-6, 11, 32, 40, 42, 44, 54 and 55), Subgenus 2 (HPVs-16, 18, 26 31, 33–35, 39, 45, 51–53, 56, 58, 59, 66–70, 73 and 82) and Subgenus 3 (HPVs-57, 61, 62, 71, 72, 81, 83, 84 and 89) infections were determined based on the phylogenetic classification of HPV types

[b] Odds ratios were adjusted for age, lifetime number of sexual partners and empirical confounders (identified using a 5 % change in estimate strategy) such as race, marital status, education, age at first intercourse, age at menarche, number of pregnancies, smoking, alcohol drinking and years since last Pap smear

with adverse or protective effects regarding cervical HPV infection, they largely did not play an appreciable role on the risk of infection in the Ludwig-McGill cohort study population.

Previous studies [5] have demonstrated various directions of effect in condom use and HPV infection, despite the underlying hypothesis of condoms being protective. In our study, condom use seemed to be a risk marker for Subgenus 3 HPV infections, which have tropism for vaginal tissue. We did not measure frequency of condom use, thus it is possible that women who reported condom use, but did not consistently use them during sexual intercourse, could still be exposed to HPV. Sexual behaviour could play a role in these associations. Upon stratifying by marital status and number of lifetime sexual partners, the risk-marker effect of condom use was stronger in women who were not in stable relationships (single, separated or widowed) and in women with three or more lifetime sexual partners at baseline (data not shown).

IUD use was associated with an overall protective effect, consistent with other studies [24, 25]. While our study did not measure differences in use between copper and hormonal IUDs, which release progestin to prevent

Table 2 Associations between reproductive health and vaginal hygiene and transient or persistent HPV infections in the Ludwig-McGill cohort study

Variable	Transient HPV infection[a]		Persistent HPV infection[b]	
	OR[c]	95 % CI	OR[c]	95 % CI
Reproductive Health Factors				
Condom Use				
Former vs. Never	1.33	0.95, 1.86	1.06	0.77, 1.46
Current vs. Never	1.47	1.00, 2.16	1.24	0.86, 1.80
Oral Contraceptives				
< 6 years vs. Never	1.16	0.76, 1.75	1.02	0.69, 1.52
6+ years vs. Never	0.90	0.56, 1.46	1.14	0.73, 1.77
Intrauterine Device				
Yes vs. No	0.65	0.48, 0.87	0.77	0.57, 1.03
Tubal Sterilization				
Yes vs. No	0.78	0.47, 1.28	0.75	0.46, 1.23
Contraceptive Injection				
Yes vs. No	1.58	1.10, 2.26	1.31	0.91, 1.89
Natural Products				
Yes vs. No	0.17	0.02, 1.31	0.46	0.14, 1.55
Vaginal Products				
Yes vs. No	0.88	0.30, 2.56	0.76	0.26, 2.21
Genital Health and Hygiene Factors				
Menstrual Cloth				
Yes vs. No	1.00	0.74, 1.36	0.79	0.58, 1.06
Hygienic Tampon				
Yes vs. No	1.48	1.00, 2.20	1.42	0.96, 2.08
Douching				
Frequent vs. Infrequent	1.10	0.60, 2.00	1.12	0.62, 2.01
Douching Products				
Natural vs. None	0.86	0.62, 1.19	0.80	0.57, 1.12
Medical vs. None	0.82	0.28, 2.40	1.70	0.72, 4.02
Unknown vs. None	0.36	0.09, 1.51	1.03	0.37, 2.87
Genital Discomfort				
Yes vs. No	0.87	0.65, 1.18	0.89	0.67, 1.20
Recent Discomfort				
Yes vs. No	1.06	0.79, 1.41	1.22	0.93, 1.59
Pain or Bleeding				
Yes vs. No	0.61	0.07, 5.03	0.90	0.18, 4.48
Gynecologic Products				
Antibiotic				
Former vs. Never	1.00	0.53, 1.89	2.09	1.10, 3.98
Current vs. Never	0.89	0.37, 2.15	2.50	1.23, 5.08
Antifungal				
Former vs. Never	1.74	0.94, 3.20	1.51	0.81, 2.82
Current vs. Never	1.52	0.67, 3.45	1.80	0.78, 4.13

Table 2 Associations between reproductive health and vaginal hygiene and transient or persistent HPV infections in the Ludwig-McGill cohort study *(Continued)*

Variable	OR[c]	95 % CI	OR[c]	95 % CI
Abrasion				
Former vs. Never	4.17	0.49, 35.27	2.47	0.40, 15.26
Current vs. Never	5.40	0.26, 113.29	-	-
External Products				
Former vs. Never	1.46	0.18, 11.99	0.91	0.08, 10.66
Current vs. Never	6.43	0.65, 63.70	-	-
Unknown Products				
Former vs. Never	1.03	0.58, 1.84	1.14	0.65, 2.02
Current vs. Never	1.31	0.62, 2.81	1.93	0.95, 3.93
Home-made Products				
Natural vs. None	1.00	0.74, 1.37	0.93	0.69, 1.26
Medical vs. None	0.97	0.47, 1.98	0.77	0.38, 1.56
Unknown vs. None	1.17	0.24, 5.73	3.20	1.00, 10.24
Vaginal Health Characteristics				
Cervical Ectropion				
Yes vs. No	1.01	0.41, 2.52	0.81	0.30, 2.19
Gynecologic Surgery				
Yes vs. No	1.22	0.72, 2.04	1.39	0.86, 2.25
Gynecologic Infection/Treatment				
Yes vs. No	0.90	0.65, 1.24	1.14	0.84, 1.54
Previous Gynecologic Infection				
HPV vs. None	3.23	1.91, 5.47	2.46	1.40, 4.31
Non-HPV vs. None	0.95	0.66, 1.37	1.15	0.82, 1.61
Cytology Observations				
Bacterial Infection				
Yes vs. No	1.16	0.69, 1.95	1.45	0.91, 2.31
Fungal Infection				
Yes vs. No	1.05	0.63, 1.75	1.24	0.77, 2.01
General Inflammation				
Yes vs. No	1.73	1.27, 2.35	1.62	1.20, 2.19

[a] Transient HPV infections were defined as one positive test result in the first four visits, followed by two subsequent negative results

[b] Persistent HPV infections were defined as two or more positive HPV test results over the first four visits, with no more than one negative result between two positive test results

[c] Odds ratios were adjusted for age, lifetime number of sexual partners and empirical confounders (identified using a 5 % change in estimate strategy) such as race, marital status, education, age at first intercourse, age at menarche, number of pregnancies, smoking, alcohol drinking and years since last Pap smear

fertilization, the protective effect on Subgenus 2 HPV infections could have resulted from a low-level immune response triggered by IUDs in the uterine endometrium and cervix. There was a general protective trend with tubal sterilization, which could be associated with behavioural factors, as tubal sterilization was more common in women in stable relationships. Moreover, due to the irreversibility of the procedure, it is more common in older women. Thus, there could be an effect of age in this interaction as protective effect was predominantly seen in women over 30 years of age (data not shown). It is also possible that the protective effects for IUD use and tubal ligation may have resulted from low viral transmission in low-risk partnerships. Although we controlled for empirical confounders, these were based on female interviews. We did not have behavior data on male partners, which would have allowed us to verify the low-risk partnership hypothesis.

Contraceptive injection use was associated with an increased prevalence of Subgenus 1, Subgenus 2 and transient HPV infections. While previous studies have shown an increased association with cervical cancer [7, 26], few studies have investigated the role of contraceptive injections in HPV infection. There is precedence for a hormonal effect of progestogen-only contraceptives in increasing susceptibility or persistence of HPV infection (compared to combined OCs containing estrogen and progestin) [27, 28]. Sexual behaviour could also be a factor as contraceptive injection/Norplant use was more prevalent in women with three or more lifetime sexual partners (16.9 % vs. 12.9 %).

Use of menstrual cloths had a slightly protective effect on HPV infections, while use of hygienic tampons had an adverse effect. Use of menstrual cloths has not previously been studied in association with HPV infection and there does not appear to be a biological mechanism for this protective effect. Very limited evidence exists for an association between tampon use and risk of HPV infection. Some studies show no association [29], while some report a positive association between tampon use and high-risk HPV infection [30]. We speculate that tampon use can lead to dryness and irritation in the vagina and cervix [31], thereby increasing susceptibility to HPV infections through possible tearing or microabrasions.

Gynecologic product use served as a proxy for vaginal health conditions. Our results suggest that bacterial infections and use of products to control these infections may play a role in increasing susceptibility to HPV infection. BV has been positively associated with HPV infections [16], which is biologically plausible. A lack of protective lactobacilli in the vaginal flora during BV can increase susceptibility to infections, such as *Chlamydia trachomatis*, *Neisseria gonorrhoeae*, HSV-1 and 2, HIV [32] and possibly HPV infections.

Previous gynecologic infections were associated with increased prevalence of Subgenus 1 infections, which we hypothesize to be related to BV. Self-reports of HPV-related infections were significantly associated with all outcomes, except for Subgenus 3 infections. Women who reported a previous HPV-related infection could have an increased risk of re-infection due to sexual behaviours or, just as plausibly, redetection of a latent HPV infection. General inflammation noted in cytology results was significantly associated with all HPV outcomes other than Subgenus 3 infections. A possible link between inflammation and cervical carcinogenesis might exist. There are indications that chronic inflammation or inflammation from other infections may play a role in increasing risk of HPV infection [13], possibly explaining this association.

Surprisingly, cervical ectropion was not associated with any HPV outcome. The location of the transformation zone can affect potential exposure to HPV infection and risk of cervical cancer [22]. Our results must be taken with reservation as this was not explicitly asked in the questionnaire. Due to mild symptoms, if any at all, women may not be aware of the condition unless diagnosed by gynecological examination, leading to potential misclassification. We found a positive association between gynecologic surgery and Subgenus 1 HPV infections. Most surgeries were dilation and curettage, a procedure sometimes used to further diagnose a suspected HPV infection in the endocervix. This might explain the observed positive association, as some cases of gynecologic surgery may be in women who were already HPV-infected.

In restricting our analysis to only women with one full year of follow-up, we may have introduced a selection bias. However, we believe that this enhanced internal validity and efficiency in defining the HPV outcome variables. Furthermore, losses to follow-up in the first year did not play a significant role as preliminary analyses of the non-restricted data yielded similar results. We classified type-specific HPV outcomes into groups based on phylogenetic relatedness to guide the statistical search for predictors on the basis of viral behavior and tropism. We were unable to study individual type-specific infections due to lack of precision.

Several limitations need to be underscored. Due to the low-income setting of the study clinics where patients were recruited from, the study population was very specific, with respect to cultural and social norms. Secondly, outside of qualitative observations from cytology reports, exposure measurements were based on self-reported responses. As this study pertains to sexual histories and behaviour, there is a possible social desirability bias where women, especially those with riskier sexual behaviours, would tend to answer questions on sensitive topics in a socially acceptable manner. Additionally, poor recall, especially on lifetime exposures, might be at play. While we anticipate that any possible exposure misclassification would be non-differential to outcome status, women with a previous history of gynecologic infections may be more conscious of the products they have previously used. In addition, the Ludwig-McGill cohort study was not designed to investigate measures of vaginal health and hygiene as a primary objective. This post hoc analysis considered exposure measures that predominantly served as proxies for vaginal conditions. Because several of these conditions are often asymptomatic or characterized by mild symptoms, women may not have been aware of these conditions. Lastly, there could still be residual confounding due to unmeasured variables, particularly related to male behaviors.

Conclusions

This study presents detailed analyses on the effects of vaginal health and hygiene factors, some of which seemed to be associated with risk of HPV infection differentially by subgenus grouping based on propensity to colonize different lower genital tract tissue subsites. Further research using hypothesis-driven designs with more accurate measures of exposure is necessary to examine the observed associations.

Additional file

Additional file 1: Table S1. Open-ended questionnaire variable category designations from the first four patient visits, including qualitative observations from cytology results in the Ludwig-McGill Cohort Study. **Table S2.** Characteristics of the Ludwig-McGill Cohort Study population by HPV infection according to phylogenetic group and transient or persistent infections. **Table S3.** Crude and restricted crude (CrudeR) odds ratios of associations between reproductive health and vaginal hygiene and the 1-year period prevalence of HPV infection according to phylogenetic group in the Ludwig-McGill Cohort Study. (DOC 331 kb)

Competing interests

The authors have no competing interests with the subject matter of this manuscript.

Authors' contributions

All authors made significant contributions to the conception, data acquisition, analysis and drafting of this manuscript and approve the final version submitted. ELF and LLV conceived and designed the parent cohort study and ELF developed the research question. ELF also contributed to the analysis design and interpretation of the data. LLV supervised the data collection and laboratory work. LG and MLB collected the data. AVR managed the data from the study and assisted in statistical analyses. FRS and MZ interpreted the data. ES performed the analysis and drafted the manuscript.

Acknowledgements

We are indebted to João Simão Sobrinho, José Carlos Mann Prado, Silvaneide Ferreira and Maria Cecilia Costa for HPV testing and genotyping.

For the Ludwig-McGill Cohort Study

Ludwig-McGill Cohort Study Team Members: Affiliated with the Ludwig Institute for Cancer Research in Sao Paulo, Brazil: Maria Luiza Baggio, Lenice Galan, João Simão Sobrinho, José Carlos Mann Prado, Silvaneide Ferreira, Lara Termini, Maria Cecília Costa, Romulo Miyamura, Andrea Trevisan, Patricia Thomann, João Candeias, Laura Sichero, Paula Rahal, Antonio Ruiz, Jane Kaiano, Monica Santos, Patricia Savio, Paulo Maciag, Tatiana Rabachini, Luisa Villa (Co-Principal Investigator). Affiliated with McGill University in Montreal, Canada: Mariam El-Zein, Marie-Claude Rousseau, Salaheddin Mahmud, Nicolas Schlecht, Helen Trottier, Alex Ferenczy, Thomas Rohan, Myriam Chevarie-Davis, Karolina Louvanto, Joseph Tota, Eileen Shaw, Agnihotram Ramanakumar, Eliane Duarte, Flavia Silva, Sophie Kulaga, Juliette Robitaille, Robert Platt, Eduardo Franco (Principal Investigator).

Funding

The Ludwig-McGill Cohort Study was funded by the Ludwig Institute for Cancer Research (intramural grant to LLV and ELF), the US National Cancer Institute (grant CA70269 to ELF) and the Canadian Institutes of Health Research (grants MA-13647, MOP-49396, CRN-83320 to ELF).

Author details

[1]Division of Cancer Epidemiology, Department of Oncology, McGill University, Montreal, Canada. [2]Department of Epidemiology, Biostatistics and Occupational Health, McGill University, 546 Pine Avenue West, Montreal, QC H2W 1S6, Canada. [3]Ludwig Institute for Cancer Research, São Paulo, Brazil. [4]Molecular Biology Laboratory, Centre of Translational Oncology, Instituto do Câncer do Estado de São Paulo, São Paulo, Brazil.

References

1. Ferlay J, Shin H, Bray F, Forman D, Mathers C, Parkin D. GLOBOCAN 2008 v2.0, Cancer Incidence and Mortality Worldwide: IARC CancerBase No. 10. 2010.
2. Kahn JA, Rosenthal SL, Succop PA, Ho GYF, Burk RD. The interval between menarche and age of first sexual intercourse as a risk factor for subsequent HPV infection in adolescent and young adult women. J Pediatr. 2002;141:718–23.
3. Burchell AN, Winer RL, de Sanjosé S, Franco EL. Chapter 6: Epidemiology and transmission dynamics of genital HPV infection. Vaccine. 2006;24 Suppl 3:S3/52–61.
4. Trottier H, Franco EL. The epidemiology of genital human papillomavirus infection. Vaccine. 2006;24 Suppl 1:S1–15.
5. Manhart LE, Koutsky LA. Do condoms prevent genital HPV infection, external genital warts, or cervical neoplasia? A meta-analysis. Sex Transm Dis. 2002;29:725–35.
6. Lam JUH, Rebolj M, Dugué P-A, Bonde J, von Euler-Chelpin M, Lynge E. Condom use in prevention of Human Papillomavirus infections and cervical neoplasia: systematic review of longitudinal studies. J Med Screen. 2014;21:38–50.
7. Appleby P, Beral V, Berrington de González A, Colin D, Franceschi S, Goodhill A, et al. Cervical cancer and hormonal contraceptives: collaborative reanalysis of individual data for 16,573 women with cervical cancer and 35,509 women without cervical cancer from 24 epidemiological studies. Lancet. 2007;370:1609–21.
8. Asiaf A, Ahmad ST, Mohammad SO, Zargar M a. Review of the current knowledge on the epidemiology, pathogenesis, and prevention of human papillomavirus infection. Eur J Cancer Prev. 2014;23:206–24.
9. Castellsagué X, Díaz M, Vaccarella S, de Sanjosé S, Muñoz N, Herrero R, et al. Intrauterine device use, cervical infection with human papillomavirus, and risk of cervical cancer: a pooled analysis of 26 epidemiological studies. Lancet Oncol. 2011;12:1023–31.
10. Kjaer SK, Mellemkjaer L, Brinton LA, Johansen C, Gridley G, Olsen JH. Tubal sterilization and risk of ovarian, endometrial and cervical cancer. A Danish population-based follow-up study of more than 65 000 sterilized women. Int J Epidemiol. 2004;33:596–602.
11. Vaccarella S, Herrero R, Dai M, Snijders PJF, Meijer CJLM, Thomas JO, et al. Reproductive factors, oral contraceptive use, and human papillomavirus infection: pooled analysis of the IARC HPV prevalence surveys. Cancer Epidemiol Biomarkers Prev. 2006;15:2148–53.
12. Nielsen A, Kjaer SK, Munk C, Iftner T. Type-specific HPV infection and multiple HPV types: Prevalence and risk factor profile in nearly 12,000 younger and older Danish women. Sex Transm Dis. 2008;35:276–82.
13. Silva J, Cerqueira F, Ribeiro J, Sousa H, Osorio T, Medeiros R. Is Chlamydia trachomatis related to human papillomavirus infection in young women of southern European population? A self-sampling study. Arch Gynecol Obstet. 2013;288:627–33.
14. Dartell M, Rasch V, Kahesa C, Mwaiselage J, Ngoma T, Junge J, et al. Human papillomavirus prevalence and type distribution in 3603 HIV-positive and HIV-negative women in the general population of Tanzania: the PROTECT study. Sex Transm Dis. 2012;39:201–8.
15. Williamson A-L. The Interaction between Human Immunodeficiency Virus and Human Papillomaviruses in Heterosexuals in Africa. J Clin Med. 2015;4:579–92.

16. Gillet E, Meys JF, Verstraelen H, Bosire C, De Sutter P, Temmerman M, et al. Bacterial vaginosis is associated with uterine cervical human papillomavirus infection: a meta-analysis. BMC Infect Dis. 2011;11:10.
17. Franco E, Villa L, Rohan T, Ferenczy A, Petzl-Erler M, Matlashewski G. Design and methods of the Ludwig-McGill longitudinal study of the natural history of human papillomavirus infection and cervical neoplasia in Brazil. Ludwig-McGill Study Group. Rev Panam Salud Publica. 1999;6:223–33.
18. Bauer HM, Ting Y, Greer CE, Chambers JC, Tashiro CJ, Chimera J, et al. Genital human papillomavirus infection in female university students as determined by a PCR-based method. JAMA, J Am Med Assoc. 1991;265:472–7.
19. Gravitt PE, Peyton CL, Alessi TQ, Wheeler CM, Coutlée F, Hildesheim A, et al. Improved amplification of genital human papillomaviruses. J Clin Microbiol. 2000;38:357–61.
20. Schiffman M, Clifford G, Buonaguro FM. Classification of weakly carcinogenic human papillomavirus types: addressing the limits of epidemiology at the borderline. Infect Agent Cancer. 2009;4:8.
21. Schiffman M, Herrero R, Desalle R, Hildesheim A, Wacholder S, Rodriguez AC, et al. The carcinogenicity of human papillomavirus types reflects viral evolution. Virology. 2005;337:76–84.
22. Castle PE, Jeronimo J, Schiffman M, Herrero R, Rodríguez AC, Bratti MC, et al. Age-related changes of the cervix influence human papillomavirus type distribution. Cancer Res. 2006;66:1218–24.
23. Schiffman M, Wentzensen N, Wacholder S, Kinney W, Gage JC, Castle PE. Human papillomavirus testing in the prevention of cervical cancer. J Natl Cancer Inst. 2011;103:368–83.
24. Roset Bahmanyar E, Paavonen J, Naud P, Salmerón J, Chow S-N, Apter D, et al. Prevalence and risk factors for cervical HPV infection and abnormalities in young adult women at enrolment in the multinational PATRICIA trial. Gynecol Oncol. 2012;127:440–50.
25. Kataja V, Syrjänen S, Yliskoski M, Hippeläinen M, Väyrynen M, Saarikoski S, et al. Risk Factors Associated with Cervical Human Papillomavirus Infections: A Case-Control Study. Am J Epidemiol. 1993;138:735–45.
26. Hildesheim A, Herrero R, Castle PE, Wacholder S, Bratti MC, Sherman ME, et al. HPV co-factors related to the development of cervical cancer: results from a population-based study in Costa Rica. Br J Cancer. 2001;84:1219–26.
27. Yuan F, Auborn K, James C. Altered Growth and Viral Gene Expression in Human Papillomavirus Type 16-Containing Cancer Cell Lines Treated with Progesterone. Cancer Invest. 1999;17:19–29.
28. Michelin D, Gissmann L, Street D, Potkul RK, Fisher S, Kaufmann AM, et al. Regulation of human papillomavirus type 18 in vivo: effects of estrogen and progesterone in transgenic mice. Gynecol Oncol. 1997;66:202–8.
29. Winer RL, Lee S-K, Hughes JP, Adam DE, Kiviat NB, Koutsky LA. Genital Human Papillomavirus Infection: Incidence and Risk Factors in a Cohort of Female University Students. Am J Epidemiol. 2003;157:218–26.
30. Richardson H, Abrahamowicz M, Tellier P-P, Kelsall G, du Berger R, Ferenczy A, et al. Modifiable risk factors associated with clearance of type-specific cervical human papillomavirus infections in a cohort of university students. Cancer Epidemiol Biomarkers Prev. 2005;14:1149–56.
31. Berkeley AS, Micha JP, Freedman KS, Hirsch JC. The potential of digitally inserted tampons to induce vaginal lesions. Obstet Gynecol. 1985;66:31–5.
32. Cherpes TL, Hillier SL, Meyn LA, Busch JL, Krohn MA. A delicate balance: risk factors for acquisition of bacterial vaginosis include sexual activity, absence of hydrogen peroxide-producing lactobacilli, black race, and positive herpes simplex virus type 2 serology. Sex Transm Dis. 2008;35:78–83.

Analysis of epidemiological trends in human papillomavirus infection among gynaecological outpatients in Hangzhou, China, 2011–2015

Lili Qian[1], Yu Zhang[1], Dawei Cui[2], Bin Lou[2], Yimin Chen[1], Ying Yu[1], Yonglin Liu[1] and Yu Chen[2*]

Abstract

Background: HPV infection is the major pathogenic factor underlying cervical cancer and precancerous lesions. The cervical HPV infection rates in gynaecological outpatients from Hangzhou, China, were studied in the period from January 2011 to December 2015.

Methods: Exfoliated cervical cells were harvested from gynaecological outpatients in Hangzhou from January 2011 to December 2015. Twenty-one HPV subtypes were detected using flow-through hybridization. The HPV infection rates in various disease groups were compared using the Chi-square test. The infection rates of different HPV subtypes in different calendar years and in different age groups were analysed using the linear-by-linear association test and gamma value.

Results: A total of 43,804 patients were recruited, of whom 9752 (22.3%) were infected with HPV. The top five among the 21 HPV subtypes detected in terms of infection rates were HPV-16, −52, −58, −53 and −18. No significant differences (linear-by-linear association test) were found in the HPV infection rates when compared over the studied years ($P > 0.05$). However, the 15–24-year-old age group showed the highest HPV infection rate, and significant differences (linear-by-linear association test) were detected among the different age groups ($P < 0.05$). The HPV infection rates exhibited an upward trend in the 15–24-year-old and >24–34-year-old groups over the past five years. There were significant differences in the HPV infection rates among the disease groups ($P < 0.05$).

Conclusions: HPV-16, −52 and −58 were the major HPV infection subtypes in Hangzhou, China. The 15–24-year-old age group had a relatively high HPV infection rate with an upward trend over the past five years and thus represented a population susceptible to HPV infection.

Keywords: Human papillomavirus, Genotype, Flow-through hybridization, Epidemiology

Human papilloma virus (HPV) contains a circular double-stranded DNA genome that exhibits strict organization and host specificity. More than 200 HPV genotypes have been characterized to date, and more than 40 HPV types can infect the genital area and result in genital lesions. HPV genotypes are classified as low-risk and high-risk types based on their potential to cause cancer [1, 2].

The incidence of cervical cancer worldwide ranks second in female malignancies and is exhibiting a trend towards younger ages [3]. Methods to prevent cervical cancer have received increasing attention from researchers. Epidemiological and biological investigations have shown that HPV infection is the major pathogenic factor underlying cervical cancer and precancerous lesions [4, 5]. The genotype distribution of HPV infection exhibits regional specificity. According to statistical data from the International Agency for Research on

* Correspondence: chenyu_zy@163.com
[2]Department of Laboratory Medicine, Center of Clinical Laboratory, the First Affiliated Hospital, School of Medicine, Zhejiang University, No. 79, Qingchun Road, Hangzhou 310003, China
Full list of author information is available at the end of the article

Cancer (IARC, 2007), the top five HPV subtypes in terms of infection frequency are HPV-16, −53, −52, −18 and −39 in North America, HPV-16, −18, −31, −33 and −58 in Europe and HPV-16, −52, −58, −18 and −56 in Asia.

The latest research showed that HPV-52, −16 and −58 were the HPV subtypes with the highest infection frequencies in China [6]. Vaccines against four HPV subtypes (HPV-6, −11, −16 and −18) have been used in clinics in developed countries. In the present study, we analysed the cervical HPV infection rates in gynaecological outpatients from Hangzhou, China, over the past five years. Additionally, we performed an age-stratified analysis and an analysis by disease type. The results provide objective evidence for epidemiological studies of HPV infection and the application of HPV vaccines in the study region.

Materials and methods

Subjects

Clinical specimens were collected from 43,804 gynaecological outpatients at the First Affiliated Hospital of Zhejiang Chinese Medical University and the First Affiliated Hospital of the Medical School of Zhejiang University from January 2011 to December 2015. A woman was considered eligible to enter the study if she a) had current or past sexual activity, b) was not pregnant at the time of enrolment, c) had never been screened or treated for cervical cancer, d) had not undergone a total uterus or cervix resection, e) agreed to undergo an HPV test and f) agreed to participate in the present study. This study was conducted in accordance with the Declaration of Helsinki and a protocol approved by the First Affiliated Hospital of Zhejiang Chinese Medical University and the First Affiliated Hospital of the Medical School of Zhejiang University (Hangzhou, China). There were 5001 cases in 2011, 6410 cases in 2012, 7863 cases in 2013, 11,402 cases in 2014 and 13 128 cases in 2015. The recruited patients were 17–88 years old, with a median age of 44 years. In accordance with a prior overseas study, [7] we organized the subjects into the following five age groups: 15–24 years, >24–34 years,>34–44 years, >44–54 years and >54 years. Regarding the disease type, the subjects were assigned to the following five groups: cervical cancer, cervical intraepithelial neoplasia grade 1 (CIN1), CIN2, CIN3 and other diseases. The other diseases included gynaecological diseases other than cervical cancer and CIN, such as uterine fibroids, ovarian cysts, endometriosis, endometrial cancer and choriocarcinoma.

Methods

HPV sample collection

The opening of the cervix was exposed using a vaginal dilator. Excess secretions at the opening of the cervix were wiped away using a cotton swab. A cervical brush was inserted into the opening of the cervix and rotated clockwise 3–5 times to acquire exfoliated cervical cells. The cells were placed into a sample tube containing cell preservation solution, stored in a refrigerator at 4 °C and analysed within 3 days of collection.

HPV genotype testing

Samples that tested positive for β-globin were analysed by PCR amplification of HPV DNA. HPV-positive samples were confirmed by PCR with universal L1 primer MY09/11 and GP5/6 systems. DNA from HeLa and Caski cell lines was used as positive controls, and mixtures without sample DNA were used as negative controls. HPV genotypes were determined using an HPV GenoArray Test Kit (Hybribio, Chaozhou, China), according to the manufacturer's instructions [8, 9]. Geno-Array is an L1 consensus primer-based PCR assay that is capable of amplifying 21 HPV genotypes, including six low-risk HPV subtypes including six low-risk HPV subtypes (HPV-6, −11, −42, −43, −44 and CP8304) and 15 high-risk HPV subtypes (HPV-16, −18, −31, −33, −35,-39, −45, −51, −52, −53, −56, −58, −59, −66 and −68) (Table 1).

The test was conducted in four steps as follows: (1) HPV DNA extraction, (2) PCR amplification, (3) flow-

Table 1 List of Probe Sequence

HPV subtype	Probe Sequence
CP8304	5′ -gcactaatagttcagttgcag-3′
HPV-6	5′ -cataagaagataccttaggacttg-3′
HPV-11	5′ -acttagcagtaacgtctcagatgt-3′
HPV-44	5′ -tagtgctcgagacacgtatcatat-3′
HPV-42	5′ -gctatcgtcatgaactatgctaga-3′
HPV-43	5′ -actgtgtcatgacacgtatcaagt-3′
HPV-16	5′ -ctatacaagtacgtcgtcgatatg-3′
HPV-52	5′ -cagagctcgagacacgtatcaact-3′
HPV-58	5′ -agcaaatgaaacagttgcagga-3′
HPV-53	5′ -ttctatcatgacacgtatcactgg-3′
HPV-18	5′ -gtatcactaagtactcgtcgaatg-3′
HPV-39	5′ -cctaagtgtagacacgtatcagtt-3′
HPV-33	5′ -ctgatcatgaactacgtcatggat-3′
HPV-31	5′ -gacttcaatagtactagtcatcgg-3′
HPV-51	5′ -tctgaatgaaacagttgctaca-3′
HPV-68	5′ -atgtgtcatgagtatcatagc-3′
HPV-66	5′ -gcatctatagtatcagttagacg-3′
HPV-56	5′ -aatggtcatgacacgtatcaagga-3′
HPV-59	5′ -gcctaatgaaacagttgcaccc-3′
HPV-45	5′ -atgtgtcatgacacgtatcatagc-3′
HPV-35	5′ -ctagtgtcatgacacgtatcatag-3′

through hybridization (a hybridized membrane coated with genotype-specific probes was placed into a hybridizer for rapid nucleic acid hybridization, and the amplification products were tested by reverse dot blotting with an enzyme label to yield a coloured reaction) and (4) result interpretation. Positive test results appeared as bluish violet dots. Samples that were positive for only one HPV subtype were defined as single HPV infections, and samples that were positive for more than one HPV subtype were defined as multiple HPV infections.

Statistical analysis

The data were analysed using SPSS 22.0 statistical software. The positive infection rate is expressed as a percentage. For multiple infection patients, the HPV-positive rate was calculated repeatedly for each genotype. The infection rates were compared based on disease group using the Chi-square test. The linear-by-linear association test and gamma value for trends were used to evaluate changes in HPV prevalence by calendar year and by age group. *P*-values were two-sided, and statistical significance was defined as $P < 0.05$.

Results

HPV infection rates and trends

In this study, 9752 of the 43,804 women examined were infected with HPV, resulting in an infection rate of 22.3%. Specifically, the rate of single infections was 17.1% (7496/43,804), and the rate of multiple infections was 5.2% (2256/43,804). Among the 21 HPV subtypes detected, the infection rate for the low-risk subtypes was 4.5% (1987/43,804), and the infection rate for the high-risk subtypes was 20.1% (8802/43,804). Regarding the infection rate, the top five HPV subtypes were HPV-16 (4.8%, 2108/43,804), HPV-52 (4.7%, 2056/43,804), HPV-58 (3.9%, 1712/43,804), HPV-53 (2.3%, 995/43,804) and HPV-18 (1.9%, 831/43,804); the top three low-risk HPV subtypes were HPV-8304 (1.9%, 822/43,804), HPV-6 (1.3-%, 585/43,804) and HPV-11 (1.2%, 524/43,804). The HPV-positive rate in 2011 was 22.7% (1133/5001), with single infections in 16.5% (823/5001) and multiple infections in 6.2% (310/5001) of the subjects. The HPV-positive rate in 2012 was 21.6% (1383/6410), with single infections in 15.8% (1015/6410) and multiple infections in 5.7-% (368/6410) of the subjects. The HPV-positive rate in 2013 was 22.2% (1745/7863), with single infections in 16.4% (1291/7863) and multiple infections in 5.8% (454/7863) of the subjects. The HPV-positive rate in 2014 was 22.6% (2575/11,402), with single infections in 16.2% (1846/11,402) and multiple infections in 6.4% (729/11,402) of the subjects. The HPV-positive rate in 2015 was 22.2% (2916/13,128), with single infections in 15.4% (2015/13,128) and multiple infections in 6.9% (901/13,128) of the subjects (Fig. 1). No significant differences (linear-by-linear association test) were found in the HPV infection rates based on the year ($P > 0.05$) (Table 2).

Infection of different age groups with the HPV subtypes

The HPV infection rates of the 15–24-, >24–34-, >34–44-, >44–54- and >54-year-old groups were 34.7% (324/933), 23.5% (2155/9159), 21.3% (2712/12,717), 20.6% (2932/14,245) and 24.1% (1629/6750), respectively. The highest infection rate appeared in the 15–24-year-old group, and

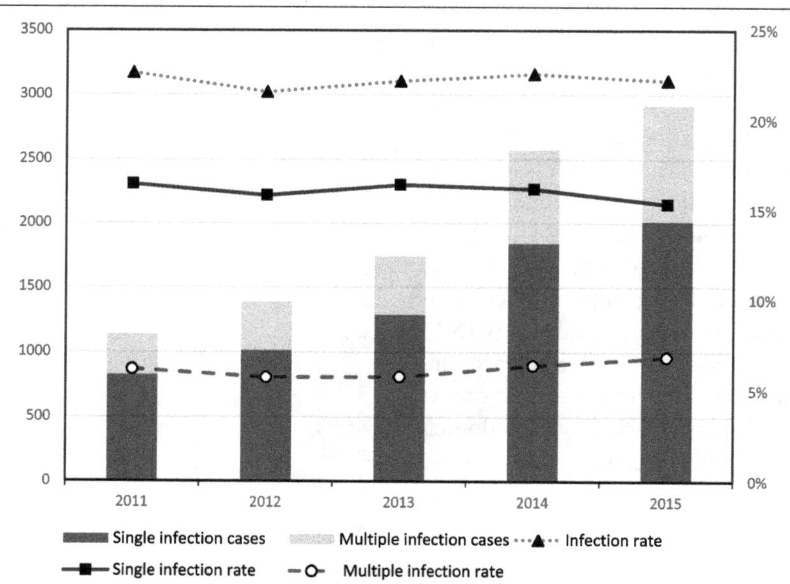

Fig. 1 Changes in the rates of single and multiple human papillomavirus infections ingynaecological outpatients, 2011–2015

Table 2 Infection of gynaecological outpatients with 21 subtypes of human papillomavirus (HPV) in different years

HPV subtype	Positive cases	2011 (*n* = 5001)	2012 (*n* = 6410)	2013 (*n* = 7863)	2014 (*n* = 11,402)	2015 (*n* = 13,128)	χ^2	*P*	gamma value
	9752	1133 (22.7%)	1383 (21.6%)	1745 (22.2%)	2575 (22.6%)	2916 (22.2%)	0.057	0.812	0.002
Low-risk									
CP8304	822	112 (2.2%)	118 (1.8%)	114 (1.5%)	197 (1.7%)	281 (2.1%)	0.228	0.633	0.028
HPV-6	585	45 (0.9%)	76 (1.2%)	140 (1.8%)	150 (1.3%)	174 (1.3%)	2.209	0.137	0.030
HPV-11	524	42 (0.8%)	83 (1.3%)	83 (1.1%)	127 (1.1%)	189 (1.4%)	7.433	0.006	-0.091
HPV-44	127	4 (0.1%)	12 (0.2%)	19 (0.2%)	43 (0.4%)	49 (0.4%)	15.253	<0.001	-0.248
HPV-42	119	13 (0.3%)	37 (0.6%)	48 (0.6%)	10 (0.1%)	11 (0.1%)	36.303	<0.001	0.410
HPV-43	35	2 (0.04%)	5 (0.08%)	4 (0.1%)	6 (0.1%)	18 (0.1%)	4.019	0.045	−0.279
High-risk									
HPV-16	2108	257 (5.1%)	311 (4.9%)	453 (5.8%)	567 (5.0%)	520 (4.0%)	15.769	<0.001	0.073
HPV-52	2056	248 (5.0%)	304 (4.7%)	328 (4.2%)	508 (4.5%)	668 (5.1%)	0.612	0.434	-0.020
HPV-58	1712	227 (4.5%)	265 (4.1%)	293 (3.7%)	454 (4.0%)	473 (3.6%)	7.423	0.006	0.046
HPV-53	995	113 (2.3%)	129 (2.0%)	148 (1.9%)	272 (2.4%)	333 (2.5%)	5.674	0.017	-0.062
HPV-18	831	91 (1.8%)	92 (1.4%)	148 (1.9%)	291 (2.4%)	209 (1.6%)	0.685	0.408	-0.007
HPV-39	765	56 (1.1%)	74 (1.2%)	78 (1.0%)	288 (2.5%)	269 (2.1%)	52.680	<0.001	-0.193
HPV-33	733	86 (1.7%)	113 (1.8%)	150 (1.9%)	187 (1.6%)	197 (1.5%)	2.691	0.101	0.049
HPV-31	611	71 (1.4%)	70 (1.1%)	141 (1.8%)	139 (1.2%)	190 (1.5%)	0.103	0.748	-0.008
HPV-51	476	11 (0.2%)	16 (0.3%)	32 (0.4%)	129 (1.1%)	288 (2.2%)	221.134	<0.001	-0.554
HPV-68	458	61 (1.2%)	75 (1.2%)	72 (0.9%)	97 (0.9%)	153 (1.2%)	0.315	0.575	0.005
HPV-66	373	44 (0.9%)	51 (0.8%)	55 (0.7%)	98 (0.9%)	125 (1.0%)	1.168	0.280	-0.049
HPV-56	270	35 (0.7%)	14 (0.2%)	43 (0.6%)	75 (0.7%)	103 (0.8%)	8.898	0.003	-0.147
HPV-59	197	11 (0.2%)	32 (0.5%)	42 (0.5%)	46 (0.4%)	66 (0.5%)	2.259	0.133	-0.068
HPV-45	122	15 (0.3%)	17 (0.3%)	33 (0.4%)	20 (0.2%)	37 (0.3%)	0.666	0.415	0.053
HPV-35	93	14 (0.3%)	16 (0.3%)	12 (0.2%)	25 (0.2%)	26 (0.2%)	0.865	0.352	0.059

significant differences (linear-by-linear association test) were found among the age groups ($P < 0.05$). Additionally, significant differences (linear-by-linear association test)-were found among the age groups in the infection rates for the 11 high-risk subtypes (HPV-18, −35, −51, −52, −53, −58, −59 and −68; $P < 0.05$) and the four low-risk subtypes (CP8304, HPV-6, −11 and −42; $P < 0.05$) (Table 3). The HPV infection rates exhibited an upward trend in the 15–24- and >24–34-year-old age groups over the past five years (Fig. 2) (Table 4).

HPV infection in the different disease groups

The HPV infection rates of the different disease groups were as follows: 97.2% (889/915) in the cervical cancer group, 88.6% (287/324) in the CIN3 group, 52.7% (143/270) in the CIN2 group, 50.8% (978/1924) in the CIN1 group and 18.5% (7455/40,371) in the other diseases group. Significant differences were found in the HPV infection rates among disease groups ($P < 0.05$) and in the single and multiple infection rates among the HPV-positive patients ($P < 0.05$) (Table 5). For each disease group, the top five HPV subtypes in terms of the infection rates were as follows: HPV-16 (46.7%, 415/889), HPV-58 (19.8%, 176/889), HPV-52 (17.5%, 155/889), HPV-18 (14.2%, 126/889) and HPV-53 (7.8%, 70/889) in the cervical cancer group; HPV-16 (44.6%, 128/287), HPV-52 (18.3%, 53/287), HPV-58 (17.1%, 49/287), HPV-33 (15.9%, 46/287) and HPV-53 (14.6%, 42/287) in the CIN3 group; HPV-16 (29.4%, 42/143), HPV-58 (23.0%, 33/143), HPV-52 (15.4%, 22/143), HPV-33 (14.1%, 20/143) and HPV-53 (11.9%,17/143) in the CIN2 group; HPV-16 (24.9%, 243/978), HPV-58 (23.3%, 228/978), HPV-52 (22.0%, 215/978), HPV-33 (9.3%,91/978) and HPV-53 (8.5%,83/978) in the CIN1 group and HPV-52 (21.6%, 1611/7455), HPV-16 (17.2%, 1280/7455), HPV-58 (16.5%, 1226/7455), HPV-53 (10.5%, 783/7455) and HPV-8304 (10.0%, 745/7455) in the other disease group (Fig. 3).

Discussion

HPV is a group of DNA viruses that specifically infect human skin and the mucosal epithelium. HPV infection can cause abnormal proliferation of the skin and mucosal epithelial cells, leading to verrucous lesions and

Table 3 Infection of gynaecological outpatients with 21 subtypes of human papillomavirus (HPV) in different age groups

HPV subtype	15–24 (*n* = 933)	>24–34 (*n* = 9159)	>34–44 (*n* = 12,717)	>44–54 (*n* = 14,245)	>54 (*n* = 6750)	χ^2	*P*	gamma value
	324 (34.7%)	2155 (23.5%)	2712 (21.3%)	2932 (20.6%)	1629 (24.1%)	13.606	<0.001	−0.027
Low-risk								
CP8304	35 (3.8%)	134 (1.5%)	208 (1.6%)	274 (2.0%)	173 (2.6%)	11.683	<0.001	0.100
HPV-6	57 (6.1%)	231 (2.5%)	137 (1.1%)	99 (0.7%)	64 (1.0%)	185.419	<0.001	-0.382
HPV-11	62 (6.7%)	208 (2.3%)	109 (0.9%)	86 (0.6%)	61 (1.0%)	186.174	<0.001	-0.393
HPV-42	1 (0.1%)	22 (0.2%)	33 (0.3%)	34 (0.2%)	29 (0.4%)	3.940	0.047	0.127
HPV-43	1 (0.1%)	7 (0.1%)	5 (0.04%)	11 (0.1%)	12 (0.2%)	3.832	0.050	0.243
HPV-44	3 (0.3%)	32 (0.4%)	28 (0.2%)	45 (0.3%)	19 (0.3%)	0.088	0.767	−0.014
High-risk								
HPV-16	74 (8.0%)	477 (5.2%)	547 (4.3%)	638 (4.5%)	381 (5.6%)	0.498	0.481	-0.006
HPV-18	31 (3.3%)	224 (2.5%)	217 (1.7%)	233 (1.6%)	132 (2.0%)	13.148	<0.001	-0.089
HPV-31	20 (2.1%)	127 (1.4%)	170 (1.3%)	189 (1.3%)	105 (1.6%)	0.002	0.962	0.003
HPV-33	34 (3.6%)	154 (1.7)	183 (1.4%)	221 (1.6%)	143 (2.1%)	0.025	0.874	0.015
HPV-35	4 (0.4%)	27 (0.3%)	32 (0.3%)	26 (0.2%)	6 (0.1%)	10.705	0.001	-0.248
HPV-39	30 (3.2%)	173 (1.9%)	217 (1.7%)	232 (1.6%)	121 (1.8%)	3.529	0.060	-0.045
HPV-45	7 (0.8%)	29 (0.3%)	30 (0.2%)	43 (0.3%)	16 (0.2%)	1.817	0.178	-0.072
HPV-51	39 (4.2%)	140 (1.5%)	105 (0.8%)	127 (0.9%)	73 (1.1%)	32.258	<0.001	-0.166
HPV-52	66 (7.1%)	459 (5.0%)	639 (5.0%)	603 (4.2%)	297 (4.4%)	15.420	<0.001	-0.065
HPV-53	45 (4.8%)	183 (2.0%)	244 (1.9%)	317 (2.2%)	215 (3.2%)	7.704	0.006	0.076
HPV-56	10 (1.1%)	68 (0.7%)	63 (0.5%)	81 (0.6%)	51 (0.8%)	0.286	0.593	-0.017
HPV-58	60 (6.4%)	320 (3.5%)	437 (3.4%)	531 (3.7%)	372 (5.5%)	17.682	<0.001	0.082
HPV-59	14 (1.5%)	53 (0.6%)	47 (0.4%)	52 (0.4%)	34 (0.5%)	6.424	0.011	-0.113
HPV-66	15 (1.6%)	97 (1.1%)	86 (0.7%)	94 (0.7%)	83 (1.2%)	0.254	0.615	-0.014
HPV-68	24 (2.6%)	116 (1.3%)	113 (0.9%)	127 (0.9%)	80 (1.2%)	5.572	0.018	−0.070

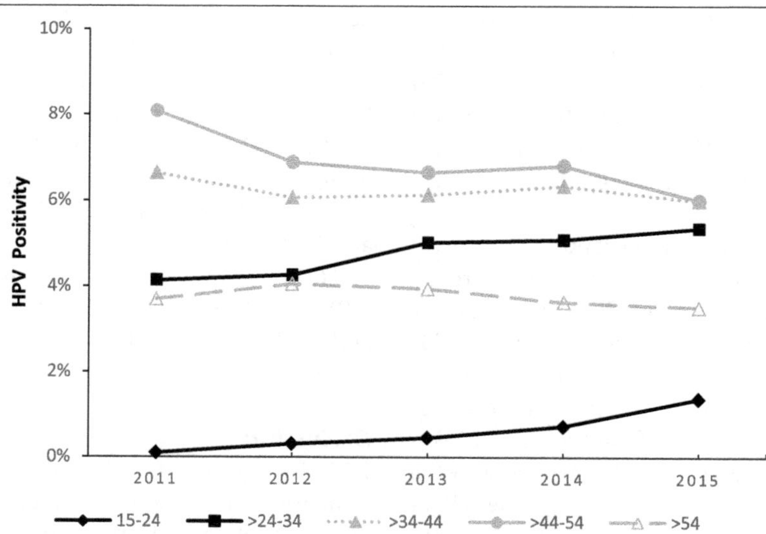

Fig. 2 Changes in the rate of human papillomavirus infection ingynaecological outpatients in different age groups, 2011–2015

Table 4 Changes in the rate of human papillomavirus infection ingynaecological outpatients in different age groups, 2011–2015

	2011 (*n* = 5001)	2012 (*n* = 6410)	2013 (*n* = 7863)	2014 (*n* = 11,402)	2015 (*n* = 13,128)	χ^2	*P*	*gamma value*
15–24	5 (0.1)	20 (0.3)	36 (0.5)	83 (0.7)	180 (1.4)	111.4	<0.001	0.464*
>24–34	207(4.1)	273(4.3)	394(5.0)	579(5.1)	702(5.4)	16.8	<0.001	0.064*
>34–44	332(6.6)	389(6.1)	482(6.1)	723(6.3)	786(6.0)	1.159	0.282	−0.015**
>44–54	404(8.1)	441(6.9)	523(6.7)	776(6.8)	788(6.0)	20.372	<0.001	−0.031**
>54	185(3.7)	260(4.1)	310(3.9)	414(3.6)	460(3.5)	2.587	0.108	−0.032**

Linear-by-linear Association test and Gamma Value for trend to evaluate changes in HPV prevalence by calendar year and by age group. *$p < 0.05$;**$p > 0.05$

papillomas in the host tissue. Epidemiological and biological investigations have shown that HPV infection and subtype distributions are closely associated with the region, age and population [10, 11]. According to statistical data obtained from the IARC, the top five HPV subtypes worldwide in terms of infection frequency are HPV-16, −18, −58, −52 and −31. The present study was conducted in Hangzhou, which is a city located on the southeast coast of China that features a developed economy and frequent population migration. Clarifying the infection rates, genetic profiles and epidemiological patterns of HPV in Hangzhou is of great significance for the prevention and control of HPV in this region.

The present study was an epidemiological study investigating HPV infection with the largest sample size in the study area to date. Both laboratories selected for the study have achieved International Standard Organization (ISO) 15,189 accreditation. The results showed that the average HPV infection rate was 22.3% in general gynaecological outpatients from Hangzhou over the past five years. This value was close to the HPV infection rate of 22.80% in gynaecological outpatients from the same region reported by Liu et al. [12, 13] and the previously reported HPV infection rate of 26% across the country of China [6]. Our result is consistent with the HPV infection rate of 20–25% reported in general gynaecological outpatients from other countries [14]; however, it was much lower the HPV infection rate of 66.7% found in a high-risk population from this region reported by Wang et al. [15] Differences in the study populations (general gynaecological outpatients vs. a high-risk population) may be the cause of the significant difference in the HPV infection rates within the same region. Over the past three years, the rate of single infections exhibited a downward trend, whereas the rate of multiple infections showed an upward trend in the study area.

The present study showed that the infection rate of the high-risk HPV subtypes was 20.1% in Hangzhou, which was 4.43 times the infection rate found for the low-risk HPV subtypes in this region (4.5%). This ratio is higher than the previously reported ratio of high-risk/low-risk HPV infection rates in China [6]. The current results showed that the top five HPV subtypes in terms of the infection rate were HPV-16, −52, −58, −53 and −18 in Hangzhou. This result is different from the subtype distribution of HPV dominated by HPV-16, −18, −31, −33 and −58 in Europe and America and from the dominant subtype distribution of HPV-53, −52, −58, −16 and −68 in South Korea in the same Asian region [16]. Moreover, our result differed from the dominant HPV subtype distributions reported in north and southwest China [17, 18]. In the cervical cancer group, the top five HPV subtypes in terms of infection frequency were HPV-16, −58, −52, −18 and −53. HPV-16 and -18 are the most prevalent HPV subtypes worldwide and are also the most common HPV subtypes in cervical cancer patients worldwide. Our result showed that the HPV-18 infection rate ranked relatively low in Hangzhou, which was in agreement with results reported in other regions of China [19, 20].

Cervical cancer has long plagued the majority of women's health care in China, particularly for rural women; every year, there are approximately 130,000 new cervical cancer cases [21]. The best choice for the

Table 5 Single and multiple infections in human papillomavirus (HPV)-positive patients in different disease groups

	Cervical cancer[a] (*n* = 915)	CIN3[b] (*n* = 324)	CIN2[c] (*n* = 270)	CIN1[d] (*n* = 1924)	Other diseases[e] (*n* = 40,371)	χ^2	*P*
HPV-positive	889 (97.2)	287 (88.6)	143 (52.7)	978 (50.8)	7455 (18.5)	4557.239	<0.001
Single infections	616 (69.3)	203(70.7)	109 (76.2)	764(78.1)	5970 (80.1)	63.613	<0.001
Multiple infections	273 (30.7)	84(29.3)	34 (23.8)	214(21.9)	1485(19.9)		

Pairwise comparisons were performed using the Bonferroni method; *α* was adjusted with $P < 0.01$ considered significant. In comparing the rates of single and multiple infections, the following results were found: the difference was significant for a + d ($\chi^2 = 18.820$, $P < 0.001$); the difference was significant for a + e ($\chi^2 = 55.598$, $P < 0.001$); the difference was significant b + e ($\chi^2 = 14.978$, $P < 0.001$)

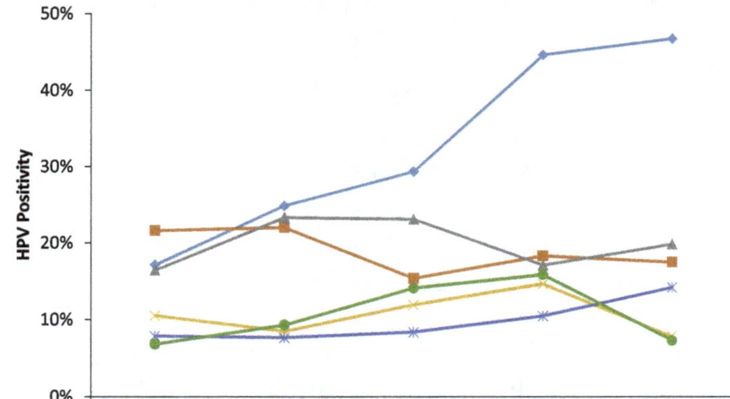

	other	CIN1	CIN2	CIN3	ICC
HPV-16	17.2%	24.8%	29.4%	44.6%	46.7%
HPV-52	21.6%	22.0%	15.4%	18.3%	17.5%
HPV-58	16.4%	23.3%	23.0%	17.1%	19.8%
HPV-53	10.5%	8.5%	11.9%	14.6%	7.8%
HPV-18	7.9%	7.7%	8.4%	10.5%	14.2%
HPV-33	6.9%	9.3%	14.1%	15.9%	7.3%

Fig. 3 Subtype distribution of human papillomavirus (HPV) in gynaecological outpatients of different disease groups

prevention of HPV infection and treatment of cervical cancer is preventive vaccination. The US Food and Drug Administration has approved two preventive vaccine products that mainly target HPV-6, −11, −16 and −18. Clinical data have shown that the specific effect is unclear despite the protective effect of the two vaccines against infection by other HPV subtypes [22–24]. Cervarix was recently approved in China mainly against HPV-16 and -18. In the current results, the top three HPV types were HPV-16, −52 and −58 in Hangzhou, which was similar to most previous surveys in China.[6] HPV-52 and -58 were more prevalent than the vaccine type HPV-18. We expect to provide objective evidence to enhance the hypothesis that second-generation HPV prophylactic vaccines including HPV-52 and -58 may offer higher protection for women in Hangzhou and other parts of China.

Age is an important factor associated with HPV infection. One point of view is that young women have frequent sex. Reports in the literature suggest that young women are more prone to have multiple partners [25]; additionally, their immune systems are susceptible to HPV infection because they are non-sensitized. Consequently, the HPV infection rate is high in women in the 15–24-year-old group, and the rate decreases with age [26, 27]. From another perspective, women in the menopausal period have reduced immune functions, with decreased viral clearance rates and increased HPV infection rates. Therefore, there are two peaks in the age distribution of HPV infection: 15–24 year olds and women >54 years [28, 29]. In the present study, the HPV infection rates in the different age groups showed the highest HPV infection rate of 34.7% in the 15–24-year-old group, followed by an infection rate of 24.1% in the >54-year-old group. The HPV infection rate in the 15–24-year-old group showed an annual upward trend over the past five years. This result suggested that HPV infection exhibited a trend towards younger patients and that the 15–24-year-old group was the population most susceptible to HPV infection. The prevalence in the >54-year-old group should also arouse attention and suggest that HPV testing is clinically valuable for perimenopausal women in cervical cancer screening programmes.

In the present study, the HPV infection rate varied in different disease groups. The highest HPV infection rate appeared in the cervical cancer group (97.2%). This rate was close to the rate reported in the literature of 99.7% [30]. Whether multiple infections with HPV can increase or promote the development of cervical cancer is currently a controversial issue. In the present study, differences were detected in the rates of single and multiple infections among the HPV-positive patients in the different disease groups. The cervical cancer group showed the highest rate of multiple infections. This result is in agreement with previous results [18, 19]. Among the five disease groups, the top three HPV subtypes in terms of infection were HPV-16, −52 and −58. The rate of HPV-16 infection was 2.7 times the rate of HPV-52 infection (46.7%/17.5%) and 2.4 times the rate of HPV-58 infection in the cervical cancer group (46.7%/19.8%).

The present study evaluated HPV infection in gynaecological outpatients in Hangzhou, China, from 2011 to 2015. This study was an investigation of HPV infection with the largest sample size in this region to date. The results showed that HPV-16, −52 and −58 were the dominant HPV infection subtypes in Hangzhou, which provided objective evidence for the application of preventative vaccines in this region. Moreover, we found that the HPV infection rate progressively increased every year in the age groups below 34 years. HPV infection exhibited a trend towards younger patients, and the 15–24-year-old group was a population susceptible to HPV infection. These findings provide objective evidence for the selection of this age group for vaccination in the study region.

Abbreviations

CIN: Cervical intraepithelial neoplasia; HPV: Human papillomavirus; IARC: International Agency for Research on Cancer; ISO: International Standard Organization

Acknowledgements

We thank all of the participants for collecting the data and testing the specimens and the Chinese Centre for Disease Control and Prevention for support during the development of this project.

Funding

This study was supported by The National Science and Technology Major Project (Infectious Disease Control and Prevention) (2012ZX10004-210).

Authors' contributions

All authors participated in interpretation of the findings. LQ and DC designed the study and drafted the manuscript. YZ, BL and YC were responsible for sample collection and patient follow-up. YY and YL performed the HPV subtype detection. YC was the principal investigator, provided all facilities necessary to complete this work and was involved in editing the manuscript. All authors read and approved the final manuscript.

Competing interests

The HPV test kit for the manuscript has a patent certificate. The WIPO-SIPO Award is bestowed upon Xie Longxu. For his invertion of Human Papillomavirus Genotyping Diagnostic Kit and Its Gene Chip Preparation Method. Chinese Patent No. :ZL200710030723.6

Consent for publication

Not applicable.

Author details

[1]Department of Laboratory Medicine, the First Affiliated Hospital of Zhejiang Chinese Medical University, Hangzhou, China. [2]Department of Laboratory Medicine, Center of Clinical Laboratory, the First Affiliated Hospital, School of Medicine, Zhejiang University, No. 79, Qingchun Road, Hangzhou 310003, China.

References

1. De Jonge M, Busecke G, Heinecke A, et al. Human papillomavirus genotype distribution in cytologically screened women from northwest Germany[J]. Acta Cytol. 2013;57(6):591–8.
2. No JH, Kim MK, Jeon YT, Kim YB, et al. Human papillomavirus vaccine: widening the scope for cancer prevention[J]. Mol Carcinog. 2011;50(4):244–53.
3. den Boon JA, Pyeon D, Wang SS, et al. Molecular transitions from papillomavirus infection to cervical precancer and cancer: role of stromal estrogen receptor signaling. Proc Natl Acad Sci U S A. 2015;112(25):E3255–64.
4. Walboomers JM, Jacobs MV, Manos MM, et al. Human papillomavirus is a necessary cause of invasive cervical cancer worldwide. J Pathol 1999 Sep; 189(1):12–9.
5. Schiffman M, Wentzensen N. Human papillomavirus infection and the multistage carcinogenesis of cervical cancer. Cancer Epidemiol Biomark Prev. 2013;22(4):553–60.
6. Zeng Z, Yang H, Li Z, He X, Griffith CC, Chen X, et al. Prevalence and genotype distribution of HPV infection in China: analysis of 51,345 HPV genotyping results from China's largest CAP certified Laboratory. J Cancer. 2016 May 25;7(9):1037–43.
7. Smith JS, Melendy A, Rana RK, et al. Age-specific prevalence of infection with human papillomavirus in females: a global review[J]. J Adolesc Health. 2008;43:S5–S25.
8. Baloch Z, Li Y, Yuan T, Feng Y, Liu Y, Tai W, et al. Epidemiologic characterization of human papillomavirus (HPV) infection in various regions of Yunnan Province of China. BMC Infect Dis. 2016 May 26;16:228. doi:10.1186/s12879-016-1562-7.
9. Yang H, Li LJ, Xie LX, Luo ZY, Lu M, Lin M, et al. Clinical validation of a novel real-time human papillomavirus assay for simultaneous detection of 14 high-risk HPV type and genotyping HPV type 16 and 18 in China. Arch Virol. 2016 Feb;161(2):449–54. doi:10.1007/s00705-015-2673-y.
10. Lee EH, et al. Prevalence and distribution of human papillomavirus infection in Korean women as determined by restriction fragment mass polymorphism assay. J Korean Med Sci. 2012;27(9):1091–7.
11. Rey-Ares L, Ciapponi A, Pichon-Riviere A. Efficacy and safety of human papilloma virus vaccine in cervical cancer prevention: systematic review and meta-analysis. Archivos argentinos de pediatria. 2012;110(6):483–9.
12. Liu XX, Fan XL, Yu YP, Ji L, Yan J, Sun AH. Human papillomavirus prevalence and type-distribution among women in Zhejiang Province. Southeast China: a cross-sectional study BMC infectious diseases. 2014;14:708.
13. Wu D, Cai L, Huang M, Zheng Y, Yu J. Prevalence of genital human papillomavirus infection and genotypes among women from Fujian province, PR China. Eur J Obstet Gynecol Reprod Biol. 2010;151(1):86–90.
14. Bruni L, Diaz M, Castellsague X, Ferrer E, Bosch FX, de Sanjosé S. Cervical human papillomavirus prevalence in 5 continents: meta-analysis of 1 million women with normal cytological findings. J Infect Dis. 2010;202:1789–99.
15. Wang X, Gu D, Lou B, et al. Hospital-based prevalence of high-risk cervical HPV types infecting the general population and female sex workers in Huzhou, China[J]. Int J Gynaecol Obest. 2013;120:37–41.
16. So KA, Hong JH, Lee JK. Human papillomavirus prevalence and type distribution among 968 women in South Korea. J Cancer Prev. 2016 Jun; 21(2):104–9.
17. Chen Z, Meng W, Du R, Zhu Y, Zhang Y, Ding Y. Genotype distribution and the relative risk factors for human papillomavirus in Urumqi. China Exp Ther Med. 2013;6(1):85–90.
18. Sun LL, Jin Q, Li H, et al. Population-based study on the prevalence of and risk factors for human papillomavirus infection in Qujing of Yunnan province, Southwest China[J]. Virol J. 2012;9(1):153.
19. Wang L, Li J, Chen L. Prevalence of human papillomavirus and its genotype among 1336 invasive cervical cancer patients in Hunan province, central south China. J Med Virol. 2015;87:516–21.
20. Jing L, Zhong X, Huang W, et al. HPV genotypes and associated cervical cytological abnormalities in women from the Pearl River Delta region of Guangdong province. China: a cross-sectional study BMC infectious diseases. 2014;14:388.
21. Shi JF, Qiao YL, Smith JS, et al. Epidemiology and prevention of human papillomavirus and cervical cancer in China and Mongolia. Vaccine. 2008; 26(Suppl 12):M53–9.
22. Harper DM, et al. Sustained efficacy up to 4.5 years of a bivalent L1 virus-like particle vaccine against human papillomavirus types 16 and 18: follow-up from a randomised control trial. Lancet. 2006;367(9518):1247–55.
23. Wheeler CM. Advances in primary and secondary interventions for cervical cancer: human papillomavirus prophylactic vaccines and testing. Nat Clin Pract Oncol. 2007;4(4):224–35.
24. Teitelman AM, et al. Human papillomavirus, current vaccines, and cervical cancer prevention. J Obstet Gynecol Neonatal Nurs. 2009;38(1):69–80.
25. Zhao FH, Tiggelaar SM, Hu SY, et al. A multi-center survey of age of sexual debut and sexual behavior in Chinese women: suggestions for optimal age

of human papillomavirus vaccination in China. Cancer Epidemiol. 2012;36(4): 384–90. doi:10.1016/j.canep.2012.01.009.
26. Slama J, Drazdakova M, Dunder P, et al. High-risk human papillomavirus DNA in the primary tumor, sentinel, and nonsentinel pelvic lymph nodes in patients with early-stage cervical cancer: a correlation with histopathology[J]. Int J Gynecol Cancer. 2009;19(4):703–7.
27. Sherpa AT, Clifford GM, Vaccarella S, et al. Human papillomavirus infection in women with and without cervical cancer in Nepal. Cancer Causes Control. 2010;21:323–30.
28. Kim MJ, Kim JJ, Kim S. Type-specific prevalence of high-risk human papillomavirus by cervical cytology and age: data from the health check-ups of 7,014 Korean women. Obstet Gynecol Sci. 2013;56(2):110–20. doi:10.5468/OGS.2013.56.2.110.
29. Wang S, Wei H, Wang N, et al. The prevalence and role of human papillomavirus genotypes in primary cervical screening in the northeast of China[J]. BMC Cancer. 2012;12(1):160.
30. Walboomers JM, Jacobs MV, Manos MM, Bosch FX, Kummer JA, Shah KV, et al. Human papillomavirus is a necessary cause of invasive cervical cancer worldwide. J Pathol. 1999;189:12–9.

12

A cross-sectional study on the concordance between vaginal HPV DNA detection and type-specific antibodies in a multi-ethnic cohort of women from Amsterdam, the Netherlands – the HELIUS study

Alexandra Kovaleva[1,2*], Catharina J. Alberts[1], Tim Waterboer[3], Angelika Michel[3], Marieke B. Snijder[4], Wilma Vermeulen[5], Liza Coyer[1], Maria Prins[1,6] and Maarten Schim van der Loeff[1,6]

Abstract

Background: Acquisition of genital human papillomavirus (HPV) infection is common among the young, sexually active population. Genital HPV infections do not always lead to seroconversion. We aimed to assess the association between cervico-vaginal high risk (hr) HPV DNA and type-specific antibodies in an ethnically diverse cohort of young women.

Methods: Women of Dutch, South-Asian Surinamese, African Surinamese, Ghanaian, Moroccan and Turkish origin participating in a large-scale multi-ethnic population-based cohort (the HELIUS study) provided vaginal self-samples and blood samples, and completed a questionnaire regarding demographics, lifestyle and sexual health. Vaginal swabs were tested for HPV using the highly sensitive SPF10-PCR DEIA/LiPA25 system (version1). Serum samples were tested for type-specific L1 antibodies against 7 hrHPV types (16,18,31,33,45,52,58) with multiplex serology. We assessed the association between vaginal HPV DNA and type-specific seropositivity with logistic and linear regression, using generalized estimating equations (GEE). We determined whether this association varies by ethnicity by adding an interaction term.

Results: We selected 532 women who completed the questionnaire, provided a vaginal swab and a blood sample. Their median age was 27 years (interquartile range 24–31 years). Prevalence of DNA of any of the 7 hrHPV was 22 %; HPV-52 was most common. Prevalence of antibodies against one or more hrHPV types was 24 %; HPV-16 seropositivity was most common. In multivariable logistic regression analysis using GEE, adjusting for other determinants, vaginal HPV DNA detection was associated with type-specific HPV seropositivity (OR 1.53, 95 % CI 1.06-2.20). In multivariable linear regression analysis using GEE, the geometric mean of type-specific antibody reactivity was 1.15 (95 % CI 1.04-1.27) times higher in women positive for HPV DNA compared to HPV DNA-negative women. There was little evidence that ethnicity modified the association between HPV DNA, and type-specific seropositivity, or with antibody reactivities ($p = 0.47$ and $p = 0.57$, respectively).

Conclusions: In this multi-ethnic group of young women in Amsterdam, cervico-vaginal hrHPV DNA detection was an independent determinant of type-specific HPV seropositivity.

Keywords: Human papillomavirus, Vaginal, Antibodies, Serology, Concordance, HELIUS study

* Correspondence: skovalev@ggd.amsterdam.nl
[1]Department of Infectious Diseases Research and Prevention, Public Health Service of Amsterdam (GGD), Nieuwe Achtergracht 100, Amsterdam 1018 WT, The Netherlands
[2]AMC Graduate School, Academic Medical Center, Meibergdreef 9, Amsterdam 1105 AZ, The Netherlands
Full list of author information is available at the end of the article

Background

Due to increased globalization, European populations are becoming more ethnically diverse, and health risks and outcomes differ between ethnic groups [1]. Acquisition of human papillomavirus (HPV) infection is common among the young, sexually active population. Oncogenic human papillomaviruses cause the majority of cervical, anal, and penile cancer, and in some countries also of oropharyngeal cancer [2]. The incidence of cervical carcinoma differs between ethnic groups in the Netherlands, with higher incidence in those of the non-Dutch origin [3].

Most infections with oncogenic HPV are cleared spontaneously and pass without malignant sequelae. Estimates of proportions of women who seroconvert after infection range from 55–85 %, depending on study design and methods employed [4–6]. The median time to seroconversion after genital infection with HPV ranged from 8.3–31.3 months between studies [4–6]. In a large multi-national study 79 % of cases of cervical HPV DNA cleared within 24 months [7]. Concordance of genital HPV detection and serum antibodies is not expected per se, because the former may constitute current infection, and the latter past infection or infection of longer duration. Some studies, examining the concordance between cervico-vaginal HPV DNA and type-specific seropositivity showed positive associations, while others showed no significant relationship [8–15].

We aimed to assess the association between prevalent cervico-vaginal HPV DNA of seven high risk HPV (hrHPV) types and type-specific antibodies in serum, and to evaluate whether this association varies by ethnicity.

Methods

Study design

The HEalthy LIfe in an Urban Setting (HELIUS) study is a multi-ethnic cohort study conducted in Amsterdam which has been described in detail elsewhere [16]. Briefly, the study was initiated in 2011 and includes people aged 18–70 years from the 6 largest ethnic groups in Amsterdam, i.e. those of Dutch, South-Asian Surinamese, African Surinamese, Ghanaian, Moroccan and Turkish origin. Participants were randomly selected per ethnicity from the Amsterdam municipal registers. Data were collected by questionnaire and physical examination; collection of biological samples took place during physical examination. Information on demographic characteristics (age, education, marital status), health-related characteristics (parity, HPV vaccination, smoking), and sexual behavior (age at sexual debut, number of lifetime male sex partners, type of sexual partner in the preceding six months) were obtained via questionnaire.

The selection process for this study has been described in detail elsewhere (Alberts et al. 2015, manuscript submitted for review). Briefly, we selected all women aged 18–34 years from the HELIUS participants who were enrolled until December 2013, who completed the questionnaire on demographics, health behavioral characteristics, and sexual behavior, provided a self-collected vaginal swab, and of whom a blood sample was available ($n = 959$). We randomly selected a maximum of 7 women per life year per ethnic group, resulting in a selection of 610 women. Participants who were not tested for HPV antibodies ($n = 60$), who reported HPV vaccination ($n = 10$) and participants with an invalid HPV DNA test result ($n = 8$) were excluded, resulting in a study sample of 532 women. The study protocol was approved by The Academic Medical Center Ethics Review Board (Amsterdam, the Netherlands), and all participants provided written informed consent (reference number METC 10/100# 17.10.1729).

HPV DNA detection and genotyping

Self-collected vaginal swabs (COPAN Italia, Brescia, Italy) were stored at 4 °C for a maximum of 5–6 days at the research location and sent to the Public Health Service of Amsterdam where they were stored at −20 °C until further analysis. Swabs were eluted in 600 μL PBS and DNA was extracted from 200 μL of each specimen using the isopropanol method [17] with an end volume of 100 mL. The presence of HPV in the swabs was assessed by using the highly sensitive SPF10-PCR DEIA/LiPA25 system version 1 (DDL Diagnostics Laboratory, Rijswijk, the Netherlands) [18]. Briefly, with this technique a 65 base-pair open reading frame of the L1 region was amplified with SPF10 primers resulting in biotinylated amplicons. The amplification products were tested for HPV DNA with a DNA enzyme immunoassay by use of hybridization with a cocktail of probes that recognized at least 54 HPV types. Optical densities were measured and compared with cut-off values from internal controls. Positive samples were genotyped by a reverse hybridization line probe assay which allows simultaneous detection of HPV-6, 11, 16, 18, 31, 33–35, 39, 40, 42–45, 51–54, 56, 58, 59, 66, 68/73, 70, and 74. Prevalence of vaginal HPV DNA in this population and determinants of vaginal HPV DNA detection have been reported elsewhere (Alberts et al. 2015, manuscript submitted for review).

HPV antibody detection

Serum samples were stored at −80 °C at the Academic Medical Center of Amsterdam until sent for analysis to the German Cancer Research Center, Heidelberg, Germany. Antibodies to the L1 proteins of HPV-16, 18, 31, 33, 45, 52 and 58 were analyzed by multiplex serology assay based on glutathione S-transferase (GST) fusion protein capture on fluorescent beads (SeroMAP

Table 1 Demographic, health and sexual behavior characteristics by ethnicity of 532 women from Amsterdam, the Netherlands

	Dutch		South-Asian Surinamese		African Surinamese		Ghanaian		Moroccan		Turkish			Total	
	N = 98		*N* = 88		*N* = 100		*N* = 68		*N* = 101		*N* = 77			*N* = 532	
	n	%	n	%	n	%	n	%	n	%	n	%	*P*-value	n	%
Age in years															
Median (IQR)	27 (23–31)	27 (23–31)	26 (22–30)	26 (21–30)	27 (23–30)	27 (23–31)	0.46	27 (23–30)							
18–22	23	23 %	19	22 %	27	27 %	22	32 %	20	20 %	16	21 %	0.98	127	24 %
23–26	24	24 %	21	24 %	25	25 %	16	24 %	28	28 %	17	22 %		131	25 %
27–30	26	27 %	26	30 %	25	25 %	15	22 %	28	28 %	24	31 %		144	27 %
31–34	25	26 %	22	25 %	23	23 %	15	22 %	25	25 %	20	26 %		130	24 %
Education[a]															
Low/Intermediate	28	29 %	56	64 %	67	68 %	50	75 %	66	65 %	58	75 %	<0.001	325	61 %
High	70	71 %	32	36 %	32	32 %	17	25 %	35	35 %	19	25 %		205	39 %
Marital status															
Married/Cohabitating	30	31 %	29	33 %	13	13 %	14	21 %	39	39 %	36	47 %	<0.001	161	30 %
Never married	68	69 %	54	61 %	86	86 %	53	78 %	52	51 %	35	45 %		348	65 %
Divorced	0	0 %	5	6 %	1	1 %	1	1 %	10	10 %	6	8 %		23	4 %
Smoking status															
Never	47	48 %	61	69 %	63	64 %	66	97 %	81	80 %	36	47 %	<0.001	354	67 %
Former	20	20 %	8	9 %	11	11 %	2	3 %	6	6 %	10	13 %		57	11 %
Current	31	32 %	19	22 %	25	25 %	0	0 %	14	14 %	31	40 %		120	23 %
Smoking in pack years															
Never	47	48 %	61	69 %	63	64 %	66	97 %	81	80 %	36	47 %	<0.001	354	67 %
< 2 pack years	24	25 %	14	16 %	22	22 %	1	1 %	9	9 %	13	17 %		83	16 %
> 2 pack years	26	27 %	13	15 %	14	14 %	1	1 %	11	11 %	27	36 %		92	17 %
Age of sexual debut in years															
Median (IQR)[b]	16 (15–18)	18 (17–20)	17 (15–18)	18 (16–19)	19 (17–22)	20 (18–22)	<0.001	18 (16–20)							
Never had sex	5	5 %	14	16 %	8	8 %	18	28 %	33	33 %	15	20 %	<0.001	93	18 %
≥ 21	9	9 %	12	14 %	3	3 %	9	14 %	29	29 %	26	34 %		88	17 %
19-20	8	8 %	16	19 %	17	17 %	5	8 %	12	12 %	16	21 %		74	14 %
18-17	27	28 %	29	34 %	27	27 %	19	30 %	13	13 %	14	18 %		129	25 %
≤ 16	49	50 %	15	17 %	45	45 %	13	20 %	13	13 %	5	7 %		140	27 %

Table 1 Demographic, health and sexual behavior characteristics by ethnicity of 532 women from Amsterdam, the Netherlands *(Continued)*

Number of lifetime male sexual partners															
Median (IQR)	6 (3–11)	2 (1–4)	5 (2–8)	2 (0–4)	1 (0–1)	1 (1–2)	<0.001	3 (1–7)							
None[c]	5	5 %	14	16 %	9	9 %	18	28 %	34	34 %	16	21 %	<0.001	96	18 %
1	8	8 %	27	31 %	6	6 %	11	17 %	44	44 %	38	50 %		134	26 %
2–5	33	34 %	34	40 %	42	42 %	25	39 %	15	15 %	12	16 %		161	31 %
6–10	25	26 %	9	10 %	26	26 %	8	13 %	4	4 %	9	12 %		81	15 %
≥11	27	28 %	2	2 %	16	16 %	2	3 %	3	3 %	1	1 %		51	10 %
Type of sexual contact past 6 months															
Never had sex	5	5 %	14	16 %	8	8 %	18	28 %	33	33 %	15	20 %	<0.001	93	18 %
No sex	17	17 %	14	16 %	11	11 %	9	14 %	16	16 %	11	14 %		78	15 %
With steady partner only	55	56 %	55	64 %	60	60 %	34	53 %	49	49 %	39	51 %		292	56 %
With casual partner[d]	21	21 %	3	3 %	21	21 %	3	5 %	2	2 %	11	14 %		61	12 %

IQR, interquartile range

P-values of categorical variables are based on Chi-squared test and p of continuous variables are based on the Kruskal-Wallis test

Missing values for: education, $n = 2$; age sexual debut, $n = 8$; lifetime male sexual partners, $n = 9$; type of sexual partner past 6 months, $n = 8$; smoking status, $n = 1$; smoking in pack years, $n = 3$. [a] Education was categorized as low or intermediate education if participant had (1) never been to school or had primary schooling only, (2) followed vocational schooling or lower secondary schooling, or (3) followed intermediate/ higher secondary education schooling; and was categorized as high education if participant had followed higher vocational schooling or university. [b]Of those women who reported ever having sex. [c]This category includes women who never had sex and those who exclusively had sexual contact with women, therefore this category has a different number than the category "Never had sex" in the variables "Age of sexual debut in years" and "Type of sexual contact past 6 months". [d]And with or without steady partner

Microspheres; Luminex) [19]. Antibody quantity was determined as the median R-phycoerythrin fluorescence intensity (MFI) from at least 100 beads of the same internal color. MFI values were dichotomized as antibody positive or negative based on predetermined cut-off values for each antibody by analyzing MFI values obtained from Korean HPV DNA-negative self-reported virgin females using an algorithm of the mean plus 5 SDs after exclusion of outliers [12]. This resulted in cut-offs varying from 394–712 MFI.

Statistical analysis

Differences in baseline characteristics between ethnic groups were assessed using the Pearson's chi-squared or the Kruskal-Wallis test as appropriate. The statistical analysis was restricted to HPV types 16, 18, 31, 33, 45, 52 and 58.

First, we assessed type-specific HPV seropositivity on a dichotomous scale among both HPV DNA positive women and HPV DNA negative women per individual HPV type by performing standard univariable logistic analyses. As a woman can be infected with multiple HPV types simultaneously we also analyzed data on all 7 HPV types with univariable and multivariable logistic regression models using generalized estimating equations (GEE). We used a binomial distribution and an exchangeable correlation structure with robust variance.

We then investigated the association between cervico-vaginal HPV DNA and type-specific antibody reactivities using linear regression. For this purpose, we transformed antibody reactivities to their natural logarithm. We first undertook standard univariable and multivariable linear regression for individual HPV types. Next, we proceeded with univariable and multivariable linear regression using GEE. Because the mean and standard deviation of antibody reactivities of the 7 hrHPV types differed, we standardized the natural logarithm of antibody reactivity levels by calculating Z-scores. We used a Gaussian distribution and an exchangeable correlation structure, with robust variance. Because we included a log-transformed outcome variable in the linear regression analysis, we back-transformed the regression coefficients in order to ease interpretation. As a result, the coefficients can be interpreted as a multiplicative factor of the geometric mean; in other words the geometric mean of an antibody reactivity in women who are positive for cervico-vaginal HPV DNA, is equal to that factor times the geometric mean of women who are HPV DNA negative.

All multivariable models were adjusted for an a priori defined set of variables, i.e. age, ethnicity, marital status, smoking in pack years, and number of lifetime male sexual partners. We included age as a continuous variable using restricted cubic splines with 4 knots. All variables other than age were included as categorical variables. No backward selection was done.

Only one sexual risk variable could be included in the model because of multicollinearity between these variables. Also, only smoking in pack years and not smoking status was included in the models because of multicollinearity. For all other variables multicollinearity did not appear to be a concern.

As a last step we investigated whether the association between HPV seropositivity and HPV DNA varied by ethnicity. To do this we tested for interaction by adding an interaction term to the multivariable model. Stata Statistical Software release 13.1 (StataCorp, College Station, TX, USA) was used for statistical analyses.

Results

A total of 532 women were included in the analyses (Table 1). The average age of the participants did not differ between ethnic groups (median 27 years, interquartile range (IQR) 23–30 years). All other baseline characteristics differed across ethnic groups; we found significant differences in education, marital status, and smoking. Furthermore, lifetime male sexual partners, age of sexual debut and type of sexual contact in in the last

Table 2 Vaginal hrHPV DNA and type-specific seropositivity[a], and association of vaginal hrHPV DNA with type-specific antibodies[b]

HPV type[c]	HPV DNA detected n (%)	HPV seropositive n (%)	Seropositive among DNA + n (%)[d]	Seropositive among DNA - n (%)[e]	Crude OR for seropositivity (95 % CI)[f]
16	32 (6 %)	73 (14 %)	6 (19 %)	67 (13 %)	1.49 (0.59,3.76)
18	20 (4 %)	59 (11 %)	4 (20 %)	55 (11 %)	2.08 (0.67,6.44)
31	28 (5 %)	68 (13 %)	6 (21 %)	62 (12 %)	1.94 (0.76,4.98)
33	7 (1 %)	36 (7 %)	2 (29 %)	34 (6 %)	5.78 (1.08,30.88)
45	8 (2 %)	51 (10 %)	1 (13 %)	50 (10 %)	1.35 (0.16,11.23)
52	43 (8 %)	54 (10 %)	9 (21 %)	45 (9 %)	2.61 (1.18,5.97)
58	9 (2 %)	46 (9 %)	3 (33 %)	43 (8 %)	5.58 (1.35,23.10)

CI, confidence interval; hrHPV, high risk human papillomavirus; IQR, interquartile range; OR, odds ratio. [a] Among 532 women from a population-based cohort (HELIUS), Amsterdam, the Netherlands. [b]Univariable analysis conducted with logistic regression. [c] Cut-offs used in this study: 422 MFI for HPV-16, 394 for HPV-18, 712 for HPV-31, 515 for HPV-33, 368 for HPV-45, 547 for HPV-52, and 371 MFI for HPV-58. [d]Among number of HPV DNA positive women in column 2. [e]Among number of HPV DNA negative women, i.e. the number cited in column 2 subtracted from 532. [f]Multivariable analysis was not undertaken because of small numbers

Table 3 Associations of risk factors and seropositivity for seven hrHPV types[a]; logistic regression using GEE

	Crude OR	95 % CI	*P*-value	Adjusted OR[b]	95 % CI	*P*-value
Cervico-vaginal HPV DNA						
No	1		0.002	1		0.02
Yes	1.70	(1.22,2.36)		1.53	(1.06,2.20)	
Age in years[c]						
19	2.76	(1.34,5.70)		4.33	(2.07,9.06)	
24	1		0.02	1		<0.001
29	1.07	(0.58,1.99)		1.10	(0.60,2.05)	
34	1.53	(0.73,3.20)		1.53	(0.72,3.24)	
Ethnicity[d]						
Dutch	1		<0.001	1		0.22
South-Asian Surinamese	0.63	(0.30,1.31)		1.39	(0.65,2.96)	
African Surinamese	1.80	(0.99,3.26)		1.96	(1.08,3.55)	
Ghanaian	0.74	(0.34,1.59)		1.11	(0.48,2.55)	
Moroccan	0.43	(0.20,0.94)		1.30	(0.57,2.96)	
Turkish	0.36	(0.14,0.88)		0.85	(0.34,2.15)	
Marital status[e]						
Ever married/Cohabitating	1		0.002	1		0.06
Never married	2.22	(1.33,3.69)		1.72	(0.98,3.03)	
Smoking status						
Never smoked	1		0.50			
Former smoker	1.42	(0.74,2.73)				
Current smoker	1.22	(0.73,2.03)				
Smoking in pack years						
Never smoked	1		0.023	1		0.04
< 2 years	1.92	(1.14,3.22)		1.45	(0.84,2.50)	
≥ 2 years	0.81	(0.43,1.52)		0.57	(0.30,1.09)	
Age of sexual debut						
Never had sex	1		<0.001			
≥ 21	1.31	(0.44,3.89)				
19-20	2.29	(0.82,6.38)				
18-17	4.03	(1.65,9.85)				
≤ 16	5.50	(2.30,13.17)				
Lifetime male sexual partners						
None	1		<0.001	1		<0.001
1	1.88	(0.73,4.85)		3.61	(1.37,9.49)	
2–5	3.44	(1.43,8.27)		4.29	(1.72,10.74)	
6–10	6.27	(2.54,15.49)		11.2	(4.13,30.33)	
≥ 11	7.08	(2.74,18.32)		12.07	(4.09,35.57)	

CI, confidence interval; GEE, generalized estimating equations; hrHPV, high risk human papillomavirus; OR, odds ratio. [a]Among 532 women from the population-based cohort HELIUS, Amsterdam, the Netherlands, 2011–2013. [b]Multivariable models adjusted for age in years, ethnicity, marital status, smoking in pack years, number of lifetime male sexual partners. [c]For analytic purposes age was modeled using restricted cubic splines with knots at the 5th, 35th, 65th and 95th percentile. The ORs of four ages from the total analysis with five years in between have been chosen for display in the table. [d]Effect estimates per ethnicity of vaginal hrHPV DNA detection for seropositivity in ORs (95 % CI): Dutch 1.74 (0.99,3.09), South-Asian Surinamese 2.13 (0.72,6.33), African Surinamese 1.43 (0.82,2.45), Ghanaian 0.93 (0.25,3.48), Moroccan 0.67 (0.13,3.51), Turkish 4.01 (1.44,11.12). [e]For marital status, the small category of divorced women was added to the category of married or cohabitating women to prevent instability of the model

six months varied significantly by ethnicity. Most women reported having one steady sexual partner in the preceding six months.

Vaginal HPV DNA of at least one of the 7 hrHPV types was detected in 115 (22 %) women of whom some had multiple infections with different HPV types; DNA of HPV-52 was detected most often (Table 2). Of the 532 women, 130 (24 %) were seropositive for at least one of the 7 hrHPV types; HPV-16 had the highest seroprevalence (14 %). Among women positive for DNA of an individual HPV type, seropositivity for the corresponding HPV type ranged from 13–33 %. Among HPV DNA negative women, seropositivity ranged from 6–13 %.

For all 7 HPV types we found that HPV DNA positive women were seropositive for the corresponding type more often than HPV DNA negative women (indicated by ORs > 1 for all), but this was only significant for HPV-33, 52 and 58 (Table 2). In univariable logistic regression analysis using GEE cervico-vaginal HPV DNA detection was significantly associated with type-specific seropositivity (OR 1.70, 95 % CI 1.22 – 2.36) (Table 3). After adjustment for age, ethnicity, marital status, smoking in pack years, and number of lifetime male sexual partners the association remained positive and statistically significant (OR 1.53, 95 % CI 1.06 – 2.20).

The geometric mean of the antibody reactivities in MFI was higher among women who were positive for cervico-vaginal HPV DNA. This was the case for all 7 hrHPV types, though only significant for HPV-31, 52 and 58 (Table 4). When we adjusted for age, ethnicity, marital status, smoking in pack years, and lifetime number of male sexual partners in multivariable linear regression models, DNA detection of HPV-31 remained significantly associated with a higher antibody reactivity for this type. For all other HPV types the back-transformed regression coefficient was >1, but the association was not significant.

Next, we investigated the association between cervico-vaginal HPV DNA and standardized antibody reactivities with linear regression analysis using GEE. In univariable linear analysis with GEE women with prevalent cervico-vaginal HPV DNA had higher type-specific antibody reactivities than women without cervico-vaginal HPV DNA (back-transformed regression coefficient 1.15 [95 % CI 1.04 – 1.27]) (Table 5). In the multivariable analysis the back-transformed regression coefficient remained unchanged (1.15 [95 % CI 1.04 – 1.27]). This indicates that women with cervico-vaginal HPV DNA have higher type-specific antibody reactivities than women without cervico-vaginal HPV DNA, independent of other determinants.

We examined whether the effect of HPV DNA on seropositivity differed by ethnicity by adding an interaction term to the models. Neither in logistic, nor in linear regression analyses using GEE did we detect significant effect modification ($p = 0.47$ and $p = 0.57$, respectively).

Discussion

Our results show that in this multi-ethnic group of young women in Amsterdam, cervico-vaginal HPV DNA detection is an independent risk factor of type-specific HPV seropositivity and that detection of cervico-vaginal HPV DNA is associated with higher antibody reactivities of type-specific antibodies.

Variables that describe sexual behavior directly or that could be considered a proxy for sexual behavior were strongly associated with higher type-specific HPV antibody reactivities and HPV seropositivity. The latter has also been shown by several other studies [8, 20, 21].

Table 4 Linear regression of antibody reactivities (MFI) and type-specific vaginal HPV detection; univariable and multivariable analyses

			Univariable			Multivariable[a]		
Vaginal HPV type detection	Geometric mean of antibody reactivities in MFI among DNA negative (95 % CI)	Geometric mean of antibody reactivities in MFI among DNA positive (95 % CI)	Back-transformed regression coefficient[b]	95 % CI	*P*-value	Back-transformed regression coefficient[b]	95 % CI	*P*-value
HPV-16	80 (70–90)	110 (72–167)	1.39	(0.83,2.31)	0.21	1.34	(0.82,2.17)	0.24
HPV-18	104 (95–112)	134 (83–216)	1.30	(0.84,2.00)	0.24	1.26	(0.81,1.93)	0.30
HPV-31	141 (126–157)	303 (203–455)	2.16	(1.34,3.48)	<0.001	1.68	(1.03,2.72)	0.04
HPV-33	80 (73–88)	128 (40–411)	1.59	(0.70,3.61)	0.26	1.17	(0.53,2.57)	0.69
HPV-45	78 (71–85)	120 (51–280)	1.54	(0.73,3.23)	0.26	1.34	(0.66,2.70)	0.42
HPV-52	90 (81–100)	147 (99–218)	1.63	(1.13,2.36)	0.01	1.30	(0.91,1.87)	0.15
HPV-58	85 (79–92)	165 (72–376)	1.93	(1.05,3.55)	0.03	1.52	(0.84,2.75)	0.16

CI, confidence interval; MFI, median fluorescence intensity. [a]Multivariable models adjusted for age in years, ethnicity, marital status, smoking in pack years, number of lifetime male sexual partners. For analytic purposes age was modeled using restricted cubic splines with knots at the 5th, 35th, 65th and 95th percentile. [b]The back-transformed regression coefficient for antibody reactivities is interpreted as being the factor by which the geometric mean of antibody reactivities of vaginal HPV DNA positive women is higher in comparison to women who do not have vaginal HPV DNA. For example, women in whom vaginal HPV-31 DNA was detected have a median antibody reactivity which is 2.16 times higher than the antibody reactivity of HPV-31 DNA negative women

Table 5 Associations of antibody reactivities for seven hrHPV[a]; linear regression using GEE[b]

	Back-transformed regression coefficient[c]	95 % CI	*P*-value	Adjusted back-transformed regression coefficient[c]	95 % CI	*P*-value
Cervico-vaginal HPV DNA						
No	1		0.005	1		0.007
Yes	1.15	(1.04,1.27)		1.15	(1.04,1.27)	
Age in years[d]						
19	1.47	(1.11,1.95)		1.54	(1.18,2.01)	
24	1		0.58	1		0.013
29	1.17	(0.95,1.43)		1.10	(0.90,1.34)	
34	1.15	(0.89,1.48)		1.08	(0.84,1.39)	
Ethnicity[e]						
Dutch	1		<0.001	1		<0.001
South-Asian Surinamese	1.09	(0.86,1.39)		1.45	(1.13,1.85)	
African Surinamese	1.57	(1.25,1.98)		1.62	(1.29,2.03)	
Ghanaian	1.14	(0.89,1.48)		1.39	(1.07,1.82)	
Moroccan	0.76	(0.60,0.96)		1.13	(0.88,1.45)	
Turkish	0.73	(0.57,0.93)		1.07	(0.82,1.40)	
Marital status[f]						
Ever married/Cohabitating	1		<0.001	1		0.05
Never married	1.30	(1.11,1.51)		1.19	(1.00,1.43)	
Smoking status						
Never smoked	1		0.73			
Former smoker	1.10	(0.86,1.40)				
Current smoker	0.99	(0.83,1.19)				
Smoking in pack years						
Never smoked	1		0.13	1		0.09
< 2 years	1.18	(0.96,1.45)		1.01	(0.82,1.24)	
≥ 2 years	0.91	(0.74,1.11)		0.81	(0.66,0.99)	
Age of sexual debut in years						
Never had sex	1		<0.001			
≥ 21	1.15	(0.90,1.47)				
19-20	1.36	(1.06,1.76)				
18-17	1.65	(1.32,2.07)				
≤ 16	1.94	(1.56,2.41)				
Lifetime male sexual partners						
None	1		<0.001	1		<0.001
1	1.23	(0.99,1.53)		1.52	(1.20,1.92)	
2–5	1.60	(1.30,1.98)		1.66	(1.32,2.09)	
6–10	1.88	(1.47,2.40)		2.14	(1.63,2.82)	
≥ 11	2.35	(1.77,3.11)		2.85	(2.06,3.95)	

CI, confidence interval; GEE, generalized estimating equations; hrHPV, high risk human papillomavirus. [a] Among 532 women from the population-based cohort HELIUS, Amsterdam, the Netherlands, 2011–2013. [b]For this analysis the antibody reactivity was transformed to its natural logarithm, and subsequently standardized by calculating Z-scores. [c]The back-transformed regression coefficient is interpreted as being the factor by which the standardized antibody reactivities of women are higher in comparison to women in the reference category, which in this analysis is the HPV DNA negative group. [d] For analytic purposes age was modeled using restricted cubic splines with knots at the 5th, 35th, 65th and 95th percentile. The back-transformed regression coefficients of four ages from the total analysis with five years in between have been chosen for display in the table. [e] Effect estimates per ethnicity of vaginal hrHPV DNA detection for antibody reactivity in back-transformed regression coefficient (95 % CI): Dutch 1.19 (0.97,1.45), South-Asian Surinamese 1.21 (0.91,1.62), African Surinamese 0.98 (0.81,1.19), Ghanaian 0.99 (0.73,1.36), Moroccan 1.29 (1.00,1.66), Turkish 1.26 (0.98,1.61). [f]For marital status, the small category of divorced women was added to the category of married or cohabitating women to prevent instability of the model. Multivariable models adjusted for age in years, ethnicity, marital status, smoking in pack years, number of lifetime male sexual partners

Since antibody formation in response to natural infection is a slow process that could extend to over a year, we expected in this young study population that concordance between cervico-vaginal DNA and antibodies would be low. Our study population however had a significant positive association even after adjustment for other well-known risk factors. Our study population most likely represents women who contracted their HPV infection relatively recently. A small proportion of these infections will become persistent and the majority will be cleared [22, 23].

With these results we aim to show that the interpretation of HPV (sero-)prevalences may not be as straightforward as sometimes is depicted, i.e. even though there is a significant positive correlation between HPV DNA and HPV seropositive participants, being HPV DNA positive does not imply that a person inevitably will be or will become HPV seropositive, while being HPV seronegative does not necessarily mean an individual has never been exposed. Concordance between HPV DNA and seropositivity therefore has little clinical application as a diagnostic tool. However it may be valuable in describing the natural history of HPV infection.

Because seropositivity to HPV is a measure of lifetime exposure to HPV we expected that age would be associated with HPV seropositivity. In our sample we found a significant positive association with age 19 and seropositivity relative to the reference age of 24 years, whereas the odds for seropositivity seem to not vary much with 29 and 34 years. A similar trend has been reported by Scherpenisse et al. (2012); seropositivity percentages rise sharply in the early twenties, then stabilize and do not vary much until 59 years of age [24].

Both significant and non-significant associations between cervical HPV DNA and type-specific seropositivity have previously been reported [8–15]. We found a significant positive association in our sample between cervico-vaginal HPV DNA and type-specific seropositivity expressed on a dichotomous scale, and further strengthened this conclusion by confirming it in an analysis with the outcome measure on a continuous scale. Our finding of a positive association between cervico-vaginal HPV DNA and type-specific antibodies is in agreement with several previous studies [9, 12–15]. We complement and expand available knowledge on HPV by including seven hrHPV types in our analysis, where most previous studies included fewer types.

Some previous studies differ in methodology to ours in several respects, in that they were conducted amongst women at higher risk for HPV infections (more sexual risk behavior or patients with cervical dysplasia or recruitment in STI clinics) [9, 13, 14]. In other publications, type-specific positive associations have also been found in young women that were recruited from populations not at high risk of HPV infection [12, 15].

The fact that we could only include women who provided a cervico-vaginal swab might have introduced some selection bias into our study. Alberts et al. (2015) have shown that women of Turkish and Moroccan origin from the same study population who declined to provide a sample exhibited less sexual risk behavior (Alberts et al., 2015, submitted for review). However, no significant differences were observed between women who did and did not provide a self-swab for the other ethnicities suggesting limited bias for these groups. The ethnic diversity of our sample, and the concurrent analysis of 7 hrHPV types are strengths of this study. Because seropositivity is a measure of lifetime exposure to HPV and not necessarily the result of a current infection, an association between cervico-vaginal HPV DNA and seropositivity can be difficult to interpret.

Conclusions

In conclusion, we observed a positive association between cervico-vaginal DNA detection and type-specific seropositivity. Moreover, we demonstrated higher type-specific antibody reactivities in women who are HPV DNA positive compared to HPV DNA negative women in a multi-ethnic urban population of young women. These associations were independent of demographic and behavioral factors. There was little evidence that ethnicity constituted a significant effect modifier in our population which suggests that effect modifiers other than genetic variation are at play that result in differing HPV infection outcomes in ethnic minorities.

Abbreviations

CI: confidence interval; GEE: generalized estimating equations; HELIUS: HEalthy LIfe in an Urban Setting; HPV: human papillomavirus; hrHPV: high-risk human papillomavirus; IQR: interquartile range; MFI: median fluorescence intensity; OR: odds ratio

Acknowledgements

We gratefully acknowledge the AMC Biobank for their support in biobank management and high-quality storage of collected samples. We are most grateful to the participants of the HELIUS study and the management team, research nurses, interviewers, research assistants and other staff who have taken part in gathering the data of this study.

Members of the HPV HELIUS study group (R. A. Vos, H. Borgdorff, J. van Bergen, S. Bruisten, S.E. Geerlings, R. van Houdt, S. Morré, H. J.C. de Vries, and J. van de Wijgert) are gratefully acknowledged for their advice and suggestions on study design.

Funding

The HELIUS study is conducted by the Academic Medical Center Amsterdam and the Public Health Service of Amsterdam. Both organizations provided core support for HELIUS. The HELIUS study is also funded by the Dutch Heart Foundation (2010 T084), the Netherlands Organization for Health Research and Development (ZonMw) (200500003), and the European Union (FP-7) (278901). This particular study was funded by grant 7115 0001 and 204005002 (Academic Collaborative for Public Health) from ZonMw and an internal grant of the Public Health for Research & Development, the Netherlands.

Authors' contributions

AK carried out statistical analyses and drafted the manuscript. LC and CJA contributed to data management and statistical analysis. MSvdL supervised statistical analyses. MBS and CJA ensured quality of the cataset. WV carried out analyses of HPV DNA in the swabs. TW and AM were responsible for the HPV serology. MBS, MP and MSvdL designed the HELIUS study. MSvdL CJA and AK designed the current study. All authors participated in review of the manuscript, and saw and approved the last version.

Competing interests

The institution of M. F. Schim van der Loeff received study funding from Sanofi Pasteur MSD; he is a co-investigator in a Merck-funded investigator-initiated study; he is an investigator on a Sanofi Pasteur MSD sponsored trial; he served on a vaccine advisory board of GSK; his institution received in-kind contribution for an HPV study from Stichting Pathologie Onderzoek en Ontwikkeling (SPOO); his institution receives research funding from Janssen Infectious Diseases and Vaccines. Other authors: no conflicts of interest.

Author details

[1]Department of Infectious Diseases Research and Prevention, Public Health Service of Amsterdam (GGD), Nieuwe Achtergracht 100, Amsterdam 1018 WT, The Netherlands. [2]AMC Graduate School, Academic Medical Center, Meibergdreef 9, Amsterdam 1105 AZ, The Netherlands. [3]German Cancer Research Center (DKFZ), Im Neuenheimer Feld 280, Heidelberg 69120, Germany. [4]Department of Public Health, Academic Medical Center, Meibergdreef 9, Amsterdam 1105 AZ, The Netherlands. [5]Public Health Laboratory, Public Health Service of Amsterdam (GGD), Nieuwe Achtergracht 100, Amsterdam 1018 WT, The Netherlands. [6]Department of Internal Medicine, Center for Infection and Immunity Amsterdam (CINIMA), Academic Medical Center, Meibergdreef 9, Amsterdam 1105 AZ, The Netherlands.

References

1. Keppel KG, Pearcy JN, Heron MP. Is there progress toward eliminating racial/ ethnic disparities in the leading causes of death? Public Health Rep. 2010; 125(5):689–97.
2. de Martel C, Ferlay J, Franceschi S, Vignat J, Bray F, Forman D, Plummer M. Global burden of cancers attributable to infections in 2008: a review and synthetic analysis. Lancet Oncol. 2012;13(6):607–15.
3. Arnold M, Aarts MJ, van der Aa M, Visser O, Coebergh JW. Investigating cervical, oesophageal and colon cancer risk and survival among migrants in The Netherlands. Eur J Public Health. 2013;23(5):867–73.
4. Carter JJ, Koutsky LA, Hughes JP, Lee SK, Kuypers J, Kiviat N, Galloway DA. Comparison of human papillomavirus types 16, 18, and 6 capsid antibody responses following incident infection. J Infect Dis. 2000;181(6):1911–9.
5. Ho GY, Studentsov YY, Bierman R, Burk RD. Natural history of human papillomavirus type 16 virus-like particle antibodies in young women. Cancer Epidemiol Biomarkers Prev. 2004;13(1):110–6.
6. Steele J, Collins S, Wen K, Ryan G, Constandinou-Williams C, Woodman CB. Measurement of the humoral immune response following an incident human papillomavirus type 16 or 18 infection in young women by a pseudovirion-based neutralizing antibody assay. Clin Vaccine Immunol. 2008;15(9):1387–90.
7. Jaisamrarn U, Castellsague X, Garland SM, Naud P, Palmroth J, Del Rosario-Raymundo MR, Wheeler CM, Salmeron J, Chow SN, Apter D, et al. Natural history of progression of HPV infection to cervical lesion or clearance: analysis of the control arm of the large, randomised PATRICIA study. PloS One. 2013;8(11), e79260.
8. Viscidi RP, Ahdieh-Grant L, Clayman B, Fox K, Massad LS, Cu-Uvin S, Shah KV, Anastos KM, Squires KE, Duerr A, et al. Serum immunoglobulin G response to human papillomavirus type 16 virus-like particles in human immunodeficiency virus (HIV)-positive and risk-matched HIV-negative women. J Infect Dis. 2003;187(2):194–205.
9. Vriend HJ, Bogaards JA, van der Klis FR, Scherpenisse M, Boot HJ, King AJ, van der Sande MA, Medical Microbiological Laboratories MHS. Patterns of human papillomavirus DNA and antibody positivity in young males and females, suggesting a site-specific natural course of infection. PloS One. 2013;8(4), e60696.
10. Paaso AE, Louvanto K, Syrjanen KJ, Waterboer T, Grenman SE, Pawlita M, Syrjanen SM. Lack of type-specific concordance between human papillomavirus (HPV) serology and HPV DNA detection in the uterine cervix and oral mucosa. J Gen Virol. 2011;92(Pt 9):2034–46.
11. Castro FA, Dominguez A, Puschel K, Van De Wyngard V, Snijders PJ, Franceschi S, Pawlita M, Ferreccio C. Serological prevalence and persistence of high-risk human papillomavirus infection among women in Santiago, Chile. BMC Infect Dis. 2014;14:361.
12. Clifford GM, Shin HR, Oh JK, Waterboer T, Ju YH, Vaccarella S, Quint W, Pawlita M, Franceschi S. Serologic response to oncogenic human papillomavirus types in male and female university students in Busan, South Korea. Cancer Epidemiol Biomarkers Prev. 2007;16(9):1874–9.
13. Bontkes HJ, de Gruijl TD, Walboomers JM, Schiller JT, Dillner J, Helmerhorst TJ, Verheijen RH, Scheper RJ, Meijer CJ. Immune responses against human papillomavirus (HPV) type 16 virus-like particles in a cohort study of women with cervical intraepithelial neoplasia. II. Systemic but not local IgA responses correlate with clearance of HPV-16. J Gen Virol. 1999;80(Pt 2):409–17.
14. Wu X, Zhang C, Feng S, Liu C, Li Y, Yang Y, Gao J, Li H, Meng S, Li L, et al. Detection of HPV types and neutralizing antibodies in Gansu province, China. J Med Virol. 2009;81(4):693–702.
15. Skjeldestad FE, Mehta V, Sings HL, Ovreness T, Turpin J, Su L, Boerckel P, Roberts C, Bryan J, Jansen KU, et al. Seroprevalence and genital DNA prevalence of HPV types 6, 11, 16 and 18 in a cohort of young Norwegian women: study design and cohort characteristics. Acta Obstet Gynecol Scand. 2008;87(1):81–8.
16. Stronks K, Snijder MB, Peters RJ, Prins M, Schene AH, Zwinderman AH. Unravelling the impact of ethnicity on health in Europe: the HELIUS study. BMC Public Health. 2013;13:402.
17. van Houdt R, Bruisten SM, Geskus RB, Bakker M, Wolthers KC, Prins M, Coutinho RA. Ongoing transmission of a single hepatitis B virus strain among men having sex with men in Amsterdam. J Viral Hepat. 2010;17(2):108–14.
18. Molijn A, Kleter B, Quint W, van Doorn LJ. Molecular diagnosis of human papillomavirus (HPV) infections. J Clin Virol. 2005;32 Suppl 1:S43–51.
19. Waterboer T, Sehr P, Michael KM, Franceschi S, Nieland JD, Joos TO, Templin MF, Pawlita M. Multiplex human papillomavirus serology based on in situ-purified glutathione s-transferase fusion proteins. Clin Chem. 2005;51(10): 1845–53.
20. Markowitz LE, Sternberg M, Dunne EF, McQuillan G, Unger ER. Seroprevalence of human papillomavirus types 6, 11, 16, and 18 in the United States: National Health and Nutrition Examination Survey 2003–2004. J Infect Dis. 2009;200(7):1059–67.
21. Nielsen A, Kjaer SK, Munk C, Iftner T. Type-specific HPV infection and multiple HPV types: prevalence and risk factor profile in nearly 12,000 younger and older Danish women. Sex Transm Dis. 2008;35(3):276–82.
22. Hildesheim A, Schiffman MH, Gravitt PE, Glass AG, Greer CE, Zhang T, Scott DR, Rush BB, Lawler P, Sherman ME, et al. Persistence of type-specific human papillomavirus infection among cytologically normal women. J Infect Dis. 1994;169(2):235–40.
23. Castle PE, Schiffman M, Herrero R, Hildesheim A, Rodriguez AC, Bratti MC, Sherman ME, Wacholder S, Tarone R, Burk RD. A prospective study of age trends in cervical human papillomavirus acquisition and persistence in Guanacaste, Costa Rica. J Infect Dis. 2005;191(11):1808–16.
24. Scherpenisse M, Mollers M, Schepp RM, Boot HJ, Meijer CJ, Berbers GA, van der Klis FR, de Melker HE. Changes in antibody seroprevalence of seven high-risk HPV types between nationwide surveillance studies from 1995–96 and 2006–07 in The Netherlands. PloS One. 2012;7(11), e48807.

13

Epidemiologic characterization of human papillomavirus (HPV) infection in various regions of Yunnan Province of China

Zulqarnain Baloch[1,2], Yuanyue Li[1,2], Tao Yuan[3], Yue Feng[1,2], Yanqing Liu[3], Wenlin Tai[3], Li Liu[1,2], Binghui Wang[1,2], A-mei Zhang[1,2], Xiaomei Wu[3*] and Xueshan Xia[1,2*]

Abstract

Background: This study was designed to determine the Human papillomavirus (HPV) prevalence and its distribution of genotypes in various regions of Yunnan Province, China.

Method: In this study, participants were recruited during routine gynecologic examination between Oct 2013 and Feb 2015. A total of 17,898 women were recruited. Polymerase chain reaction was used for detecting the HPV positive samples and HPV geno-array test was used for genotyping.

Results: The overall HPV infection rate (19.9 %) among the south-western women was significantly higher ($P = 0.001$) than that among the north-western (18.0 %), south-eastern (13.3 %), north-eastern (11.1 %) and central women (12.9 %). The high-risk (HR) (18.1 %, $P = 0.001$) and single genotype (16.7 %, $P = 0.001$) infection rates among the South-western women were also significantly higher than those of among the north-western (13.9 %, 11.3 %), south-eastern (11.6 %, 10.5 %), north-eastern (9.6 %, 9.1 %) and central women (10.5 %, 10.0 %), respectively. While, the infections with multiple HPV (4.2 %) genotypes were significantly more common ($P = 0.001$) among women in north-western Yunnan than women in the south-western (1.3 %, 3.1 %), south-eastern (1.7 %, 2.7 %), north-eastern (1.5 %, 2.0 %) and central Yunnan (2.4 %, 2.9 %). A total of 30 HPV genotypes were detected; among them 13 were HR-HPV, 3 were PHR-HPV (Potential High risk), 8 were LR-HPV (Low risk) and six were unclassified. The most common HPV genotypes were HPV-52, 16, 58, 53 in control group, HPV-16, 52, 58, 39 and 53 in CINI (Cervical intraepithelial Neoplasia), HPV-52, 16, 58, 33, 53 and 81 in CINII, HPV16, 58, 18, 52, 81 in CINIII and HPV-16 18, 58, 52 in cervical cancer (CC), respectively. Such variation has also been observed about distribution of HPV genotypes distribution among single and multiple infections.

Conclusion: This study gives an epidemiological estimate of HPV prevalence and different genotype distribution in various region of Yunnan province and further explains its prevalence in different neoplastic lesions. Overall HPV-16, 52, 58, and 18 are the leading HR-HPV genotypes.

Keywords: Yunnan, Regions, Human papillomavirus, Intercourse, Distribution, Genotype

* Correspondence: w_xiaomei@163.com; oliverxia2000@aliyun.com
[3]The First Hospital in Yunnan province, Kunming 650034, China
[1]Faculty of Life Science and Technology, Kunming University of Science and Technology, Kunming 650500, China
Full list of author information is available at the end of the article

Background

Human papillomavirus (HPV) infections are the most frequently sexually transmitted infections throughout the world. Worldwide, the prevalence of HPV is approximately 11–12 % [1], and 85 % of the infections and 88 % of the deaths caused by this virus occur in developing countries [2]. The prevalence of HPV varies substantially with respect to ethnicity and geographic location [3–5].

Papillomaviruses are non-enveloped, circular, double-stranded DNA viruses with a genome length of 8-kb. More than 200 HPV genotypes have been reported, almost 40 of which are frequently transmitted through intercourse and remain in the genital system. Genital HPV infects most sexually active females at some point during their lives and plays a vital role in the development of cervical cancer [6, 7]. HPV genotypes are classified as high risk or low risk, according to their carcinogenicity. There are about one dozen high-risk HPV genotypes, which are responsible for the formation of malignant lesions [5, 8, 9] while the low-risk genotypes may promote the development of low-grade carcinoma [9, 10]. Epidemiologically, significant geographic variation in HPV genotype distribution has been reported. Generally, the HPV-16 genotype is the most common worldwide, whereas the prevalences of the other genotypes vary from region to region [9]. Several HPV genotypes have been reported to cause cervical cancer, and geographic variation in the frequencies of these genotypes has also been reported [11]. Hence, the assessment of the regional distribution of these genotypes is extremely important for the prevention of cervical cancer.

The prevalence and genotype distributions of HPV are well documented in developed areas of China. The genotypes HPV-16, 18, 52, 58 and 59 are most commonly detected in Chinese women [12–14]. However, the pattern of HPV genotype distribution varies among different regions of the country [15]. Further, due an uneven distribution of cancer registry centres, the actual HPV prevalence is believed to be higher than the reported estimates [4].

Yunnan Province has a unique geographic location, highly complex topography, and large variations in elevation, and it has a diverse climate because of these distinctive features [16]. Yunnan is located at the threshold of the Himalayas. In north-western Yunnan, the mountains are large, the landscape is dry and rugged, and the weather is cold. It shares a border of 4060 km with Myanmar in the west, Laos in the south, and Vietnam in the south-east and the weather is hot in this region. Like its distinct topographical features, the social characteristics of Yunnan Province are also diverse [17]. Although individuals in some ethnic groups live in urban areas with racial admixture, most of them prefer to reside in individual concentrated communities with distinctive socio-cultural practices. Yunnan province is the homeland of a large number of ethnic minorities in China, including the Yi, Bai, Hani, Zhuang, Dai, Miao, Lisu, Hui, Lahu, Va, Naxi, Yao, Tibetan, Jingpo, Blang, Achang, Nu, Pumi, Jino, Benlong, Mongolian and Drung. Each of these ethnicities has its own typical customs, architectural style and unique literature. The Han population is a well-developed ethnic majority in China. It represents the largest population in this region and is equally distributed throughout Yunnan. To our knowledge, there have been no descriptions of the genotype distribution of HPV in Yunnan province. Therefore, the objective of the current study was to explore the epidemiological characteristics of the HPV genotype distributions in various regions of Yunnan Province, China and to further delineate the relationship of HPV genotype distribution with abnormal and normal cytological findings.

Methods

In this study, participants were recruited during routine gynecologic examination between Oct 2013 and Feb 2015. A Women who met the following criteria were recruited: those who (1) was mentally and physically normal, (2) was aged between above 18 years, (3) was a permanent resident of local region; (3) was not a virgin (4) had not undergone a total hysterectomy; (5) had no history of cervical surgery; (6) had never had pelvic radiation therapy. Initially 18,562 participants were recruited for this study. Sixty-three women excluded with due to invalid test result lesions and 45 were not willing for biopsy while 11 were excluded due to HPV-genotype lesions. A total of 17,898 women from the central region ($n = 7065$) north-west region ($n = 3772$), north-east region ($n = 3152$), south-west region ($n = 2164$) and south-east region ($n = 1745$) were recruited. The study designed and method has been described previously [18] with some modification.

Experimental ethics

The protocol used in this study was in accordance with the Declaration of Helsinki and was approved by the Ethics Committee at Kunming University of Science and Technology and the Center for Disease Control and Prevention (CDC) in Yunnan Province, China. Written consent was individually obtained from each participant.

Collection of data and cytological analysis

The women were interviewed at the hospital by trained interviewers using a standardized questionnaire to elicit information on socio-demographic risk factors. After the interview, all women underwent a pelvic examination performed by a senior gynecologist; two cervical scrapings were collected for cytological analysis and detection of HPV DNA. Both conventional smears and liquid-based cytology were performed.

All cytological slides were prepared by two qualified technicians individually. First Cytological slides were read locally by a junior cytopathologist from each geographical site according to the Bethesda classification system. All Pap smears with a diagnosis of atypical squamous cells of undetermined significance (ASC-US) or greater and a 10 % random sample of normal Pap smears were sent to the Research Center for Molecular Medicine, Kunming Yunnan for double cytological review by an expert senior cytopathologist who was blinded to the original diagnosis. Additionally, the slides read by the junior cytopathologist were used only for screening. The final diagnosis was the diagnosis of senior cytopathologist.

Histo-pathological analysis

During colposcopy, the cervix was divided into four parts and each part was observed individually. All visually abnormal areas were biopsied. Every part with normal colposcopic impressions had one random biopsy collected at the squamo-columnar junction. Endocervical curettage was then performed. All cervical biopsies were performed with standard 2 mm POI biopsy forceps, which allows rapid healing of the biopsy sites and minimizes patient distress. Histological slides were reviewed by two senior pathologists from Yunnan First Peoples Hospital.

The cervical intraepithelial neoplasia grading and cervical cancer was diagnosed according to the World Health Organization classification system *(CIN I–III)* [19].

HPV genotyping

Samples that tested positive for β-globin were analysed by PCR amplification of HPV DNA. HPV-positive samples were confirmed by PCR with universal L1 primer MY09/11 and GP5/6 systems [20]. DNA from HeLa and Caski cell lines was used as positive controls, and mixtures without sample DNA were used as negative controls. HPV genotypes were determined using an HPV GenoArray Test Kit (Hybribio, Chaozhou, China), according to the manufacturer's instructions. Geno-Array is an L1 consensus primer-based PCR assay [21] that is capable of amplifying 23 HPV genotypes, including 13 HR-HPV genotypes (HPV-16, 18, 31, 33, 35, 39, 45, 51, 52, 56, 58, 59, and 68), 3 PHR-HPV genotypes (HPV-53, 66, and 81) and 7 low-risk HPV (LR-HPV) genotypes (HPV-6, 11, 42, 43, 44 and 61). The assay was conducted according to the manufacturer's recommendations. PCR was performed in a reaction volume of 25 μl containing 5 μl of DNA template, 19.25 μl of the provided master mix, and 0.75 μl DNA Taq polymerase, using a Perkin-Elmer GeneAmp PCR System 9700 (Applied Biosystems) The amplification procedure was performed as follows: 9 min of denaturation at 95 °C, followed by 40 cycles of 20 s of denaturation at 95 °C, 30 s of annealing at 55 °C, 30 s of elongation at 72 °C, and a final extension for 5 min at 72 °C.

All the samples that were identified as positive through PCR were genotype with two methods. First we run Geno-Array test and secondly we performed direct sequencing. For the DNA sequencing, new PCR was run with reaction mixture 50 μL containing 6 μL of the DNA extract, 1 μL of 10 μmolar MY09 primer, 1 μL of 10 μmolar MY11 primer and 25 μL of the provided master mixture, and 15 μL dH2O. The consensus primer products were separated by electrophoresis on a 2 % agarose gel and purified with Tiangel PCR purification kit. The DNA was then directly sequenced using the ABI PRISM Big Dye Terminator Cycle Sequencing Ready Reaction (Invitrogen, Beijing, CN) on an ABI 310 DNA analyzer. The nucleotide sequences were aligned and compared with those of known HPV genotypes available through Genbank by using the BLAST 2.0 software server (http://blast.ncbi.nlm.nih.gov/Blast.cgi). The sample was identified as a particular HPV genotype if the sequence was 95 % homologous with the reference standard.

Statistical analysis

The Chi-square test was performed to compare the differences in HPV genotype distribution among the histo-pathologically normal and abnormal samples and among the various regions. Data analysis was performed using SPSS 20.0 (SPSS, Chicago, USA). All statistical tests were two-sided; P values < 0.05 were considered statistically significant.

Results

Population characteristics

All of the participants were recruited from various regions of Yunnan province, China (Table 1 and Fig. 1 show the regions inhabited by the study participants). The median age of the 17,898 women included in this study was 38 years, with a range of 18 to 93 years (mean = 40.5 years, SD = 8.79 years, 95 % CI, 40.37–40.63). A total of 75.2 % women were Han, and 24.8 % were of other ethnicities. In addition, 38.3 % of the women came from rural areas, and 61.7 % were from urban areas. Most of the women (82.3 %) were married and reported having a single sexual partner, and the mean number of years of sexual activity was 17. Only 57.7 % of the women had delivered a single baby. A summary of the participants' characteristics is shown in Table 1. Of the 17,898 women, 16,968 (94.8 %) had normal, 458 had CIN1, 247 had CIN2, 181 had CIN3, and 44 had CC (Table 3).

Table 1 The characteristics of HPV infected individuals

	Overall (*n* = 17898)	Central (*n* = 7065)	North-west (*n* = 3772)	North-east (*n* = 3152)	South-west (*n* = 2164)	South-east (*n* = 1745)
Normal	16968 (94.8)	6704 (94.9)	3570 (94.6)	2984 (94.7)	2062 (95.3)	1648 (94.4)
CINI	458 (2.5)	173 (2.4)	97 (2.8)	85 (2.7)	51 (2.3)	52 (3.0)
CINII	247 (1.4)	103 (1.4)	56 (1.5)	40 (1.3)	23 (1.1)	25 (1.4)
CINIII	181 (1.0)	64 (0.9)	37 (1.0)	36 (1.1)	25 (1.5)	19 (1.1)
CC	44 (0.2)	21 (0.3)	12 (0.3)	7 (0.2)	3 (0.1)	1 (0.05)
Ethnic						
Han	13465 (75.2)	5499 (77.8)	2841 (75.3)	2157 (68.4)	1658 (76.6)	1310 (75.1)
Others	4433 (24.8)	1566 (22.2)	931 (24.7)	995 (31.6)	506 (23.4)	435 (24.9)
Area						
Rural	6849 (38.3)	2695 (38.1)	1462 (38.8)	1176 (37.3)	820 (37.9)	696 (39.9)
Urban	11049 (61.7)	4370 (61.9)	2310 (61.2)	1976 (62.7)	1344 (62.1)	1049 (60.1)
Education						
Graduate	4399 (24.6)	1780 (25.2)	897 (23.8)	847 (26.9)	422 (19.5)	453 (25.9)
High	3841 (21.5)	1533 (21.7)	845 (22.4)	684 (21.7)	408 (18.8)	371 (21.3)
Middle	5564 (31.1)	2282 (32.3)	1114 (29.5)	892 (28.3)	733 (33.9)	543 (31.1)
Primary	2370 (13.2)	807 (11.4)	515 (13.6)	368 (11.3)	481 (22.2)	199 (11.4)
Illiterate	1724 (9.6)	663 (9.4)	401 (10.6)	361 (11.4)	120 (5.5)	179 (10.2)
Profession						
Farmer	3886 (21.7)	132[illegible] (18.7)	730 (19.3)	643 (20.4)	663 (30.7)	529 (30.3)
Government	3489 (19.5)	1407 (19.9)	663 (17.6)	602 (19.1)	496 (22.9)	321 (18.4)
Others	2410 (13.5)	968 (13.7)	547 (14.5)	351 (11.1)	307 (14.2)	237 (13.4)
Private	3918 (21.9)	1613 (22.8)	882 (23.4)	704 (22.3)	381 (17.6)	338 (19.4)
Services	2689 (15.9)	1141 (16.1)	619 (16.4)	497 (15.8)	253 (11.7)	179 (10.2)
No work	1506 (8.4)	615 (7.8)	331 (8.8)	355 (11.3)	64 (2.9)	141 (8.1)
Smoke						
Yes	7619 (42.6)	2981 (42.2)	1565 (41.5)	1409 (44.7)	903 (41.7)	761 (43.6)
No	10279 (57.4)	4084 (57.8)	2207 (58.5)	1743 (55.3)	1261 (58.3)	984 (56.4)
Drinking						
Yes	11203 (62.6)	4759 (67.4)	1613 (42.8)	2183 (69.2)	1469 (67.9)	1179 (67.6)
No	6695 (37.4)	2306 (32.6)	2159 (57.2)	969 (30.7)	695 (32.1)	566 (32.4)
Material status						
Married	14675 (82.0)	5921 (83.3)	3078 (81.6)	2478 (78.6)	1799 (83.1)	1399 (80.2)
Single	3223 (18.0)	1144 (16.2)	694 (18.4)	674 (21.3)	365 (16.9)	346 (19.8)
Pregnancy						
Single	10334 (57.7)	4511 (63.8)	2033 (53.9)	1653 (52.4)	1187 (54.8)	950 (54.4)
Multiple	7564 (42.3)	2554 (36.2)	1739 (46.1)	1499 (47.5)	977 (45.1)	795 (45.4)
Age groups						
<35 years	6582 (36.8)	2779 (39.3)	1452 (38.5)	1092 (34.6)	759 (35.1)	500 (28.6)
36–45	6941 (38.9)	3195 (45.3)	957 (25.4)	1115 (35.4)	710 (32.8)	964 (55.2)
>46 years	4375 (24.4)	1091 (15.4)	1363 (36.1)	945 (30.0)	695 (32.1)	281 (16.1)

n number

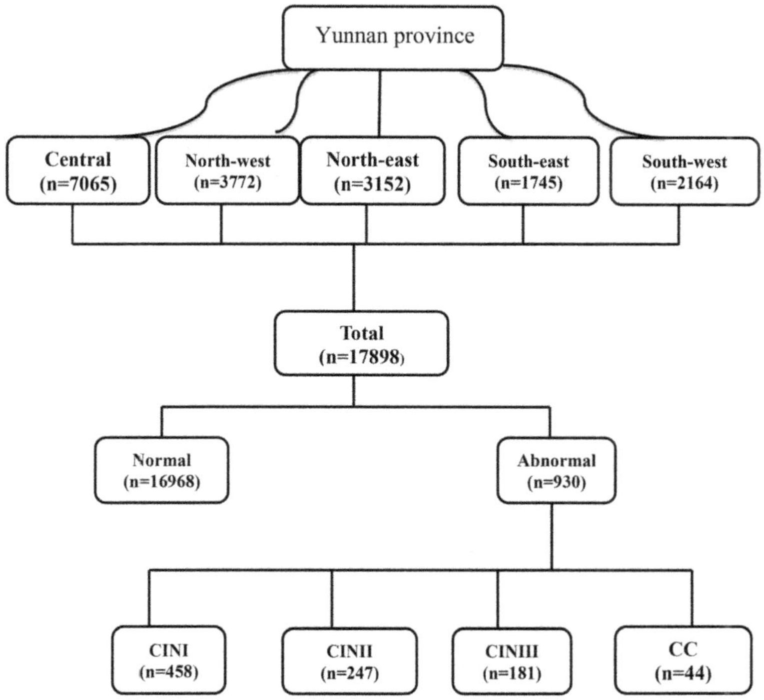

Fig. 1 Overview of study population

HPV genotype distribution by region

The overall HPV infection rate (19.9 %) among the south-western women was significantly higher than that among the north-western (18.0 %), south-eastern (13.3 %), north-eastern (11.1 %) and central women (12.9 %). The high-risk (HR) (18.1 %) and single genotype (16.7 %) infection rates among the South-western women were also significantly higher than those of among the north-western (13.9 %, 11.3 %), south-eastern (11.6 %, 10.5 %), north-eastern (9.6 %, 9.1 %) and central women (10.5 %, 10.0 %), respectively. While, the infections with other HPV (4.1 %) and with multiple HPV (4.2 %) genotypes were significantly more common ($P = 0.001$) among women in north-western than women in the south-western (1.3 %, 3.1 %), south-eastern (1.7 %, 2.7 %), north-eastern (1.5 %, 2.0 %) and central women (2.4 %, 2.9 %). The HPV genotype distribution data by region is shown in Table 4. The prevalence of HPV-16 (5.9 %) and HPV-58 (3.5 %) were significantly ($P = 0.001$, $P = 0.001$) more frequent in the southwest region compared with those in the central, north-east, south-east, and north-west regions. With the exception of the above-mentioned genotypes, no significance differences in the distributions of any of the other HPV genotypes were observed among the five regions of Yunnan province (Table 2).

HPV genotypes and histo-pathological grades

The prevalence of overall, HR-HPV, and single genotypes infection significantly increased as the infection progressed in advanced lesions. While, the prevalence of multiple genotypes infection and other genotypes were decreased as the infection progressed in advanced lesions but the difference was not significant. HPV-16, 58, 52, and 18 were significantly more frequent in advance abnormal cervical lesion that those of other genotypes (Fig. 2). The distribution of HPV genotypes according to cervical histo-pathological stage is shown in Table 2. A total of 23 HPV genotypes were detected in the histo-pathologically abnormal samples with different prevalence rates. The six most common HPV genotypes detected in the CINI samples were HPV-16, 52, 58, 53, 39, and 81. In the CINII samples, HPV-52 was the most prevalent, followed by HPV-16, 58, 33, 81, and 51. However, in the CINIII and CC samples, HPV-16 was more prevalent, followed by HPV-58, 18, and 52. A total of 30 HPV genotypes were detected in the normal group, the most common of which were HPV-52, followed by HPV-16, 58, 53, 18, 51, 68 and 81 (Table 3).

In this study, three PHR-HPV genotypes (HPV-53, 66, and 81) were also detected, and they were highly prevalent in the CIN1 and CIN2 samples. Only three CC samples were found to have a co-infection with the HPV-66 and HR-HPV genotypes. Interestingly, eight single and multiple LR-HPV infections were detected in both the normal and abnormal cytology groups. Some of the unclassified HPV genotypes, such as HPV-67, 69, 70, 71, 82 and 83, were also found in the control group. Table 3 shows the genotype distributions among the abnormal cytology and control groups.

Table 2 HPV Prevalence and genotype distribution among various regions of Yunnan province

Variable	Overall (*n* = 17898)	Central *n* = 7065	North-east *n* = 3152	North-west *n* = 3772	South-east *n* = 1745	South-west *n* = 2164	*P*-Value
Overall[a]	14.0 (13.5–14.5	12.9 (12.1–13.7)	11.1 (10.0–12.2)	18.0 (16.8–19.2)	13.3 (11.7–14.9)	19.9 (18.2–21.6)	0.001
High risk[a]	12.2 (−11.7–12.7)	10.5 (9.8–11.2)	9.6 (8.6–10.6)	13.9 (12.0–14.2)	11.6 (10.1–13.1)	18.1 (16.5–19.7)	0.001
Others[a]	1.8 (1.6–2.0)	2.4 (2.04–2.7)	1.5 (1.1–1.9)	4.1 (3.5–4.7)	1.7 (1.1–2.3)	1.3 (0.8–1.8)	0.001
Single infection[a]	11.0 (10.5–11.4)	10.0 (9.3–10.7)	9.1 (8.1–10.1)	11.3 (10.3–12.3)	10.5 (9.1–11.9)	16.7 ((15.1–18.3)	0.001
Multiple infection[a]	3.0 (2.8–3.2)	2.9 (2.5–3.3)	2.0 (1.5–2.5)	4.2 (3.6–4.8)	2.7 (1.9–3.5)	3.1 (2.4–3.8)	0.001
Unidentified[a]	1.1 (0.9–1.2)	0.7 (0.5–0.9)	0.8 (0.5–1.1)	2.2 (1.7–2.7)	0.9 (0.5–1.3)	0.9 (0.5–1.3)	0.009
HR-HPV							
HPV-52[a]	3.1 (2.9–3.3)	3.4 (3.0–3.8)	2.4 (1.9–2.9)	3.3 (2.7–3.9)	3.0 (2.2–3.8)	3.1 (2.4–3.8)	0.15
HPV-16[a]	3.4 (3.1–3.7)	3.0 (2.8–3.2)	2.4 (1.9–2.9)	3.5 (2.9–4.1)	3.4 (2.5–4.2)	5.9 (4.9–6.9)	0.001
HPV-58[a]	2.1 (1.9–2.3)	1.9 (1.6–2.2)	1.4 (1.0–1.8)	2.3 (1.8–2.8)	1.5 (0.9–2.1)	3.5 (2.7–4.3)	0.001
HPV-18[a]	1.2 (1.0–1.3)	1.1 (0.9–1.3)	1.4 (1.0–1.8)	1.4 (1.0–1.8)	13 (0.7)	1.5 (1.0–2.0)	0.16
HPV-51	120 (0.7)	49 (0.7)	18 (0.6)	23 (0.6)	-	30 (1.4)	0.2
HPV-39	118 (0.6)	45 (0.6)	13 (0.4)	34 (0.9)	17 (1.0)	9 (0.4)	0.69
HPV-33	124 (0.7)	44 (0.6)	20 (0.6)	52 (1.4)	-	8 (0.4)	0.35
HPV-68	122 (0.7)	43 (0.6)	19 (0.6)	31 (0.8)	9 (0.5)	20 (0.9)	
HPV-56	60 (0.3)	32 (0.4)	4 (0.1)	8 (0.2)	8 (0.4)	8 (0.4)	
HPV-59	56 (0.3)	27 (0.4)	3 (0.1)	19 (0.5)	5 (0.3)	2 (0.09)	
HPV-31	63 (0.3)	23 (0.3)	9 (0.3)	11 (0.3)	7 (0.4)	13 (0.6)	
HPV-35	(12) 0.07	7 (0.01)	5 (0.1)	-	-	-	
HPV-45	12 (0.07)	3 (0.04)	5 (0.1)	-	4 (0.2)	-	
PHR-HPV							
HPV-53	176 (1.0)	75 (1.1)	33 (1.0)	32 (0.8)	25 (1.4)	11 (0.5)	
HPV-81	108 (0.6)	42 (0.6)	12 (0.4)	23 (0.6)	13 (0.7)	18 (0.8)	
HPV-66		15 (0.2)	9 (0.3)	16 (0.4)	10 (0.6)	18 (0.8)	
LR-HPV							
HPV-11	68 (0.4)	14 (0.2)	-	7 (0.2)	6 (0.3)	5 (0.2)	
HPV-6	16 (0.09)	9 (0.1)	-	4 (0.1)	3 (0.2)	-	
HPV-61	30 (0.2)	-	9 (0.3)	5 (0.1)	7 (0.4)	9 (0.4)	
HPV-43	15 (0.08)	7 (0.1)	-	-	-	8 (0.4)	
HPV-55	7 (0.04)	6 (0.08)	1 (0.03)	-	-	-	
HPV-44	12 (0.07)	5 (0.07)	-	-	-	7 (0.3)	
HPV-42	9 (0.05)	4 (0.06)	-	-	3 (0.2)	2 (0.09)	
HPV-40	4 (0.02)	-	4 (0.1)	-	-	-	
HPV-67	1 (0.005)	-	1 (0.03)	-	-	-	
HPV-69	1 (0.005)	-	1 (0.03)	-	-	-	
HPV-70	2 (0.01)	2 (0.03)	-	-	-	-	
HPV-71	3 (0.002)	3 (0.04)	-	-	-	-	
HPV-82	6 (0.03)	1 (0.02)	-	-	2 (0.1)	3 (0.1)	
HPV-83	2 (0.01)	-	-	1 (0.02)	-	1 (0.05)	

n number, [a]95% Confidence interval

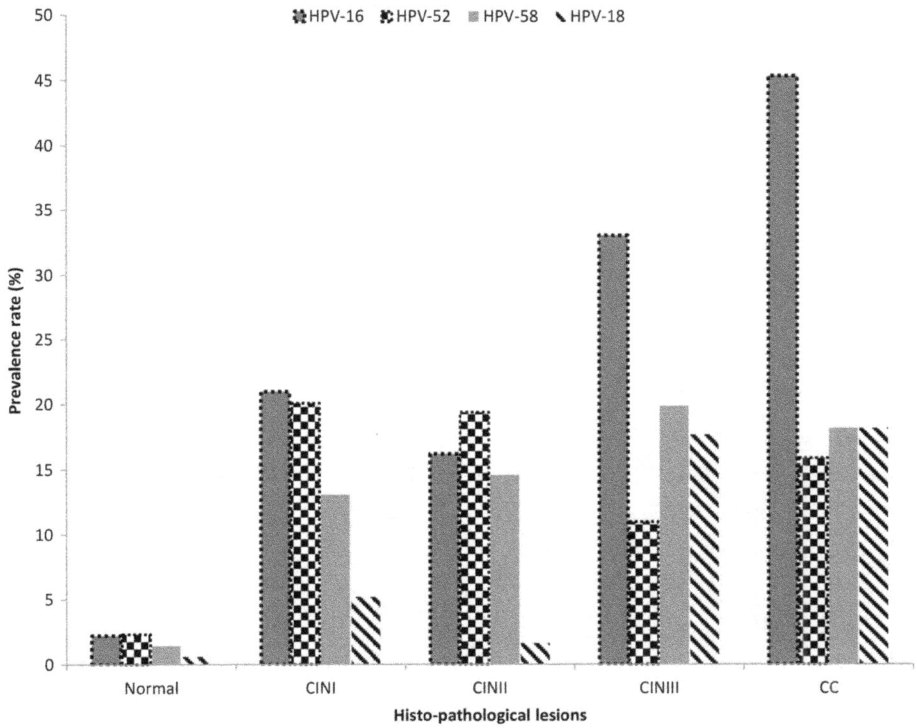

Fig. 2 Distribution of leading HPV genotypes among various histo-pathological lesions

HPV genotypes and infection

The distribution of HPV genotypes according to the type of infection is shown in Table 3. A total of 16,968 women had normal cytological (normal group) results, and of them, 8.3 % (1402/16968) were infected with a single HPV genotype. In contrast we identified the presence of HPV DNA in 60.4 % (562/930) of the women in the abnormal histo-pathological group. Multiple genotype infections were the most common, and the rate of this type of infection was significantly higher (Table 2, $P = 0.001$) in the abnormal histo-pathological group (236/930, 24.4 %) compared with that in the normal group (1.8 %, 304/16968). The proportion of uncharacterised infection was also higher in the abnormal histo-pathological group (7.1 %, 68/930) compared with that in the normal group (0.75 %, 128/16968). The distribution of HPV genotypes according to the type of infection is shown in Table 3. In cases of single infection, HPV-16 (abnormal histo-pathological group = 136/562, 24.2 %; normal group = 280/16968, 1.6 %; $P = 0.001$), 18 (abnormal histo-pathological group = 48/562, 8.5 %; normal group = 84/16968, 0.5 %; $P = 0.003$), 33 (abnormal histo-pathological group = 36/562, 6.4 %; normal group = 48/16968, 0.3 %; $P = 0.001$), and 58 (abnormal histo-pathological group = 88/562, 15.7 %; normal group = 152/16968, 0.9 %; $P = 0.001$) were detected significantly more frequently in the abnormal histo-pathological group compared with the control group. In addition, HPV-31 (abnormal histo-pathological group = 3/562, 0.5 %; normal group = 36/16968, 0.21 %; $P = 0.002$), 51 (abnormal histo-pathological group = 8/562, 1.4 %; normal group = 52/1402, 0.3 %; $P = 0.001$), 61 (abnormal histo-pathological group = 3/562, 0.5 %; normal group = 24/16968, 0.1 %; $P = 0.05$), 66 (abnormal histo-pathological group = 3/562, 0.5 %; normal group = 24/16968, 0.1 %; $P = 0.05$), and 68 (abnormal histo-pathological group = 10/562, 1.8 %; normal group = 52/16968, 0.3 %; $P = 0.001$) were significantly more common in the normal group compared with the abnormal histo-pathological group (Table 4).

To determine the possible variation in HPV genotype distribution among the various age groups, the abnormal histo-pathological and normal groups were stratified into three groups according to age. Correlation analysis revealed that HPV prevalence was more complex in the younger and older participants compared with the middle age group (Figs. 3 and 4). The highest overall, HR-HPV and multiple HPV prevalence was observed in the <35 years age group, and it declined thereafter with increasing age. A less pronounced second peak in prevalence was observed for the normal women in the older age group (>46 years). However, overall, high-risk and multiple-genotype infections among the abnormal histo-pathological women exhibited two peaks in prevalence, with the first peaks of 88.9, 63.5 and 25.5 %, respectively, occurring at <35 years and the second peaks of 95.5, 64.3 and 31.2 % occurring at >46 years. Overall, we

Table 3 Prevalence of Human Papillomavirus (HPV) and its genotype distribution among normal and histo-pathological abnormal lesion

Variable	Normal	CIN1	CIN2	CIN3	SCC	*P*-Value
	(*n* = 16968)	(*n* = 458)	(*n* = 247)	(*n* = 181)	(*n* = 44)	
overall[a]	10.0 (9.5–10.4)	81.2 (77.6–84.8)	86.2 (81.9–90.5)	94.5 (91.2–97.8)	95.4	0.001
High risk[a]	9.1 (8.7–9.5)	64.0 (59.6–68.4)	65.2 (59.3–71.1)	80.1 (74.3–85.9)	88.6 (79.2–98.0)	0.001
Others[a]	166 (1.0)	17.2 (13.8–20.6)	21.0 (15.9–26.1)	14.4 (9.3–19.5)	6.8	0.17
Single[a] infection[a]	8.3 (7.9–8.7)	56.8 (51.9–60.9)	55.5 (49.3–61.7)	72.4 (65.9–78.9)	77.3 (64.9–89.7)	0.001
Multiple infection[a]	1.8 (1.6–2.0)	24.4 (20.5–28.3)	30.8 (25.1–36.5)	22.1 (16.1–28.1)	18.2 (6.8–29.6)	0.5
Unidentified[a]	0.7	7.0 (4.7–9.3)	8.1 (4.7–11.5)	6.6 (3.0–10.2)	9.1 (0.6–17.6)	
HR-HPV						
HPV-16[a]	2.2 (1.9–2.4)	21.0 (17.3–24.7)	16.2 (11.6–20.8)	33.1 (26.3–39.9)	45.4 (30.7–60.1)	0.001
HPV-52[a]	2.3 (2.1–2.5)	20.1 (16.4–23.8)	19.4 (14.5–24.3)	11.0 (6.5–15.5)	15.9 (5.1–26.7)	0.025
HPV-58[a]	1.4	13.1 (10.0–16.2)	14.6 (10.2–20.0)	19.9 (14.1–25.7)	18.2 (6.8–29.6)	0.04
HPV-18[a]	0.6	5.2 (3.2–7.2)	1.6 (0.03–3.2)	17.7 (12.1–23.3)	18.2 (6.8–29.6)	0.001
HPV-51	92 (0.5)	16 (3.5)	12 (4.8)	-	-	
HPV-68	84 (0.5)	23 (5.0)	8 (3.2)	7 (3.9)	-	
HPV-33	80 (0.5)	20 (4.4)	20 (8.1)	4 (2.2)	-	
HPV-39	76 (0.4)	28 (6.1)	8 (3.2)	4 (2.2)	-	
HPV-31	48 (0.3)	6 (1.3)	4 (1.6)	5 (2.8)	-	
HPV-56	40 (0.2)	8 (1.7)	8 (3.2)	4 (2.2)	-	
HPV-59	40 (0.2)	8 (1.7)	-	4 (2.2)	4 (9.1)	
HPV-45	4 (0.02)	6 (1.3)	-	2 (1.1)	-	
HPV-35	9 (0.05)	3 (0.6)	-	-	-	
PHR-HPV						
HPV-53	128 (0.7)	28 (6.1)	20 (8.1)	-	-	
HPV-81	52 (0.3)	24 (5.2)	19 (7.7)	12 (6.6)	-	
HPV-66	44 (0.2)	8 (1.7)	8 (3.2)	4 (2.2)	3 (6.8)	
Others						
HPV-61	24 (0.1)	-	3 (1.2)	-	-	
HPV-11	24 (0.1)	-	4 (1.6)	4 (2.2)	-	
HPV-6	12 (0.07)	-	-	4 (2.2)	-	
HPV-43	8 (0.05)	4 (0.9)	-	3 (1.6)	-	
HPV-44	8 (0.05)	4 (0.9)	-	-	-	
HPV-42	4 (0.02)	2 (0.4)	-	3 (1.6)	-	
HPV-55	4 (0.02)	3 (0.6)	-	-	-	
HPV-40	4 (0.02)	-	-	-	-	
HPV-67	1 (0.005)	-	-	-	-	
HPV-69	1 (0.005)	-	-	-	-	
HPV-70	2 (0.01)	-	-	-	-	
HPV-71	3 (0.01)	-	-	-	-	
HPV-82	6 (0.03)	-	-	-	-	
HPV-83	2 (0.01)	-	-	-	-	

n number, [a]95 % Confidence interval

Table 4 Prevalence of Human Papillomavirus (HPV) and its genotypes among normal and histo-pathological abnormal cases with Single or Multiple genotypes infection

Variable	Single infection			Multiple infection		
	Normal	Abnormal	*P*-value	Control	Abnormal	*P*-value
	(*n* = 16968)	(*n* = 930)		(*n* = 16968)	(*n* = 930)	
Overall[a]	8.3 (7.9–8.7)	60.4 (58.8–62.0)	0.001	1.8 (1.6–2.0)	25.4 (22.6–28.2)	0.001
Unidentified[a]	0.7 (0.6–0.8)	7.3 (5.6–9.0)	0.001	-	-	
HPV-16[a]	1.6 (1.4–1.8)	14.6 (12.3–16.9)	0.001	0.6 (0.5–0.7)	9.9 (8.0–11.8)	0.001
HPV-52[a]	1.6 (1.4–1.8)	10.3 (8.4–12.2)	0.001	0.6 (0.5–0.7)	7.7 (6.0–9.4)	0.001
HPV-58[a]	0.9 (0.8–1.0)	9.5 (7.6–11.4)	0.001	0.5 (0.4–0.6)	5.6 (4.1–7.1)	0.001
HPV-18	84 (0.5)	48 (5.2)	0.001	52 (0.3)	36 (3.9)	0.001
HPV-68	52 (0.3)	10 (1.1)	0.002	32 (0.2)	28 (3.0)	0.001
HPV-51	52 (0.3)	8 (0.9)	0.012	40 (0.2)	20 (2.1)	0.001
HPV-33	48 (0.3)	36 (3.9)	0.001	32 (0.2)	8 (0.9)	0.01
HPV-39	48 (0.3)	12 (1.3)	0.001	28 (0.2)	28 (3.0)	0.001
HPV-31	36 (0.2)	3 (0.3)	0.45	12 (0.07)	12 (1.3)	0.001
HPV-59	28 (0.2)	12 (1.3)	0.001	12 (0.07)	4 (0.4)	0.008
HPV-56	20 (0.1)	-		20 (0.1)	16 (1.7)	0.001
HPV-45	4 (0.02)	-		-	8 (0.9)	
HPV-35	3 (0.02)	-		6 (0.03)	3 (0.3)	0.008
PHR-HPV						
HPV-53	88 (0.5)	24 (2.6)	0.001	40 (0.2)	24 (2.6)	0.001
HPV-66	24 (0.1)	3 (0.3)	0.16	20 (0.1)	20 (2.1)	0.001
HPV-81	20 (0.1)	11 (1.2)	0.001	32 (0.2)	44 (4.7)	0.001
LR-HPV						
HPV-61	24 (0.1)	3 (0.3)	0.16	-	-	
HPV-11	-	-		24 (0.1)	8 (0.9)	0.001
HPV-6	-	-		12 (0.07)	4 (0.4)	0.008
HPV-42	-	-		5 (0.03)	4 (0.4)	0.001
HPV-55	4 (0.02)	3 (0.3)		-	-	
HPV-40	4 (0.02)	-			-	
HPV-44	4 (0.02)	-		4 (0.02)	4 (0.4)	0.001
HPV-43	3 (0.01)	-		4 (0.02)	8 (0.9)	0.001
Unclassified						
HPV-82	7 (0.04)	-		-	-	
HPV-71	3 (0.02)	-		-	-	
HPV-70	2 (0.01)	-		-	-	
HPV-83	2 (0.01)	-		-	-	
HPV-67	1 (0.005)	-		-	-	
HPV-69	1 (0.005)	-		-	-	

n number, [a]95 % Confidence interval

did not find significant differences among the various age groups in HPV genotype distribution. Correlation analysis revealed that the HPV genotype prevalence's were highly correlated in single and multiple infections among the younger women (<35 years) and older women in both the normal and abnormal histo-pathological groups. However, HPV-16 was more frequent in the younger women (<35 years) in both the normal and abnormal histo-pathological groups. The prevalence's of other genotypes, such as HPV-52, 58, 68, 33, 53, and 66, were found vary among the different age groups and varying histo-pathological grades (Table 5).

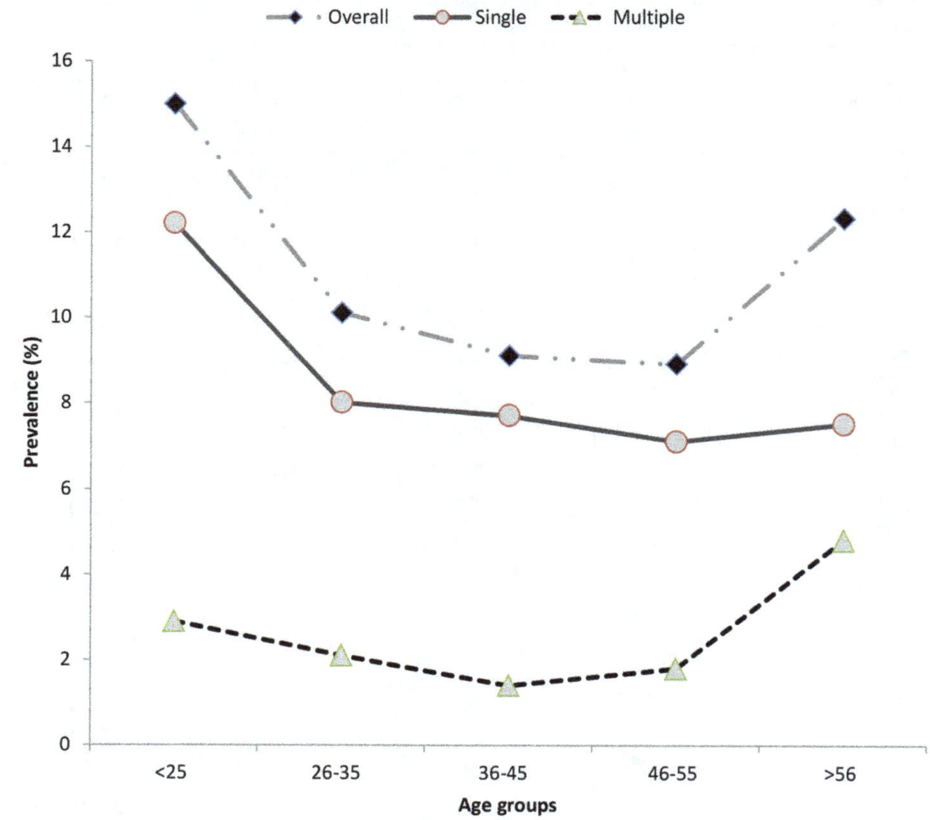

Fig. 3 Age-specific HPV prevalence among normal cases

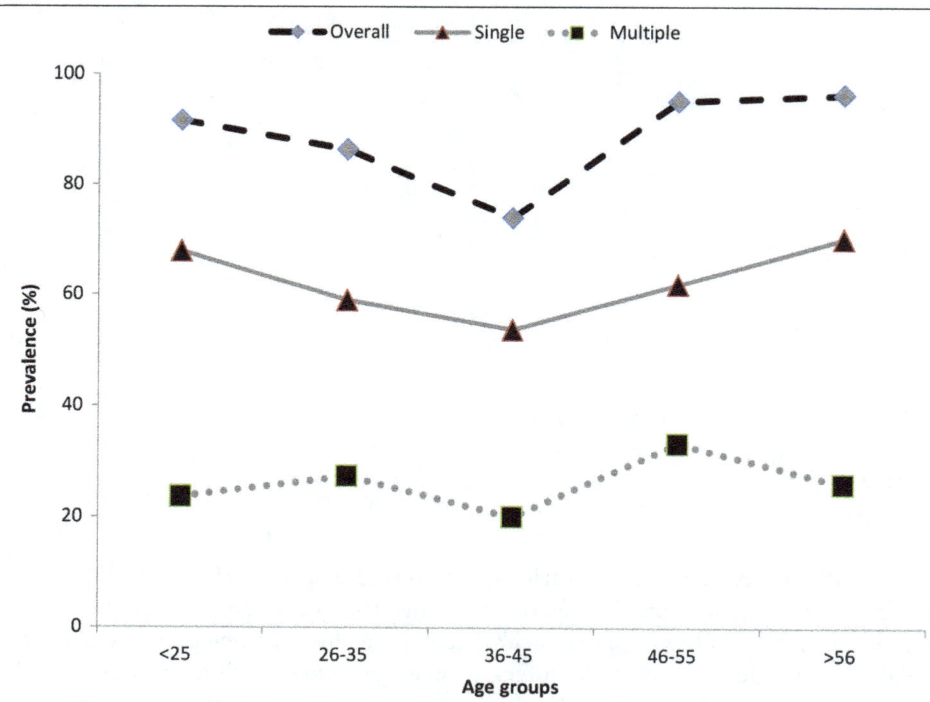

Fig. 4 Age-specific HPV prevalence among histo-pathological abnormal cases

Table 5 Prevalence of Human Papillomavirus (HPV) genotypes in according to histo-pathological result among various Age groups

Variables	Normal cases				Histo-pathologically abnormal cases			
	>35 years (*N* = 5978)	36–45 years (*n* = 6534)	<46 years (*n* = 4456)	*P*-value	>35 years (*n* = 326)	36–45 years (*n* = 318)	<46 years (*n* = 286)	*P*-Value
Overall	721 (12.1)	592 (9.1)	443 (9.9)	0.001	290 (88.9)	235 (73.9)	273 (95.4)	0.045
Single	579 (9.7)	502 (7.7)	321 (7.2)	0.001	207 (63.5)	171 (53.8)	184 (64.3)	0.9
Multiple	142 (2.4)	90 (1.4)	122 (2.7)	0.44	83 (25.5)	64 (20.1)	89 (31.2)	0.13
HR-HPV	1087							
HPV-16	160 (2.7)	132 (2.0)	88 (2.0)	0.018	100 (30.7)	80 (25.1)	48 (16.8)	0.001
HPV-52	153 (2.5)	119 (1.8)	120 (2.7)	0.003	63 (19.3)	61 (19.2)	16 (5.6)	0.001
HPV-58	98 (1.6)	69 (1.0)	65 (1.4)	0.016	52 (15.5)	80 (25.1)	36 (12.6)	0.37
HPV-18	64 (1.1)	41 (0.6)	31 (0.7)	0.022	22 (6.7)	37 (11.6)	25 (8.7)	0.35
HPV-68	40 (0.7)	31 (0.5)	13 (0.3)	0.024	10 (3.1)	25 (7.9)	3 (1.0)	0.27
HPV-33	44 (0.7)	24 (0.4)	12 (0.3)	0.001	20 (6.1)	24 (7.5)	-	
HPV-51	29 (0.5)	43 (0.6)	20 (0.4)	0.25	12 (3.7)	16 (5.0)	-	
HPV-56	12 (0.2)	16 (0.2)	10 (0.2)	0.87	8 (2.4)	-	8 (2.8)	
HPV-31	10 (0.2)	15 (0.2)	23 (0.5)	0.002	8 (2.4)	6 (1.9)	1 (0.3)	
HPV-59	10 (0.2)	21 (0.3)	9 (0.2)		5 (1.5)	3 (0.9)	8 (2.8)	
HPV-39	8 (0.1)	32 (0.5)	16 (0.3)		8 (2.4)	18 (5.7)	14 (4.9)	
HPV-35	4 (0.07)	2 (0.03)	3 (0.07)		-	3 (0.9)	-	
HPV-45	1 (0.02)	3 (0.04)	-		2 (0.6)	-	6 (2.1)	
PHR-HPV	132							
HPV-53	28 (0.5)	56 (0.8)	44 (1.0)	0.003	16 (4.9)	16 (5.0)	16 (5.6)	0.7
HPV-66	23 (0.4)	11 (0.2)	10 (0.2)	0.05	13 (4.0)	6 (1.9)	4 (1.4)	
HPV-81	20 (0.3)	12 (0.2)	20 (0.4)	0.042	-	22 (6.9)	15 (5.2)	
Others	183				-	-	-	
HPV-83	-	2 (0.03)	-		-	-	-	
HPV-69	-	1 (0.01)	-		-	-	-	
HPV-70	-	2 (0.03)	-		-	-	-	
HPV-71	-	-	3 (0.07)		-	-	-	
HPV-82	4 (0.05)	-	3 (0.07)		-	-	-	
HPV-67	1 (0.02)	-	-		-	-	-	
HPV-61	11 (0.2)	7 (0.1)	6 (0.1)	0.5	3 (0.9)	-	-	
HPV-11	10 (0.2)	7 (0.1)	7 (0.1)	0.63	-	-	8 (2.8)	
HPV-6	5 (0.08)	7 (0.1)	-		-	-	4 (1.4)	
HPV-40	4 (0.07)	-	-					
HPV-44	4 (0.07)	4 (0.06)	-		-	4 (1.2)	-	
HPV-43	2 (0.03)	-	5 (0.1)		-	3 (0.9)	5 (1.7)	
HPV-42	1 (0.02)	3 (0.04)	1 (0.02)		-	4 (1.2)	-	
HPV-55	-	4 (0.06)	-		-	3 (0.9)	-	
Unidentified	44 (0.7)	76 (1.2)	8 (0.2)	0.001	28 (8.6)	32 (10.1)	8 (2.8)	0.008

Discussion

Many studies have reported the HPV prevalence and its genotype distributions in various provinces of P. R. China [22, 23]. However, no relevant epidemiological data are available for Yunnan province. To the best of our knowledge, the current study is the first to report the epidemiological prevalence and distribution of HPV genotypes in various region of Yunnan. Samples screened in this study were obtained from different ethnic populations from different geographic regions of Yunnan province.

Therefore, the results of this study provide precise estimations of the HPV prevalence and genotype distributions in histo-pathological abnormal and normal cervical samples obtained from women throughout Yunnan province.

In this study, the overall HPV infection rate of 14.0 % was higher than the documented rates in neighbouring countries (6.2 % in Southeast Asia, 6.6 % in south central Asia and 8.0 % in other Asian countries [15, 24]. However, reports from some regions of mainland China have stated that the overall prevalence is 18.4 % in Shenzhen city [25], 13.3 % in Zhejiang province [26] and 14.8 % in Shanxi province [27], in agreement with our reported HPV prevalence. HPV prevalence has been documented to vary in different geographic regions, e.g., it is 8.1 % in Europe, 11.3 % in North America, 22.1 % in Africa and 8.0 % in Asia [15]. Here, we found that its prevalence was significantly higher among the south-western women (19.9 %) than the women from other four regions. The HPV prevalence in the south-western and north-western region was in line with the previously reported infection rate for north-western region of Yunnan (18.4 %) [27, 28]. However, the HR-HPV prevalence in the south-western women was very high compared with Zhejiang (10.2 %) and Shanxi (12.2 %) [29, 30]. The LR-HPV prevalence rates have been reported to be 3.8 and 4.4 % in Shanxi and Taiwan, respectively [29], which is in accordance with our identified LR-HPV prevalence of 4.1 % among the north-western region women. Comparatively, the calculated LR-HPV prevalence rate among the central, south-western, south-eastern and north-eastern regions women is similar to those in areas with lower LR-HPV prevalence rates in China, such as Shandong and Tibet [29, 31].

The distribution of HPV genotypes varies significantly in different geographic locations worldwide [15]. HPV-16 is the most frequently detected genotype in all regions of the world, followed by HPV-58 and 52 in Asia [24], HPV-58 in South America and HPV-31 in Europe [5]. In China, HPV-16 is the most prevalent genotype, followed by HPV-52 and 58 [26]. Moreover, HPV-33 and 31 are highly prevalent in some regions [27]. Such variation was also observed in this study, with HPV-52 being the most prevalent genotype in the central and north-east regions, followed by HPV-16 and 58. Interestingly HPV-18 is the 3rd most prevalent genotype in the north-east region only. In the north-west and south-east regions, HPV-16 is the most frequent, followed by HPV-52 and 58. Further, HPV-16 is most common in the south-west region, followed by HPV-58 and 52 (Table 5).

Our study findings do not support previously reported data that infection with multiple genotypes increases the risk of cervical cancer. Infection with multiple genotypes was significantly more frequent in the CINI and CIN2 samples. However, the prevalence this type of infection abruptly decreased with progression to CIN3 or cervical cancer. Further, infections with a single HR-HPV genotype resulted in an increase in cervical lesion progression. This finding might indicate that there is a lower risk of developing malignancy with multiple genotype infections compared with single genotype infections [32, 33] (Table 1).

Analysis of the specific HPV genotype distribution in the abnormal histo-pathological group indicated that it was highly variable in the histo-pathological abnormal lesions. HPV-16 (45.4 %) was the most frequently detected genotype in SCC, followed by HPV-58 (18.2 %), 18 (18.2 %), and 52 (15.9 %). Interestingly, 8 SCC patients were also found to have a multiple genotype infection (co-infection of HPV-59 and 66 with HPV-52 and 58, and 18). These findings are in complete agreement with previously reported data, indicating that HPV-16, 18, 52, and 58 are most frequently present in cervical cancer [9, 34]. HPV-16, 58, 18 and 52 were also frequent in the CIN3 samples, which is consistent with previous reports [25, 35]. All of these genotypes are considered to be highly oncogenic and are the most frequently detected HPV genotypes worldwide. Previous studies conducted in China and some other parts of the world have indicated that HPV-52 is the most frequent genotype in Asia, and particularly in China [25, 30]. In this study, HPV-52 was also a predominant genotype; however, its prevalence was higher in CIN1 and CIN2 samples compared with that in advanced cervical lesions. Based on these observations, infection with HPV-16, 58, and 18 might be associated with an elevated risk of cervical cancer development in the infected population. However, the declining trend in HPV-52 prevalence in advanced cervical lesions might be due to host immune factors or geographic or environmental factors [36]. In this study, we found high prevalence of other HR-HPV genotypes, such as HPV-33, 31, 39, 51, and 68, in the abnormal histo-pathological group. These genotypes were more common in the CIN1, CIN2 and CIN3 lesions than in SCC. HPV-31 and 33 are highly carcinogenic genotypes that are present worldwide [33, 37]. However, in this study, we did not find them to be highly carcinogenic, which may be due to variable geographic factors, biological factors, lifestyle, or human and viral genetic factors. Further, we found a high prevalence of PHR-HPV, particularly HPV-53 and 81 and the LR-HPV genotypes HPV-6 and 11. However, these genotypes were only identified in multiple genotype infections. These findings are in line with previously reported data [38]. In this study, the prevalence of HR-HPV was increased in samples with advanced histo-pathological grades. The incidence of HR-HPV infection, and particularly that of single genotype infection, was very high in the abnormal histo-pathological group compared with that in the normal group. These findings are in accordance with those of Castle et al. [39]. On the basis of these observations, we suggest that attention should be paid to the histopathological outcomes of CIN2, CIN3 and higher-grade lesions, even in the absence of specific genotype information.

In this study, we also evaluated the HPV genotype distributions among different age groups. HPV-16 was more frequent in women less than 35 years old in both the normal and abnormal cytology groups. However, the distributions of the other genotypes varied among the different age groups with lesions of differing cytology grades. HPV-52 and 18 showed double-peak prevalence in the normal cytology group. The prevalence of HPV-52 in the abnormal cytology group decreased with increasing age; however, that of HPV-18 increased with increasing age in this group. Such variation has also been observed for other genotypes, as shown in Table 4. These findings indicate that various age groups possess different genotypes in lesions with differing cytological grades [40]. Thus, it is very important to determine the potential roles of the different HPV genotypes in carcinogenesis development among various age groups and to further determine their potential risk and contribution to carcinogenesis in future studies.

The results of this study suggest that cervical screening is vital for women, particularly minority ethnic women, to prevent HPV-related cervical cancer [41]. An important link between HPV infection and development of cervical neoplasia has been identified in this study. Thus, the timely detection of HPV infection would be very helpful for preventing disease progression, considering that its early detection in patients with cervical lesions has been well established to result in a decrease in the rate of cancer development [42].

There are some limitations of this study that must be considered when interpreting our findings. Yunnan includes 26 state-certified ethnic minorities who live in different regions of the province. Most of them do not want to participate in epidemiological studies due to their ethnic beliefs. In this study, we focused only on those women who visited a public hospital with routine gynaecological examination.

Conclusion

This study provides epidemiological estimates of HPV genotype distributions in different regions of the province and further reports the prevalence of these genotypes in neoplastic lesions with differing cytological grades. We have found that overall, HPV-16, 52, 58, and 18 are the most common HR-HPV genotypes. However, the prevalence rates of these genotypes significantly differ in different regions of the province. PHR-HPV-53 is also a predominant genotype in some regions. These variations could be due to the large number of ethnic populations residing in the province. A vaccine currently under trial has been formulated for HPV-16, 18, 11, and 6, and it will be introduced nationally in the coming years. However, HPV-52 and 58 are the predominant genotypes in several regions. Thus, based on our observations, a new tetravalent vaccine may be more effective than a bivalent vaccine in China, and particularly in Yunnan province. Further, due to large-scale geographic variation in HPV genotype distribution, a future large-scale, multi-ethnic population-based study must be conducted to obtain comprehensive information on the prevalence and genotype distribution of HPV in various Chinese ethnic populations.

Abbreviations

HPV, human papillomavirus; HR-HPV, high risk-HPV; PHR-HPV, potential high risk-HPV; LR-HPV, low risk-HPV; CIN, cervical intraepithelial neoplasia; CC, cervical cancer.

Acknowledgments

We sincerely thank all the participants who took part in this study. We also sincerely thank Saqlain Abbas and Nafeesa Yasmeen (UVAS, Lahore) for their assistance with manuscript revision.

Funding

This study was supported by research grants from the Natural Science Foundation of China (81260248), Scientific and technological innovation talent support project (2015HC030) and the Key & New Product Development Project of Yunnan province (2013BC009). The funders had no role in the study design, data collection and analysis, decision to publish, or preparation of the manuscript.

Authors' contributions

ZB and LY designed the study, performed the data collection and genotyping, analysed the data and wrote the paper. TY, YL, and FY performed the data collection. LL, AZ, and WB contributed to collecting information from the participants. Prof. XX and XW supervised the study. All of the authors read and approved the final manuscript.

Competing interests

The authors declare that they have no competing interests.

Author details

[1]Faculty of Life Science and Technology, Kunming University of Science and Technology, Kunming 650500, China. [2]The Research Center for Molecular Medicine, Kunming 650500, China. [3]The First Hospital in Yunnan province, Kunming 650034, China.

References

1. Bruni L, Diaz M, Castellsague X, Ferrer E, Bosch FX, de Sanjose S. Cervical human papillomavirus prevalence in 5 continents: meta-analysis of 1 million women with normal cytological findings. J Infect Dis. 2010;202:1789–99.

2. Ferlay J, Shin HR, Bray F, Forman D, Mathers C. Parkin, D. M.; GLOBOCAN 2008 v2.0. Cancer incidence and mortality worldwide in 2008 IARC Cancer Base No. 10 (2010) http://www.iarc.fr/en/media-centre/iarcnews/2010/globocan2008.php. 20 Feb 2015.
3. Baloch Z, Yue L, Yuan T, Feng Y, Tai W, Liu Y, Wang B, Li X, Liu L, Zhang AM, Wu X, Xia X. Status of Human Papillomavirus Infection in the Ethnic Population in Yunnan Province, China. Biomed Res Int. 2015;2015:314815.
4. Yang L, Parkin DM, Li L. Time trends in cancer mortality in China: 1987–1999. Int J Cancer. 2003;106:771–83.
5. Clifford GM, Gallus S, Herrero R, Munoz N, Snijders PJ, et al. Worldwide distribution of human papillomavirus types in cytologically normal women in the International Agency for Research on Cancer HPV prevalence surveys: a pooled analysis. Lancet. 2005;366:991–8.
6. Liu X, Feng A, Cui Y, Tobe RG. Prevention of human papillomavirus (HPV) infection and cervical cancer in China: How does HPV vaccination bring about benefits to Chinese women? Biosci Trends. 2013;7:159–67.
7. Koutsky L. Epidemiology of genital human papillomavirus infection. Am J Med. 1997;102:3–8.
8. Li N, Franceschi S, Howell-Jones R, Snijders PJ, Clifford GM. Human papillomavirus type distribution in 30,848 invasive cervical cancers worldwide: Variation by geographical region, histological type and year of publication. Int J Cancer. 2011;128:927–35.
9. Crow JM. HPV: The global burden. Nature. 2012;488:S2–3.
10. Lacey CJ, Lowndes CM, Shah KV. Chapter 4: Burden and management of non-cancerous HPV-related conditions: HPV-6/11 disease. Vaccine. 2006;24:S35–41.
11. Munoz N, Bosch FX, Castellsague X, de Sanjose S, et al. Against which human papillomavirus types shall we vaccinate and screen? The international perspective. Int J Cancer. 2004;111:278–85.
12. Huang S, Afonina I, Miller BA, Beckmann AM. Human Papillomavirus types 52 and 58 are prevalent in cervical cancers from Chinese women. Int J Cancer. 1997;70:408–11.
13. Lo KW, Wong YF, Chan MK, Li JC, Poon JS, Wang V, Zhu SN, Zhang TM, He ZG, et al. Prevalence of human Papillomavirus in cervical cancer: a multi-center study in China. Int J Cancer. 2002;100:327–31.
14. Liu J, Rose B, Huang X, Liao G, Carter J, Wu X, Thompson C. Comparative analysis of characteristics of women with cervical cancer in high-versus low-incidence regions. Gynecol Oncol. 2004;94:803–10.
15. de Sanjose S, Diaz M, Castellsague X, Clifford G, Bruni L, Muñoz N, Bosch FX. Worldwide prevalence and genotype distribution of cervical human papillomavirs DNA in women with normal cytology: a meta-analysis. Lancet Infect Dis. 2007;7:453–9.
16. Chow CS. Cultural diversity and tourism development in Yunnan province. China Geogr. 2005;90(3):294–303.
17. Linda Stone, Kinship and Gender, 2006, Westview, 3rd ed., ch. 6. The Center for Research on Tibet Papers on Tibetan Marriage and Polyandry. https://www.coursehero.com/file/p7n9h6l/This-process-is-significant-because-it-ensures-the-continuation-of-a-specific/. Accessed 10 Jan 2015.
18. Zou H, Sun Y, Zhang G, Tu Y, Meng X, Liu T, Ping Z, Fan X, Gao Y. Positivity and incidence of human papillomavirus in women attending gynecological department of a major comprehensive hospital in Kunming, China 2012-2014. J Med Virol. 2015 Sep 12. doi: 10.1002/jmv.24377. [Epub ahead of print]
19. Kurman RJ, Norris HJ, Wilkinson EJ. Tumors of the Cervix, Vagina, and Vulva. Washington: Armed Forces Institute of Pathology; 1992.
20. Husnjak K, Grce M, Magdic L, Paveli K. Comparison of five different polymerase chain reaction methods for detection of human papillomavirus in cervical cell specimens. J Virol Methods. 2000;88:125–34.
21. Liu SS, Leung RC, Chan KK, Cheung AN, Ngan HY. Evaluation of a newly developed GenoArray human papillomavirus (HPV) genotyping assay and comparison with the Roche Linear Array HPV genotyping assay. J Clin Microbiol. 2010;48:758–64.
22. Li J, Huang R, Schmidt JE, Qiao YL. Epidemiological features of Human Papillomavirs (HPV) infection among women living in Mainland China. Asian Pac J Cancer Prev. 2013;14(7):4015–23.
23. Hou R, Xu C, Zhang S, Wu M, Zhang W. Distribution of human papillomavirus genotype and cervical neoplasia among women with abnormal cytology in Beijing, China. Int J Gynaecol Obstet. 2012;119:257–61.
24. Sukvirach S, Smith JS, Tunsakul S, Muñoz N, Kesararat V, et al. Population-based human papillomavirus prevalence in Lampang and Songkla, Thailand. J Infect Dis. 2003;187:1246–56.
25. Wu RF, Dai M, Qiao YL, Clifford GM, Liu ZH, Arslan A, et al. Human papillomavirus infection in women in Shenzhen City, People's Republic of China, a population typical of recent Chinese urbanisation. Int J Cancer. 2007;121:1306–11.
26. Li N, Dai M. Human papillomavirus infection in China: a multi-centric cross-sectional study. Chin J Dis Control Prev. 2008;12:411–5.
27. Jin Q, Shen K, Li H, Zhou XR, Huang HF, et al. Age-specific prevalence of human papillomavirus by grade of cervical cytology in Tibetan women. Chin Med J. 2010;123:2004–11.
28. Baloch Z, Yuan T, Wang B, Tai W, Feng Y, Liu Y, Li X, Liu L, Zhang AM, Wu X, Xia X. Ethnic and geographic variations in HPV prevalence and genotype distribution in north-western Yunnan, China. J Med Virol. 2015;88:532–40.
29. Dai M, Bao YP, Li N, Clifford GM, Vaccarella S, et al. Human papillomavirus infection in Shanxi Province, People's Republic of China: a population-based study. Br J Cancer. 2006;95:96–101.
30. Ye J, Cheng X, Chen X, Ye F, Lu W, Xie X. Prevalence and risk profile of cervical Human papillomavirus infection in Zhejiang Province, southeast China: a population-based study. Virol J. 2010;7:66.
31. Yuan X, Yang Y, Gu D, Liu H, Yang H, et al. Prevalence of human papillomavirus infection among women with and without normal cervical histology in Shandong Province, China. Arch Gynecol Obstet. 2011;283:1385–9.
32. Chung MY, Kim YW, Bae SM, Kwon EH, Chaturvedi PK, Battogtokh G, Ahn WS. Development of a bead-based multiplex genotyping method for diagnostic characterization of HPV infection. PLoS One. 2010;7:e32259.
33. Doménech-Peris A, Conesa-Zamora P, Sahuquillo-Frias L, Ortiz-Reina S, Moya Biosca J, Acosta-Ortega J, Pérez Guillermo M, Egea-Cortines M. Human papillomavirus genotyping in histological sections of precursor lesions of cervical carcinoma: its role as a possible adjunct for the evaluation of the oncogenic potential of specific human papillomavirus genotypes – a study in a coastal region of Southeastern Spain. Gynecol Obstet Invest. 2010;70: 113–9.
34. Smith JS, Lindsay L, Hoots B, Keys J, Franceschi S, Winer R, Clifford GM. Human papillomavirus type distribution in invasive cervical cancer and high-grade cervical lesions: a meta-analysis update. Int J Cancer. 2007;121: 621–32.
35. Chen Q, Xie LX, Qing ZR, Li LJ, Luo ZY, et al. Epidemiologic characterization of human papillomavirus infection in rural Chaozhou, eastern Guangdong Province of China. PLoS One. 2012;7:e32149.
36. Formentin A, Archambault J, Koushik A, Richardson H, Brassard P, Franco EL, Coutlee F. Human papillomavirus type 52 polymorphism and high-grade lesions of the uterine cervix. Int J Cancer. 2013;132:1821–30.
37. Clifford GM, Rana RK, Franceschi S, Smith S, Gough G, Pimenta JM. Human papillomavirus genotype distribution in low-grade cervical lesions: comparison by geographic region and with cervical cancer. Cancer Epidemiol Biomarkers Prev. 2005;14:1157–64.
38. De Sanjose S, Quint WG, Alemany L, Geraets DT, Klaustermeier JE, Lloveras B, et al. Retrospective International Survey and HPV Time Trends Study Group: Human papillomavirus genotype attribution in invasive cervical cancer: a retrospective cross-sectional worldwide study. Lancet Oncol. 2010;11:1048–56.
39. Castle PE, Fetterman B, Thoma Cox J, Shaber R, Poitras N, Lorey T, Kinney W. The age-specific relationships of abnormal cytology and human papillomavirus DNA results to the risk of cervical precanc er and cancer. Obstet Gynecol. 2010;116:76–84.
40. Ronco G, Giorgi-Rossi P, Carozzi F, Confortini M, Dalla PP, Del Mistro A, et al. Efficacy of human papillomavirus testing for the detection of invasive cervical cancers and cervical intraepithelial neoplasia: a randomised controlled trial. Lancet Oncol. 2012;11:249–57.
41. Forman D, de Martel C, Lacey CJ, Soerjomataram I, Lortet-Tieulent J, et al. Global Burden of Human Papillomavirus and Related Diseases. Vaccine. 2012;30:F12–23.
42. Laara E, Day NE, Hakama M. Trends in mortality from cervical cancer in the Nordic countries: Association with organized screening programs. Lancet. 1987;1:1247–9.

14

Human papillomavirus infections among women with cervical lesions and cervical cancer in Eastern China: genotype-specific prevalence and attribution

Lei Zhang[1], Qingqing Bi[1], Hua Deng[1], Jing Xu[2], Juan Chen[1], Meilian Zhang[3] and Xiaofeng Mu[1*]

Abstract

Background: Cervical cancer and its precursor, high-grade cervical intraepithelial neoplasia (CIN2/3), are associated with persistent high-risk human papillomavirus (HPV) infection. HPV genotype prevalence varies with severity of cervical lesions, patient age and geographical location. The aim of this study was to investigate HPV genotypes prevalence and attribution according to the severity of cervical lesions among Chinese women.

Method: A 4-year surveillance study was performed. A total of 1664 female patients were included and their cervical histological diagnosis consisted of cervical intraepithelial neoplasia grade 1 (CIN1, 376 cases), grade 2 (CIN2, 408 cases), grade 3 (CIN3, 336 cases) and invasive cervical cancers (ICC, 544 cases). HPV genotypes prevalence and attribution to cervical lesions were calculated and analyzed. The 95% confidence interval (CI) for proportion was also calculated.

Results: HPV positivity rates increased directly with cervical lesions severity (72.4% for CIN1, 81.4% for CIN2, 88.1% for CIN3 and 90.4% for ICC). Infections with multiple HPV types were inversely related to cervical lesions severity. HPV16, 52, 31, 33 and 58 were the most prevalent genotypes in ICC. 49.1% of squamous cell carcinoma, 65.1% of adenocarcinoma and 12.0–43.3% of cervical intraepithelial neoplasia could be attributed to vaccine-covered high-risk genotypes (HPV16/18). Inclusion of HPV52 and HPV31 in future vaccines would provide the highest marginal benefit in protection for individuals residing in this region.

Conclusions: These findings provide information about HPV genotypes in this region which may be important to target with future vaccination and screening programs.

Keywords: Human papillomavirus, Genotypes, Attribution, Cervical cancer

Background

Cervical intraepithelial neoplasia (CIN) is a premalignant lesion that is diagnosed by histology as CIN1, CIN2, or CIN3. If left untreated, CIN2 or CIN3 (high-grade CIN) might progress to cervical cancer. There were an estimated 527,600 new cervical cancer cases and 265,700 deaths worldwide in 2012 [1]. It is the second most commonly diagnosed cancer and third leading cause of cancer-induced death among females in less developed countries [1]. Persistent infection with one or more of carcinogenic genotypes of human papillomavirus (HPV) is a high-risk cause for cervical neoplasia [2]. At least 13 distinct high-risk HPV genotypes (HPV16, 18, 31, 33, 35, 39, 45, 51, 52, 56, 58, 59, and 68) have been identified to be associated with the risk of developing cervical cancer and defined as "carcinogenic" viral genotypes [3]. Carcinogenic HPV genotypes can be detected in more than 90% of cervical cancer specimens and in more than 60% of CIN tissues [4, 5].

For prevention of HPV infection and the potential development of cervical neoplasia, two prophylactic

* Correspondence: zxyymuxf@yeah.net
[1]Department of Laboratory Medicine, Qingdao Central Hospital, Second Affiliated Hospital of Qingdao University, Siliunan Road #127, Qingdao 266042, China
Full list of author information is available at the end of the article

vaccines (Cervarix by GlaxoSmithKline and Gardasil by Merck Sharp and Dohme) are currently available. These two HPV vaccines potentially provide protection against two most common HPV genotypes, HPV16 and 18, which cause approximately 70% of invasive cervical cancers worldwide [6]. However, prevalence of the other carcinogenic HPV genotypes varies markedly by geographic region [5, 7]. In East Asia, HPV52 and 58 are more prevalent compared to worldwide [8]. Therefore, knowledge of the regional prevalence of HPV genotypes is essential for the development of effective vaccination as well as preventative screening strategies against cervical cancer.

A recent study performed by our group reported the HPV prevalence among female outpatients from Qingdao [9], which is a major city located in eastern China with a population of over nine million where prophylactic vaccines against HPV are currently not available. In the present study, we investigated the prevalence and attribution of HPV genotypes to cervical intraepithelial neoplasia and invasive cancer among women from this region.

Methods

Study subjects and specimen collection

From January 2012 to December 2015, women who visited gynecologists or oncologists seeking for further management of abnormal cervical cytology results in Qingdao Central Hospital and Qingdao Cancer Hospital, a tertiary hospital attached to Qingdao University with 1600 beds and a tertiary hospital specializing in oncology, were enrolled with informed consents. A participant was eligible if she (a) was sexually active, (b) was a gynecological patient, (c) was no previously miscarriage nor presently pregnant, (d) had not undergone a total hysterectomy, and (e) agreed to receive HPV genotyping and cervical histopathology evaluation. A cervical scrape sample was collected for HPV genotyping. Biopsy-confirmed histopathologic findings were used to define the status of cervical neoplasia. All biopsy samples were taken by a gynecologist according to guidelines from International Agency for Research on Cancer, WHO [10]. All procedures of this study were approved by Research Ethics Boards at Qingdao Central Hospital Affiliated to Qingdao University (Ethics 2013 No. 023), in accordance with the ethical standards of the Declaration of Helsinki.

HPV genotyping and cervical histopathology

Cervical scrape samples were stored in a specimen transport medium. DNA extraction, amplification and hybridization were performed using an HPV genotyping kit (Yaneng Biotech, Shenzhen, China) according to the manufacturer's instructions. The HPV DNA chip in the kit contained 23 type-specific probes that recognize 18 high-risk (16, 18, 31, 33, 35, 39, 45, 51, 52, 53, 56, 58, 59, 66, 68, 73, 82 and 83) and 5 low-risk HPV genotypes (6, 11, 42, 43 and 81). PCR amplifications were performed in a T100 Thermal Cycler (Bio-Rad, USA) with the following parameters: enzyme activation at 50 °C for 15 min, initial denaturation at 95 °C for 10 min, followed by 10 cycles of 94 °C for 10 s, 42 °C for 90 s and 72 °C for 30 s, followed by 30 cycles of 94 °C for 10 s, 46 °C for 60 s and 72 °C for 20 s, ending with a final extension at 72 °C for 5 min. The PCR product (25 μl) was denatured at 95 °C for 10 min and immediately chilled on ice. Then, the HPV DNA hybridization reaction was performed on an automatic analyzer according to the manufacturer's instructions. The hybridization procedure was presented in Additional file 1: Figure S1. The final results were obtained by colorimetric change on the chip under direct visualization. HPV negative and positive controls, provided in the kit, were simultaneously detected in every test.

The biopsy specimens obtained from the subjects were fixed by formalin, embedded in paraffin and stained with hematoxylin-eosin for histopathology in the pathology laboratory at Qingdao Central Hospital. Cervical histological diagnosis of the specimens was reported only when three different pathologists, from Qingdao Central Hospital and Qingdao Cancer Hospital, agreed with each other. Pathology results were classified into cervical intraepithelial neoplasia grade 1 (CIN1), CIN grade 2 (CIN2), CIN grade 3 (CIN3) and invasive cervical cancer (ICC) according to cervical lesions classification criteria [11].

Statistical analysis

Frequencies of clinical data were calculated. The prevalence and attribution rates of HPV genotypes were calculated according to a previous method [8]. Crude prevalence was estimated by analyzing all studied cases as the denominator for every disease grade. The relative distribution for each disease grade was calculated only using the HPV positive samples as the denominator. The attribution of an HPV genotype to certain disease grade was calculated as follows: (percentage of samples with single-type infection) + (percentage of samples with multiple-type infection multiplied by attribution factor). The "attribution factor" for each HPV genotype was calculated based on the formula "number of samples with single-type infection of the HPV genotype concerned divided by the number of samples with single-type infection of any HPV genotype in that disease category". The 95% confidence interval (CI) for proportion was calculated by the Wilson score method [12]. Differences in HPV positivity rates and proportions of multiple-type HPV infections between disease categories were assessed by Pearson's χ^2 test and $p < 0.05$ was considered significant.

Table 1 HPV infection according to cervical pathology status

Cervical Pathology status (total no. diagnosed)	HPV positive rate no. (%)	Single-type infection no. (%)	Multiple-type infection no. (%)		
			Two HPV genotypes	Three HPV genotypes	Four or more HPV genotypes
Cervical intraepithelial neoplasia (CIN)					
CIN grade 1 (376)	272 (72.4)	156 (41.5)	68 (18.1)	36 (9.6)	12 (3.2)
CIN grade 2 (408)	332 (81.4)	208 (51.0)	80 (19.6)	24 (5.9)	20 (4.9)
CIN grade 3 (336)	296 (88.1)	236 (70.2)	40 (11.9)	20 (6.0)	0
Invasive cervical cancer					
Squamous cell carcinoma (440)	416 (94.5)	348 (79.1)	60 (13.6)	8 (1.8)	0
Adenocarcinoma (104)	76 (73.1)	68 (65.4)	8 (7.7)	0	0

Results

HPV infection according to cervical pathology status

According to the inclusive criteria, a total of 1664 women received HPV genotyping and cervical histopathology evaluation. Their cervical pathology status were as follows: 376 cases of CIN1, 408 cases of CIN2, 336 cases of CIN3, 440 cases of squamous cell carcinoma (SCC) and 104 cases of adenocarcinoma. HPV positivity rates and the proportion of single- and multiple-type infection for each cervical pathology status are presented in Table 1. HPV positivity rates of CIN1, CIN2, CIN3 and SCC samples were 72.4, 81.4, 88.1 and 94.5%, respectively, which increased directly with severity of cervical lesions. Further, the HPV positivity rate of CIN1 group was significantly lower than that of invasive cervical cancer group ($p = 6.36 \times 10^{-13}$). The HPV positivity rate of adenocarcinoma group was significantly lower than squamous cell carcinoma group ($p = 2.13 \times 10^{-11}$). In addition, patients with lower grade cervical lesions (CIN1, 42.6%) displayed a higher frequency of multiple-type HPV infections compared with those suffering from higher grade cervical lesions (CIN2 and CIN3, 29.3%, $p = 9.59 \times 10^{-5}$) and invasive cancers (15.4%, $p = 1.05 \times 10^{-16}$).

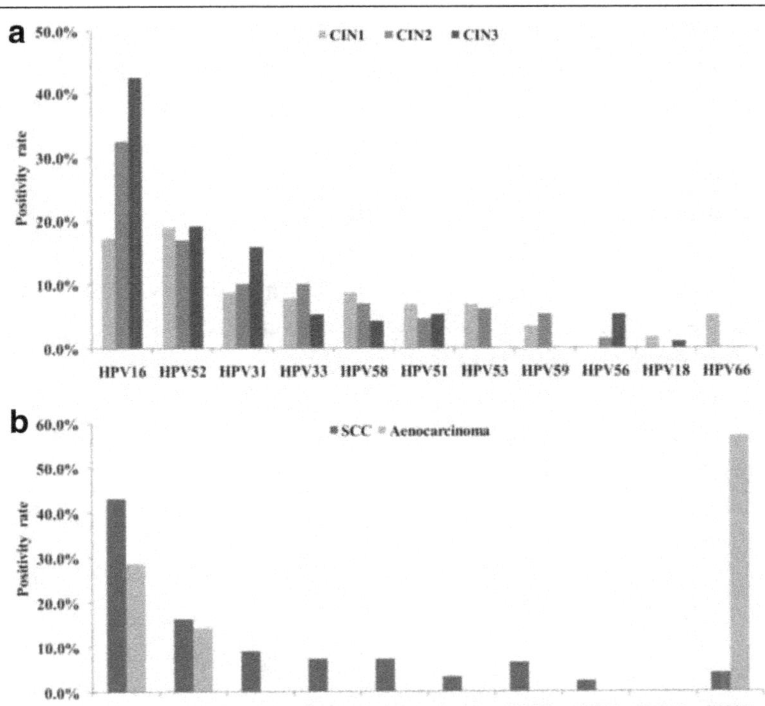

Fig. 1 Relative distribution of HPV genotypes among different grades of cervical intraepithelial neoplasia (**a**) and invasive cervical cancers (**b**). Each kind of genotype was counted separately in cases with multiple-type HPV infections. The positivity rates of genotypes were calculated using the number of HPV positive samples in each disease grade as the denominator. CIN1, cervical intraepithelial neoplasia grade 1; CIN2, CIN grade 2; CIN3, CIN grade 3. SCC, squamous cell carcinoma

Table 2 Prevalence and attribution of all HPV genotypes according to cervical pathology status

HPV Geno-types		Crude prevalence and attribution in % (95% confidence interval)				
		Squamous cell carcincma (440)	Adeno-carcinoma (104)	CIN3 (336)	CIN2 (408)	CIN1 (376)
HPV16	Prevalence	48.2 (43.5–52.8)	23.1 (16.0–32.0)	47.6 (42.3–53.0)	41.2 (36.5–46.0)	21.3 (17.4–25.7)
	Attribution	44.6 (40.0–49.3)	20.3 (13.7–29.0)	43.3 (38.1–48.6)	30.7 (26.4–35.4)	9.9 (7.3–13.3)
HPV52	Prevalence	18.2 (14.9–22.1)	11.5 (6.7–19.1)	21.4 (17.4–26.1)	21.6 (17.9–25.8)	23.4 (19.4–27.9)
	Attribution	15.2 (12.1–18.8)	4.2 (1.7–10.0)	11.1 (8.2–14.9)	14.1 (11.0–17.8)	18.8 (15.2–23.1)
HPV31	Prevalence	10.0 (7.5–13.2)	0.0 (0.0–3.6)	17.9 (14.1–22.3)	12.7 (9.9–16.3)	10.6 (7.9–14.2)
	Attribution	3.9 (2.4–6.1)	0.0 (0.0–3.6)	10.6 (7.8–14.4)	8.6 (6.2–11.7)	3.8 (2.3–6.2)
HPV33	Prevalence	8.2 (6.0–11.1)	0.0 (0.0–3.6)	6.0 (3.9–9.0)	12.7 (9.9–16.3)	9.6 (7.0–13.0)
	Attribution	1.1 (0.5–2.6)	0.0 (0.0–3.6)	3.7 (2.2–6.3)	2.4 (1.3–4.4)	5.9 (3.9–8.7)
HPV58	Prevalence	8.2 (6.0–11.1)	0.0 (0.0–3.6)	4.8 (3.0–7.6)	8.8 (6.4–12.0)	10.6 (7.9–14.2)
	Attribution	3.8 (2.4–6.0)	0.0 (0.0–3.6)	3.7 (2.1–6.2)	3.2 (1.9–5.4)	3.8 (2.3–6.2)
HPV51	Prevalence	3.6 (2.3–5.8)	0.0 (0.0–3.6)	6.0 (3.9–9.0)	5.9 (4.0–8.6)	8.5 (6.1–11.8)
	Attribution	2.7 (1.6–4.7)	0.0 (0.0–3.6)	0.0 (0.0–1.1)	0.0 (0.0–0.9)	0.0 (0.0–1.0)
HPV53	Prevalence	7.3 (5.2–10.1)	0.0 (0.0–3.6)	0.0 (0.0–1.1)	7.8 (5.6–10.9)	8.5 (6.1–11.8)
	Attribution	5.6 (3.8–8.2)	0.0 (0.0–3.6)	0.0 (0.0–1.1)	4.2 (2.6–6.6)	0.0 (0.0–1.0)
HPV59	Prevalence	2.7 (1.6–4.7)	0.0 (0.0–3.6)	0.0 (0.0–1.1)	6.9 (4.8–9.7)	4.3 (2.6–6.8)
	Attribution	2.7 (1.5–4.7)	0.0 (0.0–3.6)	0.0 (0.0–1.1)	0.0 (0.0–0.9)	3.3 (1.9–5.6)
HPV56	Prevalence	0.0 (0.0–0.9)	0.0 (0.0–3.6)	6.0 (3.9–9.0)	2.0 (1.0–3.8)	0.0 (0.0–1.0)
	Attribution	0.0 (0.0–0.9)	0.0 (0.0–3.6)	6.0 (3.9–9.1)	0.0 (0.0–0.9)	0.0 (0.0–1.0)
HPV35	Prevalence	0.9 (0.4–2.3)	0.0 (0.0–3.6)	0.0 (0.0–1.1)	0.0 (0.0–0.9)	6.4 (4.3–9.3)
	Attribution	0.0 (0.0–0.9)	0.0 (0.0–3.6)	0.0 (0.0–1.1)	0.0 (0.0–0.9)	0.0 (0.0–1.0)
HPV18	Prevalence	4.5 (3.0–6.9)	46.2 (36.9–55.7)	1.2 (0.5–3.0)	0.0 (0.0–0.9)	2.1 (1.1–4.1)
	Attribution	4.5 (2.9–6.9)	44.8 (35.6–54.3)	0.0 (0.0–1.1)	0.0 (0.0–0.9)	2.1 (1.1–4.1)
HPV45	Prevalence	0.0 (0.0–0.9)	0.0 (0.0–3.6)	0.0 (0.0–1.1)	2.0 (1.0–3.8)	0.0 (0.0–1.0)
	Attribution	0.0 (0.0–0.9)	0.0 (0.0–3.6)	0.0 (0.0–1.1)	0.0 (0.0–0.9)	0.0 (0.0–1.0)
HPV68	Prevalence	0.0 (0.0–0.9)	0.0 (0.0–3.6)	0.0 (0.0–1.1)	0.0 (0.0–0.9)	4.3 (2.6–6.8)
	Attribution	0.0 (0.0–0.9)	0.0 (0.0–3.6)	0.0 (0.0–1.1)	0.0 (0.0–0.9)	0.0 (0.0–1.0)
HPV73	Prevalence	0.0 (0.0–0.9)	0.0 (0.0–3.6)	1.2 (0.5–3.0)	0.0 (0.0–0.9)	0.0 (0.0–1.0)
	Attribution	0.0 (0.0–0.9)	0.0 (0.0–3.6)	0.0 (0.0–1.1)	0.0 (0.0–0.9)	0.0 (0.0–1.0)
HPV82	Prevalence	0.0 (0.0–0.9)	0.0 (0.0–3.6)	0.0 (0.0–1.1)	4.9 (3.2–7.4)	3.2 (1.8–5.5)
	Attribution	0.0 (0.0–0.9)	0.0 (0.0–3.6)	0.0 (0.0–1.1)	0.0 (0.0–0.9)	0.0 (0.0–1.0)
HPV66	Prevalence	0.0 (0.0–0.9)	0.0 (0.0–3.6)	0.0 (0.0–1.1)	0.0 (0.0–0.9)	6.4 (4.3–9.3)
	Attribution	0.0 (0.0–0.9)	0.0 (0.0–3.6)	0.0 (0.0–1.1)	0.0 (0.0–0.9)	1.2 (0.5–2.9)
HPV39	Prevalence	0.0 (0.0–0.9)	0.0 (0.0–3.6)	0.0 (0.0–1.1)	0.0 (0.0–0.9)	2.1 (1.1–4.1)
	Attribution	0.0 (0.0–0.9)	0.0 (0.0–3.6)	0.0 (0.0–1.1)	0.0 (0.0–0.9)	0.0 (0.0–1.0)
HPV83	Prevalence	0.0 (0.0–0.9)	0.0 (0.0–3.6)	0.0 (0.0–1.1)	0.0 (0.0–0.9)	0.0 (0.0–1.0)
	Attribution	0.0 (0.0–0.9)	0.0 (0.0–3.6)	0.0 (0.0–1.1)	0.0 (0.0–0.9)	0.0 (0.0–1.0)
HPV81	Prevalence	0.0 (0.0–0.9)	0.0 (0.0–3.6)	0.0 (0.0–1.1)	0.0 (0.0–0.9)	1.1 (0.4–2.7)
	Attribution	0.0 (0.0–0.9)	0.0 (0.0–3.6)	0.0 (0.0–1.1)	0.0 (0.0–0.9)	0.0 (0.0–1.0)
HPV6	Prevalence	0.0 (0.0–0.9)	0.0 (0.0–3.6)	0.0 (0.0–1.1)	0.0 (0.0–0.9)	0.0 (0.0–1.0)
	Attribution	0.0 (0.0–0.9)	0.0 (0.0–3.6)	0.0 (0.0–1.1)	0.0 (0.0–0.9)	0.0 (0.0–1.0)
HPV43	Prevalence	0.0 (0.0–0.9)	0.0 (0.0–3.6)	0.0 (0.0–1.1)	0.0 (0.0–0.9)	0.0 (0.0–1.0)
	Attribution	0.0 (0.0–0.9)	0.0 (0.0–3.6)	0.0 (0.0–1.1)	0.0 (0.0–0.9)	0.0 (0.0–1.0)
HPV11	Prevalence	0.0 (0.0–0.9)	0.0 (0.0–3.6)	0.0 (0.0–1.1)	0.0 (0.0–0.9)	0.0 (0.0–1.0)
	Attribution	0.0 (0.0–0.9)	0.0 (0.0–3.6)	0.0 (0.0–1.1)	0.0 (0.0–0.9)	0.0 (0.0–1.0)

Relative distribution of HPV genotypes according to cervical pathology status

Detailed HPV genotypes distribution according to the severity of cervical lesions was also investigated. Each kind of genotype was counted separately in cases with multiple-type HPV infections. As shown in Fig. 1, distribution of the 11 most frequent genotypes in this study was presented. Top five most frequent genotypes among high-grade cervical lesions (both CIN2 and CIN3) were HPV16 (336/37.7%), HPV52 (160/17.9%), HPV31 (112/12.6%), HPV33 (72/8.1%) and HPV58 (52/5.8%). In contrast, the genotypes distribution was shown to be different in CIN1, where HPV52 was the most frequent genotype detected (88/19.1%), followed by HPV16 (80/17.4%) and HPV58 (40/8.7%) (Fig.1a). As shown in Fig.1b, among squamous cell carcinoma cases, HPV16 was the most common genotype (212/43.1%), followed by HPV52 (80/16.3%), HPV31 (44/8.9%) and HPV58 (36/7.3%). As for adenocarcinoma, only three kinds of genotypes were detected and HPV18 was the most prevalent type (48/57.1%), followed by HPV16 (24/28.6%) and HPV52 (12/14.3%).

Attribution of HPV genotypes in cervical lesions

The crude prevalence and attribution rates of all HPV genotypes to each cervical pathology status were presented in Table 2. The majority (44.6%) of squamous cell carcinoma was attributed to HPV16. Subsequently, 15.2, 5.6 and 4.5% of squamous cell carcinoma were attributed to HPV52, HPV53 and HPV18, respectively. In contrast, the majority (44.8%) of adenocarcinoma was attributed to HPV18 and the following genotypes were HPV16 (20.3%) and HPV52 (4.2%).

HPV16 also accounted for the majority of high-grade lesions (CIN3 and CIN2) with attribution rate of 43.3 and 30.7%, respectively. HPV52 was the following genotype, which attributed to 11.1 and 14.1% of CIN3 and CIN2, respectively (Table 2). In contrast, HPV16 was not the most common genotype found in CIN1. Either by crude prevalence rate or attribution rate, HPV52 ranked higher than HPV16 in CIN1.

The cumulative attribution rates of 11 high-risk HPV genotypes to invasive cervical cancer and cervical intraepithelial neoplasia were presented in Figs. 2 and 3, respectively. The two high-risk types (HPV16 and HPV18) attributed to 49.1% of squamous cell carcinoma (Fig.2a), 65.1% of adenocarcinoma (Fig.2b), 43.3% of CIN3 (Fig.3a), 30.7% of CIN2 (Fig.3b) and 12.0% of CIN1 (Fig.3c) cases. The subsequent genotype, HPV52, brought the biggest marginal increase with 15.2% for squamous cell carcinoma (Fig.2a), 11.1% for CIN3, 14.1% for CIN2 and 18.8% for CIN1 lesions.

Age-specific prevalence of cervical lesions and cancers

All 1664 patients involved were classified into five groups according to age (≤25, 26–35, 36–45, 46–55,

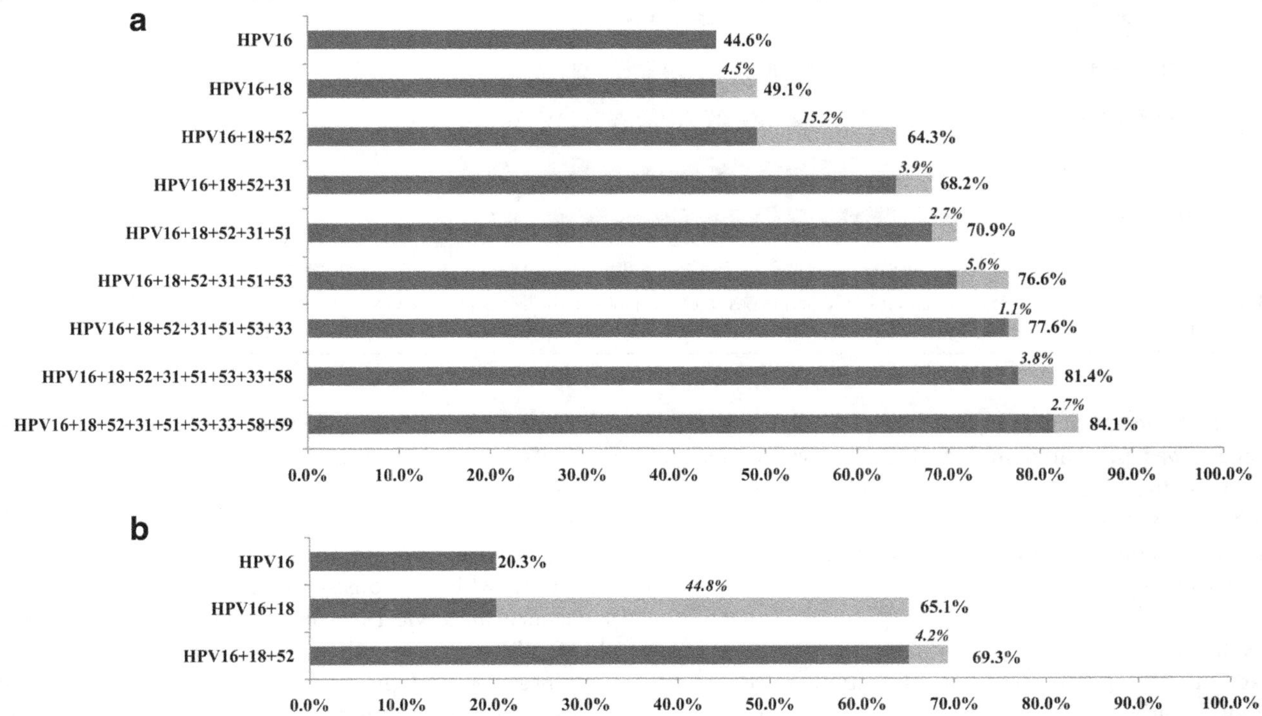

Fig. 2 Cumulative attribution rates of high-risk HPV genotypes to invasive cervical cancer. **a** Squamous cell carcinoma; **b** adenocarcinoma. Marginal attribution rates conferred by individual HPV genotypes are italicized. Bold numbers represent cumulative attribution rates

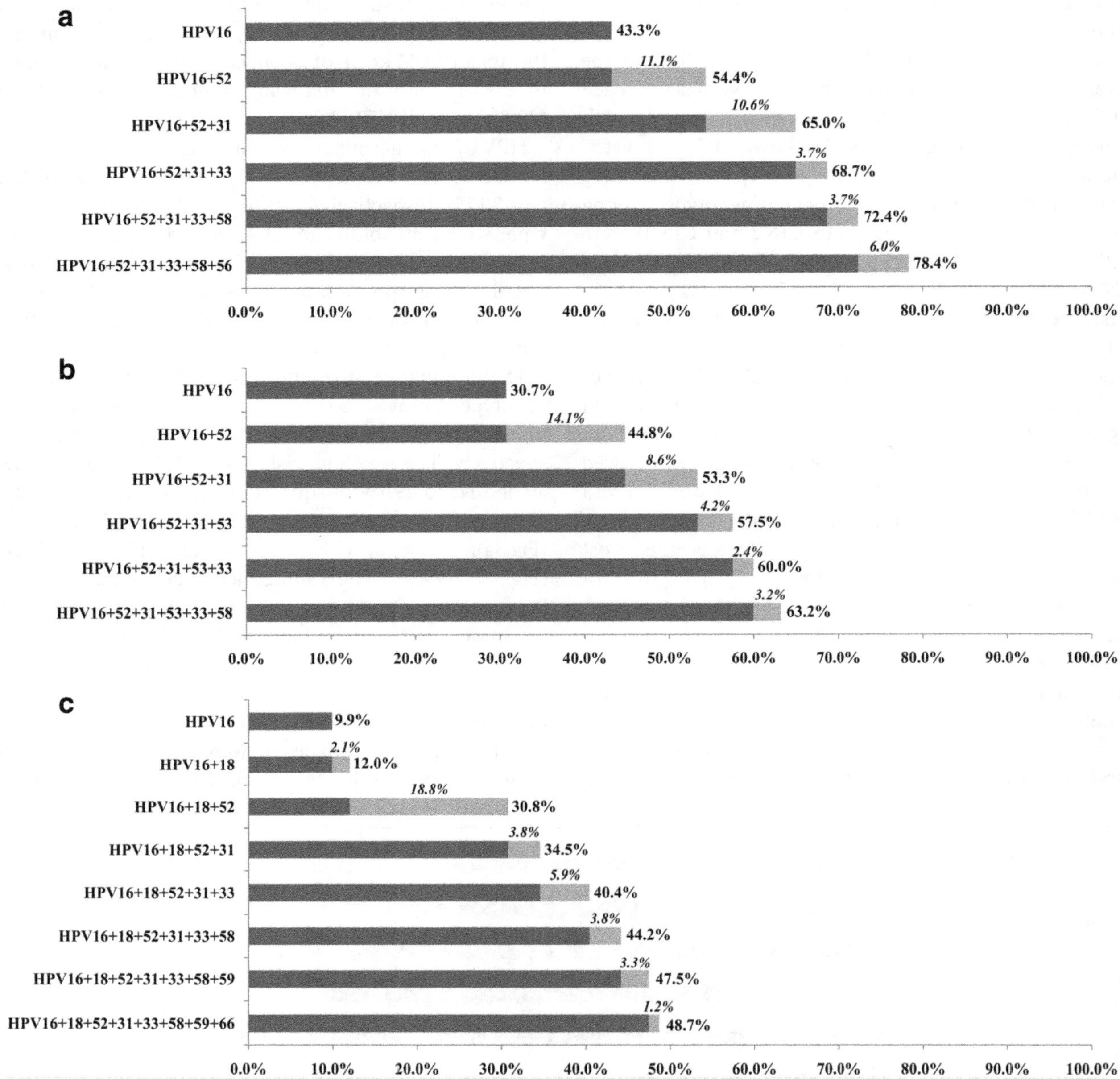

Fig. 3 Cumulative attribution rates of high-risk HPV genotypes to cervical intraepithelial neoplasia. **a** CIN grade 3; **b** CIN grade 2; **c** CIN grade 1. Marginal attribution rates conferred by individual HPV genotypes are italicized. Bold numbers represent cumulative attribution rates

≥56) and age-specific prevalence of cervical lesions and cancers was presented in Fig. 4. As shown in Fig. 4, 80.8% of the patients with adenocarcinoma and 62.7% with SCC were more than 46 years old. Moreover, 30.6% of the patients with high-grade cervical lesions (CIN2 and CIN3) were younger than 35.

Discussion

Data of HPV prevalence and attribution according to cervical pathology status presented in this study may provide guidance for HPV vaccination program and preventative strategies against cervical cancer in this region of China. Among the involved female patients, HPV positivity rates increase directly with the cervical lesion severity, which is consistent with some previous studies from different regions of China [8, 13–15]. The overall HPV prevalence among ICC patients reaches 90.4% in this study, which is consistent with the worldwide HPV prevalence in cervical cancers, ranging from 86 to 94% [4, 16, 17]. In this study, single-type HPV infection is more prevalent in high-grade CIN and ICC patients than in low-grade CIN and the single-type HPV positivity rates also increase directly with the cervical lesion severity, which is consistent with a previous study from

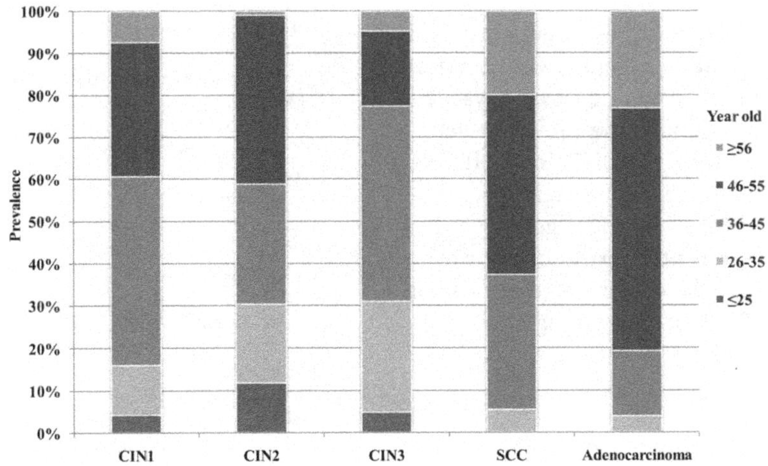

Fig. 4 Age-specific prevalence of cervical lesions and cancers

Beijing, China [18]. In this study, HPV infections are all high-risk genotypes among the high-grade CIN and ICC patients and the most prevalent genotypes are HPV16, 52, 31, 33 and 58. Another study in China reported that the most common HPV genotypes in high-grade CIN and cervical cancers are HPV16, 58, 31, 52, 33 and HPV16, 33, 18, 52, 58, respectively [13]. A multiple-center study in Beijing reported that HPV16, 58, 33, 56, and 31 are the most prevalent genotypes in cervical lesions [19]. It's observed from these results that HPV16, 52, 31, 33, 58, 56 and 18 are prevalent genotypes among women with cervical lesions in China. A worldwide meta-analysis also confirmed that eastern Asia exhibits an HPV genotype distribution pattern distinct from the other areas of the world, a relatively high contribution of HPV52 and 58 to cervical lesions [20]. In this study, HPV18 was the most prevalent genotype among adenocarcinoma patients. This is in accordance with several studies focusing on cervical adenocarcinoma. HPV18 highly correlated to adenocarcinoma worldwide including China [21, 22]. Furthermore, HPV18, 16 and 45 have been reported to be the most prevalent genotypes in adenocarcinoma worldwide [20, 23]. However, in the present study, the presence of HPV52 instead of HPV45 in adenocarcinoma was observed and consistent with studies in eastern Asia [8, 20].

In this study, we found a high rate of young women with high grade cervical lesions (CIN2 and CIN3). 30.6% of patients with high-grade cervical lesions were younger than 35. Notably, 5.0% of patients with high-grade cervical lesions were even younger than 25, which is higher than that from a neighboring area of this region (3.4%) [24]. Therefore, for this region, vaccination program and preventative screening strategies against cervical cancer are expected to pay more attention to young women.

Furthermore, an approach adopted from previous studies [8, 25], which assumed a fractional attribution of individual HPV genotypes found simultaneously in a lesion, was applied to the current data. It was estimated that the current HPV16/18-based vaccines would protect against 49.1% of squamous cell carcinoma, 65.1% of adenocarcinoma and 12.0–43.3% of CINs. In this region, HPV52 and HPV31 were determined to be the next common types in contributing to squamous cell carcinoma and CINs, which is in accordance with several studies in eastern Asia including China [20, 26, 27]. Therefore, for this region of China, vaccination program and preventative strategies against cervical cancer are expected to pay attention to HPV52, 31, 58 and 33 along with vaccine preventable HPV 16 and 18. The two prophylactic vaccines mentioned, proved to be effective in preventing cervical cancer, are available in many countries worldwide except mainland China. Even if the 2-valent (HPV16 and 18) or 4-valent (HPV6, 11, 16 and 18) is going to be commercial available in mainland China, the demand for vaccines against more particular genotypes is still strong. The newcome 9-valent HPV vaccine may provide more protections against cervical lesions for women in this region of China.

In this present work, the "attribution factor" of each HPV genotype was calculated and cumulative attribution rates of prevalent high-risk HPV genotypes were presented. The 95% confidence interval (CI) for proportion was also calculated. These methods have been rarely used to analyze HPV infections in mainland China before. There are still some limitations in this study. The total number of samples involved in this study is not large. Multi-center study, including over three tertiary hospitals, may be more valuable. In addition, interactions between different HPV genotypes still need further investigation.

Conclusions

This study presented HPV genotypes prevalence and attribution data among female patients with cervical lesions in this area, where the planning of HPV vaccination should be taken into account the prevalent genotypes of HPV16, HPV52, HPV31, HPV58 and HPV33. These data added new evidence that eastern Asia, including eastern China, exhibited an HPV genotype distribution pattern distinct from other parts of the world. Our results also could provide necessary reference for formulating a regional HPV-based screening strategy in the future.

Abbreviations

CIN: Cervical intraepithelial neoplasia; HPV: Human papillomavirus; ICC: Invasive cervical cancer; SCC: Squamous cell carcinoma

Acknowledgements

The authors acknowledge all the staff who participated in this work at Qingdao Central Hospital and Qingdao Cancer Hospital. We would like to thank Ms. Feng Yilin for her great help on data processing and statistical analysis. We also thank all the patients who agreed to participate in the study.

Funding

This study was supported by key subject grants from Qingdao Central Hospital (2013-ZDXK003). The funder had no role in the study design, data collection and analysis, decision to publish, or preparation of the manuscript.

Authors' contributions

Conceived and designed the experiments: XM, LZ and QB. Performed the experiments: QB, HD, JX and JC. Analyzed the data: XM, LZ, QB and HD. Wrote the paper: LZ and QB. Manuscript reviewing and English revision: XM and MZ. All authors read and approved the final manuscript.

Competing interests

The authors declare that they have no competing interests.

Consent for publication

Not applicable.

Author details

[1]Department of Laboratory Medicine, Qingdao Central Hospital, Second Affiliated Hospital of Qingdao University, Siliunan Road #127, Qingdao 266042, China. [2]Department of Pathology, Qingdao Central Hospital, Qingdao, China. [3]Clinical Laboratory, Qingdao Cancer Hospital, Qingdao, China.

References

1. Torre LA, Bray F, Siegel RL, Ferlay J, Lortet-Tieulent J, Jemal A. Global Cancer Statistics, 2012. CA Cancer J Clin. 2015;65:87–108.
2. Schiffman M, Castle PE, Jeronimo J, Rodriguez AC, Wacholder S. Human papillomavirus and cervical cancer. Lancet. 2007;370:890–907.
3. Schiffman M, Solomon D. Clinical practice. Cervical-cancer screening with human papillomavirus and cytologic cotesting. N Eng J Med. 2013;369: 2324–31.
4. Smith JS, Lindsay L, Hoots B, Keys J, Franceschi S, Winer R, et al. Human papillomavirus type distribution in invasive cervical cancer and high-grade cervical lesions: a meta-analysis update. Int J Cancer. 2007;121:621–32.
5. Li N, Franceschi S, Howell-Jones R, Snijders PJ, Clifford GM. Human papillomavirus type distribution in 30,848 invasive cervical cancers worldwide: Variation by geographical region, histological type and year of publication. Int J Cancer. 2011;128:927–35.
6. Roden R, Wu TC. How will HPV vaccines affect cervical cancer? Nat Rev Cancer. 2006;6:753–63.
7. Vaccarella S, Franceschi S, Zaridze D, Poljak M, Veerus P, Plummer M, et al. Preventable fractions of cervical cancer via effective screening in six Baltic, central, and eastern European countries 2017-40: a population-based study. Lancet Oncol. 2016;17:1445–52.
8. Chan PK, Cheung TH, Li WH, Yu MY, Chan MY, Yim SF, et al. Attribution of human papillomavirus types to cervical intraepithelial neoplasia and invasive cancers in southern China. Int J Cancer. 2012;131:692–705.
9. Bi Q, Zhang L, Zhao Z, Mu X, Zhang M, Wang P. Human papillomavirus prevalence and genotypes distribution among female outpatients in Qingdao, East China. J Med Virol. 2015;87:2114–21.
10. Sellors JW, Sankaranarayanan R. Colposcopy and treatment of cervical intraepithelial neoplasia: a beginner's manual. Lyon: International Agency for Research on Cancer, WHO; 2003. p. 37–44.
11. Sattar HA. Female Genital System and Breast. In: Kumar V, Abbas AK, Aster JC, editors. Robbins Basic Pathology. 9th ed. Philadelphia: Saunders Elsevier; 2013. p. 686–8.
12. Newcombe RG. Two-sided confidence intervals for the single proportion: comparison of seven methods. Stat Med. 1998;17:857–72.
13. Ding X, Liu Z, Su J, Yan D, Sun W, Zeng Z. Human papillomavirus type-specific prevalence in women referred for colposcopic examination in Beijing. J Med Virol. 2014;86:1937–43.
14. Liu X, Fan X, Yu Y, Ji L, Yan J, Sun AH. Human papillomavirus prevalence and type-distribution among women in Zhejiang Province, Southeast China: a cross-sectional study. BMC Infect Dis. 2014;14:708.
15. Zhang WY, Xue YZ, Chen M, Han L, Luo M. Prevalence of high-risk human papillomavirus infection in different cervical lesion among organized health-examination women in Shanghai, China. Chin Med J (Engl). 2008;121:1578–82.
16. de Sanjose S, Quint WG, Alemany L, Geraets DT, Klaustermeier JE, Lloveras B, et al. Human papillomavirus genotype attribution in invasive cervical cancer: A retrospective cross-sectional worldwide study. Lancet Oncol. 2010;11: 1048–56.
17. Forman D, de Martel C, Lacey CJ, Soerjomataram I, Lortet-Tieulent J, Bruni L, et al. Global burden of human papillomavirus and related diseases. Vaccine. 2012;30S:F12–23.
18. Li Y, Huang K, Ji PL, Song L, Liu HT. Cervical infection of oncogenic human papillomavirus (HPV) types in Beijing, China. Biomed Environ Sci. 2016;29: 734–41.
19. Li C, Wu M, Wang J, Zhang S, Zhu L, Pan J, et al. A population-based study on the risks of cervical lesion and human papillomavirus infection among women in Beijing, People's Republic of China. Cancer Epidemiol Biomarkers Prev. 2010;19:2655–64.
20. Chan PK, Ho WC, Chan MC, Wong MC, Yeung AC, Chor JS, et al. Meta-analysis on prevalence and attribution of human papillomavirus types 52 and 58 in cervical neoplasia worldwide. PLoS One. 2014;9(9):e107573.
21. Berrington de Gonzalez A, Green J. Comparison of risk factors for invasive squamous cell carcinoma and adenocarcinoma of the cervix: collaborative reanalysis of individual data on 8097 women with squamous cell carcinoma and 1374 women with adenocarcinoma from 12 epidemiological studies. Int J Cancer. 2007;120:885–91.
22. Li J, Zhang D, Zhang Y, Wang X, Lin Y, Hu L. Prevalence and genotype distribution of human papillomavirus in women with cervical cancer or high-grade precancerous lesions in Chengdu, western China. Int J Gynaecol Obstet. 2011;112:131–4.
23. Pirog EC, Lloveras B, Molijn A, Tous S, Guimerà N, Alejo M, et al. HPV prevalence and genotypes in different histological subtypes of cervical adenocarcinoma, a worldwide analysis of 760 cases. Mod Pathol. 2014;27: 1559–67.
24. Hu SY, Hong Y, Zhao FH, Lewkowitz AK, Chen F, Zhang WH, et al. Prevalence of HPV infection and cervical intraepithelial neoplasia and attitudes towards HPV vaccination among Chinese women aged 18–25 in Jiangsu Province. Chin J Cancer Res. 2011;23:25–32.

25. Insinga RP, Liaw KL, Johnson LG, Madeleine MM. A systematic review of the prevalence and attribution of human papillomavirus types among cervical, vaginal, and vulvar precancers and cancers in the United States. Cancer Epidemiol Biomarkers Prev. 2008;17:1611–22.
26. Sasagawa T, Maehama T, Ideta K, Irie T, Itoh F, J-HERS Study Group. Population-based study for human papillomavirus (HPV) infection in women in Japan: A multicenter study by the Japanese human papillomavirus disease education research survey group (J-HERS). J Med Virol. 2016;88:324–35.
27. Sun B, He J, Chen X, He M, He Z, Wang Y, et al. Prevalence and genotype distribution of human papillomavirus infection in Harbin, Northeast China. Arch Virol. 2014;159:1027–32.

15

The incidence, clearance and persistence of non-cervical human papillomavirus infections

Sylvia Taylor[1*], Eveline Bunge[2], Marina Bakker[2] and Xavier Castellsagué[3,4]

Abstract

Background: Human papillomavirus (HPV) vaccines were designed to prevent cervical cancer in women and their provision remains a major public health need. However, HPV is also a major cause of non-cervical anogenital and oropharyngeal cancers and the potential benefit of vaccination likely extends beyond cervical cancer.

Methods: A systematic literature search of PubMed (1995–2014) identified publications assessing the incidence, persistence, and clearance of non-cervical anogenital/oral HPV infections. Comparability with cervical HPV was assessed by identifying articles assessing the same or similar populations.

Results: Available data suggest high incidence rates of non-cervical HPV infection in men and women, with HPV-16 predominating in all sites. The incidence of high risk HPV per 100 person-years ranged from 11.4 to 72.9 for penile infections, 6.7–47.9 at other male genital sites, and 4.4–36.7 and 5.3–23.4 for anal infections in men and women, respectively. The incidence per 100 person-years of oral infection with any HPV type ranged from 5.7 to 6.7 in men and 6.8–39.6 in women. Within the limitations of the data, there was a general pattern of higher incidence and clearance of non-cervical genital HPV infections, compared to cervical infections. HIV status, circumcision, number of sex partners and partner HPV status significantly influenced high-risk HPV incidence/clearance at male anogenital sites. Few studies assessed risk factors for oral HPV.

Conclusions: Parallels appear to exist between the epidemiology of cervical and non-cervical HPV infections in terms of incidence, HPV-type distribution, and risk factors for infection. Available data suggest that non-cervical genital HPV infections may occur more frequently, with higher clearance rates, than cervical infections. More extensive studies could provide useful information for estimating vaccine impact, the wider cost-benefit of HPV vaccination, and guiding vaccination policy.

Keywords: Human papillomavirus, Cervical, Penile, Oral, Vaginal, Systematic review, Incidence, Persistence, Clearance

* Correspondence: sylvia.m.taylor@gsk.com
[1]GSK Vaccines, 20, Avenue Fleming, Parc de la Noire Epine, B-1300 Wavre, Belgium
Full list of author information is available at the end of the article

Background

Cervical cancer is the fourth most common cancer affecting women worldwide, with an estimated 528,000 new cases and 266,000 related deaths in 2012 [1]. Cervical cancer develops following persistent infection with oncogenic (or high risk) types of the human papillomavirus (HPV), that includes types 16, 18, 31, 33, 35, 39, 45, 51, 52, 56, 58, 59, 66 [2]. Approximately 70 % of cervical cancers are caused by HPV types 16 and 18, which along with several other high risk HPV types (HR-HPV), can be prevented by vaccination. However, the cancer-causing effects of HPV are not limited to the cervix; an estimated 50 % of penile, 88 % of anal, 43 % of vulvar, 70 % of vaginal, and 13–56 % of oropharyngeal cancers are attributable to HPV, primarily HPV-16 typically followed by HPV-18 [3, 4]. Sharply increasing trends in HPV-related oropharyngeal cancers have been observed in some countries [5]. The incidence of cervical cancer is far higher than that of non-genital or oropharyngeal cancers, and the provision of HPV vaccines to prevent cervical cancer remains a public health priority. However, together non-cervical and oropharyngeal cancers represented approximately 80,000 new HPV-related cancer cases worldwide in 2008, also signifying an important public health burden [6].

Available evidence from clinical trials indicates that current HPV vaccines can prevent vulval and vaginal and anal HPV infections, anogenital pre-cancers, and oral HPV infections [7] in women, and oral and anogenital infections and pre-cancer in men [7–14]. However, compared to vaccine efficacy/effectiveness data for cervical HPV infections and high-grade lesions, similar data for non-cervical HPV infections and lesions are scant. Moreover, our ability to measure the population level impact of HPV vaccination on non-cervical cancers is severely limited by a lack of systematic screening for non-cervical infections and pre-cancers, the relative rarity of these cancers, and for some, the absence of precursor lesions amenable to screening. The need to build ways of collecting such data nonetheless remains important to understand the full value of HPV vaccination, including cost-benefit, so that proper guidance can be given to vaccination policy. To this end, we conducted a systematic literature review to investigate the natural history of non-cervical HPV infections, and to identify parallels between the epidemiology of these infections and that of cervical infection. These data can inform on the design and scope of future studies of HPV vaccine effectiveness, aid in the interpretation of surveillance data, and point to knowledge gaps where further investigations may be warranted.

Methods

Objectives

The study objectives were to conduct a systematic review of the literature to describe the incidence, clearance and persistence of non-cervical HPV infections, including comparisons to cervical infections for which data were available for the same/or similar study population. We also examined risk factors for incident and persistent non-cervical HPV infections.

Search strategy and selection criteria

A systematic review of the literature in PubMed used three search strings (Supplementary material) to identify non-cervical anogenital and oral HPV infections and was limited to studies published in English between 01 January 1995 and 12 July 2014. We used specific searches to obtain articles on cervical HPV infections reporting comparable estimates of incidence, clearance, or persistence in the same or similar populations and using comparable HPV testing methods as in the articles on non-cervical HPV infections. Articles were included if they contained information on incidence, persistence, clearance or duration of non-cervical HPV infections, risk factors for non-cervical HPV infections or risk groups for incidence of non-cervical infections. Articles were excluded if they reported diagnostic test research, if they were case studies, letters to the editor, editorials or comments, literature reviews, or meta-analyses presenting no original data. Articles were also excluded if no information was listed in the inclusion criteria, or if they reported data based on testing of self-collected vaginal samples only. PRISMA guidelines were followed for the report. Independent review in duplicate was undertaken for 30 % of screened titles and abstracts and for 10 % of full text articles. Article selection, data extraction, assessment of risk factors and quality control procedures are provided in Additional file 1.

During the search for cervical cohorts, studies were found which used self-collected vaginal samples but in which the samples were referred to as 'cervical' swabs. These studies were not identified with the original non-cervical search string that did not include the term 'cervical'. We did not include studies when vaginal samples had been self-collected, because the original search may have missed studies that assessed self-collected vaginal samples, and because we could not be certain that they represented vaginal-only infections. For similar reasons cervical samples collected using cervical vaginal lavage in D'Souza et al. [15] were also excluded because we could not be certain that they represented cervical-only infections.

For ease of comparability, incidence, clearance and persistence rates were recalculated, if not provided, per 100 person-years, and all estimates of median (or mean if median not reported) time-to-clearance (or duration of infection) were calculated in terms of months. For example, conversion from 1000 person-months to 100 person-years values was done by multiplying by 12 and dividing by 10. All estimates of median time-to-clearance were calculated in terms of months (dividing days by 30.5).

When confidence intervals (CI) were not already provided and there was sufficient data, we used the exact method to calculate 95 % CI for proportions.

Ethics approval was not required for this study.

Definitions

The definition of HR-HPV was study specific. The HR-HPV types applicable to individual studies are provided in Additional file 2: Table S1.

Clearance, incidence, persistence, and duration of infection were defined broadly to capture the most studies: For individual HPV types (e.g., HPV-16), incidence was defined as at least one positive test for that HPV type following at least one negative test for that type. Clearance of infection was defined as a negative test for the individual HPV type following a positive test for that type.

Type-specific incidence of any HPV or HR-HPV was defined as a positive test for at least one HPV type or HR-HPV type not detected at baseline or other previous visit. For non-type-specific incidence, subjects were required to have tested negative for any HPV DNA or any HR-HPV DNA at baseline. We considered this to be non-type-specific incidence even if the HPV type(s) associated with the incident infection was known. In addition, for studies conducting multiple follow-up visits, incidence rates could be calculated by: 1) censoring subjects at the time of the first positive test (first acquired incidence); or 2) considering subjects to be at risk throughout the follow-up period and counting each visit where at least one new type was detected as an event (total acquired incidence).

Type-specific clearance of any HPV or HR-HPV was defined as a negative test for all HPV types or HR-HPV types detected at baseline (type-specific clearance of prevalent infection) or for all newly detected during follow-up (type-specific clearance of incident infection). Non-type-specific clearance was defined as at least one negative test for any HPV DNA or any HR-HPV DNA following a positive test for any HPV DNA or HR-HPV DNA at baseline or during follow-up.

Persistence was defined as at least two sequentially positive tests for at least one specific HPV type or HR-HPV type at least three months apart. Definitions for type-specific and non-type specific duration of infection followed those for clearance of infection.

For estimates related to any HPV and HR-HPV, calculations were required to be based on the total number of subjects rather than total number of infections as the denominator.

Results

Search results

We identified 38 articles from 25 unique study cohorts with relevant data on non-cervical anogenital or oral HPV infections (Table 1). A further 6 articles were identified that assessed cervical HPV infection in the same/similar populations. HPV-testing methods are summarised in Additional file 2: Table S1. Three articles were excluded due to unclear methods. Articles excluded due to improper testing methods or sample type were included under 'no relevant data'.

Median follow-up times varied between 6.7 and 84.5 months, with all but 8 studies conducting at least two follow-up visits at intervals ranging between 2 and 12 months. Among the 31 studies reporting data on incidence of any HPV or any HR-HPV, 10 (32 %) used type-specific definitions which counted any newly detected type as an incident infection and 17 (55 %) used non-type-specific definitions that required subjects to be negative for any HPV or any HR-HPV at baseline; an additional 4 studies reported data on incidence of individual HPV types only. A total of 31 studies were known to have multiple follow-up visits. Among the 31, 20 assessed incidence of any HPV or HR-HPV: 13/20 (65 %) estimated incidence based on time to the first acquired infection; 3/20 (15 %) considered each new infection as an event; for 2/20 it was unclear (10 %); 1/20 (5 %) used both methods; and 1/20 (5 %) did not conduct any survival analysis. Among the 29 studies reporting data on HPV clearance, type-specific definitions were used more consistently, with only 5 (17 %) using non-type-specific definitions. Three studies (10 %) required at least two consecutive negative test results to define an infection as having cleared.

Penile HPV infections

Incidence

In studies conducted in Africa, HR-HPV incidence was higher in human immunodeficiency virus positive (HIV + ve) men (42.0–72.9/100 person-years) than HIV negative (HIV-ve) men (19.7–32.9/100 person-years) (Table 2). Studies in Spain reported higher HPV incidence in HIV + ve men who have sex with men (MSM) than in men who have sex with women (MSW) (11.6 versus 5.1/100 person-years), but similar incidences of HPV-16 and HPV-18 infection. Genotype-specific incidence was highest for HPV-16 in at least one study subgroup in 7/9 studies (HIV + ve, HIV-ve, circumcised, uncircumcised and MSW) [8, 16–21].

In three articles that reported age-specific incidence of HPV infection the highest incidence was reported in the youngest age group studied (<30 or 15–24 year olds) [18, 19, 22].

Clearance and persistence

The rate of clearance of incident HR-HPV infection was 123.9/100 person-years (Table 2), with HPV-33 clearing most rapidly and HPV-58 least rapidly [22].

The clearance rate of prevalent penile infections ranged between 23.6 and 114.1/100 person-years for any HPV [19, 20, 23]. Clearance of HR-HPV was 114.7/100 person-years in HIV + ve men and 170.2/100 person-

Table 1 Summary of 38 articles included in the review

Author, study location (ref)	Study year	Population	Age	Number	Follow-up period (timing of follow-up visits)	Mean or median follow-up	Anatomical site	Outcomes (definition used for any/HR-HPV)[c]
Tobian, Uganda [19]	2003–2007	HIV + ve/-ve men	15–49	999	2 years (6, 12, 24 m)	Mean 14.4 m	Penile	Inc (TS, total) Clr (TS)
Kjaer, Denmark [63]	2000–2003	Military servicemen	18–19	374	6 m (6 m)	Range 5.4–7.8 m	Penile	Inc (NTS)
Backes, Kenya [17]	2002–2005	Uncircumcised men	17–24	966	1 year (6, 12 m)	Median 12.1 m	Penile	Inc (NTS, first)
Mbulawa, South Africa [22]	Not reported	HIV + ve/-ve men	19–67	486	2 years (6, 12, 18, 24 m)	-	Penile	Inc (TS, first) Clr (TS)[a]
Videla, Spain [23]	2005–2009	HIV + ve men	20- > 69	733	5 years (annual)	Median 24 m	Penile, anal, oral	Inc (NTS, first) Clr (NTS)
Wikström A, Sweden [21]	Not reported	MSW, sexually active without clinical HPV	18–54	235	(1–5 visits)	Mean 3.5 m between visits	Penile	Inc (TS) Clr/Pers (TS)
Gray, Uganda [18]	2003–2006	HIV-ve married men	15–49	840	24 m (6, 12, 24 m)	-	Penile	Inc Clr
Serwadda, Uganda [16]	2003–2007	HIV + ve men	15–49	210	24 m (24 m)	-	Penile	Inc (TS) Clr
Grabowski, Uganda [24]	2003–2007	HIV + ve/-ve men	15–49	936	24 m (6, 12, 24 m)	-	Penile	Pers (TS)
Giuliano, Brazil, Mexico, USA [53]	2005–2009	HIV-ve men	18–70	1159	4 years (every 6 m)	Median 27.5 m	Penile	Inc (NTS, first) Clr (TS)
Darwich, Spain [20]	2005–2009	HIV + ve men	20- > 69	606	5 years (annual)	Median 24 m	Penile, anal	Inc[b] Clr
de Pokomandy, Canada [38]	2002–2007	HIV + ve MSM	21–66	247	3 years (every 6 m)	Mean 30.8 m	Anal	Inc Clr
Nyitray, Brazil, Mexico, USA [35]	2005–2009	Men	18–70	MSM:156 MSW:954	6 m (6 m)	Median 6.7 m	Anal	Inc (TS) Clr (TS) Pers (TS)
Goodman, Hawaii, USA [36]	1998–2003	Sexually active women	18–85	431	5 years (every 4 m)	Mean 16 m	Anal	Inc (NTS, first) Clr (TS)
Shvetsov, Hawaii [39]	1998–2003	Sexually active women	18–85	431	5 years (every 4 m)	Mean 16 m	Anal	Clr (TS)
Moscicki, USA [40]	1990- > 2004	Sexually active women	13–21	75	3–9.5 years (every 4 m)	Mean 84.5 m	Anal	Clr (TS, 2+ neg)
Mullins, USA [37]	1996–2001	HIV + ve and HIV-ve at risk	12–18	496	6 years (annual)	Mean 22.4 m	Anal	Inc (NTS, first)
Glick, USA [33]	2009–2010	MSM	16–30	94	1 year (every 6 m)	-	Anal	Inc (NTS, unclear) Clr (TS)
Hernandez, USA [34]	1998–2000	HIV + ve MSM	Mean 45	369	2 years (every 6 m)	-	Anal	Inc (TS, total)

Table 1 Summary of 38 articles included in the review *(Continued)*

Lu, Arizona USA [31]	2003–2005	Men	18–44	285	2 years (every 6 m)	Median 15.5 m	Male genital (shaft, coronal sulcus, glans, scrotum)	Inc (TS, total) Clr (TS)
Hernandez, Hawaii [59]	2004–2006	Circ, UnC men	18–79	357	2.5 years (every 2 m)	Mean 14 m	Male genital (coronal sulcus, glans, shaft, scrotum)	Clr (TS, 2+ neg)
Giuliano, Arizona USA [25]	2003–2005	Men	18–44	290	2 years (every 6 m)	Mean 15.5 m	Male genital (coronal sulcus, glans, shaft, scrotum)	Inc (NTS, first & total) Pers (NTS) Clr (NTS)
Morales, Mexico [26]	2003–2004	MSW	Median 36	351	3 years (every 4 m)	Median 19.8 m	Male genital (scrotum, shaft, balano-preputial groove, urinary meatus)	Inc (NTS, unclear) Clr (TS)
Partridge, USA [29]	2003–2006	MSW university students	18–20	240	3 years (every 4 m)	Median 12.9 m	Male genital (glans &urethral meatus, shaft, scrotum)	Inc (NTS, first)
Lajous, Mexio [27]	2000–2003	Male soldiers	16–40	336	1 year (1 year)	-	Male genital (shaft, coronal sulcus, scrotum urethral meatus)	Inc (NTS) Clr (TS) Pers (TS)
Albero, Brazil, Mexico, USA [28]	2005–2009	HIV-ve men	18–70	4033	4 years (every 6 m)	Median 17.5 m	Male genital (shaft, coronal sulcus, glans, scrotum)	Inc (NTS, first) Clr (TS, 2+ neg)
Winer, USA [43]	1990–2000	Female university students	18–20	444	10 year (every 4 m)	Mean 41.2 m	Vulvovaginal	Inc (NTS, first)
Edelstein, USA [45]	2008–2010	Male university students	Median 20	212	1.5 years (every 4 m)	Median 10.7 m	Oral (rinse/OP swab)	Inc (NTS, first)
Kero, Finland [48]	Not reported	Male partners of pregnant women	19–46	131	7 years (2, 6, 12, 24, 36 m & 7 years)	Mean at visit 1: 1.8 m, visit 2: 5.9 m, visit 3: 12.1 m, visit 4: 24.7 m, visit 5: 36.8 m, visit 6: 77.0 m	Oral (scraping)	Inc
Kero, Finland [30]	2006–2008	Pregnant women and their male partners	Women: 19–46 Men: 20–52	46 women, 46 men	7 years (7 years)	-	Oral (scraping), male genital (penis/urethra)	Inc (NTS) Clr (TS)
Kero, Finland [46]	Not reported	Males partners of pregnant women	20–52	129 men	7 years (2, 6, 12, 24, 36, 7 years)	Mean in 74 HPV + ve 43.8 m	Oral (scraping)	Inc (NTS, first) Clr (TS)

Table 1 Summary of 38 articles included in the review *(Continued)*

Louvanto, Finland [51]	Not reported	Women with persistent cervical HPV (≥24 months) and HPV-ve controls	Mean 25.2–26.4	43 cases 52 controls	6 years (possibly annual)	Mean 65.2 m (cases) 38.4 m (controls)	Oral (scraping)	Clr(TS)
Rintala, Finland [50]	2006–2008	Pregnant women and their male partners	Women: 19–46 Men: 20–52	331 women, 131 men	2 years (2, 6, 12, 24 m)	Mean 26.9 m (women) 25.9 m (men)	Oral (scraping)	Inc (NTS, first) Clr (NTS)
Pickard, USA [49]	2009–2010	University students	18–30	1000	3 m (3 m)	-	Oral (rinse)	Inc (TS) Clr (TS) Pers (TS)
D'Souza, USA [15]	2004–2005	HIV + ve and high-risk HIV-ve adult women	Not reported	199	6 m (6 m)	-	Oral (rinse)	Inc (TS) Clr (NTS)
Kurose, Japan [52]	2000–2002	Healthy volunteers	3–85	662	2.5 years (2.5 years)	-	Oral (scraping)	Clr (TS) Pers (TS)
Darwich, Spain [47]	2005–2009	HIV + ve men	Median 41	733	5 years (annual)	Median 24 m	Oral (scraping/rinse)	Clr (TS)
Kreimer, Brazil, Mexico, USA [44]	2007–2009	HIV-ve men	18–70	1626	4 years (every 6 m)	Median 12.7 m	Oral (rinse)	Inc (NTS, first) Clr (TS)

Abbreviations: *IQR* interquartile range, *MSM* men who have sex with men, *MSW* men who have sex with women, *Inc* incidence, *Clr* clearance, *Pers* persistence, *Circ* circumcised, *UnC* uncircumcised, *OP* oropharyngeal

[a] If HPV types present-negative-present in sequential visits then negative result was considered false

[b] In calculation of incidence of individual HPV types, subjects were required to be negative for any HPV DNA at baseline at not just negative for that type

[c] Definitions for Any or Any HR-HPV infections: *TS* type specific. For incidence, defined as a positive test for at least one HPV type or HR type not detected at baseline (or other previous visit). For clearance, defined as a negative test for all HPV types or HR-HPV types detected at baseline or newly detected during follow-up. *NTS* non-type-specific. For incidence, defined as testing negative for any HPV DNA or any HR HPV DNA at baseline. For clearance, defined as at least one negative test for any HPV DNA or any HR-HPV DNA following a positive test at baseline or during follow-up. *2+ neg* 2+ negative test results required to define an infection as having cleared. *first* subjects censored at time of first positive test. *total* subjects not censored and each visit where new type(s) detected counted as event. *unclear* unclear if incidence based on firstacquired or total-acquired

Table 2 Incidence and clearance of penile and other male genital HPV infections

Author (ref)	Population, age (years)	Incidence					Clearance					
		Unit	Any HPV	HR	16	18	Type of Infection	Unit of clearance	Any HPV	HR	16	18
Penile												
Tobian [19]	HIV-ve, 15–49 HIV + ve,15–49	per 100py		32.9 (TS) (30.0–36.0) 66.5 (60.4–72.2)	4.2 (3.1–5.6) 10.4 (6.9–14.7)	3.7 (2.6–5.0) 8.0 (5.1–11.8)	Prevalent	per 100py		170.2 (TS) (156.7–184.4) 114.7 (103.3–129.1)	168.2 (130.0–213.9) 70.3 (47.1–101.0)	178.3 (125.6–245.8) 122.8 (83.4–174.3)
Gray [18]	HIV-ve I, 15–49 HIV-ve C, 15–49	per 100py	-	19.7 (15.3–24.9) 29.4 (24.6–34.9)	3.7 (1.0–6.3) 4.9 (3.1–7.6)	1.7 (0.6–3.7) 5.6 (3.6–8.4)	Prevalent	per 100py			190.9 (118.2–291.8) 167.6 (113.9–237.8)	285.7 (158.4–466.8) 157.9 (88.4–260.4)
Serwadda [16]	HIV + ve I, 15–49 HIV + ve C, 15–49	% at 24 m	-	42.0 (TS) (31.1–55.5) 57.0 (46.3–67.2)	5.8 (1.6–14.2) 14.9 (7.7–25.0)	4.3 (0.9–12.0) 11.1 (5.2–20.1)	Prevalent	% at 24 m			66.7 (34.9–90.1) 63.2 (38.4–83.7)	72.7 (39.0–94.0) 91.7 (61.5–99.8)
Kjaer [63]	Military, 18–29	% at 6 m	13.8 (NTS) (8.6–19.0)	-	-	-	-	-	-	-	-	-
Backes [17]	UnC, 17–24	per 100py	All: 59.2 (NTS, first) (51.6–67.6) Glans: 53.3 (46.1–60.5) Shaft: 25.9 (22.3–30.0)	All: 37.3 (32.0–43.2) Glans: 32.8 (28.1–38.0) Shaft: 15.7 (13.1–18.7)	All: 13.1 (10.7–15.6) Glans: 10.3 (8.3–12.7) Shaft: 5.3 (3.8–7.0)	All: 4.3 (3.1–5.9) Glans: 3.7 (2.6–5.3) Shaft: 1.8 (1.1–2.9)	-	-	-	-	-	-
Mbulawa [22]	All, 18–66 HIV-ve, 18–66 HIV + ve 18–66	per 100py	66.8 (TS, first) (52.3–83.0) 62.3 (47.2–79.5) 96.5 (57.1–163.2)	35.7 (28.1–45.4) 29.2 (21.9–39.1) 72.9 (47.2–112.8)	3.8 (2.2–6.5)	4.0 (2.4–6.8)	Incident	per 100py	114.1 (TS) (100.0–129.7) 128.2 (115.4–141.9) 96.4 (83.8–110.1)	123.9 (106.2–144.7)	121.5 (74.8–197.4)	160.0 (109.4–234.0)
Darwich [20], Videla [23]	HIV + ve MSM, 20- > 69 HIV + ve MSW, 20- > 69	per 100py	11.6 (NTS, first) (8.8–14.9) 5.1 (2.4–9.4)	-	1.7 (0.8–2.9) 1.4 (0.4–3.7)	0.4 (0.1–1.1) 0.4 (–)	Prevalent	per 100py	27.1 (NTS) (20.0–35.6) 23.6 (14.8–35.6)	-	29.4 (15.1–51.4) 29.5 (10.8–64.2)	40.0 (8.2–116.9) 14.6 (–)
Wikström [21]	MSW, 18–54	% at 3.5m[a]	17.1 (TS) (9.4–27.5)	11.4 (5.6–19.9)	4.5 (1.3–11.2)	0 (0–4.1)	Prevalent	% at 3.5m[a]-	41.7 (TS) (15.2–72.3)	42.9 (9.9–81.6	20 (0.5 71.6)	100 (1 case only)
Giuliano [53]	HIV-ve, 18–70	per 100py	46.1 (NTS, first) (41.2–51.6)	26.7 (23.8–29.9)	5.3 (4.3–6.4)	2.3 (1.7–3.0)	-	-	-	-	-	-

Table 2 Incidence and clearance of penile and other male genital HPV infections *(Continued)*

Genital												
Giuliano [25] (coronal sulcus, glans, shaft, scrotum)	Men, 18–44	per 100py	46.1 (NTS, Total) (41.8–61.2) 35.3 (NTS, first) (27.4–44.9)	25.0 (19.2–31.9) 18.6 (13.4–25.0)	5.8 (3.4–9.2)	1.0 (0.2–2.9)	Prevalent	% at 6 m % at 12 m % at 18 m	55.5 (NTS) 74.8 89.3	58.3 81.0 100	-	-
Morales [26] (scrotum, shaft, balano-preputial groove, urinary meatus)	MSW, median 36	per 100py	14.8 (NTS, unclear) (11.8–18.2)	6.7 (4.9–8.9)	1.7 (0.8–2.8)	0.4 (0.1–1.1)	-	-	-	-	-	-
Partridge [29] (glans &urethral meatus, shaft, scrotum)	MSW, 18–20	% at 24 m	62.4 (NTS, first) (52.6–72.2)	47.9 (38.6–58.0)	19.5 (14.0–27.2)	7.5 (4.1–13.6)	-	-	-	-	-	-
Lajous [27] (shaft, coronal sulcus, scrotum urethral meatus)	Male soldiers, 16–40	per 100py	21.5 (NTS) (15.6–28.7)	14.3 (9.8–19.9)	2.8 (1.3–5.3)	1.6 (0.5–3.6)	Prevalent	% at 12 m	70.6 (TS) (61.9–78.4)	69.0 (59.0–77.9)	68.8 (41.3–89.0)	100 (66.4–100)
Albero [28] (shaft, coronal sulcus, glans, scrotum)	HIV-ve men UnC, 18–70 HIV-ve men Circ, 18–70	per 100py	50.5 (NTS, first) (46.4–54.9) 45.6 (41–50.5)	28.4 (26.2–30.8) 28.7 (25.9–31.8)	5.8 (5–6.6) 6.6 (5.6–7.8)	2.5 (2–3) 2.9 (2.3–3.7)	-	-	-	-	-	-
Kero [30] (penis/urethra)	Male partners of pregnant women, 20–52	% at 7 years	32.3 (NTS) (16.7–51.4)	-	-	-	Prevalent	% at 7 years	88.9 % (TS) (51.8–99.7)	-	-	-

Abbreviations: *MSM* men who have sex with men, *MSW* men who have sex with women, *py* person-years, *UnC* Uncircumcised, *Circ* Circumcised, *m* months, *I* Intervention (immediate circumcision), *C* Control (circumcision delayed for 24 months), *TS* type-specific incidence defined as at least one positive test for any HPV type or HR-HPV type not detected at baseline, *NTS* non-type-specific incidence defined as at least one positive test for any HPV type or HR-HPV type among those negative for any HPV DNA or any HR-HPV DNA at baseline

[a]Mean interval between visits 3.5 m: Results at visit 1 and 2 considered here

years in HIV-ve men [19]. HPV types tending to clear the least rapidly were HPV-52 and 16 in circumcised men, 52 and 58 in uncircumcised men over a 2-year period [18], 52 and 16 in HIV + ve MSM and 18 and 51 in HIV + ve MSW up to 5 years of follow-up [20], depending on study and population. Age-specific clearance rates were highest in men aged >30 years in two studies [19, 22].

Time-to-clearance was 12.2 months for HPV-16 and 6.3 months for HPV-18 in HIV-ve men, versus 27.8–35.3 months for HPV-16 and 18 in HIV + ve men (Fig. 1).

HR-HPV persisted in 31 % of HIV-ve men and 43 % of HIV + ve men at 6 months, and in 25 %/28 %, respectively, at 12 months [24] (Table 3). Persistence of HR-HPV at 12 months was associated with higher HPV viral load at baseline in HIV + ve men [24].

Cervical infections in comparable populations

In South Africa, incidence and clearance of penile and cervical infections was assessed among 468 male–female couples aged 18–67 years (Table 4) [22]. Incidence and

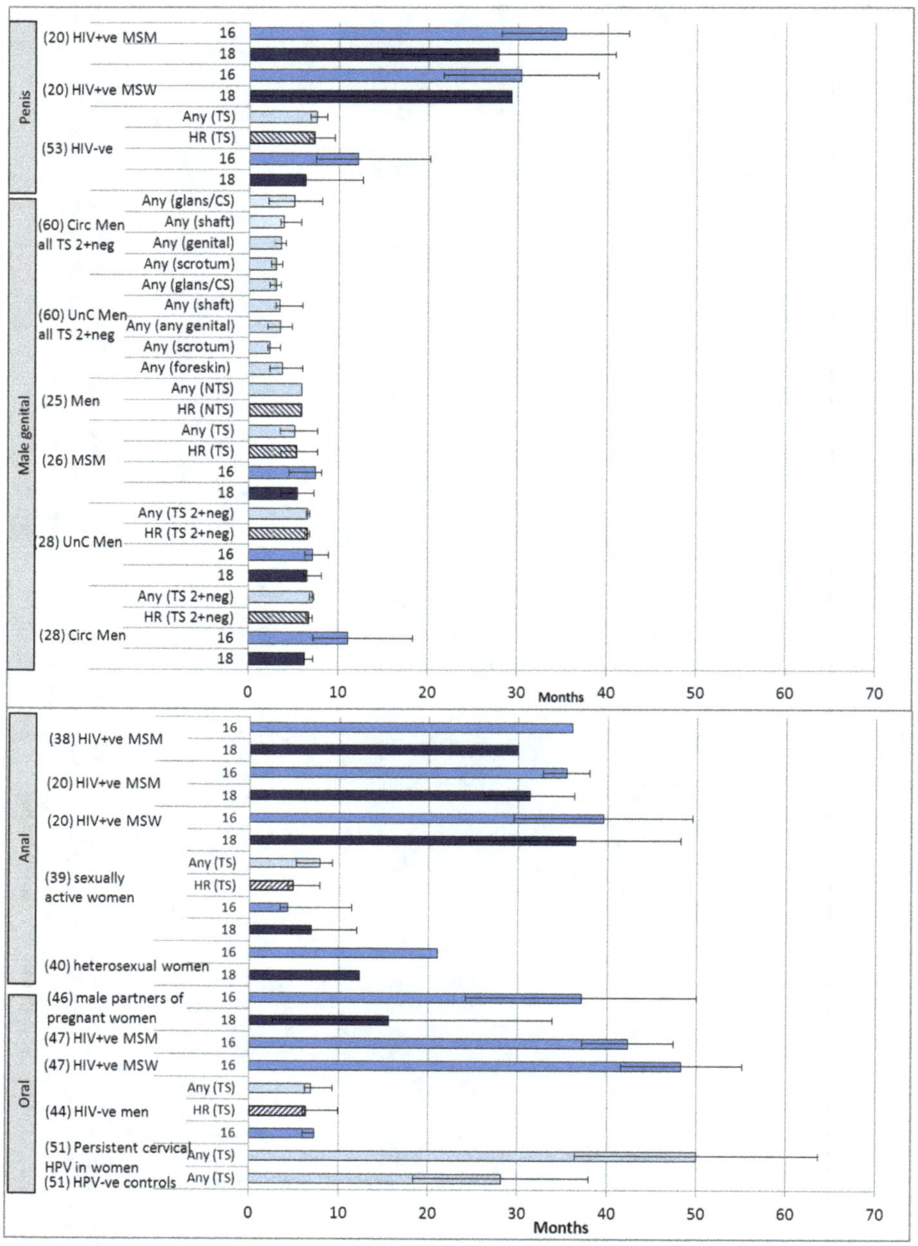

Fig. 1 Median* Time to clearance (months, 95 % CIs) of HPV from non-cervical sites in men and women. Footnote: *mean reported for [20, 46, 47, 51]. *TS* type-specific incidence defined as at least one positive test for any HPV type or HR-HPV type not detected at baseline; *NTS* non-type-specific incidence defined as at least one positive test for any HPV type or HR-HPV type among those negative for any HPV DNA or any HR-HPV DNA at baseline

Table 3 Type-specific persistence of HPV infections

Site	Reference	Population, age (years)	Infection type	Time-frame (months)	% (95 % CI) persistent at end of time frame			
					Any HPV	HR	16	18
Penile	Wikström; Sweden [21]	MSW, 18–54	Prevalent/ Incident	3.5	50 (23–77)	57 (18–90)	75 (19–99)	0 (0–98)
	Grabowski; Uganda [24]	HIV- men, 15–49	Prevalent	6		31 (27–37)		
			Prevalent	12		25 (20–30)		
		HIV+ men,		24		12 (9–16)		
		15–49		6		43 (37–48)		
				12		28 (23–34)		
				24		29 (25–34)		
Anal	Nyitray; Brazil, Mexico, USA [35]	MSM, 18–70	Prevalent	6	59 (48–70)	51 (36–66)	73 (39–94)	38 (9–76)
		MSW, 18–70	Prevalent	6	32 (24–41)	24 (14–37)	0 (0–16)	0 (0–84)
Male Genital	Lajous; Mexico [27]	Male soldiers, 16–40	Prevalent	12	29.4 (21.6–38.2)	31.0 (22.1–41.0)	31.3 (11.0–58.7)	0 (0–33.6)
Oral	Pickard; USA [49]	Male/female students, 18–30	Prevalent	3	38 (19–59)	42 (15–72)	0 (0–98)	
	Kurose; Japan [52]	Male/female volunteers, 3–85	Prevalent	30	50 (9–93)	0 (0–98)	0 (0–98)	-

Abbreviations: *MSM* men who have sex with men, *MSW* men who have sex with women

clearance rates were significantly higher among men compared with women (incidence of any HPV 66.8 versus 40.7/100 person-years; clearance of any HPV 114.1 versus 80.3/100 person-years). In regression analyses adjusting for HPV type, incidence rates remained higher in men when stratified by age-group and HIV status; clearance rates remained higher in men when stratified by age-group and among HIV + ve individuals (Table 4). HIV status was the only significant predictor of clearance in men and women, whereas in multivariate analyses, incidence was significantly predicted by HIV status and partner infection with same HPV type in men and women, and age at first sex and hormonal contraceptive use in women only.

Male genital HPV infections

Male genital sites included samples from the scrotum, coronal sulcus or combined samples of both penile and non-penile sites (Table 2).

Incidence

Incidence of any HPV ranged from 14.8 to 50.51/100 person-years in adult men and military men [25–28]. Incidence in university students (median follow-up of 12.9 months) was 62.4 % [29]. Incidence in male partners of pregnant women was 32.3 % over 7 years after the initial assessment [30]. HPV-16 was the most frequently identified type in all studies, followed by 52 and 58 [25–27, 29], or 51 and 59 [28].

Two studies reported on age-specific incidences of male genital infections, of which one was restricted to 18 or 19 year olds [29]. In an adult population the highest incidence was observed in the oldest age group studied (41–44 years) for any HPV infection (55.6/100 person-years), but the highest incidence of HR-HPV was in 26–30 year-olds (33.1/100 person-years) [31].

Clearance and persistence

Median time-to-clearance of any HPV male genital infection was 3.5–7.1 months (Fig. 1). Time-to-clearance of HPV-16 was 7.1–11.1 months, and 5.4–6.5 months for HPV-18.

The median duration of incident male genital HPV infections ranged between 5.1 and 7.1 months [25, 26, 28]. The duration of HPV-16 and/or 18 infection ranged between 5.4 and 11.1 months [25, 26, 28]. In the United States (US), HR-HPV genital infections persisted in 42 % of men at 6 months, 19 % at 12 months and had cleared in all men at 18 months [25] (Table 2).

Cervical infections in comparable populations

Incidence of male genital and cervical infections was assessed in two similar but separate cohorts of men and women from Arizona (Table 4) [25, 32]. Incidence calculated based on the first acquired infection with any HPV was similar in men and women (35.3/100 person-years [95 %CI 27.4–44.9] versus 35.3/100 person-years [95 % CI 24.7–48.8]), but the cumulative incidence of infection by 12 months was substantially higher in men than in women (41 % versus 29 % [95 % CI 22–36] for any HPV; 32 % versus 19 % [95 % CI 13–25) for HR-HPV). Median time-to-clearance for penile compared with cervical

Table 4 Comparison of non-cervical HPV infections and cervical HPV infections in same or similar study populations

Ref, site	Population, age (years)	Incidence (95 % CI)					Clearance (95 % CI)					
		Unit	Any	HR	16	18	Inf. type	Unit	Any	HR	16	18
Darwich; Spain; Penile [20]	HIV + ve MSM, 20- > 69	Per 100py	-	-	1.7 (0.8–2.9)	0.4 (0.1–1.1)	Prev	Per 100py	-	-	29.4 (15.1–51.4)	40.0 (8.2–116.9)
	HIV + ve MSW, 20- > 69	Per 100py	-	-	1.4 (0.4–3.7)	0.3 (ND)	Prev	Per 100py	-	-	29.5 (10.8–64.2)	14.6 (–)
Videla; Spain; Cervical [64]	HIV + ve women, 20–64	% at 36 m	-	-	9 (3.4–18.5)	7 (2.6–14.6)	Prev	% at 36 m	-	-	46 (26.6–66.6)	29 (3.7–71.0)
Comment: Study period 1999–2003 for women v. 2005–2009 for men												
Mbulawa; South Africa; Penile [22]	HIV + ve/-ve Men in a relationship, 19–67	Per 100py	66.8 (TS, first) (52.3–83.0)	35.7 (28.1–45.4)	3.8 (2.2–6.5)	4.0 (2.4–6.8)	Prev/Inc	Per 100py	114.1 (TS) (100–130.7)	124.9 (106.2–144.7)	121.5 (74.8–197.4)	160.0 (109.4–234.0)
Mbulawa; South Africa; Cervical [22]	HIV + ve/-ve Women in a relationship, 18–66	Per 100py	40.7 (TS) (31.7–52.2)	18.7 (13.8–25.7)	2.4 (1.3–4.7)	1.4 (0.6–3.3)	Prev/Inc	Per 100py	80.3 (TS) (68.4–94.2)	74.7 (61.3–91.4)	38.9 (16.7–90.5)	127.9 (85.2–94.2)
Comment: Incidence and clearance significantly higher in men v. women. In type- adjusted analyses, incidence remained higher in men by age group and HIV status; clearance remained higher in men by age group and HIV + ve (96.4 versus 66.0/100 person-years), but not HIV-ve (128.1 versus 132.1/100 person-years)												
Giuliano; USA (Arizona); Male genital [25]	Adult men, 18–44	Per 100py	46.1 (NTS, total) (41.8–61.2) 35.3 (NTS, first) (27.4–44.9)	25.0) (19.2–31.9) 18.6) (13.4–25.0)	5.3 (3.4–9.2)	1.0 (0.2–2.9)	-	-	-	-	-	-
Giuliano; USA (Arizona); Cervical [32]	Women attending gynecology clinic,18–35	Per 100py	35.3 (NTS, first) (24.7–48.8)	-	7.1 (3.7–12.1)	1.0 (0.1–3.5)	-	-	-	-	-	-
Comment: Study period 2003–2005 for men v. 1996–1999 for women; follow-up at 6, 12, and 24 months for men v. 4 and 10 months for women. Med time to clearance anal v. cervical: 5.9 m (5.7–6.1) v. ~9 m for any HPV; 5.8 m (5.5–6.1) v. 8.5 m for HR-HPV. PGMY09/11 assay used to detect types 61, 62, 64, 67, 69, 72, 81, IS39, and CP6108 in anal but not cervical samples												
Goodman; USA (Hawaii); Anal [36, 39]	Sexually active women, 18–85	Per 100py	56.3 (NTS, first) (48.5–65.0)	23.4 (19.2–28.3)	3.0 (1.8–4.8)	2.3 (1.2–3.9)	Inc	Per 100py	89.3 (TS) (67.8–115.4)	110.0 (83.3–142.4)	141.2 (73.0–246.7)	130.0 (47.6–282.8)
Goodman; USA (Hawaii); Cervical [41]	Sexually active women, 18–85	Per 100py	15.6 (NTS, first) (12.9–18.7)	11.1 (9.0–13.6)	2.1 (1.4–3.2)	0.6 (0.2–1.2)	Inc	Per 100py	85.1 (TS) (64.2–110.4)	92.0 (67.8–122.0)	86.4 (41.4–158.9)	69.7 (14.4–203.6)
Comment: 431 of 972 women in cervical analysis as per availability of anal sample, complete questionnaire data, and valid HPV testing results. Med time to clearance anal v. cervical: 7.8 m (5.2–9.2) v. 8.5 m (5.8–12.6) for any HPV; 4.9 m (4.3–8.0) v. 8.0 m (5.5–11.8) for HR HPV; 4.3 m (3.4–11.4) v. 9.5 m (4.4–23.8) for HPV16; 6.9 (4.6–12.0) v. 14.0 (4.8–ND) for HPV18												
Moscicki;USA; (California); Anal [40]	Sexually active women, 13–21	-	-	-	-	-	Prev	% at 12 m	-	29.7 (TS 2 + neg) (19.0–41.7)	-	-
Moscicki;USA (California); Cervical [42]	Sexually active women, 13–22	-	-	-	-	-	Prev	% at 12 m	-	~35 % (NTS)	-	-

Table 4 Comparison of non-cervical HPV infections and cervical HPV infections in same or similar study populations *(Continued)*

Comment: Anal and cervical analyses conducted on two partially overlapping cohorts of 75 and 531 women, respectively. Clearance defined as time to first of 2 consecutive negative results; data for any HPV not presented as cervical assay detected only 5 of 19 low-risk types detected by anal infection assay. HPV types 68, 69, 73, and 82 defined as HR types in analysis of anal but not cervical infection; ~35 % clearance at 12 m for cervical infections estimated from provided Kaplan-Meier curves												
Winer; USA; Vulvovaginal [43]	Female university students, 18–20	100py	16.0 (NTS, first) (13.7–18.6)	-	-	-	-	-	-	-	-	-
Winer; USA; Cervical [43]	Female university students, 18–20	100py	12.7 (NTS, first) (10.8–14.9)	-	-	-	-	-	-	-	-	-
Comment: Separate vulvovaginal and cervical swabs collected from 444 initially HPV-DNA-negative women. 35.4 % of infections were present at both sites												
Kero, Finland, Male Genital [30]	Partners of pregnant women, 20–52	% at 7 years	32.3 (NTS) (16.7–51.4)	-	-	-	Prev	% at 7 years	90 (TS) (55.5–99.7)	-	-	-
Kero; Finland; Oral [30]	Pregnant women, 19–46	% at 7 years	14.0 (NTS) (5.3–27.9)	-	-	-	Prev	% at 7 years	100 (TS) (29.2–100)	-	-	-
Kero; Finland; Cervical [30]	Pregnant women, 19–46	% at 7 years	16.7 (NTS) (6.4–32.8)	-	-	-	Prev	% at 7 years	70 (TS) (34.8–93.3)	-	-	-
Comment: Analysis based on only 46 men and 46 women returning for follow-up at 84 months. At year 7 the same infecting HPV genotype was detected in 11 % (95 % CI 0.3–48.2) and 30 % (6.7–65.2) of mean and women, respectively. HPV status during interval visits was not taken into account.												

Note: For male versus female comparison only date for penile/male genital infections versus cervical infections are presented

Abbreviations: *m* months, – data not provided, *TS* type-specific incidence defined as at least one positive test for any HPV type or HR-HPV type not detected at baseline, *NTS* non-type-specific incidence defined as at least one positive test for any HPV type or HR-HPV type among those negative for any HPV DNA or any HR-HPV DNA at baseline

infections was 5.9 months (95 % CI 5.7–6.1) versus approximately 9 months for any HPV, and 5.8 months (95 % CI 5.5–6.1) versus 8.5 months for HR-HPV. In Finland, where male genital and cervical infection data were collected at baseline and 7 years later among 46 pregnant women and their male partners, incidence and clearance of any HPV was also higher among men versus women: 32.3 % (95 % CI 16.7–51.4) versus 16.7 % (95 % CI 6.4–32.8) and 90 % (95 % CI 55.5–99.7) versus 70.0 % (95 % CI 34.8–93.3) (Table 4). Among men and women with genital HPV infections at baseline, the same infecting HPV genotype was present at the 7-year follow-up in 11 % (95 % CI 0.3–48.2) and 30 % (6.7–65.2), respectively [30].

Anal HPV infections

Ten articles reported on anal HPV infections: seven reported infections in men and four in women (Table 5).

Incidence in men

The incidence of anal HPV infection was higher in HIV + ve men (gender of partner not specified) and HIV-ve MSM (range 21.3–46.2/100 person-years), than in HIV + ve MSW (7.9/100 person-years) and MSW (HIV status not specified, 9.7/100 person-years). Among MSM, HPV-16 and 18 were among the HPV types with the highest incidence, although depending on the study, the incidences of HPV-51, 52 or 59 were similar or higher [33–35].

Incidence in women

In women, anal HPV incidence ranged from 14–56.3/100 person-years. HPV-16 and 52 were the most frequently infecting types [36]. The incidence of any and HR anal HPV infection in 12–18 year olds was higher in men than women (HIV-ve and HIV + ve), although the 95%CIs overlapped (Table 5) [37]. By contrast, in another study in women [36] the incidence (per 100 person-years) of any anal HPV infection was higher (56.3) than in all studies reported in male populations (range 7.9–46.2) (Table 5). In this study the incidence (per 100 person-years) of HR-HPV infection in women (23.4) was higher than that reported in MSW (4.4) and within the range observed in HIV + ve men or MSM (13.3–36.7).

A regression analysis conducted in a US study of sexually active women noted a statistically significant inverse relationship between acquisition of a new HR-HPV anal infection and age; with a 57 % (95 % CI 19–77) lower risk of acquisition among older women (≥45 years of age at baseline) than among younger women (<25 years at baseline) [36].

Clearance and persistence in men and women

Seven articles reported on the clearance rate of anal infections, of which five were in men who were HIV + ve and/or MSM, and two were in women (Table 5). The clearance rate of prevalent anal HPV infections in men varied between 14.6 and 66.7/100 person-years for specific HPV types. Amongst HR-HPV, the clearance rate was lowest for HPV-16 in 5/6 populations [20, 33, 35, 38]. For HPV-16 and 18 the time-to-clearance ranged between 30 and 39.5 months (Fig. 1).

In women, the clearance rate of incident anal HPV infections was 89.3/100 person-years, with a median time-to-clearance of 7.8 months [39] (Fig. 1). In another study, 56.5 % of women cleared any HR-HPV infection by year 3 [40]. In the single study that reported clearance of prevalent infections, HPV clearance in women appeared to be within the range reported in studies in men (Table 5).

HR-HPV anal infections persisted at 6 months in 51.0 % of MSW and in 24.2 % of MSM who were HR-HPV positive at baseline [35] (Table 3).

Cervical infections in comparable populations

In Hawaii, anal and cervical samples were collected in sexually active women aged 18–85 years every 4 months for an average of approximately 1.3 years [36, 39, 41]. Incidence (per 100 person-years) of anal versus cervical infections was more than three-fold higher for any HPV (56.3 [95 % CI 48.5–65.0] versus 15.6 [95 % CI 12.9–18.7]) and more than two-fold higher for HR-HPV (23.4 [95 % CI 19.2–28.3] versus 11.1 [95 % CI 9.0–13.6]); differences were similar for HPV-16 and 18 infections but not statistically significant (Table 4). Baseline cervical HPV status was not a significant risk factor for incidence of anal HPV infection. In contrast, clearance (per 100 person-years) did not significantly differ between anal versus cervical infections with either any HPV (89.3 [95 % CI 67.8–115.4] versus 85.1 [95 % CI 64.2–110.4], respectively) or with HR-HPV (109.9 [95 % CI 83.3–142.4] versus 92.0 [95 % CI 67.8–122.0], respectively).

In two partially overlapping cohorts of sexually active teenager and young adults in the US, clearance by 12 months was also similar for anal versus cervical infections (29.7 % [95 % CI 19.0–41.7] and approximately 35 %, respectively) [40, 42]. In the Hawaii cohort, there was some indication of higher clearance of anal than cervical HPV-16 and 18 infections, with more than two-fold differences in the median duration of infection (4.3 versus 9.8 months, and 6.9 versus 14 months, respectively), but CIs overlapped substantially (data not shown) [36, 39, 41].

Vaginal HPV infections

We identified one study of vulvovaginal HPV infections that employed physician-collected swabs [43]. The incidence rate for vulvovaginal HPV infections among university students was 16.0 per 100 person-years (95 % CI 13.7–18.6) compared with 12.7 per 100 person-years (95 % CI 10.8–14.9) for cervical infections (Table 4). No information on clearance or persistence was available.

Table 5 Incidence and clearance of anal HPV infections

Author (ref)	Population, age (yrs)	Incidence (per 100py)				Clearance					
		Any HPV	HR	16	18	Type of Infection	Unit of clearance	Any HPV	HR	16	18
Males											
de Pokomandy [38]	HIV + ve MSM, 21–66	-	-	13.0 (9.6–17.6)	5.3 (3.5–8.0)	Prevalent	Per 100py			14.6 (10.2–21.2)	24.5 (16.9–35.4)
Nyitray [35]	MSM, 18–70 MSW, 18–70	31.1 (TS) (16.6–53.2) 9.7 (7.2–12.8)	25.4 (14.5–41.2) 4.4 (2.9–6.6)	5.8 (1.9–13.4) 0.8 (0.2–2.0)	4.6 (1.2–11.6) 1.1 (0.4–2.3)	Prevalent	% at 6 m-	57.1 (TS) (50.1–63.8) 70.9 (63.5–77.5)	55.8 (44.1–67.2) 77.5 (66.0–86.5)	27.2 (6.0–61.0) 100 (83.9–100)	62.5 (24.5–91.5) 100 (15.8–100)
Videla [23]	HIV + ve MSM, 20- > 69 HIV + ve MSW, 20- > 69	32.4 (NTS) (23.3–43.7) 7.9 (4.9–15.7)	-	-	-	Prevalent	Per 100py	12.6 (NTS) (10.2–15.2) 18.4 (12.2–26.5)	-	-	-
Darwich [20]	HIV + ve MSM, 20- > 69 HIV + ve MSW, 20- > 69	-	-	7.1 (5.5–9.5) 5.3 (3.0–8.6)	3.6 (3.5–5.2) 0.4 (0.1–1.8)	Prevalent	Per 100py	-		22.4 (17.6–28.1) 18.6 (7.4–38.2)	31.0 (20.3–45.4) 30.0 (7.8–76.8)
Mullins [37]	HIV-ve, 12–18 HIV + ve, 12–18	24 (NTS, first) (11–52) 40 (27–61)	11 (3.4–33) 27 (17–44)	-	-	-	-	-	-	-	-
Glick [33]	MSM, 16–30	46.2 (NTS, unclear) (45.6–46.9)	36.7 (36.2–37.3)	12.4 (12.1–12.6)	5.5 (5.3–5.6)	Prevalent	% at 1 year	81.3 (TS) (67.4–91.1)	66.7 (49.0–81.4)	50.0 (26.0–74.0)	66.7 (22.3–95.7)
Hernandez [34]	HIV + ve MSM, mean 45	21.3 (TS, total) (17.7–25.4)	13.3 (10.5–16.6)	3.5 (1.8–6.1)	3.7 (2.1–6.1)	-	-	-	-	-	-
Females											
Goodman [36], Shvetsov [39]	Sexually active women, 18–44	56.3 (NTS, first) (48.5–65.0)	23.4 (19.2–28.3)	3.0 (1.8–4.8)	2.3 (1.2–3.9)	Incident	Per 100py	89.3 (TS) (67.8–115.4)	109.9 (83.3–142.4)	141.2 (73.0–246.7)	130.0 (47.6–282.8)
Moscicki [40]	Sexually active women, 13–21	-	-	-	-	Prevalent	% at 12 m	-	29.7 (TS 2 + neg) (19.0–41.7)	45.0 (27.2–62.1)	55.6 (21.2–86.3)
Mullins [37]	HIV-ve women, 12–18 HIV + ve women, 12–18	14 (NTS,first) (9.2–22) 30 (24–38)	5.3 (2.6–11) 12 (8.4–16)	-	-	-	-	-	-	-	-

Abbreviations: *MSM* men who have sex with men, *MSW* men who have sex with women, *py* person-years, *TS* type-specific incidence defined as at least one positive test for any HPV type or HR-HPV type not detected at baseline, *NTS* non-type-specific incidence defined as at least one positive test for any HPV type or HR-HPV type among those negative for any HPV DNA or any HR-HPV DNA at baseline

Oral HPV infections

Eleven articles (considering six cohorts) reported on oral HPV infections: eight in men and five in women (Table 6).

Incidence in men

The incidence of oral HPV infection was 5.7–6.1/100 person-years in HIV + ve men and 6.7/100 person-years in HIV-ve men [23, 44]. In another study conducted in university students, oral HPV incidence over 1 year was 12.3 % [45]. Finally, in the Finnish cohort, oral HPV infection was reported in 14.3–69.2 % of male partners of pregnant women 7 years after baseline. The variability in results was due to the varying sampling timetable [30, 46]. In studies reporting type-specific incidence, HPV-16 was the most frequently identified type [44, 45, 47, 48].

Two studies reported age-specific incidence rates of oral infections in men. In one study in university students the age-specific incidence was higher in the 21–24 years age-group than in the 18–20 years age-group [45]. In HIV-ve men there was no increased risk of incident HR-HPV oral infection across age groups (range 18–73 years) [44].

Incidence in women

The incidence of oral HPV infections in HIV-ve women was 6.8–20.4/100 person-years versus 39.6/100 person-years in HIV + ve women [15, 49]. In the Finnish cohort, oral infections were present in approximately 10 % of men and women after 24 months follow-up, and in 14.3 % of men and women after 7 years [30, 50]. Incidence rates in women appeared to be similar or higher than rates in men, depending on the study.

Clearance and persistence in men and women

Clearance rates of oral infections in men were reported in two study cohorts (Table 6). In HIV + ve men, the clearance rate of prevalent oral infections in MSM was 19.3/100 person-years, or 48.3 % after two-year follow-up [23, 47]. Rates for HIV + ve MSW were 15.8/100 person-years and 34 %, respectively [23, 47]. The time-to-clearance of oral HR-HPV in HIV-ve men was 6.9 months. Time-to-clearance of oral HPV-16 infection was between 7.3 and 37.1 months in HIV-ve men, and was higher (42.3–48.3 months) in HIV + ve men (Fig. 1). In the Finnish cohort, approximately 5 % of oral HR-HPV infections in 19 HR-HPV-positive men had cleared by 24 months [50].

In US studies, clearance of any oral HPV in women was 60.6 % at 3 months [49], and clearance at 6 months was 20.0 % in HIV-ve women and 40.0 % in HIV + ve women [15]. No oral HPV infections had cleared in women in the Finnish cohort at 24 months, whereas clearance at 7 years was 100 % [30, 50]. Among women with persistent cervical HPV infection the time-to-clearance of oral HPV infection was 50.0 months, versus 28.2 months in women without cervical HPV infections (Fig. 1) [51].

Persistence of oral HPV infections was reported for three cohorts (Table 3). In 662 healthy volunteers in Japan, four had a prevalent infection and two had persistent infection with the same HPV-type after 2.5 years [52]. The persistence of prevalent HR-HPV infections in male and female university students was 42 % after three months [49]..

Risk factors for non-cervical and oral HR-HPV infection

Penile and/or male genital infections with HR-HPV were significantly associated with younger age in only one study [19], although three articles reported no significant association with age [17, 31, 53]. Other significant risk factors were anal intercourse, HPV status of the partner, number of partners (current or lifetime), and HIV infection [17, 19, 22, 26, 31, 53]. Being uncircumcised was identified as a risk factor for penile HR-HPV infection in one study in HIV-ve men [19], but not in another [28].

An increased likelihood of clearance of HR-HPV penile infection was associated with an increased number of sex partners and circumcision (in HIV-ve men) [19, 31]. One study reported increased clearance in men with self-reported urethral discharge [19], but other sexually-transmitted genital infections were not associated with clearance [19, 31].

Risk factors for anal HR-HPV infection in women were younger age, condom use (possibly due to using the same condom for vaginal and anal sex), higher lifetime number of partners (≥6), and advanced HIV infection and smoking (in HIV + ve women) [36, 37]. There was decreased likelihood of clearance of anal HR-HPV infection in women with a 2–10-pack-year smoking history [39].

No risk factors were significantly associated (multivariate analyses) with anal HR-HPV infection in men.

Risk factors for persistence of oral HR-HPV were only available from one study: a history of smoking was significantly associated with longer persistence whereas a history of genital warts was associated with shorter persistence [46].

Discussion

The available data suggest a high incidence of non-cervical HPV infections in men and women, with HPV-16 most consistently ranking among the HR-HPV types with the highest incidence rates and the lowest clearance rates in all sites. Despite relatively few studies providing data for cervical and other genital infections in comparable populations, there appears to be a general pattern of both higher incidence and clearance of non-cervical versus cervical genital infections. Around one-half of the identified articles assessed HPV at male penile/other genital sites. There was a wide variation in HPV incidence reported at these sites, although the time-to-

Table 6 Incidence and clearance of oral HPV infections

Author (ref)	Population, age (years)	Incidence (95 % CI)					Clearance					
		Unit	Any HPV	HR	16	18	Infection type	Unit of clearance	Any HPV	HR	16	18
Males												
Edelstein [45]	Male students, median 20	% at 1y	12.3 % (NTS, first) (7.0–21.3)	-	0.8 (0.1–5.7)	2.7 (0.7–10.2)	-	-	-	-	-	-
Kero [48]	Male partners of pregnant women, 19–46	per 100py	-	-	6.0 (2.9–9.2)	1.2 (0.2–3.4)	-	-	-	-	-	-
Kero [30][a]	Male partners of pregnant women, 20–52	% at 7 years	14.3 % (NTS) (4.8–30.3)	-	-	-	Prevalent	% at 7 years	100 % (TS) (64.4–100)	-	-	-
Kero [46][a]	Male partners of pregnant women, 20–52	% at 7 years	69.2 % (TS) (59.5–77.2)	-	-	-	Prevalent	per 100py	3.8 (TS) (1.6–6.1)	-	4.9 (2.3–7.4)	1.4 (0–2.7)
Rintala [50]	Male partners of pregnant women, 20–52	% at 24 m	-	~10 % (NTS, first)	-	-	Prevalent	% at 24 m	-	~5 % (NTS)	-	-
Videla [23]	HIV + ve MSM, 20- > 69 HIV + ve MSW, 20- > 69	per 100py	6.1 (NTS, first) (4.2–8.4) 5.7 (3.0–9.7)	-	-	-	Prevalent	per 100py	19.3 (NTS) (12.8–27.7) 15.8 (7.6–29.0)	-	-	
Darwich [47]	HIV + ve MSM, 20- > 69 HIV + ve MSW, 20- > 69	per 100py	-	-	1.0 (0.4–2.0) 2.6 (1.1–5.4)	0.2 (0–1.0) 0.7 (0.1–2.4)	Prevalent	% at 24 m	48.3 % (TS) (35.2–61.6) 34 % (17.9–54.3)	-	22.7 per 100py (11.3–40.6)	9.1 per 100py (1.8–26.5)
Kreimer [44]	HIV-ve men, 18–70	per 100py	6.7 (NTS, first) (5.5–8.0)	3.0 (2.2–3.8)	1.0 (0.6–1.6)	0.0 (0–0.4)	-	-	-	-	-	-
Women												
Pickard [49]	Female students, 18–30	per 100py	6.8 (TS) (3.7–9.8)	-	-	-	Prevalent	% at 3 m	60.6 (TS) (42.1–77.1)	76.9 (46.2–95.0)-	100 (15.8–100)-	-
D'Souza [15]	HIV-ve women HIV + ve women	per 100py	20.4 (TS) (8.4–44.4) 39.6 (25.2–57.6)	-	-	-	Prevalent	% at 6 m	20.0 (NTS) (0.5–71.6) 40.0 (22.7–59.4)	-	-	-
Kero [30]	Pregnant women, 19–46	% at 7 years	14.3 % (NTS) (5.4–28.5)	-	-	-	Prevalent	% at 7 years	100 % (TS) (29.2–100)	-	-	-
Rintala [50]	Pregnant women, 19–46	% at 24 m	-	~10 % (NTS, first)	-	-	Prevalent	% at 24 m	-	0 % (NTS)	-	-

Table 6 Incidence and clearance of oral HPV infections *(Continued)*

Men and women												
Kurose [52]	Male/female volunteers, 3–85	-	-	-	-	-	Prevalent	% at 30 m	50.0 (TS) (6.8–93.2)	-	100 (1 sample only)	-

Abbreviations: *MSM* men who have sex with men, *MSW* men who have sex with women, *py* person-years, *y* years, *m* months, *TS* type-specific incidence defined as at least one positive test for any HPV type or HR-HPV type not detected at baseline, *NTS* non-type-specific incidence defined as at least one positive test for any HPV type or HR-HPV type among those negative for any HPV DNA or any HR-HPV DNA at baseline

[a]Study [30] considered a subset of men (46/131) included in [46]. Study [30] reported HPV status at baseline and at 7 years, whereas study [46] considered HPV status at baseline and all subsequent follow-up visits (i.e., 2 m, 6 m, 24 m, 36 m, and 7y)

clearance was comparable across all studies, with the exception of substantially longer time-to-clearance in HIV + ve men. HIV status, circumcision, number of sex partners and HPV status of the partner significantly influenced HR-HPV incidence, clearance and persistence rates at male anogenital sites in some, but not all studies. Some of these risk factors are the same as those identified for cervical HPV infection, for which the number of sex partners is the most important one [54].

Unlike cervical intraepithelial neoplasia, anal-intraepithelial neoplasia infrequently undergoes malignant transformation in immunocompetent individuals, but the risk of malignant transformation is much greater in HIV + ve individuals [55]. Corresponding with the higher incidence of anal cancer in MSM and HIV + ve men compared to the general population, we also found consistently higher incidences of anal HPV infection in these groups compared to MSW and HIV-ve men, respectively. There was a lack of similar comparison data for these risk groups for clearance. The primary exception was Nyitray et al. [35], which indicated potentially lower clearance rates for MSM versus MSW, but multivariate analyses directly comparing the two groups within the same model were not conducted.

The Hawaiian studies by Goodman et al. showed an incidence of anal HPV infection that was three-times higher than cervical HPV infection [36, 39, 41], although a recent review concluded that the prevalence of anal and cervical infections are similar in women, and that cervical HPV infection is a risk factor for anal HPV infection [56]. As prevalence is determined by the incidence rate multiplied by the average duration of infection, the similar prevalence between anal and cervical infections could be due the higher incidence of anal infections being offset by simultaneously higher clearance. The Hawaiian cohorts provided indication of higher clearance of anal infections, but despite this study having one of the largest, most carefully followed cohorts, there were limited samples sizes to assess clearance rates, especially for individual types. This was in part due to the fact that the analyses of clearance focused on infections that were acquired during the course of the study.

The incidence of oral HPV infection was within the same range in men and women, although the prevalence of oral HPV infection has been reported to be higher in men [57]. Our data were too limited to conclude whether there were differences in persistence or clearance rates between men and women. It is thought that the oncogenicity of HPV is similar in oral and cervical cancers, although numerous gaps remain in understanding the risk factors that influence progression from oral infection to oral neoplasia [57].

The factors that influence oncogenesis at non-cervical sites are not well understood, and appear to differ by site and between populations (including men versus women, immunosuppressed versus immunocompetent, circumcised versus uncircumcised) [57, 58]. Although the incidence of HPV infection at non-cervical sites appears to be high, the increased capacity for clearance of HPV observed may contribute to the lower occurrence of these types of cancers. Overall, data describing the natural history of non-cervical cancers are lacking.

A potential limitation of our study is the non-inclusion of articles in which vaginal swabs were self-collected. The single study that we identified using physician-collected vaginal swabs may not be representative for this site as it was limited to university students. However, it was one of the highest quality studies, following more than 400 women aged 18–20 years old every 4 months for 10 years and prospectively collecting sexual behavior data. The studies on cervical infections were selected from specific non-systematic searches aimed to identify comparable populations with which to compare to non-cervical infections. Thus, the results may not be applicable beyond the study setting. Most studies were not properly designed for risk factor analysis and should be interpreted cautiously.

The studies we identified were substantially different in terms of their design, including follow-up times and sampling intervals which ranged from several months to 7 years, as well as the number of types and methods used for HPV genotyping. Although it is difficult to apply a standard grading to these studies, the highest quality studies tended to be those that followed cohorts of at least 200 subjects and conducted multiple follow-up visits ≤6 months apart for at least one year. At least one such study provided data for each of the sampling sites: penile [17–19, 22, 24, 53], male genital [25, 26, 28, 31, 53, 59], anal [34, 36, 38, 39], vulvovaginal [43], oral [44].

The available published data are limited by the lack of age-specific estimates, and information on clearance/persistence of infection was frequently based on very small sample sizes, resulting in imprecise estimates. Few studies provided incidence or clearance data on oral or anal HPV infections in women versus men, and the relative burden of these infections in each sex is not clear. Specific estimates of incidence and clearance of HPV-16, which is involved in the majority of non-cervical cancers, and HPV-18 which may also be important in some sites, as well as estimation of clearance rates at 6 and 12 months, could inform on potentially important endpoints for clinical trials of vaccine efficacy. Finally, because just a few countries contributed data to this review and given the important differences in study designs, outcomes and populations, it is important to note the limited generalizability of these results to other populations.

Conclusions

Cases of cervical cancer are projected to increase, emphasising the importance of ongoing efforts to provide access of effective HPV vaccines to all [1, 60]. As yet, the implications of HPV vaccination for prevention of non-cervical cancers have not been fully explored [58]. Some countries have recommended HPV vaccination for young males on the basis that vaccination will prevent HPV-associated cancers in men, as well as theoretical benefits in preventing transmission of HPV to women [61, 62]. Programs targeting prevention of cervical HPV infection could have additional benefits on the non-cervical disease burden. This review suggests that there are parallels between the epidemiology of cervical and non-cervical HPV infections in terms of the incidence and distribution of HPV types, and of risk factors for HPV infection. However, these parallels may not be directly applicable to disease at non-cervical sites. More detailed and extensive studies could provide useful information for estimating vaccine impact, the wider cost-benefit of HPV vaccination, and for guiding vaccination policy.

Abbreviations

2+ neg, 2 or more negative test results required to define an infection as having cleared; CI, confidence intervals; HIV, human immunodeficiency virus; HPV, human papilloma virus; HR, High risk; LR, low risk; MSM, men who have sex with men; MSW, men who have sex with women; NTS, non-type specific; TS, type specific

Acknowledgements

The authors thank Attila Mihalyi (Global Medical Affairs, Vaccines Value and Health Science at GSK Vaccines) for critically reviewing the manuscript, and Joanne Wolter (independent medical writer, Brisbane, Australia on behalf of GSK Vaccines) who provided writing services and contributed to data extraction and checking. Editing and publication co-ordinating services were provided by Veronique Delpire and Mandy Payne (Words and Science, Brussels, Belgium on behalf of GSK Vaccines). All costs related to the development of this manuscript were met by GlaxoSmithKline Biologicals SA.

Funding

GlaxoSmithKline Biologicals SA was the funding source and was involved in design and conduct of the study; management, analysis, and interpretation of the data; preparation, review and approval of the manuscript and decision to submit the manuscript for publication. Pallas was involved in the design of the study, conducted the literature review, and review and approval of manuscript. GlaxoSmithKline Biologicals SA funded all costs associated with the development and the publishing of the present manuscript. The corresponding author had full access to the data and was responsible for submission of the publication.

Authors' contribution

ST conceived the review and ST, EB, MB and XC participated in the design. EB and MB collected and assembled the data, and performed the analysis. ST and XC supervised the analysis. All authors interpreted the data, and reviewed the text. All authors read and approved the final manuscript.

Author's information

Not applicable.

Competing interests

ST is an employee of, and owns share options in, the GSK group of companies. EB and MB are employees of Pallas health research and consultancy BV, a commercial entity that has received grants and carried out part of the submitted work as a supplier to GSK Vaccines. Pallas has been a supplier of literature reviews and other epidemiological services to GSK Vaccines in the past 36 months. These works cover a variety of vaccines that are in development or on the market.

XC reports having received institutional research and/or educational grants from Merck, Sanofi Pasteur MSD, GSK Vaccines, and Genticel, and occasional personal travel grants and/or speaker fees from Vianex, Merck, and Sanofi Pasteur MSD.

Consent for publication

Not applicable.

Author details

[1]GSK Vaccines, 20, Avenue Fleming, Parc de la Noire Epine, B-1300 Wavre, Belgium. [2]Pallas Health Research and Consultancy BV, Rotterdam, The Netherlands. [3]Cancer Epidemiology Research Program, Catalan Institute of Oncology (ICO), IDIBELL, L'Hospitalet de Llobregat, Catalonia, Spain. [4]CIBER Epidemiología y Salud Pública (CIBERESP), Barcelona, Spain.

References

1. Ferlay J, Soerjomataram I, Ervik M, Dikshit R, Eser S, Mathers C, et al. GLOBOCAN 2012 v1.0, Cancer Incidence and Mortality Worldwide: IARC CancerBase No. 11 [Internet]. Lyon, France: International Agency for Research on Cancer. Available from http://globocan.iarc.fr.
2. Cogliano V, Baan R, Straif K, Grosse Y, Secretan B, El Ghissassi F, et al. Carcinogenicity of human papillomaviruses. Lancet Oncol. 2005;6:204.
3. De Vuyst H, Clifford GM, Nascimento MC, Madeleine MM, Franceschi S. Prevalence and type distribution of human papillomavirus in carcinoma and intraepithelial neoplasia of the vulva, vagina and anus: a meta-analysis. Int J Cancer. 2009;124:1626–36. doi:10.1002/ijc.24116.
4. HPV Information Centre. Data Query. 2014. http://www.hpvcentre.net/dataquery.php (accessed 6 Mar 2015).
5. Mehanna H, Jones TM, Gregoire V, Ang KK. Oropharyngeal carcinoma related to human papillomavirus. BMJ. 2010;340:c1439.
6. de Martel C, Ferlay J, Franceschi S, Vignat J, Bray F, Forman D, et al. Global burden of cancers attributable to infections in 2008: a review and synthetic analysis. Lancet Oncol. 2012;13:607–15. doi:10.1016/S1470-2045(12)70137-7.
7. Herrero R, Quint W, Hildesheim A, Gonzalez P, Struijk L, Katki HA, et al. Reduced prevalence of oral human papillomavirus (HPV) 4 years after bivalent HPV vaccination in a randomized clinical trial in Costa Rica. PLoS ONE. 2013;8:e68329. doi:10.1371/journal.pone.0068329.
8. Giuliano AR, Palefsky JM, Goldstone S, Moreira ED, Penny ME, Aranda C, et al. Efficacy of quadrivalent HPV vaccine against HPV Infection and disease in males. N Engl J Med. 2011;364:401–11. doi:10.1056/NEJMoa0909537.
9. Palefsky JM, Giuliano AR, Goldstone S, Moreira ED, Aranda C, Jessen H, et al. HPV vaccine against anal HPV infection and anal intraepithelial neoplasia. N Engl J Med. 2011;365:1576–85. doi:10.1056/NEJMoa1010971.
10. Lang Kuhs KA, Gonzalez P, Rodriguez AC, van Doorn L-J, Schiffman M, Struijk L, et al. Reduced Prevalence of Vulvar HPV16/18 Infection Among Women Who Received the HPV16/18 Bivalent Vaccine: A Nested Analysis Within the Costa Rica Vaccine Trial. J Infect Dis. 2014;210:1890–9. doi:10.1093/infdis/jiu357.
11. Muñoz N, Kjaer SK, Sigurdsson K, Iversen O-E, Hernandez-Avila M, Wheeler CM, et al. Impact of human papillomavirus (HPV)-6/11/16/18 vaccine on all HPV-associated genital diseases in young women. J Natl Cancer Inst. 2010;102:325–39. doi:10.1093/jnci/djp534.
12. Kreimer AR, González P, Katki HA, Porras C, Schiffman M, Rodriguez AC, et al. Efficacy of a bivalent HPV 16/18 vaccine against anal HPV 16/18 infection among young women: a nested analysis within the Costa Rica Vaccine Trial. Lancet Oncol. 2011;12:862–70. doi:10.1016/S1470-2045(11)70213-3.
13. McCormack PL. Quadrivalent Human Papillomavirus (Types 6, 11, 16, 18) Recombinant Vaccine (Gardasil(®)): A Review of Its Use in the Prevention of Premalignant Anogenital Lesions, Cervical and Anal Cancers, and Genital Warts. Drugs. 2014;74:1253–83. doi:10.1007/s40265-014-0255-z.
14. Schiller JT, Castellsagué X, Garland SM. A review of clinical trials of human papillomavirus prophylactic vaccines. Vaccine. 2012;30 Suppl 5:F123–38. doi:10.1016/j.vaccine.2012.04.108.

15. D'Souza G, Fakhry C, Sugar EA, Seaberg EC, Weber K, Minkoff HL, et al. Six-month natural history of oral versus cervical human papillomavirus infection. Int J Cancer. 2007;121:143–50. doi:10.1002/ijc.22667.
16. Serwadda D, Wawer MJ, Makumbi F, Kong X, Kigozi G, Gravitt P, et al. Circumcision of HIV-infected men: effects on high-risk human papillomavirus infections in a randomized trial in Rakai, Uganda. J Infect Dis. 2010;201:1463–9. doi:10.1086/652185.
17. Backes DM, Snijders PJF, Hudgens MG, Bailey RC, Bogaarts M, Agot K, et al. Sexual behaviour and less frequent bathing are associated with higher human papillomavirus incidence in a cohort study of uncircumcised Kenyan men. Sex Transm Infect. 2013;89:148–55. doi:10.1136/sextrans-2012-050532.
18. Gray RH, Serwadda D, Kong X, Makumbi F, Kigozi G, Gravitt PE, et al. Male circumcision decreases acquisition and increases clearance of high-risk human papillomavirus in HIV-negative men: a randomized trial in Rakai, Uganda. J Infect Dis. 2010;201:1455–62. doi:10.1086/652184.
19. Tobian AAR, Kigozi G, Gravitt PE, Xiao C, Serwadda D, Eaton KP, et al. Human papillomavirus incidence and clearance among HIV-positive and HIV-negative men in sub-Saharan Africa. AIDS. 2012;26:1555–65. doi:10.1097/QAD.0b013e328353b83c.
20. Darwich L, Cañadas M-P, Videla S, Coll J, Molina-López RA, Sirera G, et al. Prevalence, clearance, and incidence of human papillomavirus type-specific infection at the anal and penile site of HIV-infected men. Sex Transm Dis. 2013;40:611–8. doi:10.1097/01.OLQ.0000430798.61475.08.
21. Wikström A, Popescu C, Forslund O. Asymptomatic penile HPV infection: a prospective study. Int J STD AIDS. 2000;11:80–4.
22. Mbulawa ZZA, Marais DJ, Johnson LF, Coetzee D, Williamson A-L. Impact of human immunodeficiency virus on the natural history of human papillomavirus genital infection in South African men and women. J Infect Dis. 2012;206:15–27. doi:10.1093/infdis/jis299.
23. Videla S, Darwich L, Cañadas M-P, Coll J, Piñol M, García-Cuyás F, et al. Natural history of human papillomavirus infections involving anal, penile, and oral sites among HIV-positive men. Sex Transm Dis. 2013;40:3–10. doi:10.1097/OLQ.0b013e31827e87bd.
24. Grabowski MK, Gray RH, Serwadda D, Kigozi G, Gravitt PE, Nalugoda F, et al. High-risk human papillomavirus viral load and persistence among heterosexual HIV-negative and HIV-positive men. Sex Transm Infect. 2014;90:337–43. doi:10.1136/sextrans-2013-051230.
25. Giuliano AR, Lu B, Nielson CM, Flores R, Papenfuss MR, Lee J-H, et al. Age-specific prevalence, incidence, and duration of human papillomavirus infections in a cohort of 290 US men. J Infect Dis. 2008;198:827–35. doi:10.1086/591095.
26. Morales R, Parada R, Giuliano AR, Cruz A, Castellsagué X, Salmerón J, et al. HPV in female partners increases risk of incident HPV infection acquisition in heterosexual men in rural central Mexico. Cancer Epidemiol Biomarkers Prev. 2012;21:1956–65. doi:10.1158/1055-9965.EPI-12-0470.
27. Lajous M, Mueller N, Cruz-Valdéz A, Aguilar LV, Franceschi S, Hernández-Avila M, et al. Determinants of prevalence, acquisition, and persistence of human papillomavirus in healthy Mexican military men. Cancer Epidemiol Biomarkers Prev. 2005;14:1710–6. doi:10.1158/1055-9965.EPI-04-0926.
28. Albero G, Castellsagué X, Lin H-Y, Fulp W, Villa LL, Lazcano-Ponce E, et al. Male circumcision and the incidence and clearance of genital human papillomavirus (HPV) infection in men: the HPV Infection in men (HIM) cohort study. BMC Infect Dis. 2014;14:75. doi:10.1186/1471-2334-14-75.
29. Partridge JM, Hughes JP, Feng Q, Winer RL, Weaver BA, Xi L-F, et al. Genital human papillomavirus infection in men: incidence and risk factors in a cohort of university students. J Infect Dis. 2007;196:1128–36. doi:10.1086/521192.
30. Kero KM, Rautava J, Syrjänen K, Kortekangas-Savolainen O, Grenman S, Syrjänen S. Stable marital relationship protects men from oral and genital HPV infections. Eur J Clin Microbiol Infect Dis. 2014;33:1211–21. doi:10.1007/s10096-014-2061-7.
31. Lu B, Wu Y, Nielson CM, Flores R, Abrahamsen M, Papenfuss M, et al. Factors associated with acquisition and clearance of human papillomavirus infection in a cohort of US men: a prospective study. J Infect Dis. 2009;199:362–71. doi:10.1086/596050.
32. Giuliano AR, Harris R, Sedjo RL, Baldwin S, Roe D, Papenfuss MR, et al. Incidence, prevalence, and clearance of type-specific human papillomavirus infections: The Young Women's Health Study. J Infect Dis. 2002;186:462–9. doi:10.1086/341782.
33. Glick SN, Feng Q, Popov V, Koutsky LA, Golden MR. High rates of incident and prevalent anal human papillomavirus infection among young men who have sex with men. J Infect Dis. 2014;209:369–76. doi:10.1093/infdis/jit441.
34. Hernandez AL, Efird JT, Holly EA, Berry JM, Jay N, Palefsky JM. Incidence of and risk factors for type-specific anal human papillomavirus infection among HIV-positive MSM. AIDS. 2014;28:1341–9. doi:10.1097/QAD.0000000000000254.
35. Nyitray AG, da Silva RJ C, Baggio ML, D'elle S, Abrahamsen M, Papenfuss M, et al. Six-month incidence, persistence, and factors associated with persistence of anal human papillomavirus in men: the HPV in men study. J Infect Dis. 2011;204:1711–22. doi:10.1093/infdis/jir637.
36. Goodman MT, Shvetsov YB, McDuffie K, Wilkens LR, Zhu X, Ning L, et al. Acquisition of anal human papillomavirus (HPV) infection in women: the Hawaii HPV Cohort study. J Infect Dis. 2008;197:957–66. doi:10.1086/529207.
37. Mullins TLK, Wilson CM, Rudy BJ, Sucharew H, Kahn JA. Incident anal human papillomavirus and human papillomavirus-related sequelae in HIV-infected versus HIV-uninfected adolescents in the United States. Sex Transm Dis. 2013;40:715–20. doi:10.1097/01.olq.0000431049.74390.b7.
38. de Pokomandy A, Rouleau D, Ghattas G, Vézina S, Coté P, Macleod J, et al. Prevalence, clearance, and incidence of anal human papillomavirus infection in HIV-infected men: the HIPVIRG cohort study. J Infect Dis. 2009;199:965–73. doi:10.1086/597207.
39. Shvetsov YB, Hernandez BY, McDuffie K, Wilkens LR, Zhu X, Ning L, et al. Duration and clearance of anal human papillomavirus (HPV) infection among women: the Hawaii HPV cohort study. Clin Infect Dis. 2009;48:536–46. doi:10.1086/596758.
40. Moscicki A-B, Ma Y, Farhat S, Jay J, Hanson E, Benningfield S, et al. Natural history of anal human papillomavirus infection in heterosexual women and risks associated with persistence. Clin Infect Dis. 2014;58:804–11. doi:10.1093/cid/cit947.
41. Goodman MT, Shvetsov YB, McDuffie K, Wilkens LR, Zhu X, Thompson PJ, et al. Prevalence, acquisition, and clearance of cervical human papillomavirus infection among women with normal cytology: Hawaii Human Papillomavirus Cohort Study. Cancer Res. 2008;68:8813–24. doi:10.1158/0008-5472.CAN-08-1380.
42. Moscicki AB, Shiboski S, Broering J, Powell K, Clayton L, Jay N, et al. The natural history of human papillomavirus infection as measured by repeated DNA testing in adolescent and young women. J Pediatr. 1998;132:277–84.
43. Winer RL, Lee S-K, Hughes JP, Adam DE, Kiviat NB, Koutsky LA. Genital human papillomavirus infection: incidence and risk factors in a cohort of female university students. Am J Epidemiol. 2003;157:218–26.
44. Kreimer AR, Pierce Campbell CM, Lin H-Y, Fulp W, Papenfuss MR, Abrahamsen M, et al. Incidence and clearance of oral human papillomavirus infection in men: the HIM cohort study. Lancet. 2013;382:877–87. doi:10.1016/S0140-6736(13)60809-0.
45. Edelstein ZR, Schwartz SM, Hawes S, Hughes JP, Feng Q, Stern ME, et al. Rates and determinants of oral human papillomavirus infection in young men. Sex Transm Dis. 2012;39:860–7. doi:10.1097/OLQ.0b013e318269d098.
46. Kero K, Rautava J, Syrjänen K, Willberg J, Grenman S, Syrjänen S. Smoking increases oral HPV persistence among men: 7-year follow-up study. Eur J Clin Microbiol Infect Dis. 2014;33:123–33. doi:10.1007/s10096-013-1938-1.
47. Darwich L, Cañadas MP, Videla S, Coll J, Molina-López RA, Cobarsi P, et al. Oral human papillomavirus type-specific infection in HIV-infected men: a prospective cohort study among men who have sex with men and heterosexual men. Clin Microbiol Infect. 2014;20:O585–9. doi:10.1111/1469-0691.12523.
48. Kero K, Rautava J, Syrjänen K, Grenman S, Syrjänen S. Oral mucosa as a reservoir of human papillomavirus: point prevalence, genotype distribution, and incident infections among males in a 7-year prospective study. Eur Urol. 2012;62:1063–70. doi:10.1016/j.eururo.2012.06.045.
49. Pickard RKL, Xiao W, Broutian TR, He X, Gillison ML. The prevalence and incidence of oral human papillomavirus infection among young men and women, aged 18–30 years. Sex Transm Dis. 2012;39:559–66. doi:10.1097/OLQ.0b013e31824f1c65.
50. Rintala M, Grénman S, Puranen M, Syrjänen S. Natural history of oral papillomavirus infections in spouses: a prospective Finnish HPV Family Study. J Clin Virol. 2006;35:89–94. doi:10.1016/j.jcv.2005.05.012.
51. Louvanto K, Rautava J, Syrjänen K, Grénman S, Syrjänen S. The clearance of oral high-risk human papillomavirus infection is impaired by long-term persistence of cervical human papillomavirus infection. Clin Microbiol Infect. 2014;20:1167–72. doi:10.1111/1469-0691.12700.
52. Kurose K, Terai M, Soedarsono N, Rabello D, Nakajima Y, Burk RD, et al. Low prevalence of HPV infection and its natural history in normal oral mucosa among volunteers on Miyako Island, Japan. Oral Surg Oral Med Oral Pathol Oral Radiol Endod. 2004;98:91–6. doi:10.1016/S1079210404000265.

53. Giuliano AR, Lee J-H, Fulp W, Villa LL, Lazcano E, Papenfuss MR, et al. Incidence and clearance of genital human papillomavirus infection in men (HIM): a cohort study. Lancet. 2011;377:932–40. doi:10.1016/S0140-6736(10)62342-2.
54. Chelimo C, Wouldes TA, Cameron LD, Elwood JM. Risk factors for and prevention of human papillomaviruses (HPV), genital warts and cervical cancer. J Infect. 2013;66:207–17. doi:10.1016/j.jinf.2012.10.024.
55. Scholefield JH, Castle MT, Watson NFS. Malignant transformation of high-grade anal intraepithelial neoplasia. Br J Surg. 2005;92:1133–6. doi:10.1002/bjs.4994.
56. Stier EA, Sebring MC, Mendez AE, Ba FS, Trimble DD, Chiao EY. Prevalence of anal human papillomavirus infection and anal HPV-related disorders in women: a systematic review. Am J Obstet Gynecol. 2015;213:278–309. doi:10.1016/j.ajog.2015.03.034.
57. Blitzer GC, Smith MA, Harris SL, Kimple RJ. Review of the clinical and biologic aspects of human papillomavirus-positive squamous cell carcinomas of the head and neck. Int J Radiat Oncol Biol Phys. 2014;88:761–70. doi:10.1016/j.ijrobp.2013.08.029.
58. Harper DM, Vierthaler SL. Who should be targeted for vaccination against anal cancer? Lancet Oncol. 2011;12:828–9. doi:10.1016/S1470-2045(11)70237-6.
59. Hernandez BY, Shvetsov YB, Goodman MT, Wilkens LR, Thompson P, Zhu X, et al. Reduced clearance of penile human papillomavirus infection in uncircumcised men. J Infect Dis. 2010;201:1340–3. doi:10.1086/651607.
60. Audisio RA, Icardi G, Isidori AM, Liverani CA, Lombardi A, Mariani L, et al. Public health value of universal HPV vaccination. Crit Rev Oncol Hematol. 2016;97:157–67. doi:10.1016/j.critrevonc.2015.07.015.
61. Markowitz LE, Dunne EF, Saraiya M, Chesson HW, Curtis CR, Gee J, et al. Human papillomavirus vaccination: recommendations of the Advisory Committee on Immunization Practices (ACIP). MMWR Recomm Rep. 2014;63:1–30.
62. Australian Government Department of Health and Ageing, National Health and Medical Research Council. The Australian Immunisation Handbook. 10th ed. 2015.
63. Kjaer SK, Munk C, Winther JF, Jørgensen HO, Meijer CJLM, van den Brule AJC. Acquisition and persistence of human papillomavirus infection in younger men: a prospective follow-up study among Danish soldiers. Cancer Epidemiol Biomarkers Prev. 2005;14:1528–33. doi:10.1158/1055-9965.EPI-04-0754.
64. Videla S, Darwich L, Cañadas MP, Paredes R, Tarrats A, Castella E, et al. Epidemiological data of different human papillomavirus genotypes in cervical specimens of HIV-1-infected women without history of cervical pathology. J Acquir Immune Defic Syndr. 2009;50:168–75. doi:10.1097/QAI.0b013e3181938e63.

Cost-effectiveness analysis of different types of human papillomavirus vaccination combined with a cervical cancer screening program in mainland China

Xiuting Mo[1,2], Ruoyan Gai Tobe[2*], Lijie Wang[3], Xianchen Liu[4], Bin Wu[5], Huiwen Luo[6], Chie Nagata[7], Rintaro Mori[2] and Takeo Nakayama[1]

Abstract

Background: China has a high prevalence of human papillomavirus (HPV) and a consequently high burden of disease with respect to cervical cancer. The HPV vaccine has proved to be effective in preventing cervical cancer and is now a part of routine immunization programs worldwide. It has also proved to be cost effective. This study aimed to assess the cost-effectiveness of 2-, 4-, and 9-valent HPV vaccines (hereafter, HPV2, 4 or 9) combined with current screening strategies in China.

Methods: A Markov model was developed for a cohort of 100,000 HPV-free girls to simulate the natural history to HPV infection. Three recommended screening methods (1. liquid-based cytology test + HPV DNA test; 2. pap smear cytology test + HPV DNA test; 3. visual inspection with acetic acid) and three types of HPV vaccination program (HPV2/4/9) were incorporated into 15 intervention options, and the incremental cost-effectiveness ratio (ICER) was calculated to determine the dominant strategies. Costs, transition probabilities and utilities were obtained from a review of the literature and national databases. One-way sensitivity analyses and threshold analyses were performed for key variables in different vaccination scenarios.

Results: HPV9 combined with screening showed the highest health impact in terms of reducing HPV-related diseases and increasing the number of quality-adjusted life years (QALYs). Under the current thresholds of willingness to pay (WTP, 3 times the per capita GDP or USD$ 23,880), HPV4/9 proved highly cost effective, while HPV2 combined with screening cost more and was less cost effective. Only when screening coverage increased to 60% ~ 70% did the HPV2 and screening combination strategy become economically feasible.

Conclusions: The combination of the HPV4/9 vaccine with current screening strategies for adolescent girls was highly cost-effective and had a significant impact on reducing the HPV infection-related disease burden in Mainland China.

Keywords: Cervical cancer, Cervical intraepithelial neoplasia, Incremental cost-effectiveness ratio, Vaccine

---

* Correspondence: gai-r@ncchd.go.jp
[2]Department of Health Policy, National Center for Child Health and Development, Okura 2-10-1, Setagaya-ku, Tokyo 157-8535, Japan
Full list of author information is available at the end of the article

Background

Cervical cancer is one of the most widespread gynaecological cancers worldwide and remains the second leading cause of gynaecological-related mortality. More than 85% of cases occur in developing countries, resulting in an estimated 275,000 deaths annually [1]. In mainland China, despite its decreasing incidence in recent years, cervical cancer remains among the top ten most common malignancies among women and is a leading cause of cancer-related mortality nationwide [2, 3]. Human papillomavirus (HPV) infection is the main cause of cervical cancer and can be detected in more than 95% of uterine carcinomas. Vaccinations are effective in preventing HPV infection, and a number of vaccine options have recently become available. The 2-valent HPV vaccine (HPV2), which targets HPV 16/18 and the 4-valent HPV vaccine (HPV4), which targets 6/11/16/18, have been approved in more than 100 countries worldwide. Both vaccines were highly effective in clinical trials and shown to be cost effective in health economic studies in various countries [4]. The 9-valent HPV vaccine (HPV9) targeting five additional oncogenic HPV types (31, 33, 45, 52, and 58) improved protection against 90% of cervical cancers, an increase of 20% from the previous figure, and has been licensed in more than 30 countries [5, 6]. In July 2016, a decade after international approval of the first HPV vaccine, the Chinese government approved GSK Cervarix™, a 2-valent HPV vaccine expected to become commercially available in early 2017 [7, 8]. In addition, some other HPV-related cancers (such as oropharyngeal, anal, and vulvar cancer) caused by HPV 16/18/31/33/45/52/58 may be prevented by the vaccines [9–11].

Further, as recommended by the World Health Organization (WHO), screening is a common preventative strategy targeting women of reproductive age for the early detection and treatment of HPV infection, cervical cancer, and cervical intraepithelial neoplasia (CIN). In developing countries, routine screening programs reportedly reduced the incidence of cervical cancer by up to 60% [12]. In 2005 the Ministry of Health of China formed guidelines for the screening, early detection, and treatment of cervical cancer [13]. The target demographic of these guidelines was women older than 21 years and those who engaged in sexual activity for more than three years. The guidelines recommend three different protocols each designed for a particular socioeconomic stratum: 1) primary screening by liquid-based cytology test + HPV DNA test, which has optimal sensitivity and specificity but is expensive and requires well-equipped infrastructure and ample resources; 2) primary screening by pap smear cytology test + HPV DNA test, requiring less infrastructure and resources; and 3) primary screening by visual inspection with acetic acid (VIA), a basic protocol designed for low income settings. Although a government-sponsored VIA and cytology screening program has been carried out in some regions [14], no national cervical screening program currently exists on mainland China. According to some local surveys, the coverage rate of current screening programs is approximately 10 ~ 30% [15, 16] and even when offered free of charge, remained at around 50% [17].

Although the cost-effectiveness of the HPV vaccine in China has been analysed [18–20], a thorough assessment specific to China of HPV2, 4, and 9 and the three previously mentioned screening protocols still remains to be done. Therefore, this study aims to evaluate the cost-effectiveness of different HPV vaccinations as alternatives, and as an adjunct to the three primary screening strategies currently in use in mainland China, with consideration of diversified geographical characteristics.

Methods

Overview of the model

A Markov model was used to simulate the natural history of HPV infection and to estimate the economic consequences of HPV-related diseases from a societal perspective view (Fig. 1). The rationale for using the model was the example provided by several previous natural history models of HPV simulating high and low risk HPV infections separately. In this study, the model was adapted to the Chinese context (three different screening strategies and diagnosis/treatment flow specific to the Chinese setting) in order to reflect local screening and treatment practices [21–23].

We assumed that girls under 12 years old were virgins. In our analysis, we simulated a cohort of 100,000 HPV-free girls (from 12 years old and followed up until death). In the strategies using vaccination, individuals were given the respective vaccines at the beginning of the simulation. HPV genotypes were divided into high risk (carcinogenic HPV 16/18/31/33/45/52/58, etc.) and low risk (HPV 6/11 and etc.) groups in the analysis. Health states were defined based on the natural history of HPV infection in the following manner: healthy, low risk HPV infection, high risk HPV infection, mild cervical intraepithelial neoplasia (CIN 1) caused by high risk HPV infection, moderate cervical intraepithelial neoplasia (CIN 2) caused by high risk HPV infection, severe cervical intraepithelial neoplasia or carcinoma in situ (CIN 3) caused by high risk HPV infection, CIN1/2 caused by low risk HPV infection, genital warts, invasive cervical cancer (ICC) (stages I-IV as defined by the International Federation of Gynaecology and Obstetrics, FIGO), cervical cancer survival, death from cervical cancer, and death from other causes [21]. Oropharyngeal, anal, and vulvar cancers were not included in this study because differing proportions of these cancers are caused by HPV, and it is difficult to quantify the effects of vaccination on the incidence of HPV caused by the strains

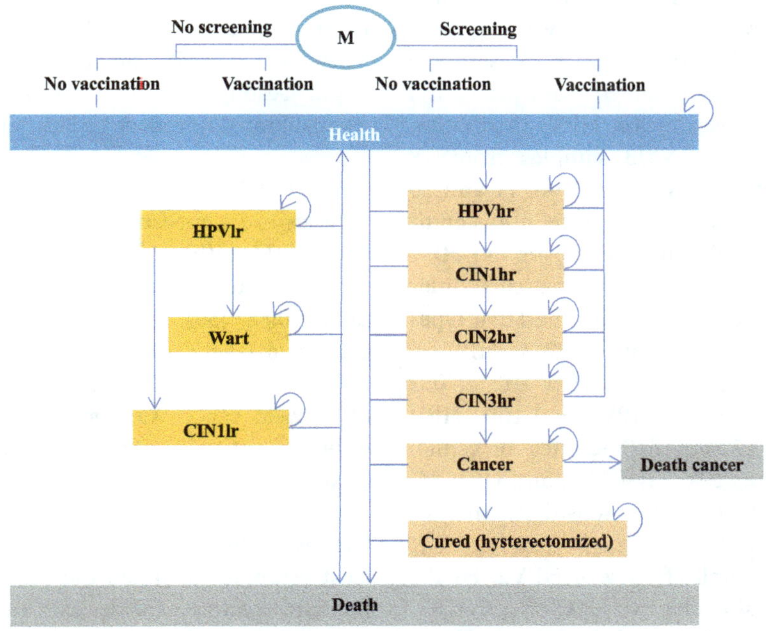

Fig. 1 Markov model of the history of high and low risk type of HPV. The *arrows* direct transitions from one state to another. hr, high-risk; lr, low-risk; CIN, cervical intraepithelial neoplasia; HPV, human papillomavirus

covered. Furthermore, the epidemiological data on HPV-related cancers other than cervical cancer caused by HPV 16/18 or HPV 16/18/31/33/45/52/58 were not available in China. Since the impact of the HPV vaccines on other non-cervical HPV-related cancers have not been included in the analysis, the projected health benefits are likely underestimated.

The Markov model developed for this study comprehensively assessed relevant and currently in-use preventative strategies including both vaccination and screening in China. The screening strategies included the three protocols recommended in the *2005 Guidelines for Screening, Early Detection and Treatment of Cervical Cancer* [13]: 1) liquid-based cytology test + HPV DNA test; 2) pap smear cytology test + HPV DNA test; 3) visual inspection with acetic acid (VIA) and a colposcopy following a positive result to make a definite diagnosis. The vaccination options were HPV2 (CERVARIX,HPV4 (GARDASIL®) and the newly developed HPV9 (GARDASIL®9). We compared 15 preventative strategies consisting of either a single modality or a combination of vaccination and screening, namely, Screening 1, Screening 2, Screening 3, HPV2, HPV4, HPV9, Screening 1 + HPV2, Screening 2 + HPV2, Screening 3 + HPV2, Screening 1 + HPV4, Screening 2 + HPV4, Screening 3 + HPV4, Screening 1 + HPV9, Screening 2 + HPV9, Screening 3 + HPV9, and no intervention.

Screening strategies

The target population for screening was women older than 21 years. Screening every three years was recommended. Based on the cervical cancer prevention guidelines of mainland China and several Chinese reports, we assumed that a liquid-based cytology test would have a sensitivity of 0.85 and a specificity of 0.90 [24]. The HPV DNA test had a sensitivity of 0.95 and specificity of 0.85 [24]. The pap smear had a sensitivity of 0.65 and specificity of 0.88 [24]. The VIA test had a sensitivity of 0.68 and specificity of 0.85 [24–26]. We assumed that the colposcopy + biopsy combination would have perfect sensitivity and specificity for the detection of CIN2+ [27].

A screening coverage rate of 20% was assumed due to the large geographical diversity in socioeconomic development, and 10%–100% was set for the sensitivity analysis [28].

Vaccine characteristics

As vaccine efficacy data specific to the Chinese population were unavailable, the data used here were obtained by multiplying the direct efficacy targeting specific HPV types by serotype coverage on mainland China. In the clinical trials, HPV2 (CERVARIX),HPV4 (GARDASIL®), and HPV9 (GARDASIL®9) all showed excellent efficacy against the relevant CIN and AIS (Adenocarcinoma in situ) in women with HPV DNA negative for oncogenic HPV types at baseline: HPV2: 96.5% (95% CI: 91.6%–98.9%) [29]; HPV4: 96.0% (95% CI: 92.3%–98.2%) [10]; HPV9: 96.0% (95% CI: 92.3%–98.2%) for HPV 6, 11, 16, or 18-related CIN or AIS, and 96.7% (95% CI: 80.9%–99.8%) for the additional five HPV types, namely, HPV 31, 33, 45, 52, and 58 [11]. The efficacy of the HPV4 and HPV9 against specific HPV-related genital warts was

99.0% (95% CI: 96.2%–99.9%) [11]. HPV2 was assumed to have the same efficacy against genital warts (99.0%, 95% CI: 96.2%–99.9%). The parameter: HPV serotype coverage of each vaccine, was obtained from a doctoral dissertation, an epidemic research on HPV distribution in genital warts, ICC and CIN2/3 samples from 18 hospitals in 7 geographic regions [30]. HPV6, 11 and 16 distribution in genital warts patients were not significantly differed by urban and rural areas. Nor did HPV prevalence in squamous cell carcinoma patients differ notably by region [30]. The following are the HPV types with their respective incidence for CIN2/3: HPV 6: 1.26%; HPV 16: 75.94%; HPV 11: 0; HPV 18: 7.70%; HPV 31: 3.14%; HPV 33: 0.94%; HPV 45: 1.10%; HPV 52: 2.20%; and HPV 58: 2.20% [30]. The rates for genital warts were HPV 6: 46.6%; HPV 11: 42.4%, and HPV 16: 11.8% [30]. The parameters for the sensitivity analysis were the baseline value ±25%.

After calculation, the overall efficacy of HPV2, HPV4, and HPV9 against cervical cancer was 80.72% (57.47%–98.9%), 81.51% (58.78%–98.2%), and 90.78% (66.54%–100%), respectively, and that against genital warts was 10.36% (7.56%–13.07%), 86.06% (62.72%–99.99%) and 86.06% (62.72%–99.99%), respectively.

Moreover, considering the reported efficacy data and demonstration of immunological memory [31], we assumed that the protection conferred by the vaccines would be life-long and obviate the need for a booster. Because of the relatively low coverage of the current prevention program, cross protective effects were not taken into account.

A vaccine coverage rate was assumed as 20%, and 10%–100% was set for the sensitivity analysis.

Transition probabilities

Each strategy (screening plus vaccination or screening only) modelled probabilities for mutually exclusive health states within a one-year cycle. At each transition, the model produced figures for the costs incurred and the QALYs according to the individual's health condition. Each year, the target population was exposed to an age-specific risk of HPV infection that could persist, progress (to CIN 1, CIN 2–3, genital warts, etc.) or resolve. In those who developed CIN 3, their disease might persist, remit, or progress to localized (FIGO stage I and IIA), regional (FIGO IIB to IVA) or metastatic invasive cancer (FIGO IVB). Given the course of cervical cancer, each individual might continue to suffer from the disease, die, or experience complete remission. Each year individuals faced age-specific risks of dying from other causes or of undergoing a hysterectomy for reasons unrelated to cervical neoplasia. Women who underwent a hysterectomy did not develop cervical cancer in our model. Table 1 summarizes the initial value and all the transition probabilities derived from the previous reports and research projects of the Cancer Institute and Hospital, Chinese Academy of Medical Sciences (CICAMS). Screening Technologies to Advance Rapid Testing for Cervical Cancer Prevention (START) was calibrated to reflect Chinese epidemiology [32].

Health utilities

Utilities are a measure of the quality of life rated on a scale of 0 (death) to 1 (optimal health), and are based on economic studies in China. CIN 2 was assigned a lower utility (0.88) [33], while CIN 3 was assigned an utility of 0.81 for a 1-year period [33]. In cases of ICC, a woman's utility was assumed to decrease to 0.69 [33]. The utility of cervical cancer survivors was 0.85 [28, 34, 35]. The utility of patients with genital warts was determined to be 0.67 based on some Chinese studies [36, 37].

Cost estimates

Cost estimates included the cost of vaccination, screening, and treatment of diseases related to HPV infection. Data were initially calculated in Chinese Yuan and then converted to US dollars in 2015 using the consumer price index (CPI) and the official exchange rate of the Chinese Yuan to US dollar (January 2015 exchange rate, USD$1 = CYN6.20). Although the three HPV vaccines mentioned above were not yet available on mainland China, *Gardasil,* a quadrivalent vaccine developed by Merck and *Cervarix,* a bivalent vaccine developed by GlaxoSmithKline, both costing about the same, were approved in Hong Kong. We estimated the costs of three doses according to the standard price in Hong Kong (2000 ~ 3000 CYN) [38], and the administration fee for each girl was estimated at USD$4.84 dollars. Cost of three doses of HPV9 vaccine was calculated by multiplying USD$ 403.23 by the ratio of cost of HPV4/HPV9 per dose ($147.78/$163.86 = 1.1088) [39]. Considering the likelihood that the costs on the mainland would be lower than in Hong Kong due to the lower economic status of the mainland population, the sensitivity analysis was performed with a value range of 0.5X-1.5X. Moreover, we approximated different screening costs using the current national tariff proposed by the Chinese Anti-Cancer Association [40]. The treatment costs were obtained from tertiary hospitals and the local health system. Treatment by FIGO staging was based on the recommendation of national and international guidelines [41]. A half cycle correction was used in order to achieve a closer approximation to proper reward/survival.

In terms of compliance, the baseline value for CIN 2/3 treatment extracted from Screening Technologies to Advance Rapid Testing for Cervical Cancer Prevention (START) was set at 90% [28]. The selection rate for a hysterectomy in the event of CIN 3 was set at 20% for those older than 35 years and 0% for all others [28]. When

Table 1 Model variables: Baseline values and ranges used in sensitivity analysis

Variable	Base case	Plausible range	References
Natural history of HPV	Age-specific table		
HPV-2	Serotypes covered*efficacy		
Efficacy for cervical cancer	0.836*0.965	0.575–0.989	[27, 30]
Efficacy for genital warts	0.107*0.990	0.756–0.131	Assumed
HPV-4			
Efficacy for cervical cancer	0.849*0.960	0.588–0.982	[28, 30]
Efficacy for genital warts	0.869*0.990	0.627–0.999	[29, 30]
HPV-9			
Efficacy for cervical cancer	0.849*0.960 + 0.096*0.967	0.665–1.000	[29, 30]
Efficacy for genital warts	0.869*0.990	0.627–0.999	[29, 30]
Pap smear			
Sensitivity	0.65	0.50–0.80	[22]
Specificity	0.88	0.85–0.90	[22]
Liquid-based cytology test			
Sensitivity	0.85	0.80–0.90	[22]
Specificity	0.90	0.85–0.95	[22]
HPV DNA test			
Sensitivity	0.95	0.80–0.98	[22]
Specificity	0.85	0.80–0.90	[22]
VIA			
Sensitivity	0.68	0.50–0.70	[22–24]
Specificity	0.85	0.66–0.96	[22–24]
Colposcopy and biopsy			
Sensitivity	1	0.50–1.0	[25]
Specificity	1	0.50–1.0	[25]
Age begin to screen	20	18–45	Assumed
Screening intervals	3	1,3,5,10	Assumed
Screening coverage	0.2	0.1–1.0	Assumed
Vaccine coverage	0.2	0.1–1.0	Assumed
Costs (USD)			
HPV 2/4 vaccine (3 does)	403.23	0.5X-1.5X	[38]
HPV 9 vaccine (3 does)	447.10	0.5X-1.5X	[38, 39]
vaccine administration (3 does)	4.84	0.5X-1.5X	Chinese Anti-Cancer Association
Pap smear	6.75	0.5X-1.5X	Chinese Anti-Cancer Association
Liquid-based cytology	43.89	0.5X-1.5X	Chinese Anti-Cancer Association
HPV DNA test	56.45	0.5X-1.5X	Chinese Anti-Cancer Association
VIA	5.06	0.5X-1.5X	Chinese Anti-Cancer Association
Colposcopy and biopsy	32.26	0.5X-1.5X	Local field study
Loop electrosurgical excision procedure (LEEP)	403.23	0.5X-1.5X	Local field study
Cold knife conisation	887.10	0.5X-1.5X	Local field study
Hysterectomy	2419.35	0.5X-1.5X	Local field study
Localized cancer	3225.81	0.5X-1.5X	Local field study
Regional cancer	4838.71	0.5X-1.5X	Local field study
Metastatic cancer	6451.61	0.5X-1.5X	Local field study

Table 1 Model variables: Baseline values and ranges used in sensitivity analysis *(Continued)*

Genital warts	161.29	0.5X-1.5X	Local field study
Utilities			
CIN1	0.9965	0.992603–1.0	[33]
CIN2	0.984	0.876–1.0	[33]
CIN3	0.984	0.806–1.0	[33]
Cancer	0.693	0.56–0.76	[33]
Genital warts	0.827	0.701–0.933	[36]
Cancer survival	0.850	0.82–0.88	[26, 34, 35]
Compliance of treatment			
CIN2+	0.9		[26]
Cancer	1.0		Assumed
Choose hysterectomy when CIN3	0.2 when >35		[26]
Discount rate of cost	3%	0–6%	Assumed
Discount rate of effectiveness	3%	0–6%	Assumed

cervical cancer was detected or symptoms appeared, compliance with treatment was assumed to be 100%.

Outcome measures

The model was programmed using TreeAge Pro 2011. We expressed the results in terms of the number of cases of cervical cancer, genital warts, and deaths from cervical cancer prevented, as well as the lifetime cost and QALYs gained. The incremental cost-effectiveness ratio (ICER) was calculated as incremental cost divided by the QALYs gained per woman by adding vaccination to the status quo (i.e., each of the three different screening strategies reflecting three different Chinese settings). According to the WHO, if the ICER is less than the per capita gross domestic product (GDP) a strategy can be considered as "very cost effective", and if less than three times the per capita GDP, as "cost effective" [42]. Three times the 2015 per-capita GDP for China amounted to USD$23,879.52 [43]. An annual discount rate of 3% was applied to both costs and benefits.

Sensitivity analyses

One-way sensitivity analysis was performed to explore the impact of the uncertainty of the parameters, taking into account simultaneous changes within the plausible ranges. The efficacy of each vaccine, the sensitivity and specificity of different tests, and the utilities associated with different health stages varied uniformly within the referred ranges. The cost parameters obtained varied uniformly in a range of +/− 50% of the deterministic estimate. The discount rate for cost and effectiveness varied uniformly between 0 to 6%. According to the results of tornado diagrams, threshold analyses were performed.

Results

Predicted cervical cancer mortality

Cervical cancer mortality in the trial (screening only without vaccination) was based on cancer statistics. The predicted cervical cancer mortality showed acceptable correspondence with data from the 2011 Chinese Cancer Registry Annual Report [44] (Additional file 1: Figure S1).

Base case analysis

The cost-effectiveness analysis and the reduction in cervical cancer and warts for each strategy under base case assumptions based on the Monte Carlo simulation of 100,000 trials showed that among the 15 options consisting either of a single strategy or one combining vaccination and screening, HPV9 combined with screening yielded the highest number of QALYs. Screening 1 and Screening 2 and their respective combination strategies showed little difference in discounted QALYs but an obvious cost difference (Table 2). In the calculation of ICERs, we first compared each single strategy (vaccine or screening) with no intervention strategy. Among three different vaccines, HPV4 cost least and gained almost the same number of QALYs as HPV9, while HPV-2 was dominated by HPV-4 due to higher costs and lower effectiveness. Screening 3, on the other hand, cost least, gained nearly the same QALYs as the other two screenings, and showed the most cost-effectiveness, while Screen1 showed no cost-effectiveness due to its ICER is over 3 times WTP. Then we compared each combination strategy in three different screening settings. HPV2 in its respective combination strategies were always ruled out by absolute dominance (higher cost and lower effectiveness) and demonstrated no cost-effectiveness while the HPV4 and HPV9 combination strategies presented significant cost-effectiveness (each

Table 2 Cost-effectiveness analysis and reduction in cervical cancer and warts of each strategy under base-case assumptions based on Monte Carlo simulation of 100,000 trails

Strategy	Discounted costs	Discounted QALYs	IC/IE ($/QALYs)	Cancer reduction incidence (%)	Cancer mortality reduction (%)	HPVhr incidence reduction (%)	Warts incidence reduction (%)
No intervention	25.359	30.858	–	1893.000	348.000	895,739.000	100,676.000
HPV-4[a]	101.631	30.872	5400.550[f]	15.850	18.200	18.130	15.570
HPV-2[a]	103.205	30.859	Dominated	13.100	13.100	4.170	14.500
HPV-9[a]	110.203	30.873	5768.350[f]	16.270	18.410	20.450	15.560
Screen1[b, c]	116.544	30.867	959,735.859[h] 9287.599[g]	18.860	19.020	10.400	5.900
Screen1 + HPV-4[c]	193.106	30.880	6070.026[f]	33.860	35.690	23.640	20.780
Screen1 + HPV-2[c]	194.301	30.869	Dominated	32.280	32.280	6.490	19.840
Screen1 + HPV-9[c]	201.724	30.881	6275.190[f]	34.390	35.950	25.820	20.800
Screen2[b, d]	82.945	30.867	20,372.19[g] 5886.421[f]	18.860	19.020	10.340	5.880
Screen2 + HPV-4[d]	159.397	30.880	6058.622[f]	33.860	35.690	23.610	20.730
Screen2 + HPV-2[d]	160.713	30.869	Dominated	32.280	32.280	6.460	19.790
Screen2 + HPV-9[d]	168.002	30.881	6262.947[f]	34.390	35.950	25.800	20.750
Screen3[b, e]	34.004	30.865	1171.435[f] 1171.435[f]	18.540	18.860	8.010	4.100
Screen3 + HPV-4[e]	110.341	30.878	5865.854[f]	32.750	35.130	21.650	19.220
Screen3 + HPV-2[e]	111.804	30.866	Dominated	31.170	31.720	3.890	18.280
Screen3 + HPV-9[e]	118.927	30.879	6098.722[f]	33.280	35.400	23.910	19.230

ICERs were calculated in 5 settings: [a]no intervention, HPV-4, HPV-2 and HPV-9; [b]no intervention, Screen3, Screen2 and Screen1; [c]no intervention, Screen1, Screen1 + HPV-4, Screen1 + HPV-2, and Screen1 + HPV-9; [d]no intervention, Screen2, Screen2 + HPV-4, Screen2 + HPV-2, and Screen2 + HPV-9; [e]no intervention, Screen3, Screen3 + HPV-4, Screen3 + HPV-2, and Screen3 + HPV-9

[f]If 0 < ICER < per capita GDP (7960 USD), it is considered very cost effective; [g]If per capita GDP (7960 USD) < ICER <3 times of per capita GDP (23,880 USD), it is considered as cost effective; [h]If ICER >3 times of per capita GDP (23,880 USD), it is considered not cost effective. Absolute dominated: An option is said to be dominated if it both costs more and is less effective than a comparator

ICER was less than per capita GDP at 7960 USD). The pathway of the most cost-effective strategy at different levels of willingness-to-pay thresholds as determined by the ICERs in different screening settings demonstrated that the dominant strategy gradually shifted from screening only to screening + HPV4, and finally screening + HPV9 (Fig. 2). When competing all strategies against each other, Screening 3, Screening 3 + HPV4 and Screening 3 + HPV9 were cost-efficient with ICERs below the threshold WTP. Screening 2 + HPV9 and Screening 1 + HPV9 were also on the cost-effective frontier but were not cost-effective as their ICERs (USD$24,867/QALY; USD$1,162,147/QALY) was over WTP (3 times of per capita USD$23,880 USD) (Additional file 1: Figure S2).

Based on the natural history (no intervention), 1893 cases got cervical cancer and 348 cases died of it. HPV and genital wart infections occurred 895,739 times and 100,676 times, respectively. Among all 15 strategies, Screening 1 + HPV9 showed the best preventative effect against HPV-related disease by reducing cervical cancer incidence by 34.39%, cancer mortality cases by 35.95%, HPV-Hr infection rate by 25.82%, and genital wart incidence by 20.80% compared to no intervention. Among the three screening protocols, Screenings 1 and 2 showed no significant difference in their preventative effects against diseases related to HPV infection but were superior to Screening 3. Among the three vaccines, HPV9 showed the strongest preventative effect against HPV-related disease compared to the other two in both the single and combination strategies (Table 2).

Sensitivity analysis

Variables with a range ≥ 1% of base case ICER (comparing each HPV9 combination strategy to HPV4 combination strategy) were listed in descending order (Fig. 3.1–3.3). The HPV4/9 combination strategies were both sensitive to efficacy of HPV4/9 for cervical cancer and genital warts, cost of HPV4/9, the discount rate of effectiveness, utility of warts, age of vaccination, screen coverage, and so on. Threshold analyses showed that when efficacy of HPV9 for genital warts/cervical cancer is smaller than 0.682/0.839, cost of HPV9 more than $567 USD, cost of HPV4 smaller than $283 USD and efficacy of HPV4 for cervical cancer greater than 0.883, ICER exceeds three times of GDP per capita (23,880 USD).

As HPV2 is the only accessible vaccine on mainland China so far, we also did a one-way sensitivity analysis for HPV2, comparing HPV2 combination strategies to

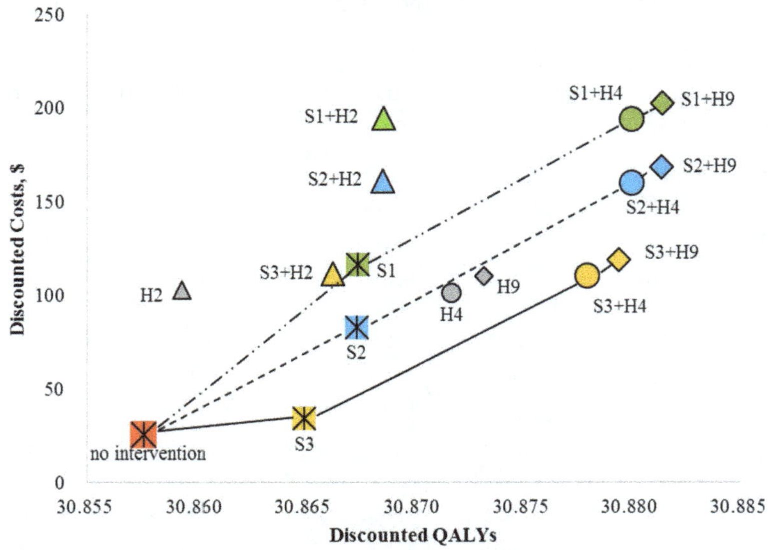

Fig. 2 Comparing Discounted cost and QALYs in different screening settings. Three lines stand for three different screening settings. S is short for screening; H is short for HPV vaccine. *Green* dot means strategies with screening1, *blue* dot means strategies with screening2 and *yellow* dot means strategies with screening3

screening alone (Additional file 1: Figure S3.1–S3.3). The results were mainly sensitive to the discount rate of effectiveness, screening coverage, discount rate of cost, utility of warts, CIN 3, age of vaccination, and so on. Since the screening coverage was important and public health meaningful among the results, we performed a threshold analysis of screening coverage from 10% to 100%, comparing it with willingness to pay (three times the GDP per capita of China). The combination of HPV2 with Screening 1 and Screening 2 showed similar values, and when screening coverage was increased to about 61%, these strategies were found to be cost-effective. When screening was increased to 78%, HPV2 combined with Screening 3 was also found to be considered acceptable (ICER doesn't exceed three times of GDP per capita).

Discussion

Past population-based screening programs demonstrated the impact of vaccination on reducing cervical cancer mortality and morbidity in both developed and developing countries [45, 46]. Despite the overall decline in its disease burden, cervical cancer still remains the most lethal gynaecological cancer in China. Before HPV vaccines were approved for use on mainland China, the chief strategy for cervical cancer prevention and control was routine screening, targeting women at reproductive age for early detection and treatment. However, well-established evidence indicates that the success of such a program depends on adequate coverage of the population, which has often proved difficult to achieve [47]. As screening alone tends to be insufficient for combating the disease, and ideally primary prevention would be integrated with secondary measures, this study provided a perspective on the potential benefits of innovative vaccination strategies as an adjunct to the current screening program in China. The results of the first economic evaluation of an integrated strategy for the prevention and control of cervical cancer in China presented here will aid in informing policy makers at both the national and local levels.

The results of this study indicated that under baseline coverage of the vaccination and the screening programs, HPV2 vaccine, recently approved in China, is not cost effective either in the single vaccine protocol or in the screening combination strategies; however, the HPV4/9 strategy showed much better cost-effectiveness compared to HPV2 (with ICER of 5400 $/QALY and 5434 $/QALY respectively), and especially the strategy combining HPV9 with screening program showed best health impact on reducing the cervical cancer incidence and mortality rate, compared to that of the HPV2 vaccine combination strategy. These results were consistent with those of studies conducted in the United States [48, 49], which showed that the HPV9 vaccine resulted in a reduction in the incidence of genital warts among different populations [26, 50, 51]. After HPV 16/18, the most common HPV types among Chinese women with either a normal or abnormal cervical diagnosis were HPV 58, 31, and 52, which have been implicated in ICC among Chinese women and have accounted for 9.59% ~ 25.7% of ICC cases [30, 52]. They have now been added to the list of oncogenic types of HPV targeted by the second-generation HPV9 (HPV-31, 33, 45, 52 and 58). Furthermore, the potential benefits of HPV9 include a reduction in the incidence of vulvovaginal, penile, and anal tumours,

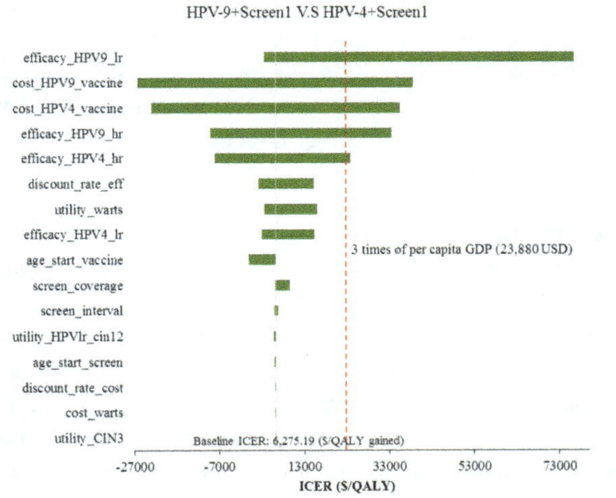

Figure 3.1 Range of ICER/Baseline ICER of HPV-9 + S1 vs HPV-4 + S1. The red dotted line is the threshold value for cost-effectiveness: 3 times of per capita CDP (23,880 USD).

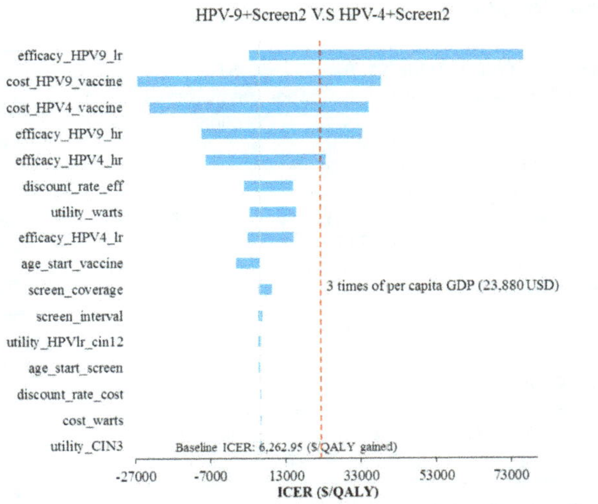

Figure 3.2 Range of ICER/Baseline ICER of HPV-9 + S2 vs HPV-4 + S2. The red dotted line is the threshold value for cost-effectiveness: 3 times of per capita GDP (23,880 USD).

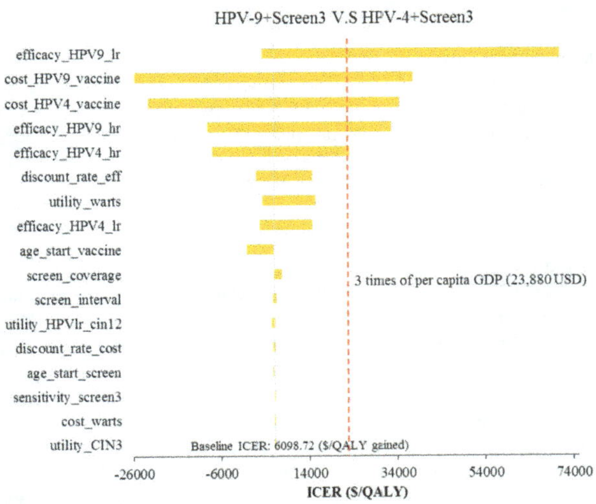

Figure 3.3 Range of ICER/Baseline ICER of HPV-9 + S3 vs HPV-4 + S3. The red dotted line is the threshold value for cost-effectiveness: 3 times of per capita GDP (23,880 USD).

Fig. 3 (3.1–3.3) Univariate sensitivity analysis to exmaine variables that impact base case

and paraneoplastic lesions arising in the lower-genital tract [53]. Among boys and male adolescents 55% of anal and penile cancers are caused by the five oncogenic HPV types listed above. HPV9 vaccination not only covers these types specifically but also 68% of all HPV types, and is thus expected to confer significant health benefits in males as well [54]. HPV9 will therefore be an invaluable adjunct to China's current vaccination program and should be considered seriously by public health policy makers.

Our results highlighted the validity of combining screening and vaccination. Combination strategies using HVP4/9 were cost-effective and able to confer greater health benefits than screening alone. Data from both developed and developing countries thus far have demonstrated that neither secondary prevention, such as screening alone, nor a conventional vaccination program can reduce the incidence of cervical cancers and warts or the disease burden [55]. Our results confirmed, in line with previous economic assessments, that integrated primary prevention (vaccination) and secondary prevention (screening program) were the most effective in terms of cost-effectiveness and health impact [55–57]. At the baseline level the HPV-9 + Screening 1 (Liquid-based cytology test + HPV DNA test) protocol was the most effective, having achieved a reduction of 34.39% in cancer incidence and of 35.95% in cancer deaths.

Vaccination is the primary preventative measure but effective only in those not yet infected by HPV [55]. Moreover, because immunity to HPV is primarily type-specific, the current generation of vaccines against a limited number of HPV types cannot provide complete protection [55]. Therefore, as a preliminary phase in the implementation of combination strategies, the current screening program should be strengthened by improving coverage for the general population [58]. Interestingly the recommended Screening 2 protocol (pap smear cytology test + HPV DNA test) showed almost the same effect as Screening 1 (liquid-based cytology test + HPV DNA test) in terms of reducing the incidence of cancer, HPV infections, and warts. The Screening 3 protocol (VIA), which cost much less and showed great cost-effectiveness, is considered the best choice in medical resource-poor settings.

The different combination strategies examined in this study were flexible enough to be adapted to the wide geographical and socioeconomic diversity found in China according to the varying income levels and availability of medical resources. The Screening 3 or 2 protocols are recommended for low income settings, and if economic conditions permit, the screening plus vaccine strategy, which is likely to achieve have greater prevention impact, is also recommended even if HPV2 vaccine alone is available in mainland China so far.

The sensitivity analysis of HPV9 showed the robustness of its cost-effectiveness. The sensitivity analysis of

HPV2, on the other hand, demonstrated that screening coverage crucially influenced the cost-effectiveness of different strategies. This study found that only when screening coverage increased to 60% ~ 70% did the HPV2 and screening combination strategies become economically feasible. In practice, coverage tends to be affected by various factors at both the social and individual level, such as affordability, the socioeconomic status of different regions, the educational level, and adherence of the target population to vaccine protocol recommendations [55]. Regarding the screening program, the current policy tends to be region driven and to focus on high risk populations, leading to a relatively low level of coverage in nonurban areas estimated to comprise approximately 20% of the population [59]. As for vaccination, most developing nations have experienced various challenges including coverage, accessibility, cold-chain transportation, and communication strategies to promote public acceptability [47]. Affordability is essential; high costs without public subsidy may restrict coverage especially among the poor and vulnerable. Educational interventions are also necessary to boost vaccination rates due to relatively poor HPV vaccine awareness among the Chinese [60]. Furthermore, because the vaccines are a relatively new development, the safety and the side effects remain a huge concern globally and affect the public's perceptions, and consequently the coverage, of any vaccination program [61, 62]. Especially for the newer HPV9 vaccine, more monitoring and surveillance are needed to establish safety and to maintain efficacy and cross-protection against oncogenic HPV types. These uncertainties should be carefully addressed in future studies for their potential impact on public health policy as well.

There were several limitations to this study. First, we did not model the transmission dynamics of HPV nor consider what protection might be conferred by HPV vaccinations against other HPV-related cancers like cervical adenocarcinoma, vulvar carcinoma, and laryngeal papillomatosis due to the lack of data. Consequently, the overall effectiveness of the vaccination program might have been underestimated, thus making the cost-effectiveness of the HPV vaccine appear even more favourable if herd immunity or protection against other diseases existed [63, 64] especially in the case of HPV9, which confers wider coverage compared to the other two vaccines. Moreover, this study did not consider the cross-protective effects of vaccines, multiple HPV infections, and unidentified HPV types, which can influence the effectiveness of vaccines; instead we set a range for vaccine efficacy in our sensitivity analysis to determine the robustness of the model, showing that these variables did not significantly affect the ICERs under the current WTP threshold. In addition, women adhering to previous cervical screening tests may have shown better compliance with subsequent tests [13]. Nevertheless, in the absence of information on local contexts, we chose not to perform individually based modelling, nor did we consider the negative indirect effects.

Conclusion

We demonstrated that HPV4/9 vaccination for adolescent girls was highly cost-effective in China when integrated into the current screening strategies. Integrated vaccination and screening is recommended. HPV9 vaccination combined with Screening 1 (liquid-based cytology test + HPV DNA test) proved to be the best preventative strategy against cervical cancer and warts.

Additional file

Additional file 1: Table S1. Transfer probability used in the Markov model. **Figure S1.** Calibration result of age-specific incidence and mortality of cervical cancer. **Figure S2.** Comparing Discounted cost and QALYs with each strategy. S is short for screening; H is short for HPV vaccine. Q is short for QALY. Blue means strategies with screening1, yellow means strategies with screening2 and green screening3. Plots with grey outline means extended dominance. **Figure S3.1.** Spread of ICER/Baseline ICER of HPV-2 + S1 V.S S1. **Figure S3.2.** Spread of ICER/Baseline ICER of HPV-2 + S2 V.S S2. **Figure S3.3.** Spread of ICER/Baseline ICER of HPV-2 + S3 V.S S3. (DOC 288 kb)

Abbreviations

AIS: Adenocarcinoma In Situ; CIN: Cervical intraepithelial neoplasia; HPV: Human papillomavirus; VIA: Visual inspection with acetic acid; FIGO: International Federation of Gynaecology and Obstetrics; QALY: Quality-adjusted life year; CPI: Consumer price index; ICER: Incremental cost-effectiveness ratio; GDP: Gross domestic product; ICC: Invasive cervical cancer; WTP: Willingness to pay; HPV2, 4, 9: 2-, 4-, 9-valent HPV vaccine

Acknowledgements

The author is grateful to valuable comments on earlier versions of this paper; many thanks to the English editors in the Department of Health Policy, National Centre for Child Health and Development; and thanks to Prof Xu Lingzhong and Prof Li Shixue in Shandong University for their generous support when the author (XM) began this study during her master's program.

Funding

This research is supported by grants from the Japan Society for the Promotion of Sciences (16H06241), the National Centre for Child Health and Development (26–5), and the Chinese Natural Sciences Foundation (81202225).

Authors' contributions

XM built the model, analysed data, and wrote the manuscript. RGT participated in the design of the study and wrote the manuscript. XL reviewed, reviewed and proofread the manuscript. LW, BW, HL, CN, RM, and TN participated in the discussion, review, and editing of the manuscript. All authors read and approved the final manuscript.

Consent for publication

All authors approved the final version of this article.

Competing interests
All authors declare there were no potential competing interests relevant to this article.

Author details
[1]Department of Health Informatics, Kyoto University School of Public Health, Kyoto, Japan. [2]Department of Health Policy, National Center for Child Health and Development, Okura 2-10-1, Setagaya-ku, Tokyo 157-8535, Japan. [3]Department of Gynecology, Qilu Hospital of Shandong University, Jinan, China. [4]College of Pharmacy, The University of Tennessee Health Science Center, Memphis, TN, USA. [5]Medical Decision and Economic Group, Department of Pharmacy, Ren Ji Hospital affiliated with Medical School of Shanghai Jiao tong University, Shanghai, China. [6]Nanjing Drum Tower Hospital affiliated Medical School of Nanjing University, Nanjing, China. [7]Department of Education for Clinical Research, National Centre for Child Health and Development, Tokyo, Japan.

References

1. de Sanjose S, Diaz M, Castellsague X, Clifford G, Bruni L, Munoz N, et al. Worldwide prevalence and genotype distribution of cervical human papillomavirus DNA in women with normal cytology: a meta-analysis. Lancet Infect Dis. 2007;7:453–9.
2. Yang L, Parkin DM, Li LD, Chen YD, Bray F. Estimation and projection of the national profile of cancer mortality in China: 1991-2005. Br J Cancer. 2004;90:2157–66.
3. Shi JF, Canfell K, Lew JB, Qiao YL. The burden of cervical cancer in China: synthesis of the evidence. Int J Cancer. 2012;130:641–52.
4. Techakehakij W, Feldman RD. Cost-effectiveness of HPV vaccination compared with pap smear screening on a national scale: a literature review. Vaccine. 2008;26:6258–65.
5. Serrano B, Alemany L, Tous S, Bruni L, Clifford GM, Weiss T, et al. Potential impact of a nine-valent vaccine in human papillomavirus related cervical disease. Infect Agents Cancer. 2012;7:38.
6. Chitnis D. Data on two-dose 9-valent HPV vaccinations encouraging, but more needed. https://www.pm360online.com/data-on-two-dose-9-valenthpv-vaccinations-encouraging-but-more-needed/. Cited date: 24 Feb 2016.
7. Liu W. China approves GSK's HPV vaccine. http://www.chinadaily.com.cn/china/2016-07/18/content_26131226.htm. Cited date: 18 July 2016.
8. GSK. GSK announces Cervarix™ approved in China to help protect women from cervical cancer. http://www.gsk-china.com/en-gb/media/press-releases/2016/gsk-announces-cervarix-approved-in-china-to-help-protect-women-from-cervical-cancer/. Cited date: 18 July 2016.
9. De Vuyst H, Clifford GM, Nascimento MC, Maceleine MM, Franceschi S. Prevalence and type distribution of human papillomavirus in carcinoma and intraepithelial neoplasia of the vulva, vagina and anus: a meta-analysis. Int J Cancer. 2009;124:1626–36.
10. Merck & CO. I. Highlights of prescribing information: GARDASIL® [Human papillomavirus quadrivalent (types 6, 11, 16, and 18) vaccine, recombinant]. https://www.fda.gov/downloads/biologicsbloodvaccines/vaccines/approvedproducts/ucm426457.pdf. Cited date: 28 Dec 2014.
11. Merck & CO. I. Highlights of prescribing information: GARDASIL®9 (Human papillomavirus 9-valent vaccine, recombinant). www.merck.com/product/patent/home.html. Cited date: 12 Mar 2015.
12. World Health Organization. Cervical cancer screening in developing countries: report of a WHO consultation. World Health Organization; 2002.
13. Dong Z. Chinese cancer screening and early detection and early treated guidelines (trail). Beijing: Peking University Medical Press; 2005.
14. Editorial. Women's health in rural China. Lancet. 2009;374:358.
15. Meng R, Ma W, Xu Y, Song X, Nie S, Xu H, et al. Screening rates of cervical cancer, breast cancer and their influential factors in Guangdong Province. South China J Pre Med. 2010:8–10.
16. Li JM, Liu ZY, Ji HW, Fan YH, Wang W. Status of screening and KAP of cervical cancer in a community of Shenzhen. Chin J Health Educ. 2008;24:542–4.
17. Liu HR. Cervical cancer screening rates of its influential factors. World of mother and infant. 2015;
18. Liu Y-J, Zhang Q, Hu S-Y, Zhao F-H. Effect of vaccination age on cost-effectiveness of human papillomavirus vaccination against cervical cancer in China. BMC Cancer. 2016;16:1–11.
19. Zhang Q, Liu Y-J, Hu S-Y, Zhao F-H. Estimating long-term clinical effectiveness and cost-effectiveness of HPV 16/18 vaccine in China. BMC Cancer. 2016;16:848.
20. Levin CE, Sharma M, Olson Z, Verguet S, Shi J-F, Wang S-M, et al. An extended cost-effectiveness analysis of publicly financed HPV vaccination to prevent cervical cancer in China. Vaccine. 2015;33:2830–41.
21. Liu PH, Hu FC, Lee PI, Chow SN, Huang CW, Wang JD. Cost-effectiveness of human papillomavirus vaccination for prevention of cervical cancer in Taiwan. BMC Health Serv Res. 2010;10:11.
22. Elbasha EH, Dasbach EJ, Insinga RP. Model for assessing human papillomavirus vaccination strategies. Emerg Infect Dis. 2007;13:28–41.
23. Myers ER, McCrory DC, Nanda K, Bastian L, Matchar DB. Mathematical model for the natural history of human papillomavirus infection and cervical carcinogenesis. Am J Epidemiol. 2000;151:1158–71.
24. Longde W, Yu P. Technical proposal for screening and early detection and treatment of cancer in China. People's medical publishing house; 2009.
25. Shi JF, Chen JF, Canfell K, Feng XX, Ma JF, Zhang YZ, et al. Estimation of the costs of cervical cancer screening, diagnosis and treatment in rural Shanxi Province, China: a micro-costing study. BMC Health Serv Res. 2012;12:123.
26. Shi JF, Xiang W, Qiao YL. A review of health economic evaluation on cervical cancer screening by visual inspection with acetic acid. Zhonghua Liu Xing Bing Xue Za Zhi. 2009;30:87–90.
27. Kulasingam SL, Myers ER. Potential health and economic impact of adding a human papillomavirus vaccine to screening programs. JAMA. 2003;290(6):781–9.
28. Jufang S. Cost-effectiveness on various modalities of cervical cancer screening in rural China: Chinese academy of medical sciences & Peking union medical college; 2009.
29. GlaxoSmithKline. Highlights of prescribing information: CERVARIX [Human papillomavirus bivalent (types 16 and 18) vaccine, recombinant]. http://us.gsk.com/products/assets/us_cervarix.pdf. Cited date: 28 Dec 2014.
30. Wen C. An epidemic study on HPV distribution in genital warts, invasive cervical cancer in China: Chinese academy of medical sciences & Peking union medical college; 2010.
31. Olsson SE, Villa LL, Costa RL, Petta CA, Andrade RP, Malm C, et al. Induction of immune memory following administration of a prophylactic quadrivalent human papillomavirus (HPV) types 6/11/16/18 L1 virus-like particle (VLP) vaccine. Vaccine. 2007;25:4931–9.
32. Zhao FH, Lin MJ, Feng C, Hu SY, Rong Z, Belinson JL, et al. Performance of high-risk human papillomavirus DNA testing as a primary screen for cervical cancer: a pooled analysis of individual patient data from 17 population-based studies from China. Lancet Oncol. 2010;11:1160–71.
33. Dongyan L. Health economic evaluation and economic feasibility research of cervical cancer screening in rural areas: medical school of Dalian; 2010.
34. Zhao ZM, Pan XF, Lv SH, Xie Y, Zhang SK, Qiao YL, et al. Quality of life in women with cervical precursor lesions and cancer: a prospective, 6-month, hospital-based study in China. Chin J Cancer. 2014;33:339–45.
35. Molassiotis A, Chan CW, Yam BM, Chan SJ. Quality of life in Chinese women with gynaecological cancers. Support Care Cancer. 2000;8:414–22.
36. Shi JF, Kang DJ, Qi SZ, Wu HY, Liu YC, Sun LJ, et al. Impact of genital warts on health related quality of life in men and women in mainland China: a multicenter hospital-based cross-sectional study. BMC Public Health. 2012;12:153.
37. Qi SZ, Wang SM, Shi JF, Wang QQ, Chen XS, Sun LJ, et al. Human papillomavirus-related psychosocial impact of patients with genital warts in China: a hospital-based cross-sectional study. BMC Public Health. 2014;14:1–8.
38. People Daily. What is HPV? http://weibo.com/rmrb?is_hot=1. Cited date: 11 Mar 2016.
39. Medscape. HPV 9: The Latest ACIP Guidance. http://www.medscape.com/viewarticle/841676. Cited date: 23 Mar 2015.
40. Chinses anti-cancer association. Early screen of cervical cancer [in Chinese] http://www.caca.org.cn/system/2008/07/31/010009930.shtml. Cited date: 15 Dec 2008.
41. National Comprehensive Cancer Network. NCCN Clinical Practice Guidelines in Oncology http://www.nccn.org/professionals/physician_gls/f_guidelines.asp. 2013.
42. World Health Organization. Macroeconomics and Health: Investing in Health for Economic Development. Report of the Commission on Macroeconomics and Health. Geneva: WHO; 2001.
43. National Bureau of Statistics of China. Gross Domestic Product http://data.stats.gov.cn/ks.htm?cn=C01&zb=A0501. Cited date: 1 Dec 2015.
44. National Office for Cancer Prevention and Control NCfCR. Disease Prevnetion and Control Bureau, MOH. Chinese Cancer Registry Annual Report (2011). Beijing: Military Medical Science Press; 2011.
45. Mandelblatt JS, Lawrence WF, Womack SM, Jacobson D, Yi B, Hwang YT, et al. Benefits and costs of using HPV testing to screen for cervical cancer. JAMA. 2002;287:2372–81.

46. Chen MK, Hung HF, Duffy S, Yen AM, Chen HH. Cost-effectiveness analysis for pap smear screening and human papillomavirus DNA testing and vaccination. J Eval Clin Pract. 2011;17:1050–8.
47. Kane MA, Serrano B, de Sanjose S, Wittet S. Implementation of human papillomavirus immunization in the developing world. Vaccine. 2012; 30(Suppl 5):F192–200.
48. Chesson HW, Markowitz LE, Hariri S, Ekwueme DU, Saraiya M. The impact and cost-effectiveness of nonavalent HPV vaccination in the United States: estimates from a simplified transmission model. Human vaccines & immunotherapeutics. 2016:1–10.
49. Brisson M, Laprise JF, Chesson HW, Drolet M, Malagon T, Boily MC, et al. Health and economic impact of switching from a 4-Valent to a 9-Valent HPV vaccination program in the United States. J Natl Cancer Inst. 2016;108
50. Sorapop K, Nicole Gastineau C, Kim JJ. Potential benefits of second-generation human papillomavirus vaccines. PLoS One. 2012;7:e48426.
51. Lee VJ, Tay SK, Teoh YL, Tok MY. Cost-effectiveness of different human papillomavirus vaccines in Singapore. BMC Public Health. 2011;11:203.
52. Bao YP, Li N, Smith JS, Qiao YL. Human papillomavirus type-distribution in the cervix of Chinese women: a meta-analysis. Int J STD AIDS. 2008;19:106–11.
53. Mariani L, Bonanni P, Castiglia P, Chiamenti G, Conforti G, Conversano M, et al. Prevention of HPV cancer related through HPV-9: state of the art, potential benefits and open issues. Igiene e sanita pubblica. 2015;71:631–52.
54. Wieland U, Brockmeyer NH, Kreuter A. A 9-Valent HPV Vaccine in Women. N Engl J Med. 2015;372:2566.
55. Liu X, Feng A, Cui Y, Tobe RG. Prevention of human papillomavirus (HPV) infection and cervical cancer in China: how does HPV vaccination bring about benefits to Chinese women? Biosci Trends. 2013;7:159–67.
56. Diaz M, Kim JJ, Albero G, Sanjosé SD, Clifford G, Bosch FX, et al. Health and economic impact of HPV 16 and 18 vaccination and cervical cancer screening in India. Br J Cancer. 2008;99:230–8.
57. Canfell K, Shi JF, Lew JB, Walker R, Zhao FH, Simonella L, et al. Prevention of cervical cancer in rural China: evaluation of HPV vaccination and primary HPV screening strategies. Vaccine. 2011;29:2487–94.
58. Zhai L, Tumban E. Gardasil-9: a global survey of projected efficacy. Antivir Res. 2016.
59. ChinaIRN. New opportunities of cervical cancer prevention and control to China in 2014 http://www.chinairn.com/news/20140506/124657368.shtml. Cited date: 30 Dec 2014.
60. Zhang Y, Wang Y, Liu L, Fan Y, Liu Z, Wang Y, et al. Awareness and knowledge about human papillomavirus vaccination and its acceptance in China: a meta-analysis of 58 observational studies. BMC Public Health. 2016;16:216.
61. Stokley S, Jeyarajah J, Yankey D, Cano M, Gee J, Roark J, et al. Human papillomavirus vaccination coverage among adolescents, 2007-2013, and postlicensure vaccine safety monitoring, 2006-2014–United States. MMWR Morb Mortal Wkly Rep. 2014;63:620–4.
62. Handler NS, Handler MZ, Majewski S, Schwartz RA. Human papillomavirus vaccine trials and tribulations: vaccine efficacy. J Am Acad Dermatol. 2015; 73:759–67. quiz 67-8
63. Chesson HW, Ekwueme DU, Saraiya M, Markowitz LE. Cost-effectiveness of human papillomavirus vaccination in the United States. Emerg Infect Dis. 2008;14:244.
64. Brisson M, Edmunds WJ. Economic evaluation of vaccination programs: the impact of herd-immunity. Med Decis Mak. 2003;23:76–82.

17

Prevalence and type-specific distribution of human papillomavirus infection among women in mid-western rural, Nepal

Niresh Thapa[1,2], Muna Maharjan[3], Girishma Shrestha[4], Narayani Maharjan[5], Marcia A. Petrini[6], Na Zuo[1], Can He[1], Jing Yang[1], Mengfei Xu[1], Caiyun Ge[1], Ziye Song[1] and Hongbing Cai[1*]

Abstract

Background: Cervical cancer is the most common cancer among women in Nepal. The prevalence of human papillomavirus (HPV) 16 and or HPV 18 among women with cervical pre-cancer and cancer is higher than the incidence of HPV in the world population. The population-based epidemiological data of HPV in the general population in most parts of the country remains unknown. The objective of this study was to assess the prevalence and type distribution of HPV infection and association of abnormal cytology with high risk HPV infection among women in mid-western rural, Nepal.

Methods: A population-based cross sectional study was conducted in Jumla, one of the most remote districts in Nepal. A total of 1050 cervical samples were collected from married and non- pregnant women aged 20–65 years during mobile Cervical Cancer Screening Clinics conducted from May 2016 to January 2017. The presence of HPV DNA was firstly confirmed by HPV consensus PCR using PGMY09/PGMY11 designed primers, then HPV positive samples were further genotyped by the membrane hybridization method to detect the 21 high-risk HPV (HR-HPV) and low-risk HPV types. The prevalence of HR-HPV among women with normal and abnormal cytology was calculated. Data were analyzed using SPSS software for Windows. $P < 0.05$ was considered statistically significant.

Results: A total of 998 women were eligible for this study with the mean age 32.6 ± 8.6 years, and the mean marital age was 16.7 ± 3.8 years. The overall prevalence of HPV infections was 19.7%. HR-HPV and low-risk HPV were 11.7 and 8.7% respectively. The six most common HR-HPV types were HPV16, 39, 58, 33, 51 and 18. HR-HPV infection among the women with abnormal and normal cytology was of 27.3 and 10.8% respectively.

Conclusions: There was a higher prevalence of HR-HPV infection among women living in Jumla than other parts of Nepal. This study provides preliminary information on overall HPV and type-specific HR-HPV prevalence, HR-HPV 16, 39, 58, 33, 51, and 18 are the most prevalent genotypes in this region. The data contribute to the epidemiological knowledge about HPV and type-specific HR-HPV genotypes prevalence in mid-Western Nepal.

Keywords: Cervical cancer, Genotype, HPV infection, Nepal, Prevalence

* Correspondence: chb2105@163.com
[1]Department of Gynecological Oncology, Zhongnan Hospital of Wuhan University, Hubei Cancer Clinical Study Center, Hubei Key laboratory of Tumor Biological Behaviors, Wuhan 430071, People's Republic of China
Full list of author information is available at the end of the article

Background

Worldwide, the prevalence of human papillomavirus (HPV) 16 and or HPV 18 among women with low grade squamous Intraepithelial Lesions (LSIL), high-grade squamous intraepithelial lesions (HSIL) and cervical cancer is 25.8, 51.9 and 69.4% respectively [1]. The burden of HPV infection is significantly high about 10 million new cases of HSIL, and 30 million new cases of LSIL are diagnosed every year. The potential risk of HPV for cervical cancer is higher than Hepatitis B virus (HBV) is for liver cancer and even smoking is for lung cancer [2]. HPV infection is regarded as the well-established cause of cervical cancer now and a risk factor for other anogenital as well as head and neck cancers [1].

Cervical cancer is the most common cancer among women in Nepal. Cervical cancer demonstrates a decreasing trend in more developed countries, but consistently remains the number one female cancer of incidence and mortality in Nepal. According to the Information Center on HPV and Cancer (ICO), Nepal reports a prevalence of HPV 16 and or HPV 18 among women with LSIL, HSIL, and cervical cancer are 30.2, 63.4, and 80.3% respectively. The prevalence of HPV infection in Nepal is higher than in the world population [3–5].

Human genital HPV types are categorized according to the epidemiologic association and potential risk of cervical cancer. The eight most common types high risk (HR) HPV (HPV-16, 18, 31, 33, 35, 45, 52, 58) and relatively less common four types (HPV-39, 51, 56, 59) found in cervical cancer were classified in group 1. Probably carcinogenic to human's HPV-68 was classified in group 2A. The remaining types of HPV 26, 53, 66, 67, 70, 73, 82 of the high-risk alpha species were classified in group 2B as "possibly carcinogenic" [6, 7].

The actual distribution of HPV is not known for some resource-limited countries, including Nepal [8]. Studies reporting the epidemiologic information on HPV in Nepal are sparse. Sherpa et al. in 2010 indicated that among the general population the overall prevalence of HPV was 8.6% including 6.1% for high-risk HPV [9]. Among the women with invasive cervical cancer, the incidence of HPV 16/18 infection was around 91% [9] and 70% [10]. Similarly, another study conducted by Shakya et al. [11] in the rural site of Kavre district found that the overall HPV prevalence was 14.4% including 7.9% of HR-HPV, whereas 9.6% of HR-HPV infection was reported in a study from far-western region of Nepal [12]. Furthermore, a study conducted by Bhatta et al. in 2017 among Nepali and Bhutanese women living in eastern Nepal reported the prevalence of 8.9% HR-HPV infection [13]. In the presence of co-factors, persistent infection with an oncogenic HPV is necessary to develop cervical cancer [14]. Therefore, the HPV test has emerged as an essential screening tool. HPV infection status is thus significant in cervical cancer screening and prevention strategy [15, 16].

Reproductive health indicators in Jumla are below the level than general Nepali women. The prevalence of female adolescent marriage is almost 83%; the total fertility rate is 4.2, literacy among women is 41% in Jumla [17, 18]. The population based epidemiological data of HPV in the general population in most parts of the country is still unknown [11]. So far, we know this was the first population-based study conducted in such remote area, Jumla. The objective of this study was to assess the prevalence and type-specific distribution of HPV infection and association of abnormal cytology with high-risk HPV infection among apparently healthy women in mid-western rural, Nepal. This study intends to give a sound basis for future strategic plans for the prevention of cervical cancer.

Methods

Study setting

A population based cross sectional study conducted in Jumla. According to National Population and Housing census 2011, the total population of Jumla is 108921, and the overall, married women registration is 27309. Jumla is one of the most remote districts in Nepal with women who have a high illiteracy rate, high poverty, low economic development, and inadequate transportation facility [17, 18].

Sample collection

Ethical approval was obtained from the Nepal Health Research Council (NHRC), Nepal and Department of Gynecological Oncology, Second Clinical College of Wuhan University, China. The study participants were recruited from the different mobile cervical cancer screening programs conducted in Jumla, in 2016 and 2017. Inclusion criteria in this study were: aged 20–65 years married, non-pregnant, apparently healthy, asymptomatic women, with no history of cervical cancer. The exclusion criteria were women who were menstruating or did not want to participate in the study. Eligible women were counseled about the research and informed that they could withdraw from the study at any time with no impact on the routine care. A written informed consent was obtained from eligible participants with either a signature or thumbprint. Cervical cells of 1050 women were collected using cytobrush (Hybribio® Limited, China) from the eligible women who were in follow up for our previous screening test (cytology) report.

Cytology was done 4 weeks earlier and reported according to the Bethesda system [19]. For the analysis purpose, the cytology report was categorized into normal and abnormal. Routine cervical cytology included negative for intraepithelial lesion or malignancy (NILM) and inflammatory changes. Abnormal cervical cytology included atypical squamous cells of undetermined significance (ASC-US), low-grade squamous intraepithelial lesion (LSIL), high-grade squamous intraepithelial lesion (HSIL) and squamous cell carcinoma (SCC).

DNA extraction PCR and HPV genotyping

DNA extracted in Intrepid Cancer Diagnostics, Kathmandu using the QIAamp DNA Mini kit (QIAGEN Germany) according to the manufacturer's instructions. Extracted DNA samples were stored at − 20 °C until transported on dry ice to the Zhongnan Hospital of Wuhan University, Hubei Cancer Clinical Study Center, Hubei Key Laboratory of Tumor Biological Behaviors, Wuhan, China for HPV DNA analyses.

The presence of HPV DNA was firstly confirmed by HPV consensus PCR using PGMY09/PGMY11 designed primers to amplify a fragment of the HPV L1 gene visible at 450 bp and Human Leukocyte Antigen (HLA) band at 230 bp as described in 'Human papillomavirus laboratory manual' published by World Health Organization [20]. Detection of HLA confirmed that DNA had been extracted in sufficient amount. Amplicons were detected after the agarose gel electrophoresis and Ethidium bromide staining under the UV transillumination. Gel electrophoresis analysis was done to limit the only HPV positive samples for further genotyping by membrane hybridization (21 HPV GenoArray Diagnostic Kit, Hybrobio® Limited, China) to detect the following 21 HPV types: HPV6, 11, 16, 18, 31, 33, 35, 39, 42, 43, 44, 45, 51, 52, 53, 56, 58, 59, 66, 68, 81 (equivalent to CP8304) according to the manufacturer's instruction. High risk HPV (HR-HPV) types included in this study were HPV16, 18, 31, 33, 35, 39, 45, 51, 52, 53, 56, 58, 59, 66, and 68 [7]. All other HPV types were considered low-risk HPV (LR-HPV).

Statistical analysis

Data were analyzed using SPSS software for Windows (version 16.0). The distribution of characteristics of participants was presented as numbers, percentage and mean. Odds ratios (ORs) and their 95% confidence intervals (CIs) were obtained using univariate analysis to assess the effect of characteristics in HPV infection. $P < 0.05$ was considered statistically significant.

Results

Altogether 1050 samples were collected; 20 samples were not adequate for DNA extraction, and 32 samples had no HLA band visible under UV transillumination after Gel Electrophoresis of PCR product suggesting invalid for further analysis. Table 1 shows the distribution of HR-HPV according to the socio-demographic and reproductive health characteristics. Among 998 eligible women, the mean age was 32.6 ± 8.6 years; the mean marital age was 16.7 ± 3.8 years. There were around 40% of women married before the age of 15 years. About 50% of women had more than three children. Forty-one percent of women were illiterate, and among the literate group more than half just had an informal education which means they can hardly read or write. Almost 16% of women were a current smoker. A significant number of women (14.3%) reported that they had sexually transmitted infection (STI) in the past and about 12% of the participant's husband had multiple marriages or multiple sexual partners. There were 5 cases of HIV positive women. HR-HPV was most prevalent in the younger age group from 20 to 29 years, and in the same way more common on those who marry before the age of 20 years. The HR-HPV Positive rate was increased correspondingly with the number of pregnancies and number of childbirths.

There were 197 (19.7%) HPV positive cases detected from 998 acceptable samples. High and low risk HPV were 115 (11.5%) and 82 (8.2%) respectively. In total, 13.6% women had single-type infections, and 6.1% had multiple-type infections. HPV 16 and HPV 39 were the most common multiple infections. The six most common HR-HPV types were HPV16 (6.7%), 39 (4.8%), 58 (2.8%), 33 (2.6%), 51 (1.4%) and 18 (1.2%). HPV 6 (0.6%) was the most common LR-HPV. There was no positive case of HR-HPV 59. The number of other uncharacterized LR-HPV type was 72 (Table 2).

Figure 1 illustrates that HR-HPV is more prevalent in the younger age group. In the age group of 20–29 years, 29.8% of HR HPV infection occurred, whereas only 3.6% of HR HPV infection presented in 50–65 years' age group. There were 'two peaks' in the prevalence pattern of the overall HPV and HPV16/18 infections; the first peak was at the age group of 25–29 years and the second small peak was at the age group of 40–44 years (Fig. 2).

Table 3 presents the association between variables and HR-HPV infection. The relationship between HR-HPV and the variables of age, marital age, number of pregnancies, number of childbirths, education status, smoking, participant's multiple marriages or multiple sexual partners, husband's multiple marriages or multiple sexual partners, contraceptive use, HIV status and STI status were analyzed with the use of odds ratio (OR). Chi-square test was used for the statistical significance. The HR-HPV was significantly associated with age, number of pregnancy, number of children, husband's multiple marriages or multiple sexual partners and participant's HIV status ($p < 0.05$).

Abnormal cytology reports were 44 in 998 women. HR-HPV infection among women with abnormal and normal cytology was 27.3 and 10.8% respectively. Positive HR-HPV was significantly higher in women with abnormal cytology. The abnormal cytology for women with LSIL, ASC-US, HSIL, and SCC had HR-HPV infection rates of 25, 13.3, 40 and 75% respectively (Table 4).

Table 1 Characteristics and distribution of high-risk Human Papillomavirus (HR-HPV) infection among women living in mid-western rural Nepal $N = 998$

Characteristics	Number (%)	HR-HPV (f/n)	HR-HPV (%)
Age			
20–29	403 (40.4)	58/403	14.4
30–39	351 (35.2)	23/351	6.5
40–49	192 (19.2)	26/192	13.5
50–59	42 (4.2)	5/42	11.9
Above 60	10 (1.0)	3/10	30
Mean ± SD	32.6 ± 8.6		
Marital age			
≤ 15	393 (39.4)	41/393	10.4
16–20	513 (51.4)	62/513	12.1
21–25	61 (6.1)	5/61	8.2
≥ 26	31 (3.1)	7/31	22.6
Mean ± SD	16.7 ± 3.8		
Number of pregnancy			
0	35 (3.5)	0/35	0
1–2	278 (27.9)	30/278	10.8
3–4	425 (42.5)	44/425	10.3
≥ 5	260 (26.1)	41/260	15.7
Number of children			
0	42 (4.2)	3/42	7.1
1–2	470 (47.1)	39/470	8.3
3–4	411 (41.2)	54/411	13.1
≥ 5	75 (7.5)	19/75	25.3
Education			
Illiterate	410 (41.1)	49/410	11.9
Literate	588 (58.9)	66/588	11.2
Education level ($n = 588$)			
Informal education	295 (50.2)	24/295	8.1
Primary level	98 (16.7)	7/98	7.1
Secondary level	101 (17.2)	21/101	20.8
Higher secondary level and above	94 (15.9)	14/94	14.9
Smoking			
Smoker	158 (15.8)	14/158	8.8
Non-smoker	840 (84.2)	101/840	12.0
Participant's multiple marriage/ sexual partners			
Present	70 (7.0)	5/70	7.1
Absent	928 (93.0)	110/928	11.8
Husband's multiple marriage / sexual partners			
Present	118 (11.8)	23/118	19.5
Absent	880 (88.2)	92/880	10.4
Oral contraceptives use			
Users	95 (9.5)	5/95	5.3
Non-users	903 (90.5)	110/903	12.2
Co-morbidity ($n = 148$)			
Sexually transmitted infection	143 (14.3)	19/143	13.3
Human immunodeficiency virus	5 (0.5)	3/5	60

Discussion

A well-established fact is that HR-HPV has a vital role in cervical cancer, which induces transformation of cervical epithelial cells into precancerous lesions and slowly into cancer [21]. About 84% of the cervical cancer burden is in the developing countries and especially in low resource areas. Though cervical cancer is the most

Table 2 Type-specific distribution of Human Papillomavirus (HPV) infection among women living in mid-western rural Nepal $N = 998$

Types	HPV infection		Total	Percentage
	Single	Multiple		
Overall HPV Positive	136	61	197	19.7
High-Risk HPV[a]				
16	19	48	67	6.7
18	5	7	12	1.2
31	1	5	6	0.6
33	7	19	26	2.6
35	3	0	3	0.3
39	11	37	48	4.8
45	1	0	1	0.1
51	5	9	14	1.4
52	1	3	4	0.4
53	3	5	8	0.8
56	3	5	8	0.8
58	6	22	28	2.8
59	0	0	0	0
66	0	3	3	0.3
68	3	0	3	0.3
Low-risk HPV[a]				
6	5	1	6	0.6
11	3	0	3	0.3
42	0	0	0	0
43	0	0	0	0
44	0	0	0	0
81	3	1	4	0.4
Other low-risk type	72	–	72	7.2

[a]Some women had multiple infections so the frequency of high-risk and low-risk HPV is not the sum of overall HPV positive

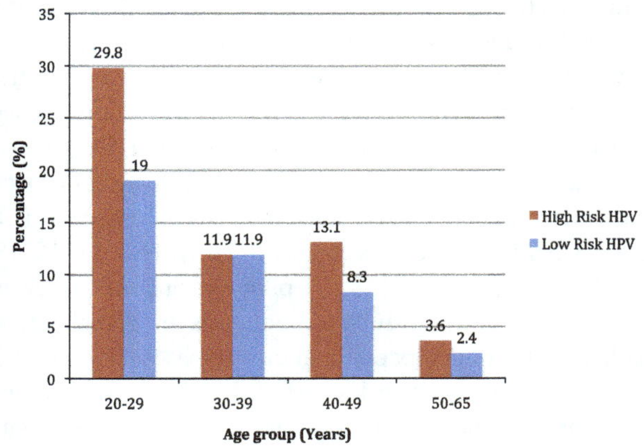

Fig. 1 Human Papillomavirus (HPV) infection according to the age group of women living in mid-western rural Nepal

common female malignancy in Nepal, a lack of proper prevention strategies exists to curb cervical cancer through screening, early treatment or vaccination. No effective screening programs have been established. However, some progress has been observed recently.

This study revealed prevalence rates of HPV infections (19.7%) and HR-HPV (11.7%). The HPV infection rate was higher in comparison to other previous studies done in Nepal which ranged from 8.6 to 14.4% [9, 11–13]. The findings of this study represent higher than the worldwide HPV prevalence of 10.4% and the corresponding estimate of 8.0% in Asia [22]. The higher incidence of HPV in Jumla may be attributed to the following risk factors: higher proportion of younger participants (age of 20–29 years participants were 40.4% of the sample), early marriage (marital age of 91% of the women was ≤20), multiple numbers of pregnancies, multiple children, risky sexual behaviors (multiple marriages, many sexual partners, higher proportion of sexually transmitted infections). Moreover, another important reason for the higher prevalence of HPV was probably due to the detection of HPV L1 gene by PGMY 09/11 primer system, which is more

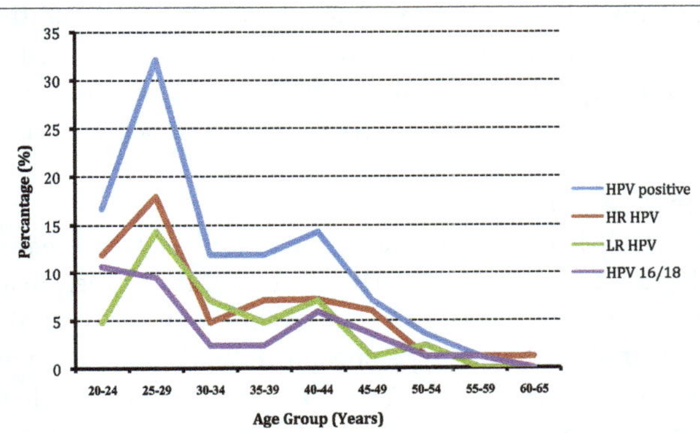

Fig. 2 Trends of Human Papillomavirus (HPV) infection according to the age group of women living in mid-western rural Nepal

Table 3 Univariate analyses of potential risk factors for high-risk Human Papillomavirus (HR-HPV) in women living in mid-western rural Nepal

Characteristics	HR-HPV		OR (95% CI)	*p*-value
	Positive	Negative		
Age				
≤ 45 years	96	803	0.50 (0.29–0.86)	0.013
≥ 46 years	19	80		
Marital age				
≤ 19 years	101	754	1.23 (0.68–2.22)	0.483
≥ 20 years	14	129		
Number of pregnancy ($n = 529$)				
≥ 4	58	392	3.74 (1.14–12.27)	0.029
0 or 1	3	76		
Number of children ($n = 630$)				
≥ 3	73	413	1.96 (1.03–3.72)	0.039
0 or 1	12	133		
Education status				
Illiterate	49	361	1.07 (0.72–1.59)	0.723
Literate	66	522		
Smoking				
Smokers	14	144	0.71 (0.39–1.27)	0.255
Non-smokers	101	739		
Participant's multiple marriage/ sexual partners				
Present	5	65	0.57 (0.22–1.45)	0.239
Absent	110	818		
Husband's multiple marriage/sexual partners				
Present	23	95	2.07 (1.25–3.43)	0.004
Absent	92	788		
Oral contraceptive use				
Users	5	90	0.40 (0.15–1.00)	0.051
Non-users	110	793		
HIV				
Present	3	2	11.82 (1.95–71.54)	0.007
Absent	112	883		
STI				
Present	19	124	1.21 (0.71–2.05)	0.476
Absent	96	759		

sensitive than GP5+/6+ or MY09/11 and able to amplify a spectrum of more than 30 genital HPV types [23]. Most of the studies conducted in China stated the prevalence of HPV was higher and varied by region ranging from 18.42 to 31.94% while in India reported a relatively lower rate (2.4 to 14%) [3, 24].

The highest prevalence of HR-HPV infection was in women of 20–29 years of age. The rate of HR-HPV

Table 4 Prevalence of high-risk Human Papillomavirus (HR-HPV) infection among women with normal and abnormal cervical cytology

Cytology result	HR-HPV		OR (95% CI)	*p*-value
	Positive	Negative		
Abnormal (*n* = 44)	12 (27.3)	32 (72.7)	3.09 (1.54–6.20)	0.001
Normal (*n* = 954)	103 (10.8)	851 (89.2)		
Total cytology (*n* = 998)	115 (11.5)	883 (88.5)		
Abnormal cytology (*n* = 44)				
LSIL (*n* = 20)	5 (25.0)	15 (75.0)		
ASC-US (*n* = 15)	2 (13.3)	13 (86.7)		
HSIL (*n* = 5)	2 (40.0)	3 (60.0)		
SCC (*n* = 4)	3 (75.0)	1 (25.0)		

infections declined with age, which is similar to a finding with a previous study [25]. In contrast to this study, a report from the rural area of China reflected HR-HPV and HPV 16/18/45 were at the peak in the age group of 55–59 years [26]. We also observed that the proportion of HR-HPV infection was higher among the women who had multiple children ($p = 0.039$) and multiple pregnancies ($p = 0.029$). Illiterate women tend to have a slightly elevated rate of HR-HPV infection compared with women who are literate, but there was no statistical significance. Previous studies have reported that high-risk sexual behavior such as multiple sexual partners is a critical factor of HPV infection in women [27], which is similar to the present study findings. Early marital age before 19 years was weakly associated with HR-HPV infection ($p = 0.483$). Though there were few cases of HIV positive participants, there was a strong association with HR-HPV infections, which was statistically significant ($p = 0.007$). The findings are similar to a previous report [28].

In Jumla, the HPV 16 is the most common genotype followed by HPV 39. HPV 18 was in 6th position in the order. The top five HR HPV genotypes in this sample were 16, 39, 58, 33 and 51. However, a study conducted by Bhusal et al. among 44 women diagnosed with invasive cervical cancer found HPV16 was the most common HR-HPV followed by HPV18 [10]. Sherpa et al. reported the most common high-risk types among women with normal cytology were HPV16, 58, 56, 18, and 52. Meanwhile, Shakya et al. reported HPV-18, 51, 59, 31 and 16 as the five most common HPV [9, 11]. So, it is clear that there are variations in the prevalence of HPV infection frequency within Nepal. Nevertheless, HPV 16 and 18 seem to be the most common. In the South Asian, HPV 16 is the most frequently detected genotype followed by HPV 58 while HPV 18 is common in Western countries. Other common HR HPV reported in the South Asian countries are 52, 18, and 31 in different orders of frequency [29, 30]. Worldwide, the most common HPV types in women are 16, 18, 31, 58, and 52, which is about 50% of all HPV infections [22].

Two types of vaccine against HPV are licensed for use in the United States by the FDA. A commonly used quadrivalent vaccine, Gardasil® covers against HPV types 6, 11, 16, and 18. A newer vaccine, Gardasil 9, was approved by the United States Food and Drug Administration (US FDA) in 2014 and protects against HPV types 6, 11, 16, 18, 31, 33, 45, 52, and 58 [31]. A pilot vaccination program was launched among 1096 school girls in Nepal giving quadrivalent human papillomavirus (types 6, 11, 16, 18) recombinant vaccine (Gardasil; Merk & Co.). A post-vaccine study reported the vaccine was safe with high acceptability in Nepali school girls but needed longer follow up to determine the long term vaccine effect [32]. Based on our findings even Gardasil 9 would cover only around 64% of women of Jumla since it does not include HPV 39, which was the second most common genotype in the present study sample. Therefore, from the 'cost and benefit' point of view, vaccination is not an ideal option in low resource countries. Thus, a simple, acceptable and sustainable screening method for cervical cancer screening provides greater efficacy.

The findings of this study suggest that abnormal cytology is strongly associated with HR-HPV infection. When the severity of disease is higher from LSIL to SCC, HR-HPV the infection rate also increased from 25 to 75%. The trend and percentage of the current findings are similar to previous studies [3, 11].

As a cross-sectional study, the prevalence of HPV infection in the rural region was obtained. Further longitudinal studies are recommended to study the relationship of the persistence HPV infection and other co-factors such as early marriage (early sexual debut), multiple pregnancies, multiple numbers of children, "chaupadi" tradition (poor harmful practice during menstruation), smoking, risky sexual behaviors and low socioeconomic status with anogenital cancers. Purposive sampling technique was used to collect a sample from the participants in a cervical cancer screening camp. Thus, the sample in this study may not be a reflection of all the Nepali women. However, the results provide valuable preliminary information on overall HPV prevalence and distribution of HR-HPV Genotype in a rural population.

Conclusions

Women living in a mid-western rural region of Nepal reflect a higher prevalence of HR-HPV infection than other areas of Nepal. This study provides preliminary information on overall HPV and type-specific HR-HPV prevalence; HR-HPV 16, 39, 58, 33, 51, and 18 are the most prevalent genotypes in this region. The data contribute to the epidemiological knowledge about HPV and type-specific HR-HPV genotypes prevalence in mid-Western Nepal.

Abbreviations

ASC-US: Atypical squamous cells of undetermined significance; HIV: Human immunodeficiency virus; HPV: Human papillomavirus; HR: High-risk; HSIL: High-grade squamous intraepithelial lesion; LR: Low-risk; LSIL: Low-grade squamous intraepithelial lesion; SCC: Squamous cell carcinoma; STD: Sexually transmitted disease

Acknowledgments

The authors acknowledge all the participants in the study. The authors would also like to acknowledge Karnali Academy of Health Sciences (KAHS) and the staff Swati Shah, Mina Rana, Satachhi Devkota, Jwala Upadhya, Nira Rai, Savina Thapa for assistance during data collection and screening. The authors are grateful to the National Natural Science Foundation of China for providing logistic support for this study.

Funding

This study was partially supported by the National Natural Science Foundation of China grant No. 81272866 (Hongbing Cai, Ph.D., Corresponding author) by providing materials and reagent. The funders had no role in the study design, data collection, and analysis, decision to publish, or preparation of the manuscript.

Authors' contributions

NT, MM, and HBC conceptualized the study. NT, MM, and NM performed the fieldwork and data collection. CH, NZ, JY, and NM were responsible for data entry. MP, MM, and NT conducted the data analysis, interpretation and manuscript writing. GS was responsible for cytology reporting. NT, CH, NZ, JY, MFX, CYG, ZYS, and NM involved in DNA extraction, PCR and HPV typing. HBC and MP critically revised the manuscript. All authors read and approved the final manuscript.

Competing interests

The authors declare that they have no competing interests.

Author details

[1]Department of Gynecological Oncology, Zhongnan Hospital of Wuhan University, Hubei Cancer Clinical Study Center, Hubei Key laboratory of Tumor Biological Behaviors, Wuhan 430071, People's Republic of China. [2]Karnali Academy of Health Sciences, Jumla, Nepal. [3]Zhongnan Hospital of Wuhan University, HOPE School of Nursing, Wuhan, Hubei, China. [4]Patan Hospital, Patan Academy of Health Sciences, Patan, Nepal. [5]Department of Clinical Laboratory Science, Zhongnan Hospital of Wuhan University, Wuhan, Hubei, China. [6]Faculty of Nursing, Chiang Mai University, Chiang Mai, Thailand.

References

1. Bruni L, Barrionuevo-Rosas L, Albero G, Serranc B, Mena M, Gómez D, Muñoz J, Bosch FX, de Sanjosé S. ICO/IARC Information Centre on HPV and Cancer (HPV Information Centre). Human Papillomavirus and Related Diseases in the World. Summary Report 27 July 2017. [cited 2017 Dec 17]. Available from: http://www.hpvcentre.net/statistics/reports/XWX.pdf.
2. Franco EL, Harper DM. Vaccination against human papillomavirus infection: a new paradigm in cervical cancer control. Vaccine. 2005;23(17-18):2388–2394. Available from: http://citeseerx.ist.psu.edu/viewdoc/download?doi=10.1.1.320.4542&rep=rep1&type=pdf.
3. Bruni L, Barrionuevo-Rosas L, Albero G, Serrano B, Mena M, Gómez D, Muñoz J, Bosch FX, de Sanjosé S. ICO/IARC Information Centre on HPV and Cancer (HPV Information Centre). Human Papillomavirus and Related Diseases in Nepal. Summary Report 27 July 2017. [cited 2017 Dec 17]. Available from: http://www.hpvcentre.net/statistics/reports/NPL.pdf.
4. Pun CB, Pradhananga KK, Siwakoti B, Subedi K, Moore MA. Malignant neoplasm burden in Nepal - Data from the seven major cancer service hospitals for 2012. Asian Pacific J Cancer Prev. 2016;16:8659–63.
5. Ferlay J, Soerjomataram I, Ervik M, Dikshit R, Eser S, Mathers C, et al. GLOBOCAN 2012: Estimated Cancer Incidence, Mortality and Prevalence Worldwide in 2012 [Internet]. GLOBOCAN 2012 v1.0. 2013 [cited 2016 Jan 10]. Available from: http://globocan.iarc.fr/Pages/fact_sheets_cancer.aspx
6. De Villiers EM, Fauquet C, Broker TR, Bernard HU, Zur Hausen H. Classification of papillomaviruses. Virology. 2004;324:17–27.
7. Bouvard V, Baan R, Straif K, Grosse Y, Secretan B, El GF, et al. A review of human carcinogens-Part B: biological agents. Lancet Oncol. 2009;10:321–2. Available from: http://linkinghub.elsevier.com/retrieve/pii/S1470204509700968
8. De Sanjose S, Quint WGV, Alemany L, Geraets DT, Klaustermeier JE, Lloveras B, et al. Human papillomavirus genotype attribution in invasive cervical cancer: a retrospective cross-sectional worldwide study. Lancet Oncol. 2010;11:1048–56.
9. Sherpa ATL, Clifford GM, Vaccarella S, Shrestha S, Nygård M, Karki BS, et al. Human papillomavirus infection in women with and without cervical cancer in Nepal. Cancer Causes Control. 2010;21:323–30. Available from: http://link.springer.com/10.1007/s10552-009-9467-z
10. Bhusal CL, Manandhar S, Singh M, Shah A, Neupane S. Evidence of HPV subtypes linked with cervical cancer in Nepal. WHO South East Asia J Public Heal. 2012;1:441–5.
11. Shakya S, Syversen U, Åsvold BO, Bofin AM, Aune G, Nordbø SA, et al. Prevalence of human papillomavirus infection among women in rural Nepal. Acta Obstet Gynecol Scand. 2017;96:29–38.
12. Johnson DC, Bhatta MP, Smith JS, Kempf MC, Broker TR, Vermund SH, et al. Assessment of high-risk human papillomavirus infections using clinician-Aand self-collected cervical sampling methods in rural women from far Western Nepal. PLoS One. 2014 [cited 2017 Jun 18];9. Available from: http://journals.plos.org/plosone/article?id=10.1371/journal.pone.0101255.
13. Bhatta MP, Johnson DC, Lama M, Aryal S, Lhaki P, Shrestha S. High-risk human papillomavirus infection and abnormal cervical cytology among Nepali and Bhutanese refugee women living in eastern Nepal. BMC Infect Dis. 2017;17(73) Available from: http://bmcinfectdis.biomedcentral.com/articles/10.1186/s12879-017-2186-2
14. Carter JR, Ding Z, Rose BR. HPV infection and cervical disease: a review. Aust. N. Z. J Obstet Gynaecol. 2011;51:103–8. Available from: https://obgyn.onlinelibrary.wiley.com/doi/abs/10.1111/j.1479-828X.2010.01269.x.
15. Tantitamit T, Termrungruanglert W, Khemapech N, Havanond P. A model approach for assessing the benefits of HPV testing against cytology in screening for cervical cancer precursors in Thailand. Asian Pacific J. Cancer Prev. 2017;18:1271–5.
16. Campos NG, Mvundura M, Jeronimo J, et al. Cost-effectiveness of HPV-based cervical cancer screening in the public health system in Nicaragua. BMJ Open. 2017;7:e015048. https://doi.org/10.1136/bmjopen-2016-015048.
17. Central Bureau of Statistics. National Population and Housing Census 2011 Central Bureau of Statistics 2012.
18. District Health Office. District Health Office Report. Jumla: District Health Office; 2011.
19. Solomon D, Davey D, Kurman R, Moriarty A, O'Connor D, Prey M, et al. The 2001 Bethesda System: Terminology for Reporting Results of Cervical Cytology. JAMA. 2002;287:2114. Available from: http://jama.jamanetwork.com/article.aspx?doi=10.1001/jama.287.16.2114
20. World_Health_Organization. Human papillomavirus laboratory manual. first. Geneva: World Health Organization; 2010.
21. Remmerbach TW, Brinckmann UG, Hemprich A, Chekol M, Kühndel K, Liebert UG. PCR detection of human papillomavirus of the mucosa: comparison between MY09/11 and GP5+/6+ primer sets. J Clin Virol. 2004;30:302–8.
22. Sanjosé S, Díaz M, Castellsagué X, Clifford G, Bruni L. Worldwide prevalence and genotype distribution of cervical HPV in women with normal cytology. Lancet Infect. 2007;7:453–9. Available from: https://www.thelancet.com/journals/laninf/article/PIIS1473-3099(07)70158-5/fulltext.
23. Coutlée F, Gravitt P, Kornegay J, Richardson H, Lapointe N, Franco E, et al. Use of PGMY primers in L1 consensus PCR improves detection of human papillomavirus DNA in genital samples use of PGMY primers in L1 consensus PCR improves detection of human papillomavirus DNA in genital samples. J Clin Microbiol. 2002;40:902–7.
24. Wang R, Lei GX, GBA W, Schuuring E, Feng WW, Yu ZZ, et al. Nationwide prevalence of human papillomavirus infection and viral genotype distribution in 37 cities in China. BMC Infect Dis. 2015;15:1–10. Available from: http://dx.doi.org/10.1186/s12879-015-0998-5
25. Hamlin-Douglas LK, Coutlée F, Roger M, Franco EL, Brassard P. Prevalence and age distribution of human papillomavirus infection in a population of

Inuit women in Nunavik, Quebec. Cancer Epidemiol Biomark Prev. 2008;17: 3141–9.

26. Kang L-N, Castle PE, Zhao F-H, Jeronimo J, Chen F, Barsil P, et al. A prospective study of age trends of high-risk human papillomavirus infection in rural China. BMC Infect Dis. 2014;14(96) Available from: http://bmcinfectdis.biomedcentral.com/articles/10.1186/1471-2334-14-96
27. Kjaer SK, Chackerian B, Van Den BAJC, Kru S, Paull G, JMM W, et al. High-Risk Human Papillomavirus Is Sexually Transmitted : Evidence from a Follow-Up Study of Virgins Starting Sexual Activity (Intercourse). Cancer Epidemiol Biomark Prev. 2001;10:101–6.
28. Camargo M, Soto-De Leon SC, Munoz M, Sanchez R, Peña-Herrera D, Pineda-Peña AC, et al. Human papillomavirus detection in women with and without human immunodeficiency virus infection in Colombia. BMC Cancer. 2014;14:1–10.
29. Bhatla N, Lal N, Bao YP, Ng T, Qiao YL. A meta-analysis of human papillomavirus type-distribution in women from South Asia: implications for vaccination. Vaccine. 2008;26:2811–7.
30. Clifford G, Smith J, Franceschi S, Plummer M, Munoz N. Human papillomavirus types in invasive cervical cancer worldwide: a meta-analysis. Br J Cancer. 2003:63–73.
31. Center for Disease Control and Prevention. HPV Vaccine Information for Clinicians; 2015. p. 1–5. Available from: https://www.cdc.gov/hpv/hcp/need-to-know.pdf. [cited 2017 Dec 23].
32. Singh Y, Shah A, Singh M, Verma S, Shrestha BM, Vaidya P, et al. Human papillomavirus vaccination in Nepal: an initial experience in Nepal. Asian Pac J Cancer Prev. 2010;11:615–7.

18

Human papillomavirus in semen and the risk for male infertility

Zhangyan Lyu[1†], Xiaoshuang Feng[1†], Ni Li[1†], Wei Zhao[2], Luopei Wei[1], Yuheng Chen[1], Wenjing Yang[1], Hongxia Ma[3,4], Bing Yao[2], Kai Zhang[5], Zhibin Hu[3,4], Hongbing Shen[3,4], Dong Hang[3*] and Min Dai[1*]

Abstract

Background: Human papillomavirus (HPV) is one of the most prevalent sexually transmitted viruses. Despite the increasing evidence of HPV prevalence in semen, the worldwide distribution of HPV types in semen and risk for male infertility remain inconclusive.

Methods: Four electronic databases were searched for English language studies conducted between January 1990 and December 2016 that reported HPV DNA prevalence in semen. Based on the PRISMA guidelines, HPV prevalence was estimated among general population and fertility clinic attendees, respectively, and heterogeneity testing was performed using Cochran's Q and I^2 statistics. The association between HPV positivity and male infertility was evaluated by a meta-analysis of case-control studies.

Results: A total of 31 eligible studies comprising 5194 males were included. The overall prevalence of HPV DNA in semen was 11.4% (95% CI = 7.8-15.0%) in general population (n = 2122) and 20.4% (95% CI = 16.2-24.6%) in fertility clinic attendees (n = 3072). High-risk type prevalence was 10.0% (95% CI = 5.9-14.0%) and 15.5% (95% CI = 11.4-19.7%), respectively. HPV16 was the most common type, with a prevalence of 4.8% (95% CI = 1.7-7.8%) in general population and 6.0% (95% CI = 3.8-8.2%) in fertility clinic attendees. A significantly increased risk of infertility was found for males with HPV positivity in semen (OR = 2.93, 95% CI = 2.03-4.24).

Conclusions: Seminal HPV infection is common worldwide, which may contribute to the risk of male infertility.

Keywords: Human papillomavirus, Semen, Prevalence, Infertility, Meta-analysis

Background

Infertility is defined as the inability of a couple to conceive after 1 year of unprotected sex. Worldwide, approximately 10% to 20% of couples at the reproductive age were affected by infertility. Among them, male factor infertility contributes to roughly 50% of cases, and the proportion is increasing rapidly [1]. Several risk factors have been proposed for male infertility, such as sexual dysfunction, varicocele, congenital dysplasia, endocrine disorders, immune factors, and sexually transmitted infections (STI) [2]. However, in approximately 50% of infertile men, the etiology remains unknown and it is termed idiopathic infertility, only showing oligospermia, asthenospermia, teratozoospermia or other sperm abnormalities.

Recent evidence suggests that HPV infection can be present in semen and is implicated in male infertility [3]. HPV is one of the most common sexually transmitted virus in both males and females worldwide. Over 170 types of HPV have been identified and among those, at least 40 types could infect the anogenital region [4]. A subset of high-risk types (HPV16, 18, etc.) have been proved to cause neoplasms at different sites, such as

* Correspondence: hangdong@njmu.edu.cn; daimin2002@hotmail.com
[†]Equal contributors
[3]Department of Epidemiology and Biostatistics, Jiangsu Key Lab of Cancer Biomarkers, Prevention and Treatment, Collaborative Innovation Center For Cancer Personalized Medicine, School of Public Health, Nanjing Medical University, Nanjing 211166, China
[1]Program Office for Cancer Screening in Urban China, National Cancer Center / Cancer Hospital, Chinese Academy of Medical Sciences and Peking Union Medical College, No.17 Panjiayuannanli, Chaoyang District, Beijing 100021, China

cervical, vulva, vagina and anus, while low-risk types (HPV6, 11, etc.) mainly result in benign papilloma or no clinical symptoms [5]. In fact, HPV is an organism with two phases, the virion and the infected cell. HPV virions, which are only assembled in non-dividing cells, can induce the infectious virion producing pathway and the clonal transforming pathway [6]. Although the clonal HPV E6/E7 transforming pathway that causes cancers has been well acknowledged, HPV virion related health consequences are greatly underestimated. Actually, HPV DNA measured in semen samples primarily originates from HPV virions and is infectious [6]. HPV virions can lie not only in the perianal region and external genitalia, including the penis foreskin, scrotum and glans penis, but also in the urethra, ductus deferens, epididymis, and testis [7].

Biological evidences indicate that HPV virions could bind two distinct equatorial regions of the sperm head and affect sperm quality, thereby increasing the risk of male infertility [8, 9]. A previous systematic review reported HPV DNA prevalence in semen varying from 0 to 100% [10]. According to a meta-analysis of seven studies focusing on populations seeking fertility evaluation or treatment, the pooled prevalence was 16% (95%CI = 10-23%) [10]. However, the worldwide distribution of seminal HPV types has not been systematically studied, and epidemiologic evidences on the association between seminal HPV infection and infertility are inconsistent. Therefore, we conducted a systematic review and meta-analysis to determine global prevalence and distribution of HPV types in semen. Moreover, we evaluated the association between seminal HPV infection and male infertility.

Methods

Literature search

Four electronic databases, including Medline, Embase, ScienceDirect and Cochrane library, were searched systematically for studies on HPV prevalence in semen, with the following MeSH terms: "Papillomaviridae", "Semen", "Spermatozoa", and "Infertility, Male", published in English during the period from January 1990 to December 2016. Relevant additional references cited in retrieved articles were also evaluated. MOOSE guidelines and the PRISMA statement were followed to conduct the search [11, 12]. The strategy used for searching PubMed is shown in the Additional file 1: Figure S1.

Eligibility criteria

Studies were included if HPV DNA prevalence in spermatozoa or whole semen of participants could be directly extracted or calculated from the original article. If data subsets were published in more than one article, only the report with the largest sample size or more detailed information was included. Studies were excluded if they were: 1) reports focusing on participants who never had intercourse, fertility clinic attendees not seeking fertility evaluation, or those with penile warts or testicular cancer; 2) case reports or reviews. The work flow is shown in the Fig. 1.

Male infertility is defined based on the following criteria: at least 1 year of unprotected sexual intercourse without conception, and/or abnormal results of semen analysis referring to the standards in the guidelines of the WHO Laboratory Manual for the Examination and Processing of Human Semen (5th edition) [13].

Study populations were separated into two groups: general population that comprised fertile men and healthy male volunteers, and fertility clinic attendees who were either confirmed infertile men or seeking ertility evaluation and assisted reproductive techniques (ART). Participants diagnosed with infertility in general population and fertile men identified in fertility clinic attendees were excluded. These two groups were created to represent low-risk and high-risk infertility populations, respectively. Only case-control studies including infertile men as cases and confirmed fertile men as controls were utilized for the meta-analysis of association between HPV positivity and male infertility.

Data extraction

The data of included articles were extracted independently by two reviewers (ZL and XF). Discrepancies were discussed and resolved by consensus (NL, DH and MD). For each study included, key extracted information included: first author, publication year, study design, population characteristics (country of region, age, sample size, general population or fertility clinic attendees), method of semen preservation (fresh or frozen), HPV detection method [polymerase chain reaction (PCR) based or not], types of primers, HPV overall and type-specific prevalence, and matching criteria if controls were present. Detailed information on all included studies is presented in Additional file 2: Table S1.

Statistical analysis

HPV prevalence was computed by dividing the number of HPV DNA positive cases by the total number of cases tested. We calculated overall and type-specific prevalence in semen, as well as corresponding two-sided 95% confidence intervals (CIs). HPV16, 18, 31, 33, 35, 39, 45, 51, 52, 56, 58, 59 and 68 were grouped as high-risk types, and HPV6, 11, 40, 42, 43, 53, 54, 56, 61, 62, 66 and 70 were grouped as low-risk types. Stratified analyses were performed with respect to potential influential parameters, and the difference in prevalence between the strata was assessed by χ^2 tests. Furthermore, the association between seminal HPV infection and male

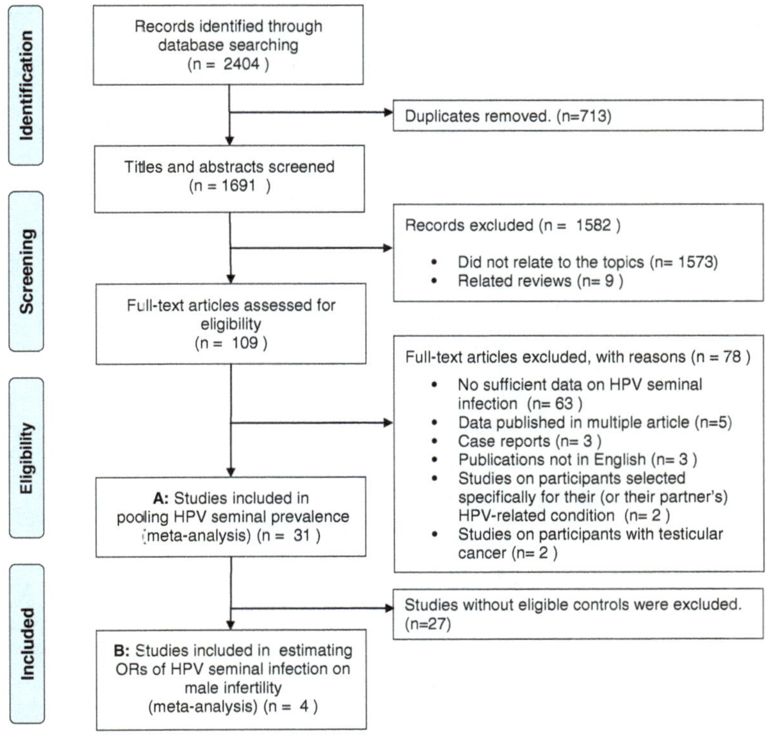

Fig. 1 Flow Diagram of the Search Strategy and Exclusion Criteria

infertility risk was estimated by odds ratio (OR) with 95% CIs in logistic regression models.

Inter-study heterogeneity was assessed with Cochran's χ^2-based Q test, and the percentage of total variation across studies was evaluated with the I^2 measure. When inter-study heterogeneity was non-significant, a fixed-effects model based on the Mantel-Haenszel method was used to pool the data; otherwise, a random-effects model based on the DerSimonian and Laird method was chosen. Sensitivity analysis was conducted to assess the influence of individual study on the strength and stability of the meta-analytic results through omitting one study at a time. Publication bias was evaluated using Egger's linear regression test [14] and Begg's rank correlation test [15]. All statistical tests were two-sided and statistical significance was defined as P value less than 0.05. Statistical analyses were performed using STATA (version 12.0) and SAS (version 9.4).

Results

Study characteristics

To estimate worldwide distribution of seminal HPV infection, a total of 31 eligible studies were identified, including 11 studies [8, 16–25] reporting HPV prevalence in general population, 16 studies [26–41] in fertility clinic attendees, and 4 studies [42–45] in both populations. In most studies, the HPV detection was based on PCR method with consensus or type-specific primers. Finally, 738 HPV DNA positive men among 5194 participants from 16 countries were pooled into the meta-analysis.

In 15 studies on the HPV prevalence of general population, 6 studies included a total of 815 confirmed fertile males and the other 9 studies included 1307 healthy male volunteers. In 20 studies on the HPV prevalence of fertility clinic attendees, 5 studies included 1002 confirmed infertile men and the other 15 studies included 2070 male partners of infertile couples who sought fertility evaluation or ART.

HPV prevalence in semen

The reported HPV DNA prevalence in semen ranged from 0.0% to 46.2% (Additional file 2: Table S1) and yielded an average of 17.1% (95% CI = 14.1-20.1%). The pooled prevalence in fertility clinic attendees (20.4%, 95% CI = 16.2-24.6%) was significantly higher than that in general population (11.4%, 95% CI = 7.8-15.0%) ($P <$ 0.001). High-risk HPV prevalence (10.0%, 95% CI = 5.9-14.0%) was similar to that of low-risk types (8.3%, 95% CI = 4.1-12.5%) in general population ($P = 0.072$). However, in fertility clinic attendees, the prevalence of high-risk HPV (15.5%, 95% CI = 11.4-19.7%) was significantly higher than that of low-risk types (10.3%, 95% CI = 6.8-13.9%) ($P < 0.001$).

A total of 24 HPV types (HPV6, 11, 16, 18, 31, 33, 35, 39, 40, 42, 45, 51, 52, 53, 54, 56, 58, 59, 61, 62, 66, 68, 70 and 81) were detected in semen samples across studies (Table 1).

Table 1 Seminal HPV prevalence by types according to population

	General Population			Fertility Clinic Attendees		
	No. of studies	No. of HPV positive	HPV DNA prevalence (%) (95%CI[a])	No. of studies	No. of HPV positive	HPV DNA prevalence (%) (95%CI[a])
Total	15	221	11.4 (7.8-15.0)	20	517	20.4 (16.2-24.6)
High-risk	10	123	10.0 (5.9-14.0)	15	314	15.5 (11.4-19.7)
Low-risk	7	97	8.3 (4.1-12.5)	10	166	10.3 (6.8-13.9)
Individual Type						
Clade 9	7	67	7.4 (3.3-11.6)	14	197	10.6 (7.3-13.9)
HPV16	7	43	4.8 (1.7-7.8)	14	122	6.0 (3.8-8.2)
HPV31	3	9	1.1 (0.0-2.5)	5	17	1.0 (0.5-1.5)
HPV33	2	5	0.8 (0.1-1.5)	4	12	0.6 (0.0-1.2)
HPV35	1	2	1.1 (0.4-2.5)	2	3	0.4 (0.0-0.8)
HPV52	2	6	1.2 (0.0-3.5)	7	27	1.2 (0.6-1.7)
HPV58	2	2	0.6 (0.0-1.6)	4	16	0.8 (0.0-2.1)
Clade 7	6	31	2.3(1.3-3.3)	8	93	4.1 (1.7-6.5)
HPV18	6	11	0.8 (0.1-1.6)	8	33	1.1 (0.1-2.1)
HPV39	1	3	0.6 (0.0-1.2)	3	9	0.5 (0.0-1.0)
HPV45	1	1	0.2 (0.0-0.6)	4	22	1.2 (0.1-2.3)
HPV59	3	7	0.9 (0.0-2.1)	4	19	1.1 (0.3-1.9)
HPV68	1	7	1.3 (0.4-2.3)	2	6	0.5 (0.1-1.0)
HPV70	1	2	0.2 (0.0-4.7)	4	4	0.2 (0.0-0.5)
Clade 10	5	18	2.6 (0.6-4.6)	10	60	2.4 (1.0-3.7)
HPV6	5	15	2.4 (0.3-4.5)	6	26	1.3 (0.3-2.3)
HPV11	2	3	0.4 (0.0-0.9)	4	29	1.9 (0.0-3.8)
HPV44	0	–	–	4	5	0.8 (0.0-1.6)
Clade 3	3	14	1.6 (0.7-2.4)	6	15	0.5 (0.1-1.0)
HPV61	2	3	1.0 (0.0-2.2)	2	2	0.3 (0.0-0.8)
HPV62	2	3	1.0 (0.0-2.2)	3	8	1.7 (0.5-2.9)
HPV81	2	8	1.0 (0.2-1.7)	3	5	0.4 (0.0-0.7)
Clade 6	6	29	2.9 (0.6-5.2)	9	61	2.8 (1.4-4.2)
HPV53	4	6	0.4 (0.0-1.0)	5	17	1.0 (0.2-1.7)
HPV56	1	8	3.8 (1.2-6.3)	4	18	1.9 (0.0-3.9)
HPV66	5	15	1.8 (0.2-3.4)	9	26	0.9 (0.5-1.4)
Clade 8	1	1	0.2 (0.0-0.6)	5	15	1.0 (0.1-1.8)
HPV40	1	1	0.2 (0.0-0.6)	3	5	0.5 (0.0-1.4)
HPV43	0	–	–	3	10	0.7 (0.0-1.9)
Clade 1						
HPV42	3	15	3.1 (0.0-7.7)	4	20	1.2 (0.5-1.9)
Clade 5						
HPV51	3	16	2.7 (0.7-4.6)	7	16	0.7 (0.2-1.3)
Clade 13						
HPV54	2	3	0.4 (0.0-0.9)	6	14	0.7 (0.1-1.3)

[a]*Abbreviations: CI* confidence interval

Two most common high-risk types in general population and fertility clinic attendees were HPV16 (4.8%, 95% CI = 1.7-7.8%; 6.0%, 95% CI = 3.8-8.2%, respectively) and HPV56 (3.8%, 95% CI = 1.2-6.3%; 1.9%, 95% CI = 0.0-3.9%, respectively). The most common low-risk type was HPV6, with the prevalence of 2.4% (95% CI = 0.3-4.5%) in general population and 1.3% (95% CI = 0.3-2.3%) in fertility clinic attendees (Table 1).

Stratified analysis

In the stratified analysis by study region, overall prevalence of HPV DNA in semen among general population was the highest in Europe (15.2%, 95% CI = 8.3-22.1%), followed by Asia (9.2%, 95% CI = 0.3-18.0%) ($P < 0.001$) and North America (4.5%, 95% CI = 2.9-6.0%) ($P < 0.001$). For fertility clinic attendees, the overall prevalence was the highest in Latin America (38.2%, 95% CI = 27.2-49.1%), followed by Ocean (29.4%, 95% CI = 7.8-51.1%) (P = 0.498), Africa (28.6%, 95% CI = 17.4-39.7%) (P = 0.234), Asia (22.0%, 95% CI = 11.4-32.5%) ($P < 0.001$), North America (19.3%, 95% CI = 0.0-49.8%) ($P < 0.001$) and Europe (17.9%, 95% CI = 13.0-22.7%) (P = 0.001).

Semen specimens were either used directly or centrifuged to collect sperms for subsequent HPV analysis. Among general population, HPV prevalence in non-centrifuged semen (12.4%, 95% CI = 6.7-18.0%) was similar to that in centrifuged semen (10.9%, 95% CI = 5.4-16.3%, P = 0.346). For fertility clinic attendees, HPV prevalence was also comparable in non-centrifuged semen (20.8%, 95% CI = 13.1-28.5%) and centrifuged semen (18.0%, 95% CI = 12.8-23.3%; P = 0.201).

As to HPV detection techniques, PCR-based methods with consensus spectrum primers or type-specific primers, and non-PCR methods including in-situ hybridization (ISH) were commonly employed. In general population, HPV prevalence was 19.0% (95% CI = 5.2-32.8%) when type-specific PCR primers were used, and it was 11.0% (95% CI = 7.3-14.7%) when consensus primers were used (P = 0.128). The analysis in fertility clinic attendees also showed relatively higher prevalence when using type-specific primers than using consensus primers (27.4%, 95% CI = 8.5-46.2%; 18.7%, 95% CI = 14.2-23.1%, respectively; P = 0.002) (Table 2).

Association between HPV positivity in semen and male infertility

To assess the association between seminal HPV infection and male infertility risk, four eligible case-control studies including 853 infertile patients and 641 fertile controls were analyzed [42–45]. According to the results of the heterogeneity test (Q = 1.63, P = 0.653, I^2 = 0.00%), the fixed-effects model was chosen to estimate the pooled OR. We found that HPV positivity was significantly associated with an increased risk of infertility (OR = 2.93, 95% CI = 2.03-4.24) (Fig. 2).

The sensitivity analysis showed that OR estimates ranged from 2.82 (95% CI: 1.93-4.12) to 3.05 (95% CI: 2.10-4.45), suggesting that no single study influenced the

Table 2 Seminal HPV prevalence by region, specimen type, and detection method

	General Population			Fertility Clinic Attendees		
	No. of studies	No. of HPV positive	HPV DNA prevalence (%) (95%CI[a])	No. of studies	No. of HPV positive	HPV DNA prevalence (%) (95%CI[a])
Region						
Europe	10	149	15.2 (8.3-22.1)	10	285	17.9 (13.0-22.7)
Asia	2	39	9.2 (0.3-18.0)	5	157	22.0 (11.4-32.5)
North America	3	33	4.5 (2.9-6.0)	2	23	19.3 (0.0-49.8)
Africa	0	–	–	1	18	28.6 (17.4-39.7)
Ocean	0	–	–	1	5	29.4 (7.8-51.1)
Latin America	0	–	–	1	29	38.2 (27.2-49.1)
Specimen type						
Non-centrifuged semen	9	133	12.4 (6.7-18.0)	7	205	20.8 (13.1-28.5)
Centrifuged semen	6	88	10.9 (5.4-16.3)	11	278	18.0 (12.8-23.3)
Unclear	0	–	–	2	34	36.4 (26.6-46.1)
Detection method						
Consensus primers	13	215	11.0 (7.3-14.7)	14	397	18.7 (14.2-23.1)
Type-specific primers	2	6	19.0 (5.2-32.8)	5	78	27.4 (8.5-46.2)
Others	0	–	–	1	42	18.6 (13.5-23.7)

[a]*Abbreviations*: *CI* confidence interval

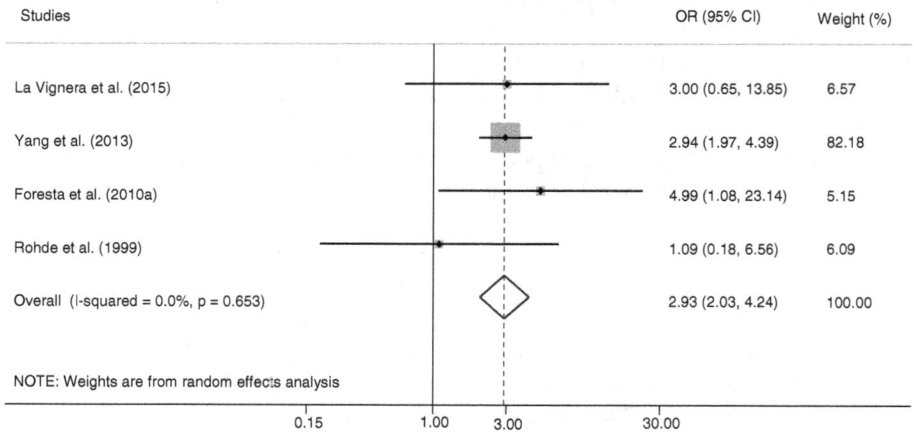

Fig. 2 Forest plots with odds ratios (ORs) of male infertility for HPV seminal infection

stability of the association (Additional file 3: Figure S2). Egger's and Begg's tests indicated no significant publication bias ($P = 0.808$ and 0.734, respectively).

Discussion

The current study provides an important overview on HPV DNA prevalence in semen and its relationship with male infertility. The results showed that the pooled HPV prevalence was significantly higher in fertility clinic attendees (20.4%, 95% CI = 16.2-24.6%) than in general population (11.4%, 95% CI = 7.8-15.0%). Moreover, a meta-analysis of case-control studies revealed a significant association between seminal HPV infection and male infertility (OR = 2.93, 95% CI = 2.03-4.24).

According to the meta-analysis by Laprise et al. in 2014, the pooled prevalence of seven studies focusing on populations seeking fertility evaluation or treatment was 16% (95% CI = 10-23%) [10],lower than 20.4% (95% CI = 16.2-24.6%) in our present study. We included six additional studies published after 2014 for fertility clinic attendees, of which four studies with relatively large sample size reported HPV prevalence higher than 16% [27, 28, 30, 42]. In addition, Laprise et al. excluded the studies that targeted less than 20 HPV types, but we made no such exclusion and analyzed type-specific HPV prevalence in semen.

In terms of HPV type distribution, mounting evidence have shown that high-risk HPV16 was predominant in male anogenital sites, prostate, bladder, and oropharynx [46, 47]. Our study indicated that HPV16 was the most common type in semen, accounting for approximately one fifth of HPV-positive samples from both general population and fertility clinic attendees. We also found that the prevalence of high-risk HPV56, which is less commonly detected in HPV-related cancers, ranked second after HPV16 in semen. In fact, clonal HPV (not infectious) is mainly responsible for cancer initiation, and infectious HPV virions could contribute to subfertility [6]. HPV virions are only assembled in non-dividing cells, and sperm and seminal plasma does not normally contain dividing cells. Thus, HPV DNA measured in semen mostly originates from virions [6]. Considering that HPV virions are mainly transmitted through sexual behaviors and HPV56 belongs to non-vaccine types, its presence in semen should be given more attention.

To the best of our knowledge, the current study was the first to examine the geographical variation of seminal HPV prevalence, showing a relatively high prevalence in fertility clinic attendees in Latin America and Africa. A previous meta-analysis of cervical HPV infection in women with normal cytology has reported a relatively high prevalence in Africa and Latin America [48]. Since HPV virions can be sexually transmitted, it is reasonable that seminal HPV prevalence exhibits a similar geographical variation to cervical HPV infection.

Type-specific PCR method was commonly used to detect HPV DNA before consensus PCR which has been widely applied since 2000. However, evidence shows that the sensitivity and specificity of consensus PCR were lower than those of type-specific PCR [49]. In addition, type-specific PCR targeting a specific region in the HPV genome (e.g. E6/E7) seems more suitable in cervical screening [50]. The present study found that seminal HPV prevalence was higher in studies using type-specific primers than in those using consensus primers. Thus, type-specific PCR may represent a better choice to detect HPV in semen, especially when HPV DNA copy number is low in semen samples.

Studies without proper control group are unable to determine the effect of HPV infection on male infertility [6]. So far, only a limited number of case-control studies have been conducted and their results are inconsistent. For example, a case-control study conducted in China showed that infertile males had significantly higher HPV prevalence in semen (17.4%) than fertile controls (6.7%) [43]; however, another study failed to confirm the association [45]. The inconsistency may be partly attributed to the relatively small sample size of individual studies. Therefore, we conducted a meta-analysis of published case-control studies to evaluate the association and its strength between HPV positivity and male infertility. Our findings suggested that men with seminal HPV infection had a two-fold increased risk of infertility compared with those without infection. To assess potential bias due to the quality of included studies, the sensitivity analysis was conducted by calculating pooled OR when omitting each one study, and the results were robust.

Several pathogenic mechanisms have been proposed to explain the effect of seminal HPV infection on male infertility. Firstly, HPV virions may lead to a significant impairment of sperm parameters (e.g. concentration, morphology, and pH), especially a reduction in sperm motility, thereby affecting male fertility [51]. Lai et al. first reported the lower performance of curvilinear velocity, straight-line velocity and mean amplitude of lateral head displacement in HPV-infected sperm [38], and the finding was confirmed in the other studies [18, 25, 43, 44]. Secondly, HPV infection is considered a risk factor for anti-sperm antibodies (ASAs) which may reduce male fertility by interfering with sperm motility and sperm-oocyte binding, and by mediating the release of cytokines that can impair sperm function. Garolla et al. demonstrated the presence of HPV DNA at sperm level is frequently associated with ASAs of IgA and IgG classes in infertile patients [52]. Thirdly, the ability of sperms to carry exogenous HPV into oocytes and viral genome into the blastocysts and its impact on fertility have been demonstrated. Lai et al. first suggested that spermatozoa can act like a vector for HPV transmission to sexual partners and to fetus through fertilized eggs [53]. The role of HPV infection in adverse pregnancy outcomes (e.g. miscarriage) has been validated by subsequent studies [3]. Finally, HPV infection might affect the integrity of sperm DNA. Connelly et al. reported that sperm cells transfected with exogenous HPV E6/E7 DNA had higher percentages of breakages characteristic of apoptosis compared to the uninfected controls [54]. However, in vivo study by Cortes et al. failed to observe the increased DNA fragmentation in semen containing HPV [55]. Future studies with large sample size and rigorous design are necessary to confirm whether HPV-positive spermatozoa are more susceptible to DNA damage.

Several limitations of the present study should be considered when interpreting the results. Firstly, though we conducted a comprehensive literature research, potential selection bias could not be completely excluded because only articles published in English were included. Secondly, it is possible that the analysis of our low-risk infertility population overestimated HPV prevalence for fertile males, and the high-risk infertility population underestimated the prevalence for infertile males, introducing a bias toward null assumption. However, the pooled prevalence in the high-risk population was still significantly higher than that in the low-risk population, supporting the role of HPV infection in male infertility. Thirdly, there was potential heterogeneity between studies different in study design, sample size, ethnicity, and number of HPV types detected. Examining possible causes of heterogeneity by the stratified analysis yielded little additional insight into sources of heterogeneity. Lastly, only four case-control studies were included to evaluate the association between seminal HPV positivity and male infertility. Additional studies with large sample size are needed to verify our current findings.

Conclusions

The current study suggests that seminal HPV infection is prevalent worldwide, which may affect male fertility. Prospective cohort studies and functional experiments are needed to increase our knowledge on the implication of HPV infection in reproductive health.

Abbreviations

ART: Assisted reproductive techniques; ASAs: Anti-sperm antibodies; CIs: Confidence intervals; HPV: Human papillomavirus; ISH: In-situ hybridization; OR: Odds ratio; PCR: Polymerase chain reaction; STI: Sexually transmitted infections

Acknowledgements

Not applicable.

Funding

This work was supported by: The National Natural Science Foundation of China [grant numbers: 81,373,079, 81,673,265 and 81,502,873]; Research Special Fund for Public Welfare Industry of Health [grant number: 201,402,003]; Natural Science Foundation of Jiangsu Province for Youth [grant number: BK20150997]; PUMC Youth Fund [grant number: 3,332,016,131]; Priority Academic Program for the Development of Jiangsu Higher Education Institutions (Public Health and Preventive Medicine); and Top-notch Academic Programs Project of Jiangsu Higher Education Institutions [grant number: PPZY2015A067].

Authors' contributions

ZL and XF drafted the manuscript. DH, MD and HS designed the study. ZL, XF and NL performed the data collection and analysis. WZ, LW, YC and WY participated in the literature search and data extraction. HM, BY, KZ and ZH contributed to result interpretation and manuscript revision. All authors have read and approved the final manuscript.

Consent for publication

Not applicable.

Competing interests

The authors declare that they have no competing interests.

Author details
[1]Program Office for Cancer Screening in Urban China, National Cancer Center / Cancer Hospital, Chinese Academy of Medical Sciences and Peking Union Medical College, No.17 Panjiayuannanli, Chaoyang District, Beijing 100021, China. [2]Reproductive Medical Center, Jinling Hospital, Nanjing 210029, China. [3]Department of Epidemiology and Biostatistics, Jiangsu Key Lab of Cancer Biomarkers, Prevention and Treatment, Collaborative Innovation Center For Cancer Personalized Medicine, School of Public Health, Nanjing Medical University, Nanjing 211166, China. [4]State Key Laboratory of Reproductive Medicine, Nanjing Medical University, Nanjing 211166, China. [5]Department of Cancer Prevention, National Cancer Center / Cancer Hospital, Chinese Academy of Medical Sciences and Peking Union Medical College, Beijing 100021, China.

References

1. Agarwal A, Mulgund A, Hamada A, Chyatte MR. A unique view on male infertility around the globe. Reprod Biol Endocrinol. 2015;13:37. doi:10.1186/s12958-015-0032-1.
2. Krausz C. Male infertility: pathogenesis and clinical diagnosis. Best Pract Res Clin Endocrinol Metab. 2011;25(2):271–85.
3. Gizzo S, Ferrari B, Noventa M, Ferrari E, Patrelli TS, Gangemi M, Nardelli GB. Male and couple fertility impairment due to HPV-DNA sperm infection: update on molecular mechanism and clinical impact–systematic review. Biomed Res Int. 2014;2014:230263.
4. de Villiers EM. Cross-roads in the classification of papillomaviruses. Virology. 2013;445(1-2):2–10.
5. Bouvard V, Baan R, Straif K, Grosse Y, Secretan B, Ghissassi FE, Benbrahim-Tallaa L, Guha N, Freeman C, Galichet L. A review of human carcinogens—part B: biological agents. Lancet Oncol. 2009;10(4):321–2.
6. Depuydt CE, Beert J, Bosmans E, Salembier G. Human Papillomavirus (HPV) virion induced cancer and subfertility, two sides of the same coin. Facts, views & vision in ObGyn. 2016;8(4):211–22.
7. Dunne EF, Nielson CM, Stone KM, Markowitz LE, Giuliano AR. Prevalence of HPV infection among men: a systematic review of the literature. J Infect Dis. 2006;194(8):1044–57.
8. Kaspersen MD, Larsen PB, Ingerslev HJ, Fedder J, Petersen GB, Bonde J, Höllsberg P. Identification of multiple HPV types on spermatozoa from human sperm donors. PLoS One. 2011;6(3) doi:10.1371/journal.pone.0018095.
9. Perez-Andino J, Buck CB, Ribbeck K. Adsorption of human papillomavirus 16 to live human sperm. PLoS One. 2009;4(6):e5847. doi:10.1371/journal.pone.0005847.
10. Laprise C, Trottier H, Monnier P, Coutlee F, Mayrand MH: Prevalence of human papillomaviruses in semen: a systematic review and meta-analysis. Human reproduction (Oxford, England) 2014, 29(4):640–651.
11. Stroup DF, Berlin JA, Morton SC, Olkin I, Williamson GD, Rennie D, Moher D, Becker BJ, Sipe TA, Thacker SB. Meta-analysis of observational studies in epidemiology: a proposal for reporting. Meta-analysis of observational studies in epidemiology (MOOSE) group. JAMA. 2000;283(15):2008–12.
12. Shamseer L, Moher D, Clarke M, Ghersi D, Liberati A, Petticrew M, Shekelle P, Stewart LA. Group P-P: preferred reporting items for systematic review and meta-analysis protocols (PRISMA-P) 2015: elaboration and explanation. BMJ (Clinical research ed). 2015;349:g7647.
13. World Health Organization (2010). WHO laboratory manual for the examination and processing of human semen Fifth edition. Cambridge, UK: Cambridge University Press. [http://www.who.int/reproductivehealth/publications/infertility/9789241547789/en/]. Accessed 4 July 2017.
14. Egger M, Davey Smith G, Schneider M, Minder C. Bias in meta-analysis detected by a simple, graphical test. BMJ (Clinical research ed). 1997; 315(7109):629–34.
15. Begg CB, Mazumdar M. Operating characteristics of a rank correlation test for publication bias. Biometrics. 1994;50(4):1088–101.
16. Luttmer R, Dijkstra MG, Snijders PJF, Jordanova ES, King AJ, Pronk DTM, Foresta C, Garolla A, Hompes PGA, Berkhof J, et al. Presence of human papillomavirus in semen of healthy men is firmly associated with HPV infections of the penile epithelium. Fertil Steril. 2015;104(4):838–844.e838. doi:10.1016/j.fertnstert.2015.06.028.
17. Kero K, Rautava J, Syrjänen K, Grenman S, Syrjänen S. Human Papillomavirus genotypes in male genitalia and their concordance among pregnant spouses participating in the Finnish family HPV study. J Sex Med. 2011;8(9): 2522–31.
18. Foresta C, Garolla A, Zuccarello D, Pizzol D, Moretti A, Barzon L, Palù G. Human papillomavirus found in sperm head of young adult males affects the progressive motility. Fertil Steril. 2010;93(3):802–6.
19. Hernandez BY, Wilkens LR, Zhu X, McDuffie K, Thompson P, Shvetsov YB, Ning L, Goodman MT. Circumcision and human papillomavirus infection in men: a site-specific comparison. J Infect Dis. 2008;197(6):787–94.
20. Giuliano AR, Nielson CM, Flores R, Dunne EF, Abrahamsen M, Papenfuss MR, Markowitz LE, Smith D, Harris RB. The optimal anatomic sites for sampling heterosexual men for human papillomavirus (HPV) detection: the HPV detection in men study. J Infect Dis. 2007;196(8):1146–52.
21. Rintala MAM, Grénman SE, Pöllänen PP, Suominen JJO, Syrjänen SM. Detection of high-risk HPV DNA in semen and its association with the quality of semen. Int J STD AIDS. 2004;15(11):740–3.
22. Rintala MA, Pollanen PP, Nikkanen VP, Grenman SE, Syrjanen SM. Human papillomavirus DNA is found in the vas deferens. J Infect Dis. 2002;185(11): 1664–7.
23. Olatunbosun O, Deneer H, Pierson R. Human papillomavirus DNA detection in sperm using polymerase chain reaction. Obstet Gynecol. 2001;97(3):357–60.
24. Inoue M, Nakazawa A, Fujita M, Tanizawa O. Human papillomavirus (HPV) type 16 in semen of partners of women with HPV infection. Lancet. 1992; 339(8801):1114–5.
25. Garolla A, Lenzi A, Palu G, Pizzol D, Bertoldo A, De Toni L, Foresta C. Human papillomavirus sperm infection and assisted reproduction: a dangerous hazard with a possible safe solution. Human reproduction (Oxford England). 2012;27(4):967–73.
26. Luttmer R, Dijkstra MG, Snijders PJ, Hompes PG, Pronk DT, Hubeek I, Berkhof J, Heideman DA, Meijer CJ. Presence of human papillomavirus in semen in relation to semen quality. Human reproduction (Oxford, England). 2016; 31(2):280–6.
27. Garolla A, Engl B, Pizzol D, Ghezzi M, Bertoldo A, Bottacin A, Noventa M, Foresta C. Spontaneous fertility and in vitro fertilization outcome: new evidence of human papillomavirus sperm infection. Fertil Steril. 2016;105(1): 65–72.e61. doi:10.1016/j.fertnstert.2015.09.018.
28. Nasseri S, Monavari SH, Keyvani H, Nikkhoo B, Vahabpour Roudsari R, Khazeni M. The prevalence of human Papilloma virus (HPV) infection in the oligospermic and azoospermic men. Med J Islam Repub Iran. 2015;29:272.
29. Golob B, Poljak M, Verdenik I, Kolbezen Simoniti M, Vrtačnik Bokal E, Zorn B. High HPV infection prevalence in men from infertile couples and lack of relationship between seminal HPV infection and sperm quality. Biomed Res Int. 2014; doi:10.1155/2014/956901.
30. Gimenes F, Medina FS, Abreu AL, Irie MM, Esquicati IB, Malagutti N, Vasconcellos VR, Discacciati MG, Bonini MG, Maria-Engler SS, et al. Sensitive simultaneous detection of seven sexually transmitted agents in semen by multiplex-PCR and of HPV by single PCR. PLoS One. 2014;9(6):e98862.
31. Schillaci R, Capra G, Bellavia C, Ruvolo G, Scazzone C, Venezia R, Perino A. Detection of oncogenic human papillomavirus genotypes on spermatozoa from male partners of infertile couples. Fertil Steril. 2013;100(5):1236–40.
32. Reich O, Auner H, Puerstner P. Should human papillomavirus testing be performed in men participating in protocols of assisted reproduction? Int J Androl. 2012;35(1):102. doi:10.1111/j.1365-2605.2011.01144.x.
33. Perino A, Giovannelli L, Schillaci R, Ruvolo G, Fiorentino FP, Alimondi P, Cefalù E, Ammatuna P. Human papillomavirus infection in couples undergoing in vitro fertilization procedures: impact on reproductive outcomes. Fertil Steril. 2011;95(5):1845–8.
34. Didelot-Rousseau MN, Diafouka F, Yayo E, Kouadio LP, Monnet D, Segondy M. HPV seminal shedding among men seeking fertility evaluation in Abidjan, Ivory Coast. J Clin Virol. 2007;39(2):153–5.
35. Bezold G, Politch JA, Kiviat NB, Kuypers JM, Wolff H, Anderson DJ. Prevalence of sexually transmissible pathogens in semen from asymptomatic male infertility patients with and without leukocytospermia. Fertil Steril. 2007;87(5):1087–97.
36. Czegledy J, Szarka K. Detection of high-risk HPV DNA in semen and its association with the quality of semen. Int J STD AIDS. 2006;17(3):211–2.
37. Tanaka H, Karube A, Kodama H, Fukuda J, Tanaka T. Mass screening for human papillomavirus type 16 infection in infertile couples. The Journal of reproductive medicine. 2000;45(11):907–11.
38. Lai YM, Soong YK, Lee JF, Yang FP, Huang HY, Pao CC. The effect of human papillomavirus infection on sperm cell motility. Fertil Steril. 1997;67(6):1152–5.

39. Kyo S, Inoue M, Koyama M, Fujita M, Tanizawa O, Hakura A. Detection of high-risk human papillomavirus in the cervix and semen of sex partners. J Infect Dis. 1994;170(3):682–5.
40. Chan PJ, BC S, Kalugdan T, Seraj IM, Tredway DR, King A. Human papillomavirus gene sequences in washed human sperm deoxyribonucleic acid. Fertil Steril. 1994;61(5):982–5.
41. Green J, Monteiro E, Bolton VN, Sanders P, Gibson PE. Detection of human papillomavirus DNA by PCR in semen from patients with and without penile warts. Genitourin Med. 1991;67(3):207–10.
42. La Vignera S, Vicari E, Condorelli RA, Franchina C, Scalia G, Morgia G, Perino A, Schillaci R, Calogero AE. Prevalence of human papilloma virus infection in patients with male accessory gland infection. Reprod BioMed Online. 2015; 30(4):385–91.
43. Yang Y, Jia CW, Ma YM, Zhou LY, Wang SY. Correlation between HPV sperm infection and male infertility. Asian journal of andrology. 2013;15(4):529–32.
44. Foresta C, Pizzol D, Moretti A, Barzon L, Palù G, Garolla A. Clinical and prognostic significance of human papillomavirus DNA in the sperm or exfoliated cells of infertile patients and subjects with risk factors. Fertil Steril. 2010;94(5):1723–7.
45. Rohde V, Erles K, Sattler HP, Derouet H, Wullich B, Schlehofer JR. Detection of adeno-associated virus in human semen: does viral infection play a role in the pathogenesis of male infertility? Fertil Steril. 1999;72(5):814–6.
46. Ndiaye C, Mena M, Alemany L, Arbyn M, Castellsague X, Laporte L, Bosch FX, de Sanjose S, Trottier H. HPV DNA, E6/E7 mRNA, and p16INK4a detection in head and neck cancers: a systematic review and meta-analysis. The Lancet Oncology. 2014;15(12):1319–31.
47. Yang L, Xie S, Feng X, Chen Y, Zheng T, Dai M, Zhou CK, Hu Z, Li N, Hang D. Worldwide prevalence of human Papillomavirus and relative risk of prostate cancer: a meta-analysis. Sci Rep. 2015;5:14667. doi:10.1038/srep14667.
48. de Sanjose S, Diaz M, Castellsague X, Clifford G, Bruni L, Munoz N, Bosch FX. Worldwide prevalence and genotype distribution of cervical human papillomavirus DNA in women with normal cytology: a meta-analysis. Lancet Infect Dis. 2007;7(7):453–9.
49. Depuydt CE, Boulet GA, Horvath CA, Benoy IH, Vereecken AJ, Bogers JJ. Comparison of MY09/11 consensus PCR and type-specific PCRs in the detection of oncogenic HPV types. J Cell Mol Med. 2007;11(4):881–91.
50. Tjalma WA, Depuydt CE. Cervical cancer screening: which HPV test should be used–L1 or E6/E7? Eur J Obstet Gynecol Reprod Biol. 2013;170(1):45–6.
51. Foresta C, Noventa M, De Toni L, Gizzo S, Garolla A. HPV-DNA sperm infection and infertility: from a systematic literature review to a possible clinical management proposal. Andrology. 2015;3(2):163–73.
52. Garolla A, Pizzol D, Bertoldo A, De Toni L, Barzon L, Foresta C. Association, prevalence, and clearance of human papillomavirus and antisperm antibodies in infected semen samples from infertile patients. Fertil Steril. 2013;99(1):125–31.
53. Lai YM, Yang FP, Pao CC. Human papillomavirus deoxyribonucleic acid and ribonucleic acid in seminal plasma and sperm cells. Fertil Steril. 1996;65(5): 1026–30.
54. Connelly DA, Chan PJ, Patton WC, King A. Human sperm deoxyribonucleic acid fragmentation by specific types of papillomavirus. Am J Obstet Gynecol. 2001;184(6):1068–70.
55. Cortes-Gutierrez EI, Davila-Rodriguez MI, Fernandez JL, de la OPLO, Garza-Flores ME, Eguren-Garza R, Gosalvez J. The presence of human papillomavirus in semen does not affect the integrity of sperm DNA. Andrologia. 2017; doi:10.1111/and.12774.

Prevalence of oncogenic human papillomavirus genotypes in patients diagnosed with anogenital malignancies in Botswana

Patricia S. Rantshabeng[1,2*], Sikhulile Moyo[1,3,4], Natasha O. Moraka[3], Andrew Ndlovu[1], Iain J. MacLeod[3,4], Simani Gaseitsiwe[3,4] and Ishmael Kasvosve[1]

Abstract

Background: Human papillomavirus (HPV) associated malignancies are the leading cause of cancer death in Botswana. We sought to determine causative HPV types in patients with anogenital malignancies in Botswana to inform vaccine strategy.

Methods: We used formalin-fixed and paraffin-embedded (FFPE) tissue blocks from patients diagnosed with anal, penile and vulvar squamous cell carcinomas between the years, 2014 and 2016. Presence of HPV 16, 18, or other high-risk (HR) types was detected using Abbott *m*2000 real-time PCR platform. Tissues with other high-risk types were subsequently analysed using a multiplex qPCR assay that includes 15 validated fluorophore probes.

Results: A total of 126 tissue specimens, comprising of 21 anal (9 males, 12 females), 31 penile and 74 vulvar were studied. Ninety-three (73.8%) patients had their HIV status documented in the records while the rest did not. Eighty-three (83) out of 93 were HIV positive, a prevalence of 89.4% (95% CI: 81–94). HPV was detected in 68/126 (54%) tissues, of which 69% (95% CI: 54–79) had HPV 16 only, 28% (95% CI: 19–40) had other hr.-HPV types and 2.9% (95% CI, 3.5–10.1) were co-infected with HPV 16 and other hr.-types. Other high-risk types detected included HPV 26, 31, 33, 35, 39, 45, 51, 52, 66 and 68. HPV 18 was not detected. Multiple-type HPV infection was detected in 44 of 47 (93.6%) HIV positive participants co-infected with HPV. In HIV-negative individuals, only HPV 16 was detected.

Conclusion: In our study, anogenital carcinomas were associated with HPV 16 and other hr.-HPV types besides HPV 16 and 18. HIV co-infected patients had multiple hr.-HPV types detected whereas in HIV-negative patients only HPV 16 was detected. Our study suggests that multivalent vaccines may be more suitable in this setting, especially for HIV-infected individuals.

Keywords: Human papillomavirus, Squamous cell carcinoma, Anogenital, Penile cancer, Anal cancer, Vulvar cancer

* Correspondence: trishrant@gmail.com; patricia.rantshabeng@mopipi.ub.bw
[1]Department of Medical Laboratory Sciences, Faculty of Health Sciences, University of Botswana, Private Bag UB072, 4775 Notwane Rd., Gaborone, Botswana
[2]Department of Pathology, Faculty of Medicine, University of Botswana, Gaborone, Botswana
Full list of author information is available at the end of the article

Background

Human papillomavirus (HPV) is a common sexually transmitted infection and is one of the major causes of infection-related cancer worldwide [1]. Globally, the prevalence of HPV infection in women with normal cytology is 11–12% and sub-Saharan Africa (SSA) has the highest prevalence rate, 24% [2]. There is regional variation in HPV-related disease burden in SSA with Eastern and Western regions of the continent having the highest burden [2]. In 2008, 12.7 million new cancer cases were reported globally and of these, 610,000 were attributable to HPV infection [3]. The incidence and mortality was significantly higher in developing countries compared to developing countries.. HPV-related disease burden is expected to rise in the next 20 years in this SSA because of the aging population and growth, which is compounded by the HIV epidemic, especially in the Southern African region [3, 4].

High-risk HPV (hr-HPV) prevalence rate remains highest in HIV-infected individuals despite the increasing coverage of combination antiretroviral therapy (cART) [4–8]. HIV infection leads to a reduction in CD4 T-cells, which are important for the resolution of HPV infection [5, 6]. HPV infection has been reported to persist longer in HIV-infected patients and this often leads to development of cancerous lesions' [9, 10]. Other studies suggest that anogenital HPV infection is associated with increased acquisition of HIV [11–16]. In a study conducted on HIV-positive patients with vulvar cancer in Botswana, oncogenic viruses were associated with vulvar cancer [17]. However, younger women with HPV infection have been found to be at a lower risk of developing vulvar cancer as HPV infection appears to be self-limiting [18].

More than 120 HPV genotypes have been identified and these are categorized as either high-risk/oncogenic or low-risk HPV types, based on their aetiological association with squamous cell carcinoma (SCC) of the cervix [19, 20]. High-risk HPVs have received the most attention in many countries in the past decade especially HPV types 16 and HPV 18. This is because many studies have found these two types to be associated with about 99.7% of cervical cancers, 91% of anal cancers and 71% of vaginal cancers especially in the developed world [21, 22]. In SSA, there is limited data on HPV-related diseases such as; vulvar, vagina, anus and penis cancer due to other hr.-HPV types besides HPV 16 and HPV 18, as compared to cervical cancer.

It is also reported that, although HPV types 16 and 18 are the most common, others hr.-HPV types such as HPV 45, 35 and 58 are being detected more frequently in SSA [2]. HPV prevalence has also been reported to be high amongst men in SSA and this could the reason for high cervical and penile cancer rates in this part of the world [23]. The low-risk HPV types are mainly associated with genital warts and oral papilloma [24].

To date, there is no known cure for HPV infection and prevention via vaccination remains the bulwark against some of the hr.-HPV types. The quadrivalent Gardasil vaccine (Merck Company, USA) protects against HPV types 6, 11, 16 and 18. However, Cervarix vaccine (GlaxoSmithKline, USA) provides cross-protection against HPV types; 26, 18, 31, 33 and 45 [25]. A new 9-valent HPV vaccine Gardasil (Merck Company, USA) that provides cross-protection against HPV types 6, 11, 16, 18, 31, 33, 45, 52, and 58 is now available [25]. The most prevalent HPV type worldwide is HPV 16 and there is less variation in the geographical distribution of HPV 16 than other types [22]. Variations in HPV types present in different regions could affect regional vaccine effectiveness.

Studies comparing invasive cervical cancers in Botswana, Kenya and United States have demonstrated differences in HPV type distribution, which may be driven by HIV infection [26, 27]. Data on the association between anogenital cancers and HPV diversity in Botswana is limited [28]. Our study sought to determine the prevalence of oncogenic HPV genotype in patients with anogenital malignancies in Botswana. Previous studies have documented HPV genotypes in cervical cancer and precursor lesions mostly amongst HIV infected individuals [26, 27, 29, 30].

The incidence of HPV-associated cancers is increasing by an estimated 3.9% per year in Botswana and this increase has been primarily associated with HIV co-infection [4]. Treatment with HAART does not seem to decrease the cancer incidence in the HIV infected population and as life expectancy improves, cancer incidence seems to be also increasing due to the aging population [4]. The importance of HPV types in the development of cancer lesions needs further investigation in Botswana in order to better understand the epidemiology of HPV infections. To our knowledge, this study is the first to report prevalence of oncogenic HPV types in anogenital cancers in Botswana.

Methods

Study design and population

This was a retrospective cross-sectional study that used residual Formalin Fixed Paraffin Embedded (FFPE) tissue material from 137 patients diagnosed with anogenital cancers who attended public health facilities for diagnostic and treatment services in the southern part of Botswana during the years, 2004 to 2006 and 2013 to 2016. Anogenital cancer diagnosis was made by the Anatomical Pathologist at the Botswana's Ministry of Health and Wellness National Health Laboratory: a reference laboratory providing pathology services to southern

Botswana. Demographic data, and clinical data on the anatomical site of the tissue sampled, HIV status, histopathology result, and year of diagnosis was obtained from the patients' pathology reports. The specimens were de-identified for the purposes of this study. The Ethical Review board of University of Botswana, and the Ministry of Health's Research and Development Committee (HRDC) approved this study. We obtained permission to access the specimens from the National Health Laboratory.

DNA extraction

Each tissue block was cooled at −3.5 °C before a 20 µm thick section were cut and processed for DNA extraction. The first 20 µm tissue section for each block was discarded to ensure consecutive cleaner sections were collected. To avoid contamination between different participants, specimens during sectioning, the microtome stage and blade were cleaned with xylene followed by absolute alcohol and DNA/RNA AWAY solution after each tissue block section.

The tissue samples were incubated overnight in 15 ml of xylene to ensure complete removal of paraffin wax from the tissue, followed by three one-hour washes in absolute alcohol to clear xylene. Gradual re-hydration of the tissue sections was done by successional one-hour incubations in 95%, 80%, and 70% alcohol.

Tissue sections were incubated in distilled water overnight before digestion. Tissue digestion was achieved by adding 600 µL of Nuclisens lysis buffer (bioMerieux SA, France) and 200 µL of proteinase-K enzyme (Thermo Fisher Scientific, USA) to the tissue section. This was mixed by vortexing, followed by pulse centrifugation and overnight incubation at 56 °C. Tissue digests were incubated at 100 °C to de-activate the Proteinase-K enzyme before centrifugation at 3, 500 rpm for 5 min. After centrifuging, 700 µL of the lysate was transferred into Abbott RealT*ime* HR HPV assay reaction vessel for DNA isolation using the *m*Sample Preparation System DNA kit on the Abbott *m*2000*sp* instrument, following the manufacturer's instructions.

HR HPV genotyping

The Abbott RealT*ime* HR HPV assay (Abbott GmbH & Co. KG, Wiesbaden, Germany) qualitatively detects DNA from 14 high-risk human papillomavirus genotypes using modified GP5+/6+ primer mix consisting of three forward primers and two reverse primers targeting the conserved L1 region of HPV and an internal control (IC) primer pair targets a human β-globin sequence. The Abbott RealT*ime* HR HPV assay provides specific probes that are differentially labelled qualitatively detect of HPV16 and HPV18, and an evaluation of the human beta-globin internal control. Probes for hr.-HPV types 31, 33, 35, 39, 45, 51, 52, 56, 56, 59, 66 and 68 are labelled with the same dye, and presence of any of these genotypes is reported as Other HR detected [31].

All tissues with other hr.-HPV types detected using the Abbott RealT*ime*, were subsequently analysed using an in-house multiplex qPCR assay. This assay uses 15 validated fluorophoreprobes in order to differentiate specific hr.-HPV types. To validate our methods and results, 26 h-HPV positive and 10 h-HPV negative known samples from previous HPV studies were included as controls from extraction to genotyping. Their previous results were confirmed by our methods. The in-house hr.-HPV testing was performed as a triplex where each well of a 96 well PCR plate contained primers and probes for two HPV types in addition to human genomic DNA control (β-globin). The real-time PCR reactions were setup in 20 µL total volumes containing 10 µL KAPA Probe Force qPCR Master Mix (KAPA Biosystems, MA, USA) and HPV primer and probe mix, as well as 10 µL of the extracted DNA template. The PCR reactions were run on the ABI 7500 Real-Time PCR System (Applied Biosystems, Foster City, CA); starting with the pre-PCR hold at 98 °C for 10 min, followed by 5 cycles at 95 °C for 10 s, 50 °C for 20 s and 72 °C for another 20 s. The last stage was 95 °C for 10 s, followed by 45 cycles in 1 min at 60 °C before holding indefinitely at 60 °C. Two or three replicates with concordant detection of the HPV types being tested were considered true positives. Results were considered valid only if the human genomic DNA control (β-globin) was positive.

Statistical analysis

Prevalence estimates were presented with 95% confidence intervals calculated using the binomial exact methods. Fisher's exact tests were used to compare prevalence by selected categorical variables such as HIV status, HPV DNA extraction and HPV type. Data was first managed using the Microsoft Excel spreadsheets and all analysis was conducted using STATA version 14.2 (College Station, TX).

Results

A total of 126/137 (92%) FFPE tissue blocks had amplifiable DNA as measured by the successful detection of the human ß-globin gene. Samples were obtained from individuals with squamous cell carcinoma, of which 21 (16.7%), 31 (24.6%) and 74 (58.7%) were from anal, penile, and vulvar biopsies, respectively. The median age was 44 years (IQR: 39, 56) (Table 1). Among the anal specimens, 9 (43%) were from males and 12(57%) were from females (Table 1). Ninety-three (73.8%) patients had their HIV status documented in the records while the rest did not. 83 out of 93 were HIV positive, a prevalence of 89.4% (95% CI: 81–94).

Table 1 Demographic and laboratory characteristics of the study population

Age (median; IQR)	44 years (39–56)
Gender	
Female, n (%)	87 (69)
Male, n (%)	39 (31)
Anatomical sites	$n = 126$
Anal, n (%)	21 (16.7)
Penile, n (%)	31 (24.6)
Vulvar, n (%)	74 (58.7)
HIV status	
HIV negative, n (%)	10 (7.9)
HIV positive, n (%)	83 (65.9)
Unknown status, n (%)	33 (26.2)

High-risk HPV was detected in 68/126 tissues, a prevalence of 54% (95% CI: 44.9–62.9), Table 2. High-risk HPV was most frequently detected in anal SCC (62%), followed by vulvar SCC (58%) and penile SCC (42%), Table 3. There was no statistically significant difference observed in hr.-HPV prevalence in the different anatomical sites ($P = 0.274$; Fisher's exact). Overall HPV 16 prevalence was 69% (95% CI: 58–80). The highest HPV 16 prevalence was observed in vulvar SCC at 81% (34/42), followed by anal SCC at 62% (8/13) and the lowest prevalence was observed in penile SCC at 39% (5/13). The presence of HPV 16 was statistically marginally associated with anatomical site ($P = 0.0160$; Table 3). Other hr.-HPV (i.e. non-HPV 16/18) types were detected in 28% of tissue samples (95% CI: 18–40) and these included HPV 26, 31, 33, 35, 39, 45, 51, 52, 66 and 68 (Fig. 1, Table 3). The highest prevalence of other hr.-HPV types was observed in penile SCC at 46% (6/13), followed by anal SCC at 39% (5/13) and the lowest in vulvar SCC at 19% (8/42). Co-infection with HPV 16 and other hr.-HPV types was only observed in patients with penile SCC (15%; 2/13).

Multiple-type hr.-HPV infection was detected in 44 of 47 (93.6%) HIV-positive participants co-infected with hr.-HPV. In HIV-negative individuals, only HPV 16 was detected. HPV 18 was not detected in this study.

Discussion

To our knowledge this is the first report on the prevalence of oncogenic HPV infection in patients with anogenital squamous cell carcinoma (SCC) in Botswana. As expected, the prevalence of HIV co-infection was high, with 89% of the patients with documented HIV status being positive for HIV. This is higher than the HIV prevalence in the general population, which is estimated to be at 24.3% in 15 to 49 years age group in Botswana. The observed high HIV and HPV co-infection in our study is consistent with findings from other studies that have reported an underlying HIV infection as a predisposing factor to acquisition and persistence of oncogenic HPV infection [11–14, 16] in both men and women [32, 33] but the risk is much higher in men having sex with men (MSM) compared to heterosexual men [12, 34, 35]. In another study, up to 60% of women with cervical cancer had HIV co-morbidity [36]. HIV co-infection significantly increases the incidence, prevalence and persistence of HPV infection, and is associated with multiple HPV types [37]. HIV immunosuppression has also been linked to multiple HPV infections [37, 38] and the inability to clear HPV infections leading to higher rates of reactivation of latent HPV infections [39]. This has been attributed to the impaired cell-mediated immunity [37, 40–42].

Although the prevalence of hr.-HPV in this study was high in this population with SCC (54%), it is lower than what has been estimated by cervical cancer studies in Botswana. This could be due to the fact that the previous studies focused on the individuals with HIV infection in Botswana. Ramogola-Masire et al., [29] reported a 93% prevalence of hr.-HPV in HIV-infected women with cervical intraepithelial neoplasia 2 and 3 (CIN 2 and 3) lesions.

MacLeod et al., [30] reported 64% hr.-HPV prevalence in HIV-infected women with similar cervical lesions, and in another study, of HIV positive women with invasive cervical cancer (ICC), the prevalence of hr.-HPV was 95% [27].

Across all anatomical sites, the most frequently observed hr.-HPV type was HPV 16 at 69% and other hr.-HPVs at 28%. This is in keeping with previous studies that have reported HPV 16 as the most commonly isolated genotype in anogenital cancers. The

Table 2 Laboratory characteristics of the study participants stratified according tumor anatomical site. Results are expressed as count and proportion ($N = 126$)

Anatomical site/ HPV	Anal			
	Males $n = 8$	Females $n = 13$	Penile $n = 31$	Vulvar $n = 74$
HPV prevalence	4/8 (50.0%)	9/13 (69.2%)	13/31 (41.9%)	42/74 (56.8%)
HIV prevalence	3/8 (37.5%)	9/13 (69.2%)	15/31 (48.4%)	56/74 (75.7%)
HPV-HIV Co-infection rates, %	2/3 (66.7%)	6/9 (66.7%)	8/15 (53.3%)	41/56 (55.4%)

Table 3 Prevalence of high risk-HPV in the study population according to anatomical sites ($N = 126$)

		Anatomical Site/HPV type				
		Anal $n = 21$	Penile $n = 31$	Vulvar $n = 74$	All sites $n = 126$	*P*-value[b]
All hr.-HPV*	HPV+	13	13	42	68	0.274
	HPV-	8	18	32	58	
	Total	21	31	74	126	
	%	61.9	41.9	56.8	54.0	
HPV 16 only	HPV 16+	8	5	34	47	
	HPV 16-	5	8	8	21	
	Total	13	13	42	68	0.016
	%	61.5	38.5	81.0	69.1	
Other hr.-HPV Only	Other hr.-HPV+	5	6	8	19	
	Other hr.-HPV-	8	7	34	49	
	Total	13	13	42	68	0.115
	%	38.5	46.2	19.0	27.9	
HPV 16 + Other hr.-HPV Co-Infection	Co-Infection	0	2	0	2	
	No Co-Infection	13	11	42	66	
	Total	13	13	42	68	0.068
	%	0	15.4	0	2.9	

*HPV 18 was not detected in this study population
[a]Fisher's exact *p*-value for comparison of proportion with hr.-HPV by anatomical site
[b]Fisher's exact *p*-value for comparison of proportion with HPV 16 only by anatomical site

prevalence of HPV 16 was much higher compared to previous studies [26, 29, 30]. Conversely, other hr.-HPV types had a lower prevalence in our study compared to the previous studies; [26, 29].

Unlike in the previous studies done on cervical cancer, [27, 29, 30], HPV 18 was not detected in our study. We also observed HPV types; 26, 31, 45, 51, 66 and 68, which have not been previously reported. Observed differences may be explained in part by the variation in anatomical sites. Statistically, there was no significant difference observed in the oncogenic HPV prevalence amongst the different anatomical sites except that of HPV 16.

A similar study conducted in Myanmar reported an overall hr.-HPV prevalence of 34% in anogenital SCC [43] whereas in our study hr.-HPV prevalence was 54%, which is much higher. The study found a prevalence of 36.1% for vulvar and 27% for penile SCC respectively [43]. In contrast to our study, Mu Mu et al., [43] found that HPV type 16 was the most commonly isolated HPV

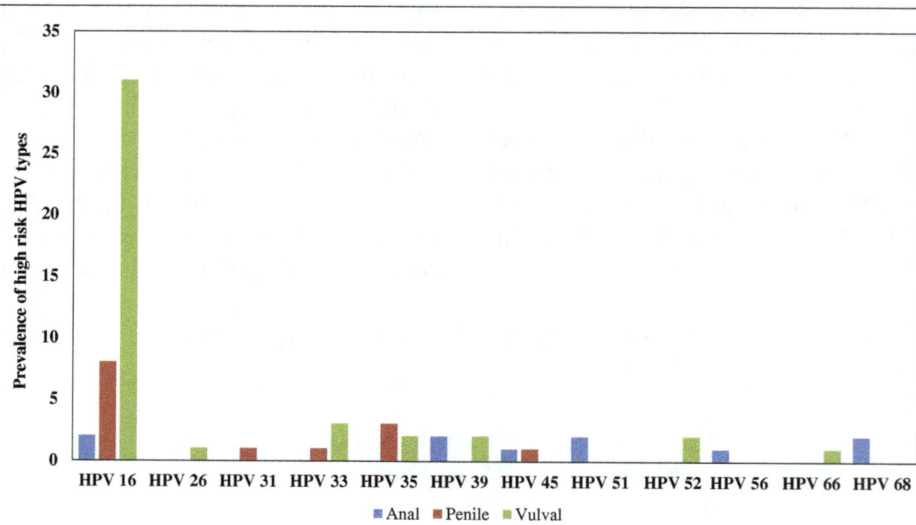

Fig. 1 Prevalence of high rsik HPV types in anogenital carcinoma by anatomical site

type in penile SCC whereas in our study other hr.-HPV types were the most common in penile SCC. HPV 18 was not detected in our study.

Prevalence of penile carcinomas carrying hr.-HPV has been reported to range from 30 to 100% [44] and this is corroborated by our findings. HPV type 16 has been shown to be involved in the pathogenesis of a subset of penile cancer [45]. This has also been reported by a study in the US that found a high prevalence of HPV 16 among participants with penile cancer [46] Another study in Uganda found that the most common oncogenic HPV genotypes were 16, 18 and 45 with a prevalence of 46% among penile cancer cases [47]. A review study of HPV prevalence in SSA also found that South African men had higher rates of HPV 16 in penile cancers [48].

A proportion of penile cancer cases have also been found to be not associated with HPV 16, as compared to anal and vulvar cancer cases [49]. This information correlates well with our study findings, as HPV 16 was not the most common HPV type isolated in penile SCC as compared to anal and vulvar SCC. The low HPV 16 prevalence in penile SCC may be due to lower numbers of penile cancers studied and may not reflect the true difference in the proportion of penile SCC attributable to hr.-HPV infection [50]. Men are also said to clear off HPV infection faster than women [51].

Women are reported to have higher anal cancer rates than men in the entire population [52, 53]. This could be the reason why there are more women participants with anal cancer in our study than males. In our study 62% of the anal cancer cases had hr.-HPV genotypes isolated and of these, only 62% had HPV type 16.

However, this information does not correlate with earlier findings by [49] who reported that about 88% of the anal, vulvar and vaginal cancers are HPV-associated and that 73% of them are attributable to HPV type 16.

HPV 16 and 18 are reported to be the most common genotypes associated with anogenital cancers worldwide. Our findings show that HPV 16 is the most common but HPV 18 is rare.

HPV 16 remains the most prevalent genotype in sub-Saharan Africa with HPV 18 showing lower prevalence than other hr.-HPVs as compared to developed countries [54]. The availability of bivalent or quadrivalent vaccines that include the low-risk HPV types 6 and 11, represent significant progress in cervical cancer prevention in HIV-negative women. However, our data supports growing epidemiological evidence to suggest that in HIV positive populations, HPV 16 is more frequent, but not predominantly seen in most HIV negative populations [40, 55]. Therefore there is merit in advancing the development and distribution of polyvalent HPV vaccines that reflects the diversity of HPV genotypes peculiar to African populations as advocated by other studies [56]. A study in France reported a potential impact of 93% by nonavalent vaccine in preventing hr.-HPV associated anal cancers [57]. A similar study in Spain also advocated for the new generation vaccine with additional of HPV types as it has potential to prevent almost 90% of hr.-HPV associated female cancers worldwide [58]. In Botswana, Emerl et al., [27] has reported a theoretical coverage of 77.8% from 61.8% by the nonavalent vaccine in cervical cancers.

In our study HPV type 16 was the most commonly isolated genotype at 59% but there were other significant hr.-HPV types, which are not covered by the HPV vaccine currently in use in Botswana. Quadrivalent Gardasil© protects against HPV 6, 11, 16 and 18 is currently in use in Botswana but it is only given to young girls aged 9–13 years [59, 60]. The second-generation HPV vaccines with expanded genotype coverage should be advocated for use in Botswana population.

Our study had limitations; we used available tissue samples in a national reference laboratory bio-repository serving southern region of Botswana population, and this may limit generalization. However, it contributes the first set data in anogenital SCC in Botswana.

HIV status was not available for a small fraction of the samples obtained and although DNA amplification rate was high 92%, using archived FFPE for genotyping requires further investigation. It is plausible that stratifying our data according to age categories could have epidemiological insights. Due to the small sample size per anatomical site, a sub-analysis according to anatomical site and age could not performed.

Conclusions

Anogenital carcinomas in our study were associated with HPV 16 and other hr.-HPV types. HIV-positive participants had multiple hr.-HPV types detected as compared to HIV-negative participants where only HPV 16 detected. Our study suggests that multivalent vaccines may be more suitable especially for HIV positive individuals. Further studies on possible other causes of anogenital SCC that is not hr.-HPV-associated should be explored, as there were some patients with hr.-HPV negative penile and vulvar SCC.

Abbreviations

cART: combination antiretroviral therapy; DNA: Deoxy-ribonucleic acid; FFPE: Formalin Fixed Paraffin Embedded; HIV: Human Immune-deficiency virus; HPV: Human papillomavirus; HRDC: Health Research and Development Council; HR-HPV: High risk-Human papillomavirus; IC: Internal control; ICC: Invasive squamous cell carcinoma; RNA: Ribonucleic acid; SCC: Squamous cell carcinoma; SSA: Sub-Saharan Africa

Acknowledgements

We would like to acknowledge the generous donation of testing reagents from Abbott Molecular South Africa. We would like to thank National Health Laboratory, Ministry of Health and Wellness, Botswana-Harvard HIV Reference Laboratory, and Pathology Department University of Botswana staff for their assistance.

Funding
The Wellcome Trust DELTAS Initiatives/Sub-Saharan Africa Network for TB/HIV Research Excellence (SANTHE) (107,752/Z/15/Z) funded the study.

Authors' contributions
Study concept and design: PSR, SM, AN and IK; Acquisition of data (sample retrieval from the bio-repository, DNA extraction, testing and database maintenance): PSR. Oversaw experimental methods and acquisition of data; PSR, NOM, SM and IK. Analysis and interpretation of results: PSR, AN, IK, NOM and SM. Drafting of the initial manuscript: PSR. Contributed to the design of the in-house method and HPV type specific probes; IM. Critical revision of the manuscript for important content: PSR, IK, SM, AN, IM, SG. Critical revision of the manuscript for important content: PSR, IK, SM, AN, IM, SG. All authors approved the manuscript before submission.

Consent for publication
Not Applicable.

Competing interests
The authors declare that they have no competing interests.

Author details
[1]Department of Medical Laboratory Sciences, Faculty of Health Sciences, University of Botswana, Private Bag UB072, 4775 Notwane Rd., Gaborone, Botswana. [2]Department of Pathology, Faculty of Medicine, University of Botswana, Gaborone, Botswana. [3]Botswana Harvard AIDS Institute Partnership, Gaborone, Botswana. [4]Harvard T. H. Chan School of Public Health, Department of Immunology and Infectious Diseases, Boston, MA, USA.

References

1. Bosch FX, Broker TR, Forman D, Moscicki A-B, Gillison ML, Doorbar J, Stern PL, Stanley M, Arbyn M, Poljak M, et al. Comprehensive Control of Human Papillomavirus Infections and Related Diseases. Vaccine. 2013;31(0 8):I1–31.
2. De Vuyst H, Alemany L, Lacey C, Chibwesha CJ, Sahasrabuddhe V, Banura C, Denny L, Parham GP. The Burden of Human Papillomavirus Infections and Related Diseases in Sub-Saharan Africa. Vaccine. 2013;31(0 5):F32–46.
3. Forman D, de Martel C, Lacey CJ, Soerjomataram I, Lortet-Tieulent J, Bruni L, Vignat J, Ferlay J, Bray F, Plummer M, et al. Global burden of human papillomavirus and related diseases. Vaccine. 2012;30(Suppl 5):F12–23.
4. Dryden-Peterson S, Medhin H, Kebabonye-Pusoentsi M, Seage GR 3rd, Suneja G, Kayembe MK, Mmalane M, Rebbeck T, Rider JR, Essex M, et al. Cancer incidence following expansion of HIV treatment in Botswana. PLoS One. 2015;10(8):e0135602.
5. Coleman N, Birley HD, Renton AM, Hanna NF, Ryait BK, Byrne M, Taylor-Robinson D, Stanley MA. Immunological events in regressing genital warts. Am J Clin Pathol. 1994;102(6):768–74.
6. Strickler HD, Burk RD, Fazzari M, Anastos K, Minkoff H, Massad LS, Hall C, Bacon M, Levine AM, Watts DH, et al. Natural history and possible reactivation of human papillomavirus in human immunodeficiency virus-positive women. J Natl Cancer Inst. 2005;97(8):577–86.
7. Stanley M. Immunobiology of HPV and HPV vaccines. Gynecol Oncol. 2008; 109(2 Suppl):S15–21.
8. Buonaguro FM. HIV/HPV coinfection: state-of-the-art. Retrovirology. 2010; 7(1):I22.
9. Moscicki AB, Ellenberg JH, Farhat S, Xu J. Persistence of human papillomavirus infection in HIV-infected and -uninfected adolescent girls: risk factors and differences, by phylogenetic type. J Infect Dis. 2004;190(1):37–45.
10. Konopnicki D, Manigart Y, Gilles C, Barlow P, de Marchin J, Feoli F, Larsimont D, Delforge M, De Wit S, Clumeck N. High-risk human papillomavirus infection in HIV-positive African women living in Europe. J Int AIDS Soc. 2013;16(1):18023.
11. Auvert B. Association of oncogenic and nononcogenic human papillomavirus with HIV incidence. J Acquir Immune Defic Syndr. 2010;53(1):111–6.
12. Averbach SH, Gravitt PE, Nowak RG, Celentano DD, Dunbar MS, Morrison CS, Grimes B, Padian NS. The association between cervical human papillomavirus infection and HIV acquisition among women in Zimbabwe. AIDS. 2010;24(7):1035–42.
13. Smith JS, Moses S, Hudgens M, Parker CB, Agot K, Maclean I, Ndinya-Achola JO, Snijders PJF, Meijer C, Bailey RC. Increased risk of HIV acquisition among Kenyan men with human papillomavirus infection. J Infect Dis. 2010;201(11): 1677–85.
14. Veldhuijzen NJ, Vyankandondera J, van de Wijgert JH. HIV acquisition is associated with prior high-risk human papillomavirus infection among high-risk women in Rwanda. AIDS. 2010;24(14):2289–92.
15. Phanuphak N. HPV and HIV coinfection. Int J Infect Dis. 2012;16:e62.
16. Phanuphak N, Teeratakulpisarn N, Pankam T, Kerr SJ, Barisri J, Deesua A, Rodbamrung P, Hongchookiat P, Chomchey N, Phanuphak P, et al. Anal human papillomavirus infection among Thai men who have sex with men with and without HIV infection: prevalence, incidence, and persistence. J Acquir Immune Defic Syndr. 2013;63(4):472–9.
17. Simbiri KO, Jha HC, Kayembe MK, Kovarik C, Robertson ES. Oncogenic viruses associated with vulva cancer in HIV-1 patients in Botswana. Infect Agent Cancer. 2014;9:28.
18. Castle PE, Stoler MH, Wright TC Jr, Sharma A, Wright TL, Behrens CM. Performance of carcinogenic human papillomavirus (HPV) testing and HPV16 or HPV18 genotyping for cervical cancer screening of women aged 25 years and older: a subanalysis of the ATHENA study. Lancet Oncol. 2011; 12(9):880–90.
19. Bosch FX, Lorincz A, Munoz N, Meijer CJ, Shah KV. The causal relation between human papillomavirus and cervical cancer. J Clin Pathol. 2002; 55(4):244–65.
20. Bernard HU. The clinical importance of the nomenclature, evolution and taxonomy of human papillomaviruses. J Clin Virol. 2005;32(Suppl 1):S1–6.
21. Ault KA, Giuliano AR, Edwards RP, Tamms G, Kim LL, Smith JF, Jansen KU, Allende M, Taddeo FJ, Skulsky D, et al. A phase I study to evaluate a human papillomavirus (HPV) type 18 L1 VLP vaccine. Vaccine. 2004; 22(23–24):3004–7.
22. Parkin DM. The global health burden of infection-associated cancers in the year 2002. Int J Cancer. 2006;118(12):3030–44.
23. Olesen TB, Munk C, Christensen J, Andersen KK, Kjaer SK. Human papillomavirus prevalence among men in sub-Saharan Africa: a systematic review and meta-analysis. Sex Transm Infect. 2014;90(6):455–62.
24. Bouvard V, Baan R, Straif K, Grosse Y, Secretan B, El Ghissassi F, Benbrahim-Tallaa L, Guha N, Freeman C, Galichet L, et al. A review of human carcinogens–part B: biological agents. Lancet Oncol. 2009;10(4):321–2.
25. Malagon T, Drolet M, Boily MC, Franco EL, Jit M, Brisson J, Brisson M. Cross-protective efficacy of two human papillomavirus vaccines: a systematic review and meta-analysis. Lancet Infect Dis. 2012;12(10):781–9.
26. Ermel A, Ramogola-Masire D, Zetola N, Tong Y, Qadadri B, Azar MM, Brown DR. Invasive cervical cancers from women living in the United States or Botswana: differences in human papillomavirus type distribution. Infect Agent Cancer. 2014;9:22.
27. Ermel A, Qadadri B, Tong Y, Orang'o O, Macharia B, Ramogola-Masire D, Zetola NM, Brown DR. Invasive cervical cancers in the United States, Botswana and Kenya: HPV type distribution and health policy implications. Infect Agent Cancer. 2016;11:56.
28. DiAngi YT, Panozzo CA, Ramogola-Masire D, Steenhoff AP, Brewer NT. A cross-sectional study of HPV vaccine acceptability in Gaborone, Botswana. PLoS One. 2011;6(10):e25481.
29. Ramogola-Masire D, McGrath CM, Barnhart KT, Friedman HM, Zetola NM. Subtype distribution of human papillomavirus in HIV-infected women with cervical intraepithelial neoplasia stages 2 and 3 in Botswana. Int J Gynecol Pathol. 2011;30(6):591–6.
30. MacLeod IJ, O'Donnell B, Moyo S, Lockman S, Shapiro RL, Kayembe M, van Widenfelt E, Makhema J, Essex M, Wester C. Prevalence of human papillomavirus genotypes and associated cervical squamous intraepithelial lesions in HIV-infected women in Botswana. J Med Virol. 2011;83(10):1689–95.
31. Poljak M, Ostrbenk A. The Abbott RealTime high risk HPV test is a clinically validated human papillomavirus assay for triage in the referral population and use in primary cervical cancer screening in women 30 years and older: a review of validation studies. Acta dermatovenerologica Alpina, Pannonica, et Adriatica. 2013;22(2):43–7.
32. Mbulawa ZZ, Marais DJ, Johnson LF, Coetzee D, Williamson AL. Impact of human immunodeficiency virus on the natural history of human papillomavirus genital infection in south African men and women. J Infect Dis. 2012;206(1):15–27.
33. Delany-Moretlwe S, Bello B, Kinross P, Oliff M, Chersich M, Kleinschmidt I, Rees H. HIV prevalence and risk in long-distance truck drivers in South

Africa: a national cross-sectional survey. Int J STD AIDS. 2014;25(6):428–38.
34. Houlihan CF, Larke NL, Watson-Jones D, KK S-MC, Shiboski S, Gravitt PE, et al. HPV infection and increased risk of HIV acquisition: a systematic review and meta-analysis. AIDS. 2012;26(17):2211–22.
35. Lissouba P, Van de Perre P, Auvert B. Association of genital human papillomavirus infection with HIV acquisition: a systematic review and meta-analysis. Sex Transm Infect. 2013;89(5):350–6.
36. Grover S, Raesima M, Bvochora-Nsingo M, Chiyapo SP, Balang D, Tapela N, Balogun O, Kayembe MK, Russell AH, Monare B, et al. Cervical cancer in Botswana: current state and future steps for screening and treatment programs. Front Oncol. 2015;5:239.
37. Levi JE, Kleter B, Quint WG, Fink MC, Canto CL, Matsubara R. High prevalence of human papillomavirus (HPV) infections and high frequency of multiple HPV genotypes in human immunodeficiency virus-infected women in Brazil. J Clin Microbiol. 2002;40(9):3341–5.
38. Menon S, van den Broeck D, Rossi R, Ogbe E, Mabeya H, Multiple HPV. Infections in female sex workers in western Kenya: implications for prophylactic vaccines within this sub population. Infect Agent Cancer. 2017;12(1):2.
39. Palefsky JM, Minkoff H, Kalish LA, Levine A, Sacks HS, Garcia P, Young M, Melnick S, Miotti P, Burk R. Cervicovaginal human papillomavirus infection in human immunodeficiency virus-1 (HIV)-positive and high-risk HIV-negative women. J Natl Cancer Inst. 1999;91(3):226–36.
40. Ahdieh L, Klein RS, Burk R, Cu-Uvin S, Schuman P, Duerr A, Safaeian M, Astemborski J, Daniel R, Shah K. Prevalence, incidence, and type-specific persistence of human papillomavirus in human immunodeficiency virus (HIV)-positive and HIV-negative women. J Infect Dis. 2001;184(6):682–90.
41. Ng'andwe C, Lowe JJ, Richards PJ, Hause L, Wood C, Angeletti PC. The distribution of sexually-transmitted human papillomaviruses in HIV positive and negative patients in Zambia, Africa. BMC Infect Dis. 2007;7:77.
42. Russomano F, Paz BR, Camargo MJ, Grinstejn BG, Friedman RK, Tristao MA, Oliveira CA. Recurrence of cervical intraepithelial neoplasia in human immunodeficiency virus-infected women treated by means of electrosurgical excision of the transformation zone (LLETZ) in Rio de Janeiro, Brazil. Sao Paulo Med J. 2013;131(6):405–10.
43. Mu Mu S, Hlaing Myat T, Khin Saw A, Aye Aye M, Mya T, Khin Shwe M, Khin Khin O, Khin Sandar A, Okada S, Kyaw Zin T. Determination of oncogenic human papillomavirus (HPV) genotypes in Anogenital cancers in Myanmar. Acta Med Okayama. 2016;70(2):103–10.
44. Rubin MA, Kleter B, Zhou M, Ayala G, Cubilla AL, Quint WG, Pirog EC. Detection and typing of human papillomavirus DNA in penile carcinoma: evidence for multiple independent pathways of penile carcinogenesis. Am J Pathol. 2001;159(4):1211–8.
45. Heideman DA, Waterboer T, Pawlita M, Delis-van Diemen P, Nindl I, Leijte JA, Bonfrer JM, Horenblas S, Meijer CJ, Snijders PJ. Human papillomavirus-16 is the predominant type etiologically involved in penile squamous cell carcinoma. J Clin Oncol. 2007;25(29):4550–6.
46. McCance DJ, Kalache A, Ashdown K, Andrade L, Menezes F, Smith P, Doll R. Human papillomavirus types 16 and 18 in carcinomas of the penis from Brazil. Int J Cancer. 1986;37(1):55–9.
47. Newton R, Bousarghin L, Ziegler J, Casabonne D, Beral V, Mbidde E, Carpenter L, Parkin DM, Wabinga H, Mbulaiteye S, et al. Human papillomaviruses and cancer in Uganda. Eur J Cancer Prev. 2004;13(2):113–8.
48. Lebelo RL, Boulet G, Nkosi CM, Bida MN, Bogers JP, Mphahlele MJ. Diversity of HPV types in cancerous and pre-cancerous penile lesions of south African men: implications for future HPV vaccination strategies. J Med Virol. 2014; 86(2):257–65.
49. Daling JR, Madeleine MM, Johnson LG, Schwartz SM, Shera KA, Wurscher MA, Carter JJ, Porter PL, Galloway DA, McDougall JK, et al. Penile cancer: importance of circumcision, human papillomavirus and smoking in in situ and invasive disease. Int J Cancer. 2005;116(4):606–16.
50. Daling JR, Sherman KJ. Relationship between human papillomavirus infection and tumours of anogenital sites other than the cervix. IARC Sci Publ. 1992;119:223–41.
51. Van Doornum GJ, Prins M, Juffermans LH, Hooykaas C, van den Hoek JA, Coutinho RA, Quint WG. Regional distribution and incidence of human papillomavirus infections among heterosexual men and women with multiple sexual partners: a prospective study. Genitourin Med. 1994;70(4): 240–6.
52. Palefsky JM, Gillison ML, Strickler HD. Chapter 16: HPV vaccines in immunocompromised women and men. Vaccine. 2006;24(Suppl 3):S3/140–6.
53. Frisch M. On the etiology of anal squamous carcinoma. Dan Med Bull. 2002; 49(3):194–209.
54. Bruni L, Diaz M, Castellsague X, Ferrer E, Bosch FX, de Sanjose S. Cervical human papillomavirus prevalence in 5 continents: meta-analysis of 1 million women with normal cytological findings. J Infect Dis. 2010;202(12):1789–99.
55. Didelot-Rousseau MN, Nagot N, Costes-Martineau V, Valles X, Ouedraogo A, Konate I, Weiss HA, Perre P, Mayaud P, Segondy M. Human papillomavirus genotype distribution and cervical squamous intraepithelial lesions among high-risk women with and without HIV-1 infection in Burkina Faso. Br J Cancer. 2006;95(3):355–62.
56. Akarolo-Anthony SN, Al-Mujtaba M, Famooto AO, Dareng EO, Olaniyan OB, Offiong R, Wheeler CM, Adebamowo CA. HIV associated high-risk HPV infection among Nigerian women. BMC Infect Dis. 2013;13:521.
57. Riethmuller D, Jacquard AC, Lacau St Guily J, Aubin F, Carcopino X, Pradat P, Dahlab A, Pretet JL. Potential impact of a nonavalent HPV vaccine on the occurrence of HPV-related diseases in France. BMC Public Health. 2015;15:453.
58. Serrano B, de Sanjose S, Tous S, Quiros B, Munoz N, Bosch X, Alemany L. Human papillomavirus genotype attribution for HPVs 6, 11, 16, 18, 31, 33, 45, 52 and 58 in female anogenital lesions. Eur J Cancer. 2015;51(13):1732–41.
59. Grover S, Raesima M, Bvochora-Nsingo M, Chiyapo SP, Balang D, Tapela N, Balogun O, Kayembe MKA, Russell AH, Monare B, et al. Cervical cancer in Botswana: current state and future steps for screening and treatment programs. Front Oncol. 2015;5:239.
60. Raesima MM, Forhan SE, Voetsch AC, Hewitt S, Hariri S, Wang SA, Pelletier AR, Letebele M, Pheto T, Ramogola-Masire D, et al. Human papillomavirus vaccination coverage among school girls in a demonstration project - Botswana, 2013. MMWR Morb Mortal Wkly Rep. 2015;64(40):1147–9.

Prevalence and genotype distribution of human papillomavirus infection among women in northeastern Guangdong Province of China

Pingsen Zhao[1,2,3,4,5*†], Sudong Liu[1,2,3,4,5†], Zhixiong Zhong[2,3,4], Jingyuan Hou[1,2,3,4,5], Lifang Lin[1,2,3,4,5], Ruiqiang Weng[1,2,3,4,5], Luxian Su[1,2,3,4,5], Nanxiang Lei[6], Tao Hou[6] and Haikun Yang[6]

Abstract

Background: Human papillomavirus (HPV) DNA testing is an important method in cervical cancer screening. However, the studies on prevalence and genotype distribution of HPV among women in northeastern Guangdong Province of China are very limited.

Methods: A total of 28,730 women attending the Department of Gynecology of Meizhou People's Hospital (Huangtang Hospital), Meizhou Hospital Affiliated to Sun Yat-sen University between January 1st, 2013 and June 1st, 2015 were enrolled in this study. HPV type-specific distribution was tested using flow-through hybridization and gene chip.

Results: The overall prevalence of HPV infection was 19.81%, among which 79.09% were infected with high-risk HPV subtypes in the subjects. The 5 most predominant genotypes were HPV16, 52, 58, 18 and 81. Most HPV infections were observed in women aged 41–50 and women aged 30–59 accounted for a proportion of over 80%.

Conclusions: Our findings suggested a high burden of HPV infection among women in northeastern Guangdong Province of China. We identified the top 5 HPV genotypes as well as the age-specific distribution of HPV infections in this area.

Keywords: Human papilloma virus (HPV), Cervical cancer, Genotypes, Infection, Southern China

Background

Human papilloma virus (HPV) is a kind of double-stranded DNA virus without enveloped icosahedral capsids. This virus infects epithelium of cutaneous or mucosal tissues [1]. HPV infection is known as the major causes of cervical cancers, some vaginal, vulvar, and penile cancers. Furthermore, recent evidence has demonstrated that HPV infection at least responsible for 25% of head and neck cancers (HNCs), among which are up to 60% of the oropharyngeal carcinoma (OPC) [2].

As the third most common type of cancers in women, cervical cancer accounts for 9% of the total new diagnosed cancer cases and 8% of the total cancer deaths among females respectively. Notedly, more than 85% of these new cases and deaths occurred in developing countries [3]. Incidence of cervical cancer of females in China is estimated to be about 8.7–11.3/100,000 and the mortality of women with cervical cancer is up to 45.0% [4–6]. It has been established that most cervical cancers are caused by HPV infections [7]. HPV infections are so common that approximately 75% to 80% of sexually active individuals would be infected in their lifetime [8]. The highest prevalence was observed in women under age 25 [9]. The HPV infection rate and HPV genotypes

* Correspondence: zhaopingsen01@163.com; zhaopingsen@hotmail.com
†Equal contributors
[1]Clinical Core Laboratory, Meizhou People's Hospital (Huangtang Hospital), Meizhou Hospital Affiliated to Sun Yat-sen University, Meizhou 514031, People's Republic of China
[2]Center for Precision Medicine, Meizhou People's Hospital (Huangtang Hospital), Meizhou Hospital Affiliated to Sun Yat-sen University, Meizhou 514031, People's Republic of China
Full list of author information is available at the end of the article

are varied among different countries [10], and even varied in different regions of one countries [11]. It is reported that the global prevalence of HPV infection in women without cervical abnormalities is 11% to 12%, while in Asia as whole and China, this data goes to 8% and 11.4%–20.3%, respectively [10, 12]. This highlights that China is a country with a high burden of HPV infections. As the most important province in southern China, Guangdong has a high HPV burden as its infection rate of high-risk HPV reaches to about 21.07% [4].

Liquid-based cytology is still the most common screening test for HPV infection. Concerns about cytology test lie in its subjective and significant interlaboratory variation, as well insufficient sensitivity and high false-negative [7, 13]. Currently more and more molecular testing methods have been applied to HPV detection in cervical specimen, with the advantage of higher sensitivity and capable of HPV genotyping [14]. Genotyping has an important role in triaging patients for colposcopy in women who are high-risk HPV positive but have normal cytology [7].

Until now more than 200 HPV genotypes have been identified with more than 2% different homology between each two types [7]. HPVs are commonly divided into high-risk or low-risk based on their capacity to drive the development of cancer. There are at less 12 HPV subtypes, i.e. HPV16, HPV18, HPV31, HPV33, HPV35, HPV39, HPV45, HPV51, HPV52, HPV56, HPV58, and HPV59, that are evidently considered as high-risk and one less evident high-risk is HPV68 [7]. These 13 HPV subtypes have been proved to cause more than 96% cervical cancers [15]. Additionally, another 12 HPV subtypes that have been associated with rare cases of cervical cancer are also defined as high-risk [16]. Low-risk genotypes infection, such as HPV6 and HPV11, cause benign or low-grade changes in cervical cells of genital warts [17]. The process from HPV infections to development of cervical cancer usually takes a long period and only the continued infection of high-risk HPV might result in cervical cancer as well as high-risk HPV raise different risk to cervical cancer [18]. This highlights the importance of HPV genotyping in early detection, treatment as well as prognosis of cervical cancer.

It was shown that a HPV vaccine provides potent protections against HPV infection [19]. To date, there are four prophylactic vaccines targeting various high-risk HPV types, including monovalent vaccine (HPV16), the bivalent vaccine (HPV 16/18), the quadrivalent vaccine (HPV16/18/6/11) and the nonavalent vaccine (HPV 16/18/6/11/31/33/45/52/58) [20]. Therefore, detection and genotyping of HPV is of high importance since it provides valuable information for proper HPV vaccine development.

In the present study, we detected and genotyped HPV infection among women attending Department of Gynecology of Meizhou People's Hospital (Huangtang Hospital), Meizhou Hospital Affiliated to Sun Yat-sen University during 2013–2015. Our study aimed to assess the prevalence of HPV infection and identify the predominant HPV genotypes in women in northeastern Guangdong Province of China.

Methods

Study subjects

Twenty-eight thousand seven hundred thirty women attending Department of Gynecology of Meizhou People's Hospital (Huangtang Hospital),Meizhou Hospital Affiliated to Sun Yat-sen University between January 1st, 2013 and June 1st, 2015 were enrolled in our study. All of the participants enrolled in this study came from the eight counties of Meizhou city, which is located in the northeastern Guangdong Province of China. Patients were enrolled according to the including criteria: (i) aged 15–89; (ii) didn't have HPV screen before; (iii) provided enough cervical specimen for HPV DNA testing. This study was approved by the Human Ethics Committees of Meizhou People's Hospital (Huangtang Hospital), Meizhou Hospital Affiliated to Sun Yat-sen University, Guangdong Province, China. All patients provided written informed consent to participate. For the sake of privacy, data were de-identified before analysis.

Specimen collection and storage

Cervical specimens were collected by a gynecological practitioner using plastic cervical brushes. All cervical brushes and store bottles with specimen transport medium were from the manufacturer (Hybrobio Biotechnology Corp., Chaozhou, Guangdong, China). In brief, specimen was obtained by inserting the cytobrush into the endocervical canal and rotating four times in a clockwise direction to collect the cervical epithelial cells which adhered to the flat sides of the bristles. The tip of brush was then placed into a vial containing transport medium and stored at 4 °C.

DNA extraction

DNA from exfoliated cervical cells collected in transport medium was extracted using DNA extraction kit (Hybrobio Biotechnology Corp., Chaozhou, Guangdong, China). Briefly, specimen was added with proteinase K and BL buffer for digestion, followed by ethanol precipitation and column collection. Nanodrop 2000 (Thermo-Fisher Scientific, CA, USA) was used to determine the concentration and purification of DNA productions.

Detection and genotyping of HPV

HPV DNA amplification and genotyping were performed using HPV genotyping Kit (Hybrobio Biotechnology Corp., Chaozhou, Guangdong, China) according to the manufacturer's instructions. Amplification of

HPV-DNA was done with the L1 consensus HPV PGMY09/PGMY11 primer set. In brief, the amplification system was consisting of 1 μl HPV-DNA and 24 μl reaction system (Hybribio Biotechnology PCR Kit, Chaozhou, Guangdong, China). HPV was amplified using Roche LightCycler 480 instrument (Roche, USA) following a specific program provided by manufacturer. HPV genotyping was done by flow-through hybridization and gene-chip which contained type-specific oligonucleotides (Hybribio Biotechnology Corp., Chaozhou, Guangdong, China). The gene-chip includes 21 type-specific oligonucleotides designed to detect 15 high-risk(HR) HPV genotypes (HR: 16, 18, 31, 33, 35, 39, 45, 51, 52, 53, 56, 58, 59, 66 and 68) together with 6 low-risk(LR) HPV genotypes (LR: 6, 11, 42, 43, 44 and 81) The final results were determined by colorimetric change on the chip under direct visualization. Quality controls were performed throughout the experiments, including DNA extracting, amplification and hybridization by applying positive and negative controls for PCR reaction.

Data analysis

Proportion of women in different age groups in each year was presented. Single, double and multiple HPV infection was defined as infected by one, two or more than two subtypes of HPV infections. Type-specific HPV positivity and corresponding 95% confidence interval (CI) was calculated. Descriptive and inferential statistical analysis of the data was done using Statistical Package for the Social Sciences version 22 (SPSS Inc., Illinios, USA). Data were compared by Pearson χ^2 or Fisher exact tests as appropriate. $P < 0.05$ was considered to be statistically significant.

Results

Participants and prevalence of HPV infection

As shown in Fig. 1, between January 1st, 2013 and June 1st, 2015, there were 30,039 women attending Department of Gynecology of Meizhou People's Hospital (Huangtang Hospital), Meizhou Hospital Affiliated to Sun Yat-sen University that accepted HPV DNA testing. One thousand three hundred nine women were excluded from our study because they were either under the age of 15 or without age information. Finally, this study included 28,730 participants for analysis.

A total of 5690 (19.81%) women were infected with HPV in this period. 4500 (15.66%) women had HR infection and 678 (2.36%) women have LR infection and 512 (1.78%) women had both HR and LR HPV infection. Meanwhile, double and multiple HPV infections were observed with infection rates of 3.84% and 0.66%, respectively (Table 1).

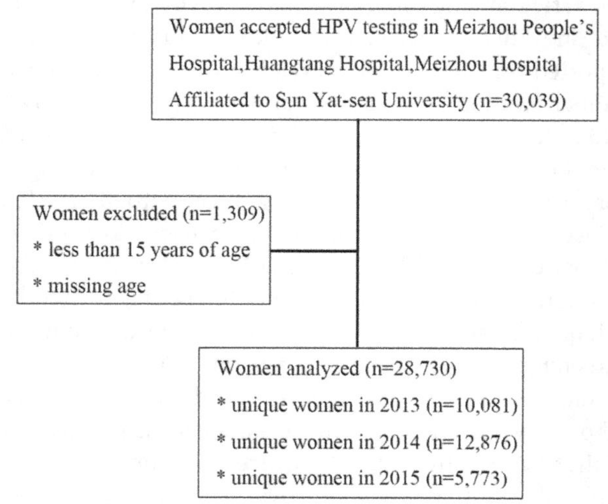

Fig. 1 Flow chart of study subject inclusion and exclusion

HPV genotype distribution

Twenty-one different HPV subtypes were identified in this study. HPV16,52 and 58 were the three most predominant subtypes, with proportions of 27.81%, 14.60% and 10.58%, respectively. Other genotypes that ranked top ten were HPV18, 81, 53, 33, 31, 51 and 39, with corresponding proportions of 6.01%, 5.45%, 5.10%, 4.94%, 3.80%, 3.69% and 3.28% (Table 2). To be noted, HPV81 is the only LR subtype that has a relative high infection rate in women. Double or multiple HPV infections were common, especially among the HR subtypes like HPV16, 18 and 33.

It was shown in Table 3 the HPV type-specific positivity in each year from 2013 to 2015. It is obviously that there is an increasing trend of HPV positivity, as well as HR and LR HPV infections during this period.

HPV positivity and age

Here we identified the age distribution of HPV infection in a population in northeastern Guangdong Province of China. As shown in Table 4, most HPV infections occurred in women with the age groups of 40–49, 30–39 and 50–59, which in total account for over 80% of the positivity. Besides, the young women aged 20–29 also

Table 1 Prevalence of HPV infection in study participants in northeastern Guangdong Province of China

	Single	Double	Multiple	Total
Negative	–	–	–	23,040 (80.19%)
Positive	4396 (15.30%)	1104 (3.84%)	190 (0.66%)	5690 (19.81%)
HR only	3747 (13.04%)	621 (2.16%)	132 (0.46%)	4500 (15.66%)
LR only	649 (2.26%)	27 (0.09%)	2 (0.00%)	678 (2.36%)
HR&LR	–	456 (1.59%)	56 (0.20%)	512 (1.78%)

HR:high-risk; LR:low-risk

Table 2 Genotypes of the HPV infection in study participants in northeastern Guangdong Province of China

HPV Type	Single	Double	Multiple	Total
6	136 (2.63%)	11 (0.21%)	1 (0.02%)	148 (2.86%)
11	136 (2.63%)	4 (0.08%)	1 (0.02%)	141 (2.72%)
16	1121 (21.65%)	245 (4.73%)	74 (1.43%)	1440 (27.81%)
18	237 (4.58%)	60 (1.16%)	14 (0.27%)	311 (6.01%)
31	143 (2.76%)	48 (0.93%)	6 (0.12%)	197 (3.80%)
33	201 (3.88%)	42 (0.81%)	13 (0.25%)	256 (4.94%)
35	23 (0.44%)	7 (0.14%)	2 (0.04%)	32 (0.62%)
39	136 (2.63%)	28 (0.54%)	6 (0.12%)	170 (3.28%)
42	23 (0.44%)	3 (0.06%)	0	26 (0.5%)
43	7 (0.14%)	2 (0.04%)	0	9 (0.17%)
44	66 (1.27%)	6 (0.12%)	1 (0.02%)	73 (1.41%)
45	34 (0.66%)	5 (0.10%)	2 (0.04%)	41 (0.79%)
51	145 (2.80%)	40 (0.77%)	6 (0.12%)	191 (3.69%)
52	662 (12.78%)	90 (1.74%)	4 (0.08%)	756 (14.60%)
53	237 (4.58%)	26 (0.50%)	1 (0.02%)	264 (5.10%)
56	47 (0.91%)	8 (0.15%)	1 (0.02%)	56 (1.08%)
58	534 (10.31%)	12 (0.23%)	2 (0.04%)	548 (10.58%)
59	37 (0.71%)	1 (0.02%)	0	38 (0.73%)
66	89 (1.72%)	5 (0.10%)	0	94 (1.82%)
68	141 (2.72%)	4 (0.08%)	1 (0.02%)	146 (2.82%)
cp8304	281 (5.43%)	1 (0.02%)	0	282 (5.45%)

emerged as a main population that threatened by HPV prevalence of 12.1%.

On the other hand, the positivity of HPV types varied in different age groups. As shown in Fig. 2, U-shaped curves were seemed in HPV prevalence that correlated with age group. The positive of combined HPV infection peaked among women aged 15–19 years, then decreased with age, stabilized among women aged 25–49, and then surged again among women aged 50 years and older.

Discussion

The present study investigated the prevalence of HPV infection and genotypes of HPV in women attending Department of Gynecology of Meizhou People's Hospital (Huangtang Hospital), Meizhou Hospital Affiliated to Sun Yat-sen University from January 1st, 2013 to June 1st, 2015. To our knowledge, this is the first large-scale study on prevalence and genotype distribution of HPV participants in northeastern Guangdong Province of China.

Type-specific persistent infection, such as HPV16 and 18, has been recognized as a major risk factor for cervical cancer [21]. Cervical cancer is the third common cancer in women worldwide and cause most deaths in developing countries [3]. It was reported previously that cervical cancer was the second leading cause of cancer mortalities among 15- to 44-year-old females in China [22]. In the present study, our data shows that more than 80% HPV infections occurred in women aged 20- to 59-years. This highlights the emergent necessity for these women to be protected from HPV infections. Recent years a predominant reduction of cervical cancer has been achieved in developed countries with the application of effective cervical screening programs [23, 24]. Molecular testing of hrHPV in cervical specimen have served as a complement approach for the early diagnosis of cervical cancer with the advantages of higher sensitivity and specificity [23]. It has been reported that several European countries would carry on hrHPV testing as the primary screen for cervical cancer in view of clinical trials [25].

In addition to HPV screening, HPV vaccination has been shown to be an effective strategy against HPV infection and has been recently implemented in most western countries [20]. To date, there are four HPV vaccines available to protect against HPV, including monovalent vaccine (HPV16), bivalent vaccine (HPV16/18), quadrivalent vaccine (HPV16/18/6/11) [26] and nonavalent vaccine (HPV16/18/6/11/31/33/45/52/58) [27]. Although bivalent vaccine (HPV16/18) and quadrivalent vaccine (HPV6/11/16/18) protect against infection by HPV16 and HPV18, they have little effect on other hrHPVs found in at least 25% of cervical cancers [28].

Our study revealed a 19.81% prevalence of cervical HPV infection among women who presented for cervical cancer screening in Meizhou City of southern China. Wang et al. have studied the nationwide HPV prevalence and HPV genotype distribution in China and found that total hrHPV infection rate in Guangdong Province was 21.07% [4]. However, even in Guangdong Province, the prevalence of HPV infection varied greatly in different cities. The available data showed that the prevalence of HPV infection in Guangzhou, Shenzhen and Chaozhou was 10% [29], 18.4% [30] and 12.6% [31], respectively. Meanwhile, a latest study reported that the HPV prevalence in Hakka women in Heyuan City which is not far away from Meizhou is 12.27% [32]. Several risk factors contribute to the prevalence of HPV, like genetic variation, sexual behavior and biological predisposition [33]. A limitation of our study is that the samples were collected from women attending gynecological department of the hospital. Thus, the rate of HPV positivity might be higher than those in general population. Therefore, our findings might overestimate the prevalence of HPV infection in general population in northeastern region of Guangdong Province in China. Meanwhile, of the 21 HPV types we detected, HPV 16, 52 and 58 were observed to be the most predominant high-risk types among women in this area, which totally accounted for over a half

Table 3 Positivity of HPV infection in study participants in northeastern Guangdong Province of China

HPV type	2013(*N* = 10,081)		2014(*N* = 12,876)		2015(*N* = 5773)		*P*
	n	%(95%CI)	n	%(95%CI)	n	%(95%CI)	
6	38	0.38 (0.26–0.50)	57	0.44 (0.33–0.56)	54	0.94 (0.69–1.18)	< 0.001
11	45	0.45 (0.32–0.58)	65	0.50 (0.38–0.63)	38	0.66 (0.45–0.87)	0.085
16	401	3.98 (3.60–4.36)	626	4.86 (4.49–5.23)	404	7.00 (6.34–7.66)	< 0.001
18	91	0.90 (0.72–1.09)	136	1.06 (0.88–1.23)	113	1.96 (1.60–2.31)	< 0.001
31	54	0.54 (0.39–0.68)	93	0.72 (0.58–0.87)	80	1.39 (1.08–1.69)	< 0.001
33	94	0.93 (0.74–1.12)	132	1.03 (0.85–1.20)	89	1.54 (1.22–1.86)	0.001
35	6	0.06 (0.01–0.11)	13	0.10 (0.05–0.16)	20	0.35 (0.16–0.50)	< 0.001
39	41	0.41 (0.28–0.53)	115	0.89 (0.73–1.06)	69	1.20 (0.91–1.48)	< 0.001
42	4	0.04 (0.00–0.08)	7	0.05 (0.01–0.09)	18	0.31 (0.17–0.46)	< 0.001
43	0	0.00	3	0.02 (0.00–0.05)	7	0.12 (0.03–0.21)	< 0.001
44	15	0.15 (0.07–0.22)	32	0.25 (0.16–0.33)	29	0.50 (0.32–0.68)	< 0.001
45	22	0.22 (0.13–0.31)	25	0.19 (0.12–0.27)	10	0.17 (0.07–0.28)	0.529
51	10	0.10 (0.04–0.16)	104	0.81 (0.65–0.96)	131	2.27 (1.89–2.65)	< 0.001
52	254	2.52 (2.21–2.83)	388	3.01 (2.72–3.31)	248	4.30 (3.77–4.82)	< 0.001
53	99	0.98 (0.79–1.17)	165	1.28 (1.09–1.48)	103	1.78 (1.44–2.13)	< 0.001
56	14	0.14 (0.07–0.21)	42	0.33 (0.23–0.42)	27	0.47 (0.29–0.64)	< 0.001
58	214	2.12 (1.84–2.40)	359	2.79 (2.50–3.07)	200	3.46 (2.99–3.94)	< 0.001
59	18	0.18 (0.10–0.26)	29	0.23 (0.14–0.31)	18	0.31 (0.17–0.46)	0.096
66	31	0.31 (0.20–0.42)	54	0.42 (0.31–0.53)	59	1.02 (0.76–1.28)	< 0.001
68	89	0.88 (0.70–1.07)	87	0.68 (0.53–0.82)	39	0.68 (0.46–0.89)	0.095
cp8304	76	0.75 (0.59–0.92)	117	0.91 (0.74–1.07)	103	1.78 (1.44–2.12)	< 0.001
6/11	83	0.82 (0.65–1.00)	120	0.93 (0.77–1.10)	89	1.54 (1.22–1.86)	< 0.001
16/18	484	4.80 (4.38–5.22)	755	5.86 (5.46–6.27)	510	8.83 (8.10–9.57)	< 0.001
4vHPV	567	5.625.17–6.07)	875	6.80 (6.36–7.23)	599	10.38 (9.59–11.16)	< 0.001
9vHPV	1123	11.14 (10.53–11.75)	1706	13.25 (12.66–13.84)	1080	18.71 (17.70–19.71)	< 0.001
HR HPV	1106	10.97 (10.36–11.58)	1651	12.82 (12.24–13.40)	964	16.70 (15.74–17.66)	< 0.001
LR HPV	169	1.68 (1.43–1.93)	267	2.07 (1.83–2.32)	216	3.74 (3.25–4.23)	< 0.001
ANY HPV	1433	14.21 (13.54–14.90)	2248	17.46 (16.80–18.11)	1499	25.97 (24.83–27.10)	< 0.001

4vHPV: 4-valent HPV types including HPV 6, 11, 16, and 18; 9vHPV: 9-valent HPV types including HPV 6, 11, 16, 18, 31, 33, 45, 52, and 58; HR HPV: high risk HPV types including HPV 16, 18, 31, 33, 35, 39, 45, 51, 52, 53, 56, 58, 59, 66, 68, and cp8304; LR HPV: low risk HPV types including HPV 6, 11, 42, 43, and 44. Any HPV: any of the 21 HPV types mentioned above

Table 4 Age distribution in study participants in northeastern Guangdong Province of China

Age (year)	2013(N = 10,081)		2014(N = 12,876)		2015(N = 5773)		HPV positivity(*N* = 5180)	
	n	%	n	%	n	%	n	%(95%CI)
15–19	21	0.21	37	0.29	30	0.51	24	0.46 (0.28–0.64)
20–29	1015	10.07	1226	9.52	587	10.17	627	12.10 (11.21–12.99)
30–39	2801	27.79	3407	26.46	1500	25.98	1187	22.92 (21.78–24.06)
40–49	4456	44.20	5758	44.72	2578	44.65	2085	40.25 (38.91–41.59)
50–59	1366	13.55	1867	14.50	817	14.15	906	17.49 (16.46–18.52)
60–69	302	3.00	443	3.44	194	3.35	260	5.02 (4.43–5.61)
70–79	101	1.00	120	0.93	50	0.86	78	1.51 (1.18–1.84)
80–89	18	0.18	21	0.16	18	0.32	13	0.25 (0.11–0.39)

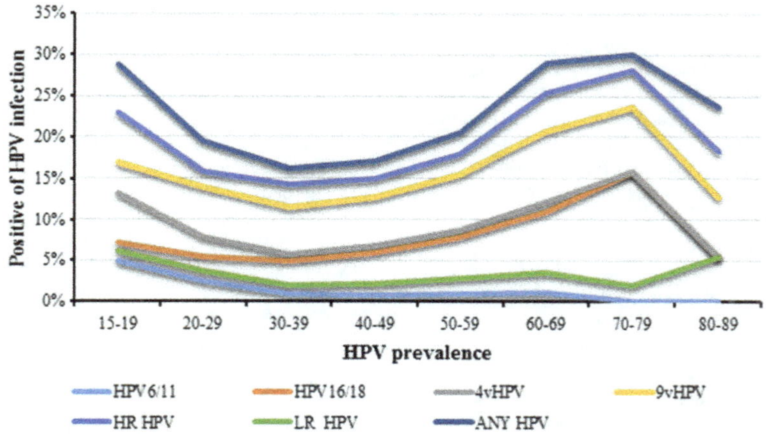

Fig. 2 Positivity of type-specific cervical HPV infection in study participants in northeastern Guangdong Province of China. By age group 4vHPV: 4-valent HPV types including HPV 6, 11, 16, and 18; 9vHPV: 9-valent HPV types including HPV 6, 11, 16, 18, 31, 33, 45, 52, and 58; HR HPV: high risk HPV types including HPV 16, 18, 31, 33, 35, 39, 45, 51, 52, 53, 56, 58, 59, 66 and 68; LR HPV: low risk HPV types including HPV 6,11, 42, 43, 44 and 81. Any HPV: any of the 21 HPV types mentioned above

of the HPV infections. This is consistent with the studies generated by some Chinese population-specific investigations [4, 34]. These findings suggested that in addition to HPV16 and HPV18, HPV vaccines against HPV52 and HPV58 would be valuable for population in northeastern Guangdong Province of China.

Meta-analysis showed that global HPV prevalence was higher in the younger and older women [7]. Also, previous studies showed that HPV prevalence in cities of China like Kunming, Hongkong and Heyuan presented the similar pattern. In the present study, we observed peaks of prevalence in subjects aged 15–19 or 60–79 years and steady decrease in mid-aged women. The exact mechanism underlying the relation between HPV infection and age remains unclear. A possible reason may be that the women of these ages have a lower level of hormone as well as weaker immune function and therefore less capable to resist HPV infection [32]. Also, younger women that shortly after becoming sexually active are susceptible to HPV infection because they don't know how to protect themselves [7]. Besides, this study presented the age-specific HPV prevalence in women. The results showed that more than 40% of HPV infections occurred in women aged 40–49. On one hand, this may be attributed to largest number of participants of these ages. On the other, this also suggested that women of these ages suffer severely from HPV infection As the first study to report year- and age-specific HPV positivity in such a large number of participants in Meizhou, southern China, the information presented in this study would be instructive to protect women against HPV virus.

The prevalence of HPV infection and viral genotypes are different in different nations [4]. Common risk factors that correlate the prevalence of HPV infection include genetic variation, sexual activity (earlier age at first sexual activity, two or more sex partners), coinfection with other pathogens like herpes simplex virus, and human immunodeficiency virus (HIV) [33, 35]. Meizhou is located in northeastern Guangdong Province of China, with a total area of 15,836 km^2 and a population of 5.05 million. More than 95% people lived in Meizhou are Hakka, which is a special Han Chinese population that have a long history and unique culture, such as language, behavior and traditional food [36, 37]. Currently, few data are available on the prevalence and genotype distribution of HPV infection in Hakka population of Meizhou. Hence, the present study would be instructive to assess the clinical benefits of screening and vaccination strategies against HPV for in this area.

Conclusions

In conclusion, this study presented the heavy burden of HPV infection and the viral genotype distribution in women in northeastern Guangdong Province of China. HPV16, 52 and 58 are the dominant high-risk genotypes and over 80% of HPV infections occurred in women aged 20–49. The findings in this study provide important information for cervical screening and vaccination in population in northeastern Guangdong Province of China.

Abbreviations

HIV: Human immunodeficiency virus; HNC: Head and neck cancers; HPV: Human papillomavirus; HR: High-risk; LR: Low-risk; OPC: Oropharyngeal carcinoma

Acknowledgements

The authors would like to thank other colleagues whom were not listed in the authorship of Clinical Core Laboratory and Center for Precision Medicine, Meizhou People's Hospital (Huangtang Hospital), Meizhou Hospital Affiliated to Sun Yat-sen University for their helpful comments on the manuscript.

Funding
This study was supported by the grants from The National Key Research and Development Program of China (No. 2016YFD0050405), The National Key Research and Development Program of China (No. 2017YFD0501705), Medical Scientific Research Foundation of Guangdong Province, China (No. A2016306), Natural Science Foundation of Guangdong Province, China (No. 2016A030307031), Natural Science Foundation of Guangdong Province, China (No. 2014A030307042) and Key Scientific and Technological Project of Meizhou People's Hospital, Guangdong Province, China (No. MPHKSTP-20170102).

Authors' contributions
PZ conceived and designed the experiments; SL contributed to the data collection and the manuscript draft. SL, ZZ, JH, LL, RW, LS, HT, NL and HY helped to recruit patients, collected clinical data, conducted the clinical performances and researches; PZ and SL analyzed the data; PZ and SL wrote the paper. PZ, SL and ZZ reviewed the paper. All authors provided final approval of the version to be published and agree to be accountable for all aspects of the work in ensuring that questions related to the accuracy or integrity of any part of the work are appropriately investigated and resolved.

Competing interests
The authors declare that they have no competing interests.

Author details
[1]Clinical Core Laboratory, Meizhou People's Hospital (Huangtang Hospital), Meizhou Hospital Affiliated to Sun Yat-sen University, Meizhou 514031, People's Republic of China. [2]Center for Precision Medicine, Meizhou People's Hospital (Huangtang Hospital), Meizhou Hospital Affiliated to Sun Yat-sen University, Meizhou 514031, People's Republic of China. [3]Guangdong Provincial Engineering and Technology Research Center for Molecular Diagnostics of Cardiovascular Diseases, Meizhou 514031, People's Republic of China. [4]Meizhou Municipal Engineering and Technology Research Center for Molecular Diagnostics of Cardiovascular Diseases, Meizhou 514031, People's Republic of China. [5]Meizhou Municipal Engineering and Technology Research Center for Molecular Diagnostics of Major Genetic Disorders, Meizhou 514031, People's Republic of China. [6]Department of Gynaecology, Meizhou People's Hospital (Huangtang Hospital), Meizhou Hospital Affiliated to Sun Yat-sen University, Meizhou 514031, People's Republic of China.

References
1. Spence T, Bruce J, Yip KW, Liu FF. HPV associated head and neck Cancer. Cancers (Basel). 2016;8:75.
2. Cancer Genome Atlas N. Comprehensive genomic characterization of head and neck squamous cell carcinomas. Nature. 2015;517(7536):576–82.
3. Jemal A, Bray F, Center MM, Ferlay J, Ward E, Forman D. Global cancer statistics. CA Cancer J Clin. 2011;61(2):69–90.
4. Wang R, Guo XL, Wisman GB, Schuuring E, Wang WF, Zeng ZY, Zhu H, Wu SW. Nationwide prevalence of human papillomavirus infection and viral genotype distribution in 37 cities in China. BMC Infect Dis. 2015;15:257.
5. Wang Y, Wang S, Shen J, Peng Y, Chen L, Mai R, Zhang G. Genotype distribution of human papillomavirus among women with cervical cytological abnormalities or invasive squamous cell carcinoma in a high-incidence area of esophageal carcinoma in China. Biomed Res Int. 2016; 2016:1256384.
6. Ferlay J, Shin HR, Bray F, Forman D, Mathers C, Parkin DM. Estimates of worldwide burden of cancer in 2008: GLOBOCAN 2008. Int J Cancer. 2010; 127(12):2893–917.
7. Burd EM. Human papillomavirus laboratory testing: the changing paradigm. Clin Microbiol Rev. 2016;29(2):291–319.
8. Syrjanen K, Syrjanen S. Epidemiology of human papilloma virus infections and genital neoplasia. Scand J Infect Dis Suppl. 1990;69:7–17.
9. Weaver B, Shew M, Qadadri B, Tu W, Tong Y, Denski C, Fortenberry JD, Ermel A, Brown D. Low-level persistence of human papillomavirus 16 DNA in a cohort of closely followed adolescent women. J Med Virol. 2011;83(8):1362–9.
10. de Sanjose S, Diaz M, Castellsague X, Clifford G, Bruni L, Munoz N, Bosch FX. Worldwide prevalence and genotype distribution of cervical human papillomavirus DNA in women with normal cytology: a meta-analysis. Lancet Infect Dis. 2007;7(7):453–9.
11. Krul EJ, Van De Vijver MJ, Schuuring E, Van Kanten RW, Peters AA, Fleuren GJ. Human papillomavirus in malignant cervical lesions in Surinam, a high-risk country, compared to the Netherlands, a low-risk country. Int J Gynecol Cancer. 1999;9(3):206–11.
12. Forman D, de Martel C, Lacey CJ, Soerjomataram I, Lortet-Tieulent J, Bruni L, Vignat J, Ferlay J, Bray F, Plummer M, et al. Global burden of human papillomavirus and related diseases. Vaccine. 2012;30(Suppl 5):F12–23.
13. Spence AR, Goggin P, Franco EL. Process of care failures in invasive cervical cancer: systematic review and meta-analysis. Prev Med. 2007;45(2–3):93–106.
14. Poljak M, Kocjan BJ, Ostrbenk A, Seme K. Commercially available molecular tests for human papillomaviruses (HPV): 2015 update. J Clin Virol. 2016; 76(Suppl 1):S3–S13.
15. Arbyn M, Tommasino M, Depuydt C, Dillner J. Are 20 human papillomavirus types causing cervical cancer? J Pathol. 2014;234(4):431–5.
16. Halec G, Alemany L, Lloveras B, Schmitt M, Alejo M, Bosch FX, Tous S, Klaustermeier JE, Guimera N, Grabe N, et al. Pathogenic role of the eight probably/possibly carcinogenic HPV types 26, 53, 66, 67, 68, 70, 73 and 82 in cervical cancer. J Pathol. 2014;234(4):441–51.
17. Munoz N, Bosch FX, de Sanjose S, Herrero R, Castellsague X, Shah KV, Snijders PJ, Meijer CJ, International Agency for Research on Cancer multicenter cervical Cancer study G. Epidemiologic classification of human papillomavirus types associated with cervical cancer. N Engl J Med. 2003; 348(6):518–27.
18. Cogliano V, Baan R, Straif K, Grosse Y, Secretan B, El Ghissassi F, Cancer WHOIAfRo. Carcinogenicity of human papillomaviruses. Lancet Oncol. 2005;6(4):204.
19. Palefsky JM, Giuliano AR, Goldstone S, Moreira ED Jr, Aranda C, Jessen H, Hillman R, Ferris D, Coutlee F, Stoler MH, et al. HPV vaccine against anal HPV infection and anal intraepithelial neoplasia. N Engl J Med. 2011;365(17):1576–85.
20. Patel H, Jeve YB, Sherman SM, Moss EL. Knowledge of human papillomavirus and the human papillomavirus vaccine in European adolescents: a systematic review. Sex Transm Infect. 2016;92(6):474–9.
21. Zur Hausen H. Papillomaviruses in human cancers. Mol Carcinog. 1988; 1(3):147–50.
22. de Sanjose S, Serrano B, Castellsague X, Brotons M, Munoz J, Bruni L, Bosch FX. Human papillomavirus (HPV) and related cancers in the Global Alliance for Vaccines and Immunization (GAVI) countries. A WHO/ICO HPV Information Centre Report. Vaccine. 2012;30(Suppl 4):D1–83.
23. Priebe AM. 2012 cervical cancer screening guidelines and the future role of HPV testing. Clin Obstet Gynecol. 2013;56(1):44–50.
24. Smith M, Lew JB, Simms K, Canfell K. Impact of HPV sample self-collection for underscreened women in the renewed cervical screening program. Med J Aust. 2016;204(5):1941e–1947.
25. Castle PE, de Sanjose S, Qiao YL, Belinson JL, Lazcano-Ponce E, Kinney W. Introduction of human papillomavirus DNA screening in the world: 15 years of experience. Vaccine. 2012;30(Suppl 5):F117–22.
26. Lowndes CM. Vaccines for cervical cancer. Epidemiol Infect. 2006;134(1):1–12.
27. Joura EA, Giuliano AR, Iversen OE, Bouchard C, Mao C, Mehlsen J, Moreira ED Jr, Ngan Y, Petersen LK, Lazcano-Ponce E, et al. A 9-valent HPV vaccine against infection and intraepithelial neoplasia in women. N Engl J Med. 2015;372(8):711–23.
28. Herrero R. Human papillomavirus (HPV) vaccines: limited cross-protection against additional HPV types. J Infect Dis. 2009;199(7):919–22.
29. Liu SS, Chan KY, Leung RC, Chan KK, Tam KF, Luk MH, Lo SS, Fong DY, Cheung AN, Lin ZQ, et al. Prevalence and risk factors of human papillomavirus (HPV) infection in southern Chinese women - a population-based study. PLoS One. 2011;6(5):e19244.
30. Wu RF, Dai M, Qiao YL, Clifford GM, Liu ZH, Arslan A, Li N, Shi JF, Snijders PJ, Meijer CJ, et al. Human papillomavirus infection in women in Shenzhen City, People's Republic of China, a population typical of recent Chinese urbanisation. Int J Cancer. 2007;121(6):1306–11.
31. Chen Q, Luo ZY, Lin M, Lin QL, Chen CY, Yang C, Xie LX, Li H, Zheng JK, Yang LY, et al. Prevalence and genotype distribution of human papillomavirus infections in women attending hospitals in Chaozhou of Guangdong province. Asian Pac J Cancer Prev. 2012;13(4):1519–24.

32. Zeng XX, Yan LX, Huang XX, He CH, Liu WG, Yuan WQ, Qiu YP, Liu ZX. Prevalence and genotype distribution of human papillomavirus among Hakka women in China. Ann Transl Med. 2016;4(15):276.
33. Kliucinskas M, Nadisauskiene RJ, Minkauskiene M. Prevalence and risk factors of HPV infection among high-risk rural and urban Lithuanian women. Gynecol Obstet Investig. 2006;62(3):173–80.
34. Jing L, Zhong X, Huang W, Liu Y, Wang M, Miao Z, Zhang X, Zou J, Zheng B, Chen C, et al. HPV genotypes and associated cervical cytological abnormalities in women from the Pearl River Delta region of Guangdong province, China: a cross-sectional study. BMC Infect Dis. 2014;14:388.
35. Oakeshott P, Aghaizu A, Reid F, Howell-Jones R Hay PE, Sadiq ST, Lacey CJ, Beddows S, Soldan K. Frequency and risk factors for prevalent, incident, and persistent genital carcinogenic human papillomavirus infection in sexually active women: community based cohort study. BMJ. 2012;344:e4168.
36. Wang WZ, Wang CY, Cheng YT, Xu AL, Zhu CL, Wu SF, Kong QP, Zhang YP. tracing the origins of Hakka and Chaoshanese by mitochondrial DNA analysis. Am J Phys Anthropol. 2010;141(1):124–30.
37. Zhu Y, Shennan M, Reynolds KK, Johnson NA, Herrnberger MR, Valdes R Jr, Linder MW. Estimation of warfarin maintenance dose based on VKORC1 (−1639 G>A) and CYP2C9 genotypes. Clin Chem. 2007;53(7):1199–205.

Evaluation of vaccination herd immunity effects for anogenital warts in a low coverage setting with human papillomavirus vaccine—an interrupted time series analysis from 2005 to 2010 using health insurance data

Kathrin Thöne[1,2], Johannes Horn[3] and Rafael Mikolajczyk[3,4,5*]

Abstract

Background: Shortly after the human papillomavirus (HPV) vaccine recommendation and hence the reimbursement of vaccination costs for the respective age groups in Germany in 2007, changes in the incidence of anogenital warts (AGWs) were observed, but it was not clear at what level the incidence would stabilize and to what extent herd immunity would be present. Given the relatively low HPV vaccination coverage in Germany, we aimed to assess potential vaccination herd immunity effects in the German setting.

Methods: A retrospective open cohort study with data from more than nine million statutory health insurance members from 2005 to 2010 was conducted. AGW cases were identified using ICD-10-codes. The incidence of AGWs was estimated by age, sex, and calendar quarter. Age and sex specific incidence rate ratios were estimated comparing the years 2009–2010 (post-vaccination period) with 2005–2007 (pre-vaccination period).

Results: Incidence rate ratio of AGWs for the post-vaccination period compared to the pre-vaccination period showed a u-shaped decrease among the 14- to 24-year-old females and males which corresponds well with the reported HPV vaccination uptake in 2008. A maximum reduction of up to 60% was observed for the 16- to 20-year-old females and slightly less pronounced (up to 50%) for the 16- and 18-year-old males. Age groups outside of the range 14–24 years demonstrated no decrease. The decrease of incidence occurred in both sexes early after the vaccine recommendation and stabilized at lower levels in 2009–2010.

Conclusions: A relative reduction of up to 50% among males of approximately similar age groups as that of females receiving the HPV vaccination suggests herd protection resulting from assortative mixing by age. The early decrease among males can be reduced over time due to partner change.

Keywords: Human papillomavirus (HPV) vaccine, Anogenital warts (AGWs), Vaccine coverage, Herd immunity, Indirect vaccination effect

* Correspondence: Rafael.Mikolajczyk@helmholtz-hzi.de
[3]Helmholtz Centre for Infection Research, Inhoffenstr. 7, 38124 Braunschweig, Germany
[4]Hannover Medical School, Carl-Neuberg-Str. 1, 30625 Hannover, Germany
Full list of author information is available at the end of the article

Background

Infections with the human papillomavirus (HPV) are the most frequent sexually transmitted viral infections worldwide affecting both men and women [1]. HPV types 6 and 11 account for over 90% of anogenital warts (AGWs) [2]; HPV types 16 and 18 are responsible for 70% of all cervical cancers [3].

In 2006, a quadrivalent vaccine against HPV 6, 11, 16, and 18 was approved by the European Medicines Agency (EMA) for the prevention of cervical cancer. In Germany, both, the bivalent as well as the quadrivalent HPV vaccination have been recommended for girls between 12 and 17 years of age by the German Standing Vaccination Committee (STIKO) since March 2007. In Germany, both, the bivalent as well as the quadrivalent HPV vaccination have been recommended for girls between 12 and 17 years of age by the German Standing Vaccination Committee (STIKO) since March 2007. The decision, which of the two vaccines to use, is jointly made by the physicians and their patients. In reality, the German market is strongly dominated by the quadrivalent HPV vaccine (90% of the market share) [4].

Clinical trials have shown HPV vaccine efficacy of 90–100% for preventing persistent and incident HPV infections [5] and AGWs (quadrivalent vaccine only) [6]. The latter develop rapidly after HPV infection [7, 8], which enables to monitor trends in AGW incidence rates as an indicator of the HPV vaccine impact, while the incidence estimation indicating a protection against cervical cancer requires longer follow-up times [7].

Recent studies in Australia [7, 9–11], Europe [2, 8, 12–15], and the United States [16] reported a AGW incidence reduction of up to 90% in the vaccine-recommended age group, but most of them were conducted in countries with a high vaccine coverage of 70 to 90% [2, 7, 9–11, 14, 15]. Some studies also reported decreasing incidence in older age groups of females [7, 9–12, 15, 16] as well as in males [7, 10, 11, 14–16], suggesting effects of herd immunity dependent on vaccine coverage.

Since HPV vaccine introduction in Germany, controversial discussions on effectiveness and safety may have led to uncertainty among young women, their parents and maybe also among physicians [17] resulting in a limited HPV vaccine uptake [18]. It has been reported, that vaccination recommendations by physicians have a great influence on the pros and cons of the decision making process of their patients [19]. Furthermore, the German health care system includes only recommendation of HPV vaccination and the individual decision is made by the physicians and the patients. While HPV vaccination is covered by health insurance companies, an immunization program conducted by e.g. school-based health centers, primary care centers or community centers which has led to higher vaccination rates in other countries does not exist in Germany. One year after the STIKO recommendation, HPV vaccine uptake in Germany with at least one vaccine dose was about 32.2% in 12- to 17-year-old females [20]. In 2012, a similarly low vaccine uptake was reported ranging from 6.1% in 12-year-old females to 47.6% in 16-year-old females [21]. These numbers are low compared to other countries with introduced HPV vaccinations. While changes in incidences of AGWs shortly after the HPV vaccine introduction were previously studied in Germany [13], effects on herd immunity were not yet investigated, and it is not clear to what extent such effects are present in a German low coverage setting. The purpose of this study is to investigate changes in AGW incidence and potential herd immunity effects of HPV vaccination over the years 2005 to 2010 in Germany.

Methods

Data source

This study was conducted using data from the German Pharmacoepidemiological Research Database (GePaRD) which has been described elsewhere [22–24]. Briefly, GePaRD consists of records of four statutory health insurance providers (SHIs), including data of 17 million insurants of all ages (nearly one fourth of the population in Germany) and covering all geographical regions of Germany. In the current analysis, claims data of one of the four SHIs was used, including more than nine million insurants, covering about 8.5% of the German population. The membership in an SHI is compulsory for employees with an annual income below a predefined threshold (approximately 44,000€ in 2009). The majority of the German population is insured in SHIs (approximately 85%). There may be some overrepresentation of patients with middle to higher socio-economic status than in the average population in our data of one big countrywide SHI which is more likely to insure these patients. The database contains demographic data, in- and outpatient diagnoses recorded according to the International Classification of Diseases (ICD-10-GM), in- and outpatient diagnostic and therapeutic procedures, and outpatient drug prescriptions. Outpatient diagnoses can only be allocated to a quarter of a year and not to an exact date. Utilization of health insurance data for scientific research is regulated by the Code of Social Law in Germany. The use of the data for this study was approved by the contributing SHI and the regulatory authority. Informed consent was not required by law.

Study design

To estimate the incidence rates of AGWs, an open cohort design was applied. Cohort entry was on January 1, 2005 or on the first day after a patient had a continuous insurance time of 12 months without an AGW diagnosis during this period and had at least his/her 11th birthday in the year of cohort entry. For the calculation of person-time under risk, cohort exit was defined as the end of the study period (i.e. December 31st, 2010), December 31st of the year in which the patient had his/her 80th birthday, interruption of insurance time for more than 3 days, end of insurance (incl. Death), or the date of an AGW diagnosis. Cohort re-entry was not possible. Age at diagnosis was calculated by subtracting the year of birth from the year of the incident diagnosis - 1: e.g. for a person born in 1979 and diagnosed with AGW in 2008: 2008–1979 – 1 = 28. According to this definition, in 2008 this person was at least 28 years old and had his/her 29th birthday.

Case definition

Incident AGW diagnoses (ICD-10-GM A63.0) were identified via both inpatient and outpatient diagnoses, that were not proceeded by an earlier AGW diagnosis in previous 12 months. For inpatient data, all admission and discharge diagnoses were considered. For outpatient data all diagnoses coded as 'certain' and 'suspected' were taken into account.

Statistical analysis

The incidence of AGWs for each calendar quarter was estimated for the years 2005 to 2010 by dividing the number of incident cases in each stratum by the total person time of the respective stratum, expressed as per 100,000 person-years (PY). A narrower time interval was not possible, as outpatient diagnoses representing the majority of AGW diagnoses were only reported quarterly. 95% confidence intervals (CIs) for incidence rates were calculated by the substitution method [25]. Based on a previous analysis, in which we studied changes in AGW incidence immediately following the recommendation of vaccination [13], we defined two time intervals: 1) before the recommendation of vaccination (1st quarter 2005 to 2nd quarter 2007) and 2) after uptake of vaccination was established (1st quarter 2009 to 4th quarter 2010). For the two time intervals, we estimated average incidence of AGW in a given age group and calculated the relative incidence ratio for the period after establishing the vaccination compared to the pre-vaccination period, and its 95% CI. For testing and calculation of confidence intervals, we used Poisson regression model. This analysis was restricted to males and females aged 11 to 30 years. All statistical analyses were conducted using SAS statistical software, version 9.3.

Results

About 5 million insurance members aged 11 to 79 years were included in the cohort for each study year. Overall, 49,214 incident AGW cases were identified, ranging from 7288 in 2005 to 9352 in 2010 (Table 1). Overall incidence rates were approximately stable throughout the study years except in 2009 where overall incidences were slightly lower.

Table 1 Crude incidence rates (IRs) of anogenital warts per 100,000 person-years (PY) for 10- to 79-year-olds by sex from 2005 to 2010

Year	Sex	AGW cases	PY	IRs	CI (95%)
2005	Total	7288	43.7	166.7	162.9–170.6
2006		7972	47.8	166.7	163.0–170.4
2007		8068	47.6	169.6	195.9–173.3
2008		8644	51.2	168.8	165.3–172.4
2009		7890	50.9	155.0	151.6–158.5
2010		9352	56.2	166.5	163.1–169.9
2005	Male	3118	23.3	133.6	128.9–138.4
2006		3460	25.2	137.3	132.7–141.9
2007		3540	25.1	141.1	136.5–145.8
2008		3.826	26.6	144.0	139.5–148.6
2009		3605	26.5	136.2	131.8–140.7
2010		4510	29.4	153.3	148.8–157.8
2005	Female	4170	20.4	204.6	198.5–211.0
2006		4512	22.6	199.4	193.6–205.3
2007		4528	22.5	201.4	195.6–207.3
2008		4818	24.6	195.6	190.1–201.2
2009		4285	24.4	175.4	170.1–180.7
2010		4842	26.8	181.0	175.9–186.1

Abbreviations: AGW anogenital warts, *PY* person-years, *IRs* incidence rates, *CI (95%)* 95% confidence intervals

Incidence and its changes varied strongly by age (Additional file 1: Table S1), making analyses stratified into 1-year age groups necessary (Fig. 1). In all age-groups, incidence was approximately stable between the 1st quarter of 2005 and the 2nd quarter of 2007. With an exception of the 21-year-old females where a statistically non-significant decrease was found, the incidence decreased between the 2nd quarter of 2007 and the 4th quarter of 2008 among 16- to 26-year-old females and 16- and 18-year-old males and stabilized at a lower level afterwards. At the same time, in most other age groups, the incidence was approximately stable or increased slightly over the studied period.

When comparing the post-vaccination period with the pre-vaccination period, the relative incidence ratio indicated a u-shaped reduction of AGWs after the recommendation of vaccination in the group of 14- to 24-year-olds (Fig. 2a). The reduction was strongest for 16- to 20-year-old females (up to 60% reduction) and slightly less pronounced for 16- and 18-year-old males (up to 50% reduction (Fig. 2b and c)). In females 21 to 26 years of age a reduction of 10–20% was seen which was also found for males but estimates did not achieve

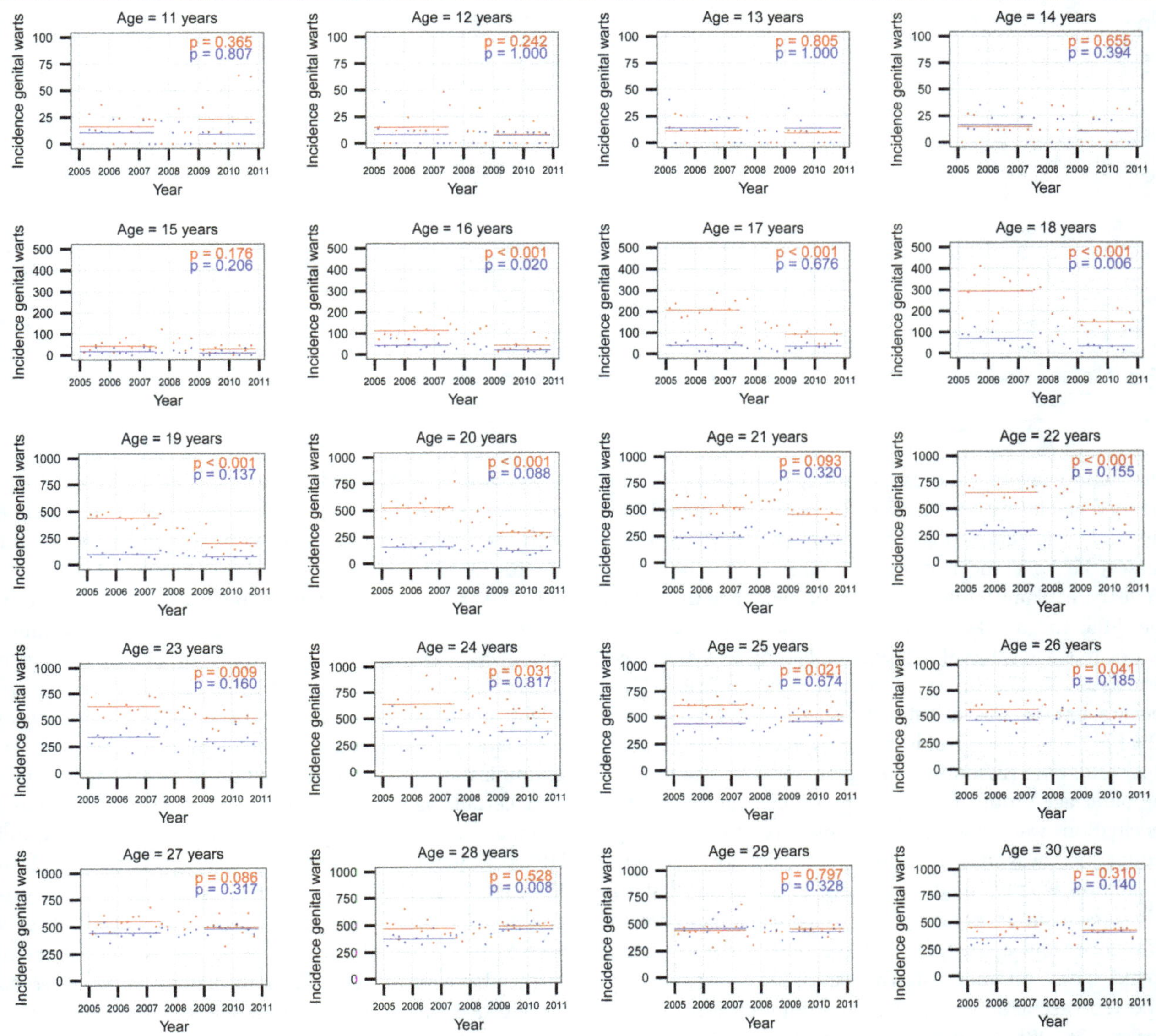

Fig. 1 Changes in the incidence rates per 100,000 person-years (PY) of AGWs among 11- to 30-year-olds by one-year age-groups and sex (*solid lines* indicate estimated incidence in two time intervals: up to 2nd quarter of 2007 and after 1st quarter of 2009, *p*-values indicate Wald-test from Poisson regression for the indicator variable coding the two time intervals (upper (*red*) for females, lower (*blue*) for males)

significance. The reduction in the age groups 12- to 15-year-olds was about 20–30% but confidence intervals were wide.

Discussion

The present study analyzed changes in the incidence of AGWs following the HPV vaccine recommendation in Germany and particularly the effects of herd protection among males in a low vaccine coverage setting. We found a u-shaped decrease among the 14- to 24-year-olds with a maximum reduction up to 60% observed for the 16- to 20-year-old females and a similar, but slightly less pronounced reduction for 16- and 18-year-old males.

In our analysis, the decrease of incidence occurred early after the vaccine recommendation in 2007 and stabilized after reaching a lower level in the first quarter of 2009. This reflects the finding that those who are going to be vaccinated do so in a relatively short time window. The decrease in incidence in this respective group reflects the increasing proportion of those getting vaccinated. This appears also plausible, e.g., for females aged 16, 17, or 18 years, as they had only one to 2 years in the recommended age range of vaccination and are the age groups with the most pronounced reduction in our analysis.

The u-shaped incidence reduction within the age groups of 14 to 24 years can be explained by the fact that HPV

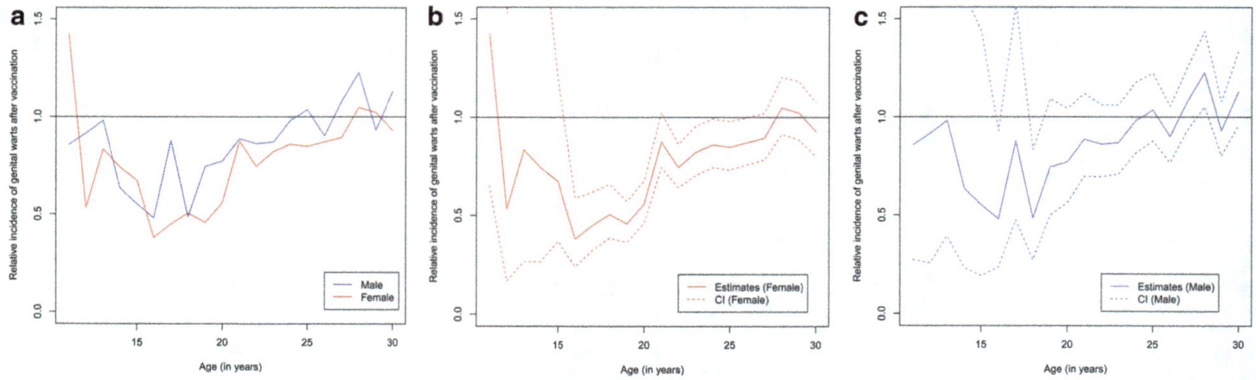

Fig. 2 Relative incidence of AGWs by sex and age **a** overall, **b** females, **c** males (incidence 2005–2007* compared to incidence 2009–2010). (*Dotted lines* indicate 95% confidence interval). *up to 2nd quarter of 2007

vaccination coverage increases with age within the recommended age interval from 12 to 17 years [20]. In addition, the study population originated from an SHI which reimburses the HPV vaccination in females up to the age of 26 years, explaining the reduction of incidence up to that age. Still, the uptake of vaccination closer to the upper end of this age interval is lower explaining why the effect diminishes. In the first year after recommendation, HPV vaccine uptake was about 30% for 12- to 17-year-olds, 12% for 18- to 26-year-olds, and only about 2% in 26-year-olds) [20]. One reason for low uptake or coverage rates in the older age groups (18 to 26) might be that neither the vaccination was officially recommended for these age groups nor was it stated in the vaccination schedule. Therefore, women might not have been aware that the reimbursement is possible. The maximum reduction of 60% is broadly consistent with the observed vaccination uptake based on administrative data [20, 21] or with the reported vaccination coverage based on data from several surveys [26–28], or from private insurance companies [18] in Germany. The most prominent decrease of incidence among females 16 to 20 years of age corresponds to the highest uptake in 14- to 17-year-old females of about 37% in 2008 [20]. Also the reduction in younger age groups (13 to 15 years of age) of 20 - 30% as well as in older age groups (18- to 26-year-olds) corresponds well with the reported HPV vaccination uptake in 2008 [20].

Despite the fact that the recommendation for HPV vaccination only includes females in Germany, we observed parallel effects among males of nearly the same age. Here, the most pronounced decrease was seen in 16- to 18-year-olds which is plausible as females have, on average, similarly aged or one to 2 years older sexual partners during adolescence. Other studies reported decreasing incidences of AGWs in males of the same age as vaccinated females, in a high vaccine coverage setting of about 80% or higher [10, 11, 14, 15, 29]. But also some studies with low age-specific vaccine coverage of about 50% or lower reported a decrease in AGW incidence or prevalence [30] for males younger than 20 [31] or 25 [16] years of age. This is in line with the incidence reduction of AGWs in our study for 16- to- 20-year-old females and less pronounced for 16- and 18-year-old males. A prior review including some of the above mentioned studies concluded that herd immunity effects were demonstrated only in populations with vaccine coverage of 50% or higher [32]. However, there might be differences with respect to homogeneity of vaccination coverage, for example in countries with an immunization program against HPV a percentage of girls of a certain age is vaccinated. In contrast, in Germany vaccination in general is recommended but voluntary and HPV vaccination can occur at any age between 12 to 17 years. In consequence, coverage is low for the full age-group of 12- to 17-year-olds, but in females aged 18 years vaccine coverage approaches 50%. Such heterogeneity might also explain why effects in males can be observed despite overall low coverage. While the relative changes were similar in both sexes, changes in the absolute incidence among males between pre-vaccination and post-vaccination period were less prominent. However, this might rather be a diagnostic bias than a true epidemiological difference, resulting from the fact, that females usually consult gynaecologists routinely about once a year, while males are not enrolled in a comparable system and are diagnosed only by actively consulting a physician or via an incidental finding. Thus, a higher fraction of the true incidence might be reported for females than for males, resulting in a higher incidence. In some of the age groups among males the incidence was so low, that relative reduction did not achieve significance.

The only slightly lower herd immunity effects in males than the direct protection effects in females of the same age suggest strongly assortative mating by age. The relatively short time period since the recommendation of vaccination most likely covers a single sexual relationship, which reportedly lasts for a median time of 26 months for males (interquartile range (IQR), 8.5–42) and 32 months (IQR, 9–49) for females in the relevant age groups [33]. HPV infectivity is high and in heterosexual serially monogamous partnerships, the protection of males by having a vaccinated female partner will decrease with change of partners, particularly as the reported median gap between different partners of 14 to 24 days is shorter than an HPV infection period [34]. Consequently, studies covering longer study periods particularly in low vaccination coverage settings would possibly observe diminishing protection among males while direct effects among females would remain constant. On the other hand, in high coverage settings, overall herd immunity effects may reduce the cumulative effects of change of female partners among males. In accordance with findings of other studies [2, 8, 9, 11–16], the incidence of AGWs among older age groups did not display a decreasing trend. Potential herd immunity effects in older age groups are based on sexual mixing with partners from vaccinated age groups. In a low coverage setting, the influence of such indirect protection might be too small to be detected.

In our study, the incidence of AGWs started to decrease among the 16- to 26-year-olds approximately 3 months after the vaccine recommendation by STIKO in Germany in March 2007. The short delay with which the effects of vaccination on AGW incidence were observed is consistent with the biology of infection. As HPV immunity is reported already after one vaccine dose [35] and AGWs develop after a medium incubation time of about 3 months [6–8], the corresponding time lag of decreasing incidence of one to two quarters of a year after the vaccine recommendation for females is plausible. A decreasing incidence in the target vaccination group soon after vaccine introduction has been also reported from several other ecologic studies conducted in Australia, Europe, and the US [2, 8, 9, 11–16].

We could not find herd immunity effects in older age groups (> 24 years of age) which could be explained by a limited sample size and less exclusive sexual mixing patterns of older age groups with much younger partners.

Limitations of our study are mainly related to the underlying administrative data used for analyses. For example, it was not possible to validate the diagnoses of AGWs, because we had to rely on what was used for reimbursement. Also, not all relevant variables were available in the desired detail. In particular, exact diagnosis dates in the outpatient sector are not available in the database, making the estimation of incidence less precise. It was not possible to determine the vaccine coverage of non-vaccinated persons per age cohort within the database as the vaccination status before the study period would have to be known, but was not available in our data. However, HPV vaccine uptake has been estimated in 2008 [20] and recently confirmed in a newer study in 2014 [36]. Both sources point towards a coverage of about 40–50%, or even higher if also single vaccine dose is considered. Due to data protection reasons, only the birth year but not the exact date of birth is contained in the database, which might lead to some non-differential misclassification of persons by age as some persons may already be 1 year older according to the definition of age. For the analysis of trends over time, the age of one patient is kept the same throughout all four quarters of the year, which leads to an average aging cohort from the 1st to the 4th quarter of a year resulting in higher incidences in the 4th quarter than in the 1st quarter of each year most prominently for 16- to 20-year-olds. Another limitation is that only patients who see a physician for AGWs could be identified in the database. AGWs do not necessarily cause discomfort or pain, and some patients might be embarrassed and not consult a physician. This would result in a possible underestimation of incidences of AGWs. Furthermore, AGWs may be coded as an unspecific disease, for example, as viral warts or as a sexually transmitted infection not otherwise specified, which would also result in an underestimation of AGW incidence. Finally, because of practical reasons related to data availability and permissions to use, we were unfortunately limited to analyze only data up to 2010. Particularly assessing longer trends would be of interest and should be conducted in the future.

Strengths of the study are the large population size which was not restricted to specific regions or settings in Germany and the almost complete lack of selection effects among participants, as a routine care situation is reflected in the data.

Conclusions

In conclusion, soon after the vaccine recommendation in Germany in 2007, the incidence of AGWs decreased among 14- to 24-year-old females. In the same time there was a slightly less pronounced decrease among males of approximately the same age. The only slightly weaker effect among males suggests protection effects due to assortative sexual mixing with respect to age. The strength of this indirect protection effect might decrease over time due to partner change.

Abbreviations

AGW: Anogenital wart; CI: Confidence interval; EMA: European Medicines Agency; GePaRD: German Pharmacoepidemiological Research Database; HPV: Human papillomavirus; ICD-10-GM: International Classification of Diseases, Version 10, German modification; IQR: Interquartile range; PY: Person years; SHI: Statutory Health Insurance; STIKO: German Standing Vaccination Committee

Acknowledgements

The authors would like to thank the statutory health insurance for providing data for this study (namely the Techniker Krankenkasse (TK)). They also want to thank Dr. Tania Schink, Nils Fabian Gesing, and Inga Schaffer for contributing to the statistical analyses. The authors would also like to thank Dr. Géraldine Dominiak-Felden for her support on the study.

Funding
This study was funded by Sanofi Pasteur MSD and conducted by KT et al. as employee of the BIPS. RM and JH (past employees of the BIPS and involved in earlier related studies) contributed based on their internal funding from the Helmholtz Center for Infection Research. The authors had complete autonomy for the process of establishing the protocol, carrying out the analyses and interpreting the results. This also includes the full right to publish the results without limitation.

Authors' contributions
KT, JH and RM analyzed and interpreted the data. KT drafted the manuscript and JH and RM critically reviewed the manuscript. All authors read and approved the final manuscript version for submission.

Consent for publication
Utilization of health insurance data for scientific research is regulated by the Code of Social Law in Germany. The use of the data for this study was approved by the contributing statutory health insurance provider and the regulatory authority. Informed consent was not required by law.

Competing interests
As employees of the Leibniz Institute for Prevention Research and Epidemiology – BIPS the authors have performed research studies paid by pharmaceutical companies (Bayer Pharma AG (RM), Sanofi-Pasteur MSD (RM, JH, KT), and Takeda (KT), outside of the current work.

Author details
[1]Leibniz-Institute for Prevention Research and Epidemiology – BIPS, Achterstr. 30, 28359 Bremen, Germany. [2]Hubertus Wald Tumor Center, University Cancer Center Hamburg (UCCH)/ University Medical Center Hamburg-Eppendorf (UKE), Martinistr. 52, 20246 Hamburg, Germany. [3]Helmholtz Centre for Infection Research, Inhoffenstr. 7, 38124 Braunschweig, Germany. [4]Hannover Medical School, Carl-Neuberg-Str. 1, 30625 Hannover, Germany. [5]Institute for Medical Epidemiology, Biometrics, and Informatics, Medical Faculty of the Martin-Luther University Halle-Wittenberg, 06112 Halle (Saale), Germany.

References
1. Gross G, Pfister H. Role of human papillomavirus in penile cancer, penile intraepithelial squamous cell neoplasias and in genital warts. Med Microbiol Immunol. 2004;193:35–44. doi:10.1007/s00430-003-0181-2.
2. Baandrup L, Blomberg M, Dehlendorff C, Sand C, Andersen KK, Kjaer SK. Significant decrease in the incidence of genital warts in young Danish women after implementation of a national human papillomavirus vaccination program. Sex Transm Dis. 2013;40:130–5. doi:10.1097/OLQ.0b013e31827bd66b.
3. Smith J, Lindsay L, Hoots B, Keys J, Franceschi S, Winer R, et al. Human papillomavirus type distribution in invasive cervical cancer and high-grade cervical lesions: a meta-analysis update. Int J Cancer. 2007;121:621–32. doi:10.1002/ijc.22527.
4. Schwabe U, Paffrath D. Arzneiverordnungsreport 2009. Aktuelle Daten, Kosten, Trends und Kommentare. Berlin Heidelberg: Springer-Verlag. 2009.
5. Harper DM, Franco EL, Wheeler CM, Moscicki A-B, Romanowski B, Roteli-Martins CM, et al. Sustained efficacy up to 4·5 years of a bivalent L1 virus-like particle vaccine against human papillomavirus types 16 and 18: follow-up from a randomised control trial. Lancet. 2006;367:1247–55.
6. FUTURE I/II Study Group, Dillner J, Kjaer SK, Wheeler CM, Sigurdsson K, Iversen O-E, et al. Four year efficacy of prophylactic human papillomavirus quadrivalent vaccine against low grade cervical, vulvar, and vaginal intraepithelial neoplasia and anogenital warts: randomised controlled trial. BMJ. 2010;341:c3493.
7. Donovan B, Franklin N, Guy R, Grulich AE, Regan DG, Ali H, et al. Quadrivalent human papillomavirus vaccination and trends in genital warts in Australia: analysis of national sentinel surveillance data. Lancet Infect Dis. 2011;11:39–44.
8. Blomberg M, Dehlendorff C, Munk C, Kjaer SK. Strongly decreased risk of genital warts after vaccination against human Papillomavirus: Nationwide follow-up of vaccinated and unvaccinated girls in Denmark. Clin Infect Dis. 2013;57:929–34. doi:10.1093/cid/cit436.
9. Fairley CK, Hocking JS, Gurrin LC, Chen MY, Donovan B, Bradshaw CS. Rapid decline in presentations of genital warts after the implementation of a national quadrivalent human papillomavirus vaccination programme for young women. Sex Transm Infect. 2009;85:499–502. doi:10.1136/sti.2009.037788.
10. Read TRH, Hocking JS, Chen MY, Donovan B, Bradshaw CS, Fairley CK. The near disappearance of genital warts in young women 4 years after commencing a national human papillomavirus (HPV) vaccination programme. Sex Transm Infect. 2011;87:544–7.
11. Ali H, Donovan B, Wand H, Read TRH, Regan DG, Grulich AE, et al. Genital warts in young Australians five years into national human papillomavirus vaccination programme: national surveillance data. BMJ. 2013;346:f2032. doi:10.1136/bmj.f2032.
12. Leval A, Herweijer E, Arnheim-Dahlström L, Walum H, Frans E, Sparén P, et al. Incidence of genital warts in Sweden before and after quadrivalent human papillomavirus vaccine availability. J Infect Dis. 2012;206:860–6. doi:10.1093/infdis/jis405.
13. Mikolajczyk RT, Kraut AA, Horn J, Schulze-Rath R, Garbe E. Changes in incidence of anogenital warts diagnoses after the introduction of human papillomavirus vaccination in Germany-an ecologic study. Sex Transm Dis. 2013;40:28–31. doi:10.1097/OLQ.0b013e3182756efd.
14. Howell-Jones R, Soldan K, Wetten S, Mesher D, Williams T, Gill ON, et al. Declining genital warts in young women in england associated with HPV 16/18 vaccination: an ecological study. J Infect Dis. 2013;208:1397–403. doi:10.1093/infdis/jit361.
15. Sandø N, Kofoed K, Zachariae C, Fouchard J. A reduced national incidence of anogenital warts in young danish men and women after introduction of a national quadrivalent human papillomavirus vaccination programme for young women - an ecological study. Acta Derm Venereol. 2014;94:288–92.
16. Bauer HM, Wright G, Chow J. Evidence of human papillomavirus vaccine effectiveness in reducing genital warts: an analysis of California public family planning administrative claims data, 2007-2010. Am J Public Health. 2012;102:833–5. doi:10.2105/AJPH.2011.300465.
17. Perkins RB, Clark JA. What affects human Papillomavirus vaccination rates? A qualitative analysis of providers' perceptions. Womens Heal Issues. 2012;22(4):e379–86.
18. Wild F. Impfung gegen humane Papillomaviren (HPV); Eine Analyse der Verordnungsdaten Privatversicherer. 2011; WIP-Diskussionspapier 3/2011.
19. Bundeszentrale für gesundheitliche Aufklärung (BZgA). Elternbefragung zum Thema "Impfen im Kindesalter". http://www.bzga.de/forschung/studien-untersuchungen/studien/?sid=10. Accessed 16 Feb 2017.
20. Hense S, Hillebrand K, Horn J, Mikolajczyk R, Schulze-Rath R, Garbe E. HPV vaccine uptake after introduction of the vaccine in Germany: an analysis of administrative data. Hum Vaccines Immunother. 2014;10:1729–33.
21. Rieck T, Feig M, Deler Y, Wichmann O. Utilization of administrative data to assess the association of an adolescent health check-up with human papillomavirus vaccine uptake in Germany. Vaccine. 2014;32:5564–9.
22. Pigeot I, Ahrens W. Establishment of a pharmacoepidemiological database in Germany: methodological potential, scientific value and practical limitations. Pharmacoepidemiol Drug Saf. 2008;17:215–23. doi:10.1002/pds.1545.
23. Ohlmeier C, Frick J, Prütz F, Lampert T, Ziese T, Mikolajczyk R, et al. Use of routine data from statutory health insurances for federal health monitoring purposes. Bundesgesundheitsblatt Gesundheitsforschung Gesundheitsschutz. 2014;57:464–72.
24. Garbe E, Suling M, Kloss S, Lindemann C, Schmid U. Linkage of mother–baby pairs in the German Pharmacoepidemiological research database. Pharmacoepidemiol Drug Saf. 2011;20:258–64.
25. Daly LE. Confidence limits made easy: interval estimation using a substitution method. Am J Epidemiol. 1998;147:783–90.
26. Deleré Y, Böhmer MM, Walter D, Wichmann O. HPV vaccination coverage

among women aged 18-20 years in Germany three years after recommendation of HPV vaccination for adolescent girls: results from a cross-sectional survey. Hum Vaccin Immunothe. 2013;9:1706–11.
27. Blödt S, Holmberg C, Müller-Nordhorn J, Rieckmann N. Human Papillomavirus awareness, knowledge and vaccine acceptance: a survey among 18-25 year old male and female vocational school students in Berlin, Germany. Eur J Pub Health. 2012;22:808–13.
28. Samkange-Zeeb F, Spallek L, Klug SJ, Zeeb H. HPV infection awareness and self-reported HPV vaccination coverage in female adolescent students in two German cities. J Community Health. 2012;37:1151–6.
29. Chow EP, Read TR, Wigan R, Donovan B, Chen MY, Bradshaw CS, Fairley CK. Ongoing decline in genital warts among young heterosexuals 7 years after the Australian human papillomavirus (HPV) vaccination programme. Sex Transm Infect. 2015;91(3):214-9. doi:10.1136/sextrans-2014-051813. Epub 2014 Oct 10.
30. Flagg EW, Schwartz R, Weinstock H. Prevalence of anogenital warts among participants in private health plans in the United States, 2003-2010: potential impact of human papillomavirus vaccination. Am J Public Health. 2013;103:1428–35.
31. Oliphant J, Perkins N. Impact of the human papillomavirus (HPV) vaccine on genital wart diagnoses at Auckland sexual health services. N Z Med J. 2011; 124:51–8.
32. Drolet M, Bénard É, Boily M-C, Ali H, Baandrup L, Bauer H, et al. Population-level impact and herd effects following human papillomavirus vaccination programmes: a systematic review and meta-analysis. Lancet Infect Dis. 2015;15:565–80. doi:10.1016/S1473-3099(14)71073-4.
33. Widdice L, Ma Y, Jonte J, Farhat S, Breland D, Shiboski S, et al. Concordance and transmission of human papillomavirus within heterosexual couples observed over short intervals. J Infect Dis. 2013;207:1286–94.
34. Mercer CH, Aicken CRH, Tanton C, Estcourt CS, Brook MG, Keane F, et al. Serial monogamy and biologic concurrency: measurement of the gaps between sexual partners to inform targeted strategies. Am J Epidemiol. 2013;178:249–59.
35. Kreimer AR, Struyf F, Del Rosario-Raymundo MR, Hildesheim A, Skinner SR, Wacholder S, et al. Efficacy of fewer than three doses of an HPV-16/18 AS04-adjuvanted vaccine: combined analysis of data from the Costa Rica vaccine and PATRICIA trials. Lancet Oncol. 2015;16:775–86. doi:10.1016/S1470-2045(15)00047-9.
36. Robert-Koch-Institut. Impfquoten der Rotavirus-, Masern-, HPV-und Influenza- Impfung in Deutschland. Epidemiol Bull. 2017;1–16. https://www.rki.de/DE/Content/Infekt/EpidBull/Archiv/2017/Ausgaben/01_17.pdf?__blob=publicationFile. Accessed 16 Feb 2017.

Good concordance of HPV detection between cervico-vaginal self-samples and general practitioner-collected samples using the Cobas 4800 HPV DNA test

Mette Tranberg[1,2*], Jørgen Skov Jensen[3], Bodil Hammer Bech[4], Jan Blaakær[5,6], Hans Svanholm[7] and Berit Andersen[1,2]

Abstract

Background: Studies comparing self-samples and clinician-collected samples for high-risk human papillomavirus (HPV) detection using clinically validated PCR-based HPV DNA assays are limited. We measured the concordance of HPV detection between home-based self-sampling and general practitioner (GP) sampling using the Cobas 4800 HPV DNA test and studied women's accept of home-based self-sampling.

Methods: Paired GP-collected samples and cervico-vaginal self-samples were obtained from 213 women aged 30–59 years diagnosed with ASC-US within the cervical cancer screening program. After undergoing cervical cytology at their GP, the women collected a self-sample with the Evalyn Brush at home and completed a questionnaire. Both samples were HPV-tested using the Cobas 4800 test. Histology results were available for those who tested HPV positive in GP-collected samples.

Results: We observed good concordance for HPV detection between self-samples and GP-collected samples (κ: 0.70, 95% CI: 0.58–0.81). No underlying CIN2+ cases were missed by self-sampling. Women evaluated that self-sampling was easy (97.2%, 95% CI: 93.9–98.9%) and comfortable (94.8%, 95% CI: 90.9–97.4%).

Conclusions: Home-based self-sampling using the Evalyn Brush and the Cobas 4800 test is an applicable and reliable alternative to GP-sampling.

Keywords: Self-sampling, Human papillomavirus testing, Cervical cancer screening, Acceptability

Background

DNA tests for HPV testing in cervical cancer screening have been developed due to the strong causal relationship between persistent cervical infection caused by high-risk human papillomavirus (HPV) types and cervical cancer and its pre-cancer lesions [1, 2].

Screening based on HPV testing is more sensitive in detecting cervical intraepithelial neoplasia of grade 3 (CIN3) and cancer than cytology-based screening [3, 4], and women with a negative HPV test have a lower 5-year risk of CIN3 and cancer than women with a negative cytology [5]. An advantage of HPV testing is that, unlike cytology, it enables women to self-sample cervico-vaginal material at home (HPV self-sampling), which may improve cervical cancer screening participation [6].

Studies comparing self-samples and clinician-collected samples for HPV detection show moderate to very good concordance in referral populations [7, 8], whereas one study conducted in a screening population reported a very high level of agreement [9]. Yet, studies on HPV concordance derive mainly from studies using Hybrid Capture II (HC2) or in-house Polymerase Chain Reaction (PCR)-based assays [7, 8], while only few studies have used established, clinically validated PCR-based HPV DNA assays [9, 10].

* Correspondence: mettrani@rm.dk
[1]Department of Public Health Programmes, Randers Regional Hospital, Skovlyvej 15, 8930 Randers NØ, Denmark
[2]Department of Clinical Medicine, Aarhus University, Palle Juul-Jensens Boulevard 82, 8200 Aarhus N, Denmark
Full list of author information is available at the end of the article

A systematic review demonstrated that self-sampling is a well-accepted screening method. The main reported concerns were pain, discomfort touching themselves, and uncertainty as to whether the sample was collected correctly [11]. However, in most studies assessing acceptability, the women obtained the samples in clinics after face-to-face oral information from healthcare professionals, which is not the set-up if self-sampling is to be implemented in a routine screening program where self-sampling is to be home-based [11].

Aims

This study aimed to measure concordance in HPV detection between paired self-samples collected at home using the Evalyn Brush device and general practitioner (GP)-collected samples, when using the clinically validated Cobas 4800 HPV DNA test. Further, we wanted to measure women's accept of home-based self-sampling.

Methods

Setting

This study was conducted in the Central Denmark Region (CDR), which covers 23% of the Danish population [12]. Like the rest of the country, this region has been covered by a nationwide, organized, free-of-charge cervical cancer screening program since the late 1990s [13, 14].

Currently, 23–49-year-old women are invited for cervical cancer screening every third year, 50–64-year-old women every fifth year. A liquid-based cervical cytology sample is taken at their GP (GP-collected sample). The primary screening method is microscopic examination of the cytology sample for 23–59-year-old women; a primary HPV-DNA check-out test for 60–64-year-old women [13].

In the CDR, the Department of Pathology at Randers Regional Hospital handles all cytology and HPV analyses. As per routine, GPs obtain the sample using a cervical brush and the brush head is placed in 10 ml SurePath medium (BD Diagnostics, Burlington, NC) and mailed to the Pathology Department for further processing and testing according to guidelines, which for women aged 30–59 is microscopic examination. Women with high-grade cytological lesions (threshold ASC-H or HSIL or, AGC, or AIS or malignant tumor cells) are referred directly for colposcopy. Women diagnosed with ASC-US undergo routine reflex HPV DNA triage testing using the cell pellet from 1 mL SurePath medium. ASC-US/HPV-positive women are referred for colposcopy within 3 months. ASCUS/HPV-negative women are referred back to the routine screening program. Women with LSIL are monitored by repeated cytology testing [13].

For HPV DNA analyses, the Cobas 4800 assay (Roche Diagnostic, Switzerland) is used. This test is a real-time PCR fully automated method separately detecting HPV16, HPV18, and 12 other high-risk HPV types (HPV 31, 33, 35, 39, 45, 51, 52, 56, 58, 59, 66, and 68) using the β-globin gene as an extraction and amplification control [15].

Inclusion of participants

Paired GP-collected samples and cervico-vaginal self-samples were obtained from 30 to 59-year-old women diagnosed with low-grade cytological lesions (ASC-US) within the screening program. As per routine, GP-collected samples from these women are all analyzed by both microscopy and HPV, which is not the case for younger and older women, or women with other cytological diagnoses [13].

Between June 2015 and December 2016, eligible women were consecutively identified daily through patient lists provided by the Department of Pathology. They received written information about the study and then contacted the investigator for oral information if they wanted to participate. A written and signed informed consent form had to be mailed back to the investigator before inclusion.

The exclusion criteria were pregnancy, giving birth less than < 3 months previously, and collecting the self-sample after colposcopy.

Self-sampling collection, storage, and analysis

The women were sent a self-sampling kit comprising a brush device (Evalyn® Brush, Rovers Medical Devices B.V., Oss, Netherlands), written and picture-based user instructions showing how to collect the cervico-vaginal sample using the device, a questionnaire, and a pre-addressed return envelope.

Upon arrival at the laboratory, the brush head was placed in 10 ml of SurePath medium (BD Diagnostics, Burlington, NC), stored overnight at 4 °C, and then vortexed for 5 min. A 6.4 ml volume of the self-sample material was centrifuged at 3000 x RPM for 20 min at room temperature. After centrifugation, with supernatant removed, the cell pellet was placed in 1 mL 25% ethanol-buffered (TRIS) and stored at -80 °C, until further processing. A volume of 6.4 ml was chosen to adjust for the material volume used for cytology examination performed on the GP-collected samples.

The self-samples were thawed overnight at 4 °C before the day of analysis. For analysis, the self-sample (1 ml volume) was vortexed for 15 s before being placed in test tubes, being the starting point for the HPV testing. Each run included four water samples to measure contamination. All HPV testing was performed following the manufacturers' instructions using a protocol without a sample pre-heating step which was also the case for the GP-collected samples. The investigator and the laboratory personnel performing the HPV testing were blinded to the HPV results of the GP-collected samples.

Questionnaire

The questionnaire included three questions on self-sampling experience and one on the clarity of the user instructions. To avoid low frequencies, the responses were grouped into three groups "Agree" (totally agree or agree), "Disagree" (disagree or totally disagree), and "Do not know". Multiple response answers were not allowed. The women were asked to record the date they had taken the self-sample, whether they had had sexual intercourse in between the two samplings, and their partner status (i.e., regular partner). Open feedback was possible. The data were double-entered into REDCap [16].

Data on test results

Information on the HPV self-sample test results was obtained through patient lists provided by the Department of Pathology. Data on the GP-collected HPV test results and the histological results were retrieved from the nationwide Danish Pathology Data Bank (DPDB), which has been complete since the late 2000s [17]. Histological results were available only for women who had tested HPV-positive in their GP-collected sample and were classified using the CIN classification, which was grouped into normal, CIN, CIN1, and CIN2+ (including CIN2, CIN3/AIS, and carcinoma). To ascertain the histological result, the most severe diagnosis was used if more were available.

Sample size

The study was designed to estimate a 95% confidence interval (CI) with a width of +/− 5%. With an expected 86% sensitivity and 85% specificity of HPV detection (high-risk HPV types) using the Evalyn Brush and a PCR-based HPV DNA test, a minimum of 198 women had to be included [10].

Statistical analyses

The HPV concordance between the paired samples was assessed using the Kappa statistic (Cohen's Kappa, κ) and defined as "Poor" ($\kappa \leq 0.20$), "Fair" ($0.21 \leq \kappa \leq 0.40$), "Moderate" ($0.41 \leq \kappa \leq 0.60$), "Good" ($0.61 \leq \kappa \leq 0.80$), or "Very good" ($\kappa \geq 0.81$) [18]. The overall percentage of agreement between the paired samples was calculated as the proportion of concordant sample sets divided by the total number of samples. We calculated the sensitivity and specificity of HPV detection in the self-samples with corresponding 95% CIs based on the binomial distribution using the GP-collected samples as reference standard. When assessing the HPV concordance regarding specific genotypes (HPV16/18 and HPV other), the genotypes were defined as "HPV16/18" (HPV16 and/or HPV18 including those having co-infections with other HPV types) and "HPV other" (HPV of other types including those having co-infections with HPV16/18). Concordance was determined as at least one identical genotype in both samples; discordance was determined as no genotype similarities. For continuous data, medians and interquartile ranges (IQR) were calculated; the Mann Whitney rank sum test was used to test for differences. Descriptive statistics (proportions and 95% CIs) were used to measure the women's accept of self-sampling. The χ^2-test was used to test for differences in categorical data.

P-values < 0.05 were considered statistically significant. All statistical analyses were performed using STATA, version 14 (STATA College).

Ethical approval

The study was approved by the local Ethical Committee of the Central Denmark Region (journal no.: 1–16–02-209-15) and by the Danish Data Protection Agency (journal no.:1–10–72-69-15).

Results

Participant characteristics

From a total of 1110 eligible women, 216 (19.5%) returned a self-sample. Three women (0.3%) were excluded because the self-sample was taken after the biopsy, leaving 213 (19.2%) women for analysis.

The included women's median age was 44 years (IQR: 38–49 years). The majority were aged 40 to 49 years (n = 113, 53.0%) followed by women aged 30 to 39 years (n = 59, 27.7%) and 50 to 59 years (n = 41, 19.3%). All paired GP-collected samples and self-samples were valid for HPV testing.

The median number of days between the GP-collected sample and the self-sample was 43 days (IQR: 34–53 days, range: 13–95 days). Histological results were available for 46 women, of whom 19 (41.3%) had a normal biopsy, 4 had CIN (not specified) (8.7%), 11 had CIN1 (23.9%), and 12 (26.1%) had CIN2+ (2 CIN2, 9 CIN3, 1 adenocarcinoma).

HPV prevalence and concordance between self-sampling and GP-sampling

For self-samples, the HPV prevalence (any type) was 24.4% (95% CI: 18.8–30.8%); for GP-collected samples 22.1% (95% CI: 16.7–28.2%) (Table 1). There was good concordance for HPV detection between the self-samples and the GP-collected samples (κ: 0.70, 95% CI: 0.58–0.81). The overall level of agreement was 89.2% (95% CI: 84.2–93.0%) (Table 1). For HPV detection in self-samples, the sensitivity was 80.9% (95% CI: 66.7–90.9%) and the specificity 91.6% (95% CI: 86.3–95.3%) when the GP-collected sample was used as reference.

A total of 23 women (10.7%) had disconcordant results. In nine cases, the women were GP-collected sample HPV-positive/self-sample HPV-negative. For these women, the median number of days between the two

Table 1 Concordance and agreement for HPV detection (any type) between self-samples and GP-collected samples

	GP-collected samples						κ[b] (95% CI)	Agreement (%) (95% CI)	Sensitivity (%) (95% CI)	Specificity (%) (95% CI)
	HPV any positive[a]		HPV negative		Total					
	n	%	n	%	n	%				
Self-samples										
HPV any positive[a]	38	17.8	14	6.6	52	24.4	0.70 (0.58–0.81)	89.2 (84.2–93.0)	80.9 (66.7–90.9)	91.6 (86.3–95.3)
HPV negative	9	4.2	152	71.4	161	75.6				
Total	47	22.1	166	77.9	213	100.0				

[a]HPV any positive: HPV16 and/or HPV18 and/or HPV31, 33, 35, 39, 45, 51, 52, 56, 58, 59, 66, and 68. % = Row percentage
[b]Cohen's Kappa. "Poor" (κ ≤ 0.20), "Fair" (0.21 ≤ κ ≤ 0.40), "Moderate" (0.41 ≤ κ ≤ 0.60), "Good" (0.61 ≤ κ ≤ 0.80), or "Very good" (κ ≥ 0.81) (18)

samples was insignificantly higher than in women with concordant sample results (n = 38) (40 versus 35 days, respectively) (p = 0.20). None of these nine women reported having trouble taking the self-sample, although one woman responded feeling insecure if she had collected the self-sample correctly. Histological results were available for eight out of the nine women, of whom five (62.5%) had no CIN, one (12.5%) had CIN (not specified), and two women (25.0%) had CIN1. The 12 women diagnosed with CIN2+ all had HPV detected in their self-sample.

Fourteen women were GP-collected sample HPV-negative/self-sample HPV-positive; two of whom (14.2%) reported no sexual intercourse in the time span separating the two samples.

The HPV prevalence was insignificantly higher in self-samples than in GP-collected samples for HPV16/18 (9.4%, 95% CI: 5.8–14.1%) versus (8.0%, 95% CI: 4.7–12.5%) and HPV of other types (21.1%, 95% CI: 15.8–27.2) versus (18.3%, 95% CI: 13.4–24.2%) (Table 2). Concordance for HPV16/HPV18 detection between self-samples and the GP-collected samples was good (κ: 0.73, 95% CI: 0.57–0.90) with overall 95.7% agreement (95% CI: 92.1–98.0%) (Table 2). For HPV16/18, the sensitivity and specificity in self-samples as compared with GP-collected samples was 82.4% (95% CI: 56.7–96.2%) and 96.9% (95% CI: 93.5–98.8%), respectively. For HPV of other types, a good concordance was seen between self-samples and GP-collected samples (k = 0.64, 95% CI: 0.51–0.78), with an overall agreement of 88.7% (95% CI: 83.7–92.6%) (Table 2). The corresponding sensitivity was 76.9% (95% CI: 60.7–88.9%); the specificity 91.4% (95% CI: 86.2–95.1%).

Women's accept of self-sampling

A total of 212 out of 213 women answered the questionnaire. Self-sampling with the Evalyn Brush was recorded as easy by 97.2% (95% CI: 93.9–98.9%) (Fig. 1), while 6 (2.8%, 95% CI: 1.0–6.1%) recorded that self-sampling was not easy. Most women reported that self-sampling was comfortable (94.8%, 95% CI: 90.9%–97.4%). A total of 21 (9.9, 95% CI: 6.2–14.7%) women reported uncertainty about performing the self-sample correctly, with three women reporting that they felt insecure because it

Table 2 Concordance and agreement between self-samples and GP-collected samples according to specific genotypes

	GP-collected samples						κ[a] (95% CI)	Agreement (%) (95% CI)	Sensitivity (%) (95% CI)	Specificity (%) (95% CI)
	HPV 16/18[b] positive		HPV16/18[b] negative		Total					
	n*	%	n*	%	n	%				
Self-samples										
HPV 16/18[b] positive	14	6.6	6	2.8	20	9.4	0.73 (0.57–0.90)	95.7 (92.1–98.0)	82.4 (56.7–96.2%)	96.9 (93.5–98.8%)
HPV 16/18[b] negative	3	1.4	190	89.2	193	90.6				
Total	17	8.0	196	92.0	213	100				
	HPV other[c] positive		HPV other[c] negative		Total					
Self-samples	n*	%	n*	%	n					
HPV other[c] positive	30	14.1	15	7.0	45	21.1	0.64 (0.51–0.78)	88.7 (83.7–92.6)	76.9 (60.7–88.9%)	91.4 (86.2–95.1%)
HPV other[c] negative	9	4.2	159	74.6	168	78.9				
Total	39	18.3	174	81.7	213	100				

n* = Women with co-infections with HPV16/18 and HPV of other types appear in both sub-analyses
[a]Cohen's Kappa. "Poor" (κ ≤ 0.20), "Fair" (0.21 ≤ κ ≤ 0.40), "Moderate" (0.41 ≤ κ ≤ 0.60), "Good" (0.61 ≤ κ ≤ 0.80), or "Very good" (κ ≥ 0.81) (18)
[b]HPV16/18: HPV16 and/or HPV18 including co-infections with HPV of other types (HPV31, 33, 35, 39, 45, 51, 52, 56, 58, 59, 66, and 68)
[c]HPV other: HPV31, 33, 35, 39, 45, 51, 52, 56, 58, 59, 66, and 68 including co-infections with HPV16/18. % = Row percentage

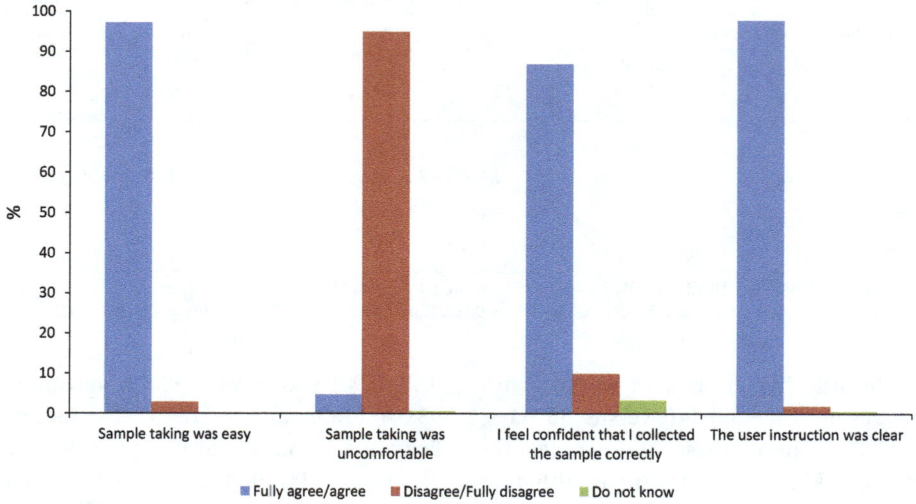

Fig. 1 The women's accept of self-sampling

was difficult to hear the click when rotating the brush. In 86.8% (95% CI: 81.5–91.0%) of the cases, the women felt confident that they collected the self-sample correctly. Most women responded that the user instructions were clear (97.6%, 95% CI: 94.6–99.2%). There were no statistically differences between the age groups ($p = 0.33$) for any of the questions.

Discussion

Main findings

Our study showed good concordance in HPV detection between paired self-samples and GP-collected samples. Home-based self-sampling using the Evalyn Brush was a well-accepted screening method. Compared with GP-sampling, no cases of underlying CIN2+ were overlooked by self-sampling.

Strengths and limitations

A key strength of our study was that we used a combination of a clinically validated self-sampling device and a clinically validated automated PCR-based HPV DNA test assay on paired samples [10, 19]. Furthermore, women collected the self-sample at home without supervision by healthcare professionals, which is the most relevant setting for testing self-sampling before its rollout in a routine screening program.

The main limitation is the time span between the GP-collected samples and self-samples, making the results not directly comparable. Still, the questionnaire data helped us to interpret discordant results. Another explanation for the discordant results could be that the self-samples had been subjected to freezing at -80 °C prior to the HPV testing which potentially could have affected the amount of HPV DNA in the self-samples, unlike the GP-collected samples which have not been frozen. However, since DNA is generally considered to be stable at -80 °C, we assume that this has not significantly affected the results and conclusions of this study. Our study population comprised women with ASC-US of whom one fourth was referred for colposcopy due to concurrent HPV infection; thus, histological results were not available for women with HPV-negative GP-collected samples. Ideally, histological results should have been available from all women. This was not possible in our set-up. Still, the available histological results allowed us to make the important conclusion that no cases of underlying CIN2+ had been overlooked by self-sampling which is important when implementing self-sampling in routine screening practice.

Even though our study population can be considered a "low-risk" population compared with the referral populations that have typically been targeted in similar studies [7], our population is still not representative of a screening population. Consequently, this study cannot be generalized to such populations.

Interpretation and comparison with previous studies

The concordance in our study (k = 0.70) was comparable with the mean k (k = 0.71) reported for brush devices combined with PCR-based HPV DNA tests in the review by Schmeink et al. [7], but higher than the mean k (k = 0.66) in the review by Petignat et al. [8]. This difference might be explained by differences in self-sampling devices, HPV tests, laboratory protocols, and study populations (screening or referral population). In our study, some of the discrepancy in the HPV concordance between self-sampling and GP-sampling could plausibly also be explained by spontaneous clearance or a new HPV exposure due to the time span separating the samples.

In our study, the sensitivity and specificity of HPV detection (of any type) was 80.9% and 91.6% in self-samples, respectively, when using the GP-collected samples as reference standard. These results are comparable to those by Van Baars et al. [10] who found a sensitivity of 82.7% and a specificity of 89.5% for HPV detection using the Evalyn Brush together with the clinically validated PCR-based GP5+/6+ HPV DNA test in a referral population. Thus, self-sampling using validated HPV DNA analyses seems feasible, but the optimal combination of self-sample device and HPV DNA test remains unknown.

Ketelaars et al. [9] found no significant differences in HPV16/18 prevalence between samples, whereas the prevalence of HPV of other types was significantly higher in self-samples (8.0%) than in GP-collected samples (6.3%). We observed no significant differences in the HPV prevalence between samples, but the same trend was seen, especially for the prevalence of HPV of other types (21.1% versus 18.3%, respectively). The higher HPV prevalence in self-samples compared with GP-collected samples increases referral rates, especially because reflex cytology triage is not possible on self-sampled material. To avoid excessive referral rates in women with HPV-positive self-samples without underlying CIN2+, a direct triage method like DNA methylation [20] could be considered to reduce referral rates and prevent overtreatment.

Most importantly, we showed that no underlying CIN2+ cases were overlooked by self-sampling. Some of the women in the GP-collected HPV negative/self-sample HPV-positive group might possibly have had underlying CIN2+, but this cannot be explored further in this study since referral for colposcopy was based on the result of the GP-collected sample.

The self-sampling device and user instructions must be acceptable if we wish to improve screening participation by this method. In our study, more than 85% expressed confidence in having collected the self-sample correctly, and only 5% expressed discomfort with collecting the sample. Hence, home-based self-sampling using the Evalyn Brush appeared to be a well-accepted screening method. Yet, almost 10% reported uncertainty regarding sample collection and some stated the lack of a click when rotating the brush as their reason. Despite small numbers, this finding is higher than reported by Van Baars et al. [10] (3.0%) and Ketelaars et al. [9] (0.8%) who used the same device in a referral and screening population, respectively. This difference might be explained by the fact that the women in our study performed home-based self-sampling, whereas in the study by Van Baars et al. [10] the women performed clinic-based self-sampling allowing them to ask questions and receive guidance. Nevertheless, our results suggest that if home-based self-sampling were to be rolled out in a routine setting, it should be considered giving women the opportunity to contact healthcare professionals for guidance.

Conclusions

We report a high acceptability of home-based self-sampling and good concordance between self-samples and GP-collected samples in terms of HPV detection using the clinically validated Cobas 4800 HPV DNA test. Our findings demonstrate the feasibility of offering self-sampling as an alternative to GP-sampling in cervical cancer screening.

Abbreviations

AGC: Atypical Glandular Cells; AIS: Adenocarcinoma In Situ; ASC-H: Atypical Squamous Cells cannot exclude HSIL; ASC-US: Atypical Squamous Cells of Undetermined Significance; CDR: Central Denmark Region; CI: Confidence interval; CIN: Cervical Intraepithelial Neoplasia; CIN1: Cervical Intraepithelial Neoplasia of grade 1; CIN2 + : Cervical Intraepithelial Neoplasia of grade 2 or worse; CIN3: Cervical Intraepithelial Neoplasia of grade 3; DPDB: Danish Pathology Data Bank; GP: General Practitioner; HC2: Hybrid Capture II; HPV: Human Papilloma Virus; HSIL: High-grade Squamous Intraepithelial Lesion; IQR: InterQuartile Ranges; LSIL: Low-grade Squamous Intraepithelial Lesion; PCR: Polymerase Chain Reaction

Acknowledgments

We take this opportunity to extend our gratitude to the laboratory staff at Department of Pathology, Randers Regional Hospital, for their great work in the laboratory and for their collaboration during this study. A special thanks to Pia Nørregaard and Rikke Andersen for helping set up the study in the laboratory. We would also like to thank Camilla Rasmussen and Marianne Rævsbæk Pedersen, Department of Public Health Programmes, for their assistance with the development of the user instructions and for sending out invitations to potential participants, respectively.

Funding

This study was funded by the Health Research Fund of the Central Denmark Region (no ref. no was provided), the Health Foundation (ref.no: 15-B-0160), the LSB Foundation (no ref.no was provided), the Family Hede Nielsen's Foundation (no ref.no was provided), the Krista and Viggo Petersen's Foundation (no ref.no was provided), and the Aragon Foundation (no ref.no was provided). The funding body had no role in the design of the study and collection, analysis, and interpretation of data and in writing the manuscript.

Authors' contributions

MT was the principal investigator of the study and was responsible for the scientific coordination of the study, the statistical analyses, and manuscript preparation. MT was supervised by BA, JSJ, BHB, and JB. MT drafted the first version of the article, which was subsequently further developed by BHB, JB, JSJ, HS, and BA. MT, JSJ, BHB, JB, and BA are primarily responsible for the design of the study and received input on the study design from all of the authors. HS validated the histological diagnosis codes. JSJ provided laboratory advice during the study. All authors reviewed the manuscript and approved the final version.

Consent for publication

Not applicable.

Competing interests
Axlab, the Danish manufacturer of the Evalyn® Brush, provided self-sampling devices for the study. In accordance with the contract between the manufacturers and the Department of Public Health Programmes, Randers Regional Hospital, Axlab had no influence on the scientific process and no editorial rights pertaining to this manuscript. The authors retained the right to submit the manuscript. None of the authors were compensated for their work on this study, have any shares in the manufacturers' companies, or received bonuses from any of the manufacturers. The authors declare that they have no competing interests.

Author details
[1]Department of Public Health Programmes, Randers Regional Hospital, Skovlyvej 15, 8930 Randers NØ, Denmark. [2]Department of Clinical Medicine, Aarhus University, Palle Juul-Jensens Boulevard 82, 8200 Aarhus N, Denmark. [3]Research Unit for Reproductive Microbiology, Statens Serum Institut, Artillerivej 5, 2300 Copenhagen S, Denmark. [4]Section for Epidemiology, Department of Public Health, Aarhus University, Bartholins Allé 2, 8000 Aarhus C, Denmark. [5]Department of Obstetrics and Gynecology, Odense University Hospital, Sdr. Boulevard 29, 5000 Odense C, Denmark. [6]Department of Clinical Medicine, University of Southern Denmark, J.B. Winslows Vej 25, 5000 Odense C, Denmark. [7]Department of Pathology, Randers Regional Hospital, Østervangsvej 48, 8930 Randers NØ, Denmark.

References

1. Walboomers JM, Jacobs MV, Manos MM, Bosch FX, Kummer JA, Shah KV, Snijders PJ, Peto J, Meijer CJ, Munoz N. Human papillomavirus is a necessary cause of invasive cervical cancer worldwide. J Pathol. 1999;189(1):12–9.
2. Bosch FX, Lorincz A, Munoz N, Meijer CJ, Shah KV. The causal relation between human papillomavirus and cervical cancer. J Clin Pathol. 2002; 55(4):244–65.
3. Arbyn M, Ronco G, Anttila A, Meijer CJ, Poljak M, Ogilvie G, Koliopoulos G, Naucler P, Sankaranarayanan R, Peto J. Evidence regarding human papillomavirus testing in secondary prevention of cervical cancer. Vaccine. 2012;30:F88–99.
4. Cuzick J, Arbyn M, Sankaranarayanan R, Tsu V, Ronco G, Mayrand M, Dillner J, Meijer CJ. Overview of human papillomavirus-based and other novel options for cervical cancer screening in developed and developing countries. Vaccine. 2008;26:K29–41.
5. Dillner J, Rebolj M, Birembaut P, Petry KU, Szarewski A, Munk C, de Sanjose S, Naucler P, Lloveras B, Kjaer S, Cuzick J, van Ballegooijen M, Clavel C, Iftner T, Joint European Cohort Study: Long term predictive values of cytology and human papillomavirus testing in cervical cancer screening: joint European cohort study. BMJ 2008, 337:a1754.
6. Verdoodt F, Jentschke M, Hillemanns P, Racey C, Snijders P, Arbyn M. Reaching women who do not participate in the regular cervical cancer screening programme by offering self-sampling kits: a systematic review and meta-analysis of randomised trials. Eur J Cancer. 2015;51(16):2375–85.
7. Schmeink CE, Bekkers RL, Massuger LF, Melchers WJ. The potential role of self-sampling for high-risk human papillomavirus detection in cervical cancer screening. Rev Med Virol. 2011;21(3):139–53.
8. Petignat P, Faltin DL, Bruchim I, Tramer MR, Franco EL, Coutlee F. Are self-collected samples comparable to physician-collected cervical specimens for human papillomavirus DNA testing? A systematic review and meta-analysis. Gynecol Oncol. 2007;105(2):530–5.
9. Ketelaars P, Bosgraaf R, Siebers A, Massuger L, van der Linden J, Wauters C, Rahamat-Langendoen J, van den Brule A, IntHout J, Melchers W. High-risk human papillomavirus detection in self-sampling compared to physician-taken smear in a responder population of the Dutch cervical screening: results of the VERA study. Prev Med. 2017;101:96–101.
10. van Baars R, Bosgraaf RP, ter Harmsel BW, Melchers WJ, Quint WG, Bekkers RL. Dry storage and transport of a cervicovaginal self-sample by use of the Evalyn Brush, providing reliable human papillomavirus detection combined with comfort for women. J Clin Microbiol. 2012;50(12):3937–43.
11. Nelson EJ, Maynard BR, Loux T, Fatla J, Gordon R, Arnold LD. The acceptability of self-sampled screening for HPV DNA: a systematic review and meta-analysis. Sex Transm Infect. 2017;93(1):56–61.
12. Statistics Denmark. www.statistikbanken.dk. Accessed January. 2018.
13. The Danish Health and Medicines Authority [Sundhedsstyrelsen] Screening for livmoderhalskræft-anbefalinger 2012 [In English: Cervical cancer screening-recommendations]. Copenhagen [in Danish with English summary]. 2012.
14. Lynge E, Clausen LB, Guignard R, Poll P. What happens when organization of cervical cancer screening is delayed or stopped? J Med Screen. 2006; 13(1):41–6.
15. Rao A, Young S, Erlich H, Boyle S, Krevolin M, Sun R, Apple R, Behrens C. Development and characterization of the cobas human papillomavirus test. J Clin Microbiol. 2013;51(5):1478–84.
16. Harris PA, Taylor R, Thielke R, Payne J, Gonzalez N, Conde JG. Research electronic data capture (REDCap)—a metadata-driven methodology and workflow process for providing translational research informatics support. J Biomed Inform. 2009;42(2):377–81.
17. Dugué P, Lynge E, Bjerregaard B, Rebolj M. Non-participation in screening: the case of cervical cancer in Denmark. Prev Med. 2012;54(3):266–9.
18. Altman DG. Practical statistics for medical research: Chapman and Hall/CRC; 1991.
19. Heideman DA, Hesselink AT, Berkhof J, van Kemenade F, Melchers WJ, Daalmeijer NF, Verkuijten M, Meijer CJ, Snijders PJ. Clinical validation of the cobas 4800 HPV test for cervical screening purposes. J Clin Microbiol. 2011; 49(11):3983–5.
20. Verhoef VM, Bosgraaf RP, van Kemenade FJ, Rozendaal L, Heideman DA, Hesselink AT, Bekkers RL, Steenbergen RD, Massuger LF, Melchers WJ. Triage by methylation-marker testing versus cytology in women who test HPV-positive on self-collected cervicovaginal specimens (PROHTECT-3): a randomised controlled non-inferiority trial. Lancet Oncol. 2014;15(3):315–22.

Trends in genital warts by socioeconomic status after the introduction of the national HPV vaccination program in Australia: analysis of national hospital data

Megan A. Smith[1,2,7*], Bette Liu[3,4], Peter McIntyre[5], Robert Menzies[5,6,8], Aditi Dey[5] and Karen Canfell[1,2,7]

Abstract

Background: Human papillomavirus (HPV) vaccination targeting females 12–13 years commenced in Australia in 2007, with catch-up of females 13–26 years until the end of 2009. No analyses of HPV vaccination program impact by either socioeconomic or geographic factors have been reported for Australia.

Methods: Hospital admissions between July 2004-June 2011 involving a diagnosis of genital warts were obtained from a comprehensive national database. We compared sex- and age-specific admission rates in July 2006–June 2007 (pre-vaccination period) and July 2010–June 2011 (post-vaccination period) according to Index of Relative Socio-economic Disadvantage, nationally and stratified by remoteness area relating to the individual's area of residence, using Poisson/ negative binomial models.

Results: Admission rates per 100,000 population in females aged 10–19 years (predominantly vaccinated at school), reduced from 42.2 to 6.0 (rate reduction 86.7 %; 95 % CI:82.2–90.0 %) in more disadvantaged areas and from 26.8 to 4.0 (85.0 %; 95 % CI:79.7–88.9 %) in less disadvantaged areas. In females aged 20–29 years (predominantly vaccinated in the community), the decreases were from 73.9 to 26.4 (66.0 %; 95 % CI:57.7–72.6 %) and from 61.9 to 23.8 (61.6 %; 95 % CI:52.9–68.7 %) in more and less disadvantaged areas, respectively. The reductions were similar in more vs less disadvantaged areas both inside major cities (88.6 %; 95 % CI: 82.2–92.7 % vs 87.9 %; 95 % CI:82.6–91.6 % in females aged 10–19 years; 64.0 %; 95 % CI:57.0–69.9 % vs 63.8 %; 95 % CI:52.9–72.1 % for females aged 20–29 years) and outside major cities (88.8 %; 95 % CI: 83.7–92.3 % vs 85.8 %; 95 % CI:73.5–92.4 % in females aged 10–19 years; 71.1 %; 95 % CI:58.8–79.7 % vs 67.6 %; 95 % CI:48.2–79.8 % for females aged 20–29 years). Admission rates in males aged 20–29 years also reduced, by 23.0 % (95 % CI:4.8–37.8 %) and 39.4 % (95 % CI:28.9–48.3 %) in more versus less disadvantaged areas respectively.

Conclusions: The relative reduction in genital warts appears similar in young females across different levels of disadvantage, including within and outside major cities, both for females predominantly vaccinated at school and in the community.

Keywords: Human papillomavirus, HPV, Vaccination, Genital warts, Impact, Socioeconomic, SES, Remoteness, Geographic, Immunization

* Correspondence: megan.smith@nswcc.org.au
[1]School of Public Health, University of Sydney, Sydney, NSW 2006, Australia
[2]Prince of Wales Clinical School, UNSW Australia, Sydney, NSW 2052, Australia
Full list of author information is available at the end of the article

Background

A publicly-funded vaccination program against human papillomavirus (HPV) commenced in Australia in 2007, initially targeting 12–13 year old females and from 2013 including males aged 12–13 years. The National HPV Vaccination Program (NHVP) included catch-up programs for school-aged girls (12–17 years; delivered through schools in 2007 and 2008), young women (18–26 years; delivered in community settings until end-2009) and school-aged boys (14–15 years, delivered through schools in 2013 and 2014). The quadrivalent vaccine listed for use within the NHVP (Gardasil®, Merck&Co., Whitehouse Station, NJ USA) provides protection against HPV 16, 18, 6 and 11. HPV 16 and 18 are associated with approximately 78 % of cervical cancers in Australia [1], and HPV 6 and 11 are associated with approximately 90 % of genital warts [2].

Comparisons of vaccine uptake from the first target age-group of young females (aged 12–13 years in 2007) across different socioeconomic groups and remoteness areas of Australia estimated three-dose vaccine uptake was 71.5 % in the most disadvantaged areas versus 75.6 % in the least disadvantaged areas, and ranged from 70.1 % in remote areas to 73.6 % in major cities [3]. Less is known about the school or community-based catch-up programs. However initial studies from two Australian jurisdictions suggest uptake in young women was lower in more disadvantaged areas than in less disadvantaged areas [4, 5], and lower in inner regional areas than in either major cities or outer regional and remote areas [5].

To date there are no corresponding data on NHVP impact in Australia by socioeconomic status (SES) or geographic factors. Therefore, the aim of this study was to compare the impact of the NHVP in Australia on genital warts hospitalisations according to socioeconomic and geographic factors, both in females vaccinated at school and in the community. The indirect impact on genital warts hospitalisations in males according to socioeconomic and geographic factors was also examined.

Material and methods

Data sources

Data from the National Hospital Morbidity Database (NHMD), a comprehensive census of admissions to virtually all public and private hospitals in Australia, were obtained from the Australian Institute of Health and Welfare. Recorded data include information on the age, sex, geographic area of residence and Indigenous status of the individual; date of admission; primary and any contributing diagnoses; and any procedures performed. The current analysis includes all admissions with a primary or contributing diagnosis coded with the International Classification of Diseases (ICD-10) code A63.0 (anogenital warts) between 1 July 2004 and 30 June 2011, in females and males aged 10–39 years at admission. Population estimates were sourced from the Australian Bureau of Statistics website [6].

Age groups

Admissions and population estimates were stratified by sex and classified into three age groups based on likely exposure to HPV vaccination and delivery method in females from 2007 onwards, with those 10–19 years corresponding to those predominantly offered vaccination at school, those 20-29 years predominantly offered vaccination in the community, and those 30–39 years not offered vaccination through the public program.

Socioeconomic status (SES)

Data from the Australian Census are used to create a standard suite of indices which rank geographic areas according to different measures of socioeconomic disadvantage based on characteristics of residents within that area, for example measures of income, unemployment, occupation skill level and aspects of housing [7, 8]. Admissions and population data were classified based on the Statistical Local Area (SLA; the smallest area for which socioeconomic, health and population are available) of usual residence and that area's corresponding Index of Relative Socioeconomic Disadvantage (IRSD) ranking, using published data [7]. Areas within IRSD deciles 1–5 were categorised as more disadvantaged, while areas within IRSD deciles 6–10 were categorised as less disadvantaged.

Remoteness area of residence

Admissions and population data were also classified as resident inside or outside major cities, according to a published mapping between SLA and the Remoteness Area structure of the Australian Standard Geographical Classification [9], which is based on the physical road distance of the location to urban centres of different sizes [10]. As there is some correlation between the remoteness and socioeconomic index of areas (people living in more disadvantaged areas are under-represented in major urban areas but over-represented in smaller towns and remote areas) [11], this classification was used for stratifying analyses of SES.

Statistical analyses

Consistent with previous analyses of this data [12], Poisson and negative binomial regression were used to assess overall change in admission rates between the last pre-vaccination year (July 2006–June 2007; hereafter 2006/2007) and the most recent data available (July 2010–June 2011; hereafter 2010/2011), by age group and sex.

Interaction terms were used to examine whether any observed variation in admission rates since 2006/2007 differed by socioeconomic status.

A secondary analysis was performed, using admission rate ratios, comparing admission rates in each successive twelve-month period from 1 July 2007 onwards to the three-year average pre-vaccination admission rate (1 July 2004–30 June 2007). Due to the comparatively high level of missing data for remoteness area in July 2004–June 2005 (~22 %; <1 % thereafter) and SES in July 2004–June 2006 (~25 %; <1 % thereafter), the admission rate ratio was not used as the main analysis.

In order to assess whether missing data for remoteness area and SES might have biased the results, in both cases an overall analysis was done by age as in previous work [12], but restricted only to those admissions where remoteness area/ SES data were not missing.

Additional subgroup analyses

Cervical screening: Approximately 23 % of warts admissions in females aged 10–39 years involved a procedure related to investigation or treatment of screen-detected cervical abnormalities ("screening follow-up"; Additional file 1: Table S1). Participation in cervical screening in Australia varies by SES (but relatively little by remoteness area) [13]; to exclude the possibility that variations in cervical screening behaviour between subgroups influenced the findings, we undertook a sensitivity analysis where "screening follow-up" admissions were excluded.

Men who have sex with men (MSM): As in a previous analysis [12] we examined trends in male admissions stratified according to whether the admission involved a diagnosis or procedure code associated with anal warts, or whether only non-anal sites were recorded (Additional file 1 Table S1), since anal HPV infections

Table 1 Admissions involving a diagnosis of genital warts by sex, age, socioeconomic status and area of residence, July 2004–June 2011

	More disadvantaged[a]		Less disadvantaged[a]	
Females				
10–19 years	947		746	
(excl. screening follow-up[b])	784		573	
20–29 years	2,061		2,610	
(excl screening follow-up[b])	1,594		1,955	
30–39 years	1,034		1,308	
(excl screening follow-up[b])	834		1,020	
Males				
10–19 years	118		144	
20–29 years	956		1,636	
(anal site involved[c])	429		798	
(anal site NOT involved[c])	436		645	
30–39 years	654		1,146	
	Major cities[d]		Other areas[d]	
	More disadvantaged	Less disadvantaged	More disadvantaged	Less disadvantaged
Females				
10–19 years	349	563	598	183
20–29 years	984	2,171	1,077	439
30–39 years	561	1,123	473	185
Males				
20–29 years	506	1,402	450	234
(anal site involved[c])	257	699	172	99
(anal site NOT involved[c])	196	532	240	113
30–39 years	376	1,004	278	142

[a]Based on the Index of Relative Socioeconomic Disadvantage of the admitted individual's area of residence [7, 8]. [b]Admissions involving a procedure related to follow-up of cervical screening were excluded from this sub-analysis (see Additional file1: Table S1) [c]Admissions were stratified according to whether the admission involved a diagnosis or treatment procedure code associated with anal warts, or whether only non-anal sites were recorded (Additional file1: Table S1); admissions where the warts site could not be ascertained were excluded from this sub-analysis [d]Based on the Australian Standard Geographical Classification (ASGC) remoteness area of the admitted individual's area of residence [10]. "Other areas" includes the ASGC categories Inner Regional, Outer Regional, Remote and Very Remote. In cases where the NHMD did not record remoteness area (RA) for an admission, this was assigned based on a standard Australian Bureau of Statistics (ABS) mapping for the admitted individual's SLA [9]. In cases where that SLA contained locations with different levels of remoteness, the admission was assigned according to the standard ABS weighting for each remoteness area within the SLA [9]

and HPV-related disease generally are more common in MSM [14, 15]. Admissions where the warts site could not be ascertained were excluded from this sub-analysis.

Results

Table 1 shows the distribution of admissions included in the analysis by sex, age group, SES and remoteness area.

Socioeconomic status

Annual admission rates by age, sex and SES are shown in Fig. 1 (national) and Fig. 2 (inside versus outside major cities). Significant reductions in admissions involving a diagnosis of genital warts since 2006/2007 were observed for females aged 10–19 and 20–29 years, and males aged 20–29 years, with the greatest reductions observed in females aged 10–19, followed by those 20–29 and then males 20–29 years (Table 2).

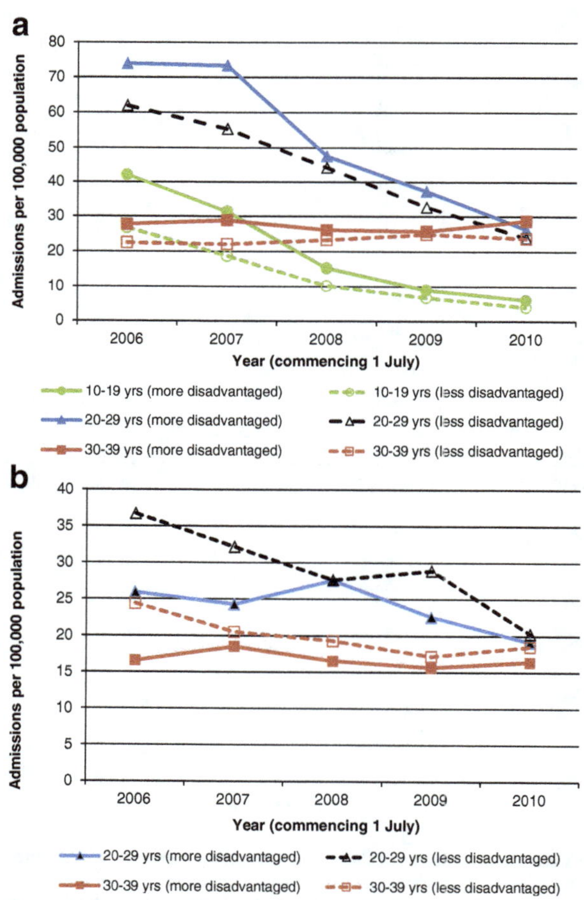

Fig. 1 Admissions involving a diagnosis of genital warts (per 100,000 population), by age and socioeconomic status, in **a**) females and **b**) males. Males aged 10–19 years were excluded due to the small number of admissions

In females, percentage reductions did not differ significantly between those living in more versus less disadvantaged areas, either for females aged 10–19 years at admission (predominantly vaccinated at school) or 20–29 years at admission (predominantly vaccinated in the community) (Table 2). Similar patterns were observed when admissions were stratified by residence inside versus outside major cities, with significant reductions in admissions observed across all subcategories of females aged 10–19 years and 20–29 years, but not in females 30–39 years. There was no evidence of an interaction between SES and the change in admission rates over time in females in any age group, inside or outside major cities.

In males aged 20–29 years, admission rates decreased since 2006/2007 both in more and less disadvantaged areas, with no evidence of an interaction between SES and the change in admission rates (Table 2). The findings varied for 20–29 year old males residing in major cities, however, where there was evidence of an interaction between SES and the change in admission rates ($P_{interaction} = 0.02$), with a significant reduction observed in less disadvantaged, but not more disadvantaged areas of major cities. There were some significant reductions in estimated admission rates for males by particular subgroupings (for example males aged 20–29 years living outside major cities in more disadvantaged areas) but there was no consistent pattern and no other evidence of interaction between SES groups.

The findings based on the admission rate ratio were very similar to the main analysis findings (Figs. 3 and 4). Significant reductions were observed in all subcategories for females aged 10–19 years and 20–29 years (but not in females or males aged 30–39 years). Nationally, reductions in males aged 20–29 years were significant in both more and less disadvantaged areas.

Additional analyses

The observed patterns in females aged 10–19 and 20–29 years did not alter when admissions relating to cervical screening follow-up were excluded from the analysis. The estimated reductions within an age group did not differ significantly by SES, and the estimated reductions for each subgroup were broadly similar regardless of whether admissions relating cervical screening follow-up were included or not (Additional file 1: Table S2).

When admissions in males aged 20–29 years were stratified based on whether or not anal site was involved, the estimated reductions in admissions not involving anal site were substantial and significant, and did not differ by SES; however admissions involving anal site did differ by SES and only reduced in less disadvantaged areas (Additional file 1: Table S2). As

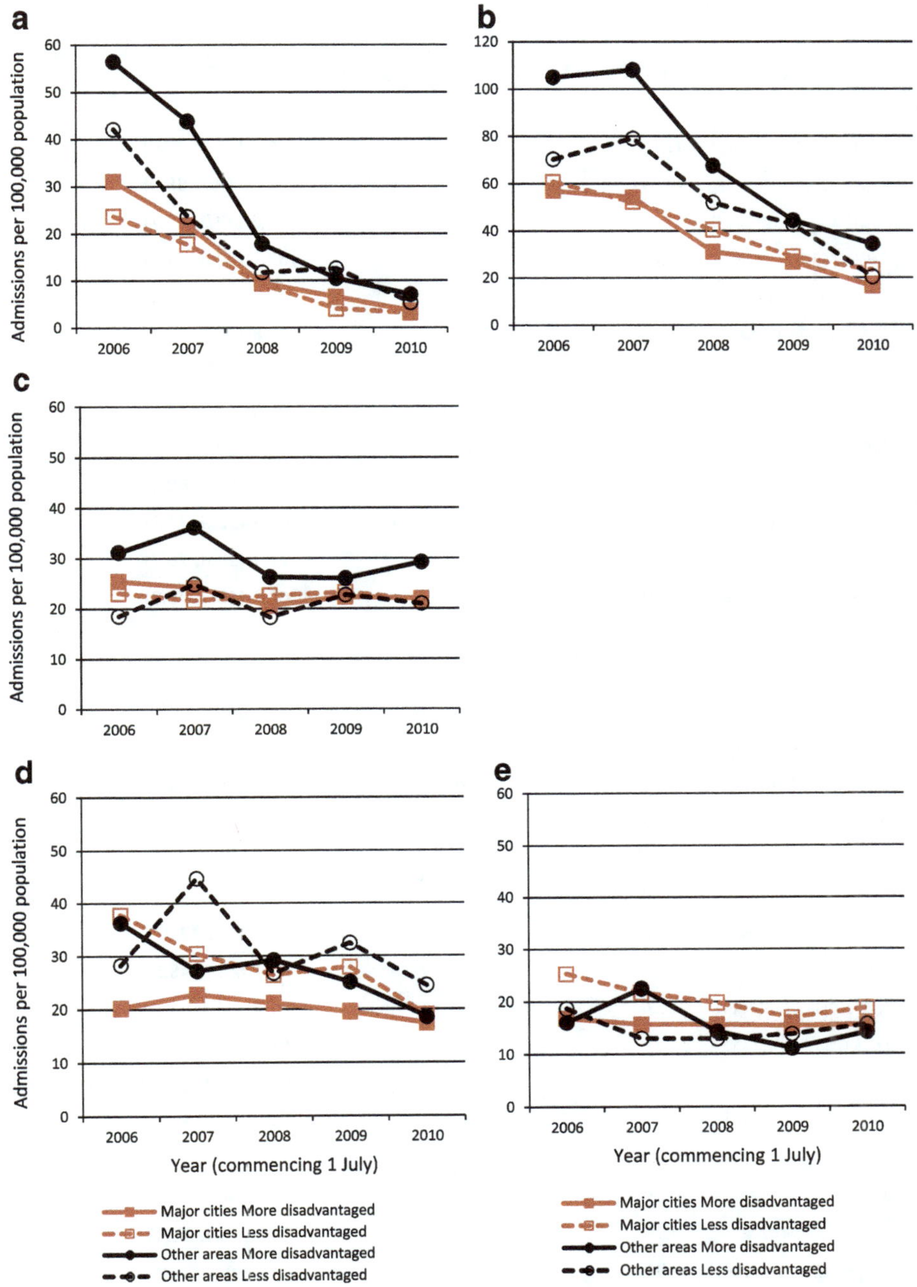

Fig. 2 Admissions involving a diagnosis of genital warts (per 100,000 population), by age, socioeconomic status and remoteness area of residence. **a** Females 10–19 years; **b** Females 20–29 years; **c** Females 30–39 years; **d** Males 20–29 years; **e** Males 30–39 years

there were apparent interactions by SES in males aged 20–29 years both in major cities and for anal warts, an additional analysis examined admissions in this age group in major cities, stratified by site. The interaction by SES for males this age residing in major cities appeared to be driven by differences in anal warts ($P_{interaction} < 0.01$), whereas there was a substantial and significant reduction in admissions involving only non-anal sites which did not differ by SES (Additional file 1: Table S2).

In overall analyses by age, as undertaken in previous work [12] but restricted to those admissions where SES/ remoteness area data were not missing, we found that the estimated reductions in the admission rate did not significantly differ from the original estimates based on the full set and reported in the previous analysis [12], but both the remoteness subset and the SES subset tended to result in lower point estimates of the reduction (Additional file 1: Figure S1).

Table 2 Admission rates and estimated post-vaccination program reductions, by sex, age, socioeconomic status and area of residence

Group		Admission rate per 100,000[a]		Overall reduction July 2006-June 2007 to July 2010-June 2011 % (95% CI)	Interaction term P value[b]
		July 2006-June 2007	July 2010-June 2011		
Females 10–19 years					
National[c]	More disadvantaged	42.16	6.03	**86.7 (82.2, 90.0)**	
	Less disadvantaged	26.75	3.96	**85.0 (79.7, 88.9)**	0.57
Major cities[d]	More disadvantaged	31.13	3.62	**88.6 (82.2, 92.7)**	
	Less disadvantaged	23.73	3.16	**87.9 (82.6, 91.6)**	0.83
Other areas[d]	More disadvantaged	56.47	7.05	**88.8 (83.7, 92.3)**	
	Less disadvantaged	42.11	5.36	**85.8 (73.5, 92.4)**	0.52
Females 20–29 years					
National	More disadvantaged	73.93	26.39	**66.0 (57.7, 72.6)**	
	Less disadvantaged	61.37	23.82	**61.6 (52.9, 68.7)**	0.61
Major cities[d]	More disadvantaged	57.05	16.62	**64.0 (57.0, 69.9)**	
	Less disadvantaged	60.81	23.35	**63.8 (52.9, 72.1)**	0.09
Other areas[d]	More disadvantaged	105.01	34.28	**71.1 (58.8, 79.7)**	
	Less disadvantaged	70.29	20.34	**67.6 (48.2, 79.8)**	0.71
Females 30–39 years					
National	More disadvantaged	27.72	28.67	1.7 (−20.4, 19.7)	
	Less disadvantaged	22.50	23.72	−9.4 (−30.9, 8.5)	0.44
Major cities[d]	More disadvantaged	25.50	22.04	14.1 (−13.9, 35.1)	
	Less disadvantaged	23.11	21.80	1.8 (−19.4, 19.2)	0.45
Other areas[d]	More disadvantaged	31.18	29.25	17.2 (−13.5, 39.6)	
	Less disadvantaged	18.52	21.02	−5.6 (−77.2, 37.1)	0.43
Males 20–29 years					
National	More disadvantaged	25.95	19.17	**23.0 (4.8, 37.8)**	
	Less disadvantaged	36.69	20.28	**39.4 (28.9, 48.3)**	0.08
Major cities[d]	More disadvantaged	20.27	17.47	16.5 (−11.1, 37.3)	
	Less disadvantaged	37.81	18.96	**43.7 (33.0, 52.6)**	0.02
Other areas[d]	More disadvantaged	36.28	18.61	**42.6 (19.4, 59.1)**	
	Less disadvantaged	23.23	24.38	23.5 (−19.5, 51.0)	0.32
Males 30–39 years					
National	More disadvantaged	16.63	16.44	7.5 (−19.8, 28.5)	
	Less disadvantaged	24.44	18.56	**26.0 (10.1, 39.1)**	0.18
Major cities[d]	More disadvantaged	16.94	15.75	6.4 (−30.9, 33.1)	
	Less disadvantaged	25.32	18.84	**29.0 (12.7, 42.3)**	0.17
Other areas[d]	More disadvantaged	16.14	14.22	32.2 (−5.0, 56.2)	
	Less disadvantaged	18.76	15.75	13.0 (−61.8, 53.3)	0.52

Significant reductions between July 2006–June 2007 and July 2010-June 2011 in bold. [a]Admission rate per 100,000 individuals in the population [b]P value for whether the effect of time on admission rates (if any) differed by SES (ie P value for model interaction term) [c]SES: socioeconomic status, based on the Index of Relative Socioeconomic Disadvantage of the admitted individual's area of residence [7, 8] [d] Remoteness of admitted individual's area of residence, based on the Australian Standard Geographical Classification [10]

Discussion

In a previous analysis of this data, we found that the rate of genital warts admissions had decreased in school-aged girls (12–17 years), and in both young women and men (18–26 years) since the introduction of the NHVP [12]. In this further analysis, we found these reductions appear to be similar across different socioeconomic groups for teenaged-girls (10–19 years) and young women (20–29 years), and generally also for young men (20–29 years), residing both inside and outside major cities. This is the first study in Australia to examine HPV vaccine impact within subgroups based on socioeconomic

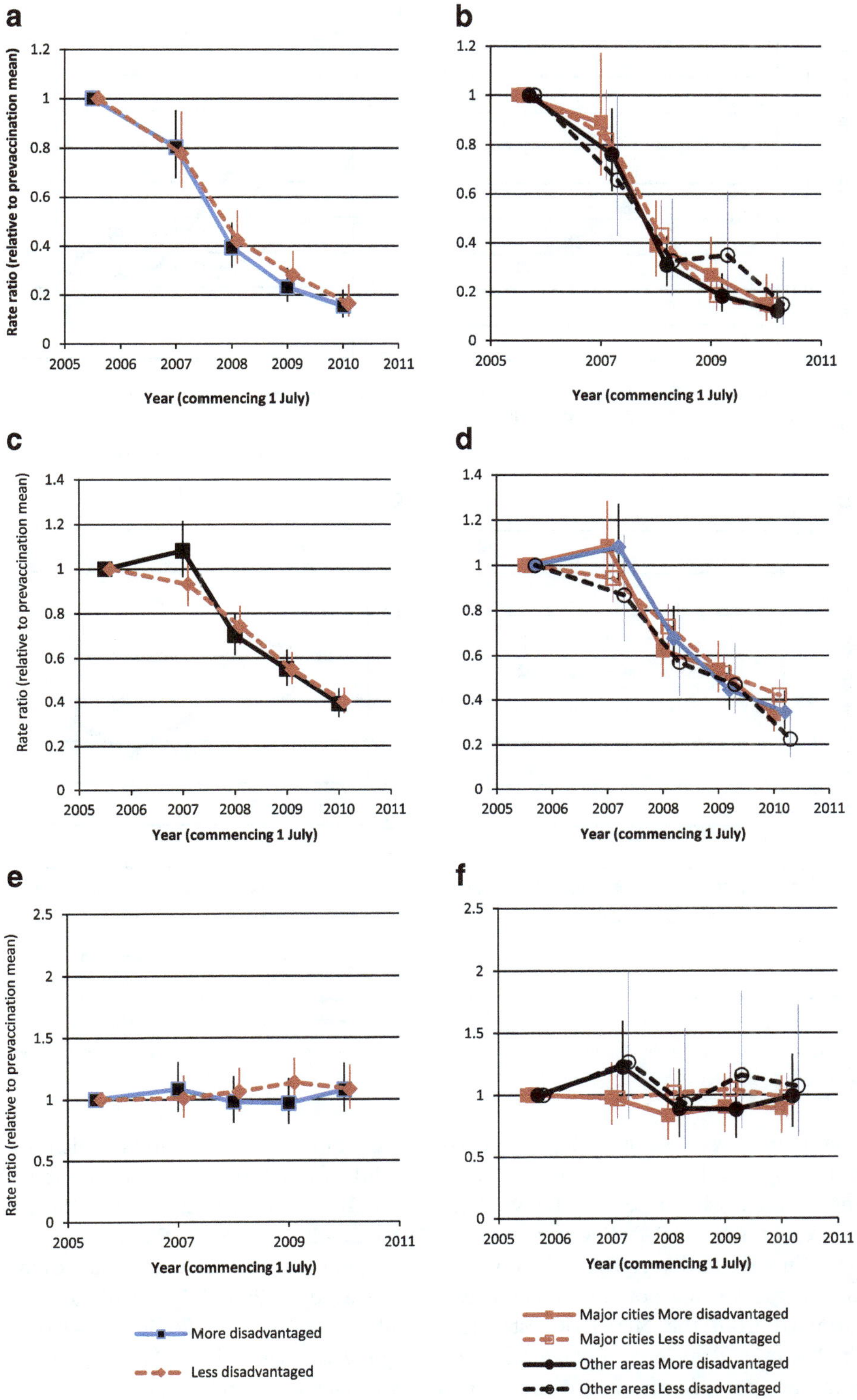

Fig. 3 Admission rate ratio (relative to pre-vaccination mean) by age, SES and remoteness area of residence (females). **a** and **b** 10–19 years; **c** and **d** 20–29 years; **e** and **f** 30–39 years

or geographic factors, and one of only a small number of studies internationally to have examined vaccine impact within sociodemographic subgroups of females [12, 16]. Our findings that reductions in teenaged-females were very similar across different socioeconomic areas, including inside and outside major cities, is consistent with initial estimates of vaccine uptake from the first target age-group of young females (aged 12–13 years in 2007)

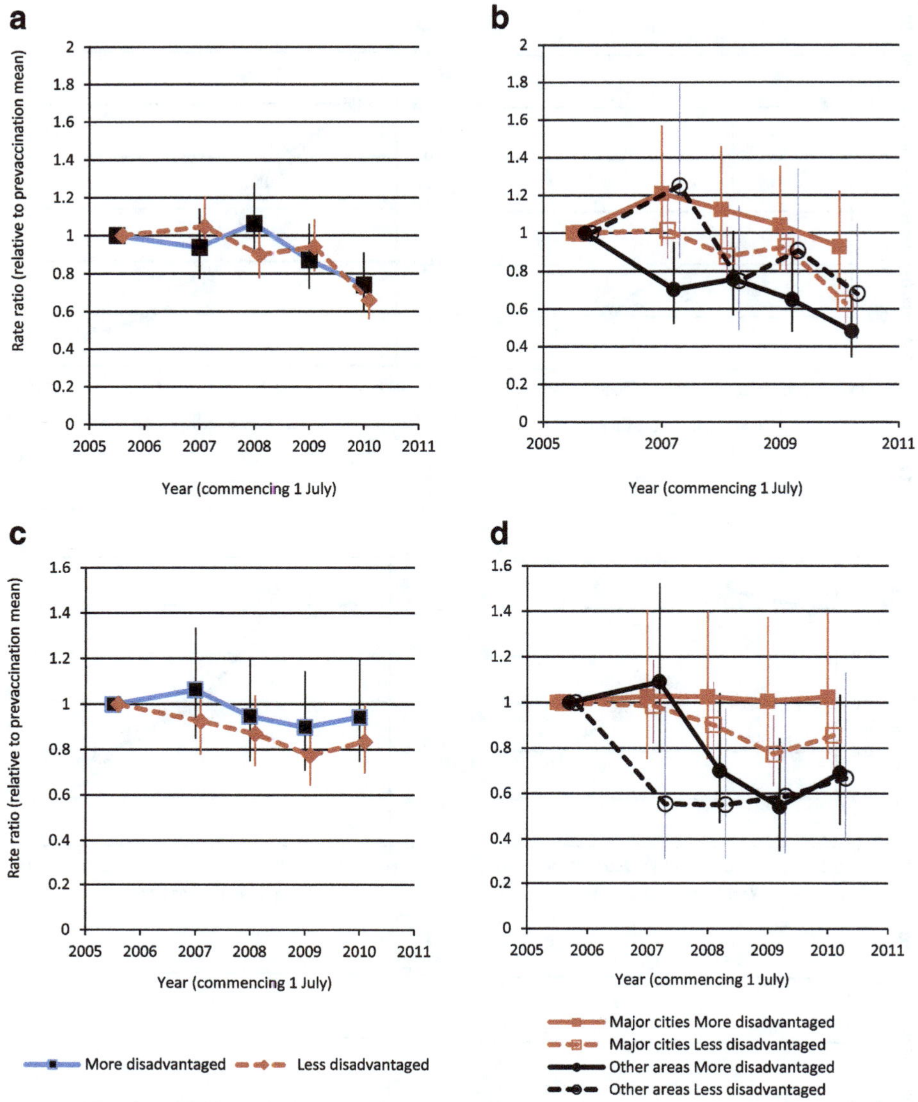

Fig. 4 Admission rate ratio (relative to pre-vaccination mean) by age, SES and remoteness area of residence (males). **a** and **b** 20–29 years; **c** and **d** 30–39 years

which reported that uptake was relatively equal across these different groups [3]. Similar national data are not available for young women who accessed the vaccine through primary care, as the NHVP Register data is known to under-report uptake in this group [17], however data from two states suggest some potential differences. Based on data extracted from the NHVP Register for women residing in Victoria, three-dose uptake was reported as 33.4 % in the most disadvantaged areas and 38.0 % in the least disadvantaged areas [4], and in a NSW-based study of young women with a recent negative cervical screening test, self-reported uptake of one or more vaccine doses was associated with higher socioeconomic status and living outside inner regional areas [5]. We found no significant difference in the estimated reductions between women living in more versus less disadvantaged areas, although the cohorts which we examined differ slightly from those examined in the Victorian (females aged 18–26 years in 2007) and the NSW (females both aged 20–29 in 2008–2009 and 26 years or younger in mid-2007) studies. The last year of data examined here includes those aged 20–29 in July 2010-June 2011, who were potentially aged from 16–26 in mid-2007. The inclusion of slightly younger cohorts (aged 16–17 in 2007; predominantly offered vaccination at school) may potentially weaken differences in uptake between more and less disadvantaged areas if these differences were smaller in the school-based catch-up than in the community (in the youngest age group vaccinated at school, dose 1 uptake differed by only 1.2 % which is smaller than differences in the Victorian and NSW studies) [3–5]. Additionally the SES associated with the area of residence of these younger cohorts of women at the time of their hospital admission may not be the same as it was when they were vaccinated, as young women could have moved since that time. Furthermore as our results are for impact, they may not reflect exactly the same patterns as uptake, due to indirect protection effects [18]. Our finding that reductions in young men were also very similar across different socioeconomic areas, including inside and outside major cities, is also reassuring. An identified difference in the relative reduction in young men by SES within major cities appeared to be driven by differences in anal warts. No difference was observed in admissions involving only non-anal sites, which may more closely reflect indirect protection from female-only vaccination if MSM are over-represented in admissions involving anal warts.

A major strength of this study is that it uses data from a large, comprehensive and routinely-collected national dataset.

A limitation of this study is that is ecological, and vaccination status of admitted individuals is not known. However, an analysis of the same data over a longer period found the substantial reductions in admissions involving genital warts since mid-2007 were confined to young females and males, and the observed reduction did not appear to be a continuation of a pre-existing decline in either group [12]. This study is also ecological in relation to measuring socioeconomic status, since this represents the socioeconomic characteristics of the admitted individual's area of residence, rather than the personal characteristics of the admitted individual (which were not available). However this is a widely-used approach and SLAs are the smallest area for which socioeconomic, health and population are available. Differences could also have been masked by classifying women into two SES groups rather than smaller groups such as quintiles; however an initial analysis by SES quintile also found very little difference between groups (data not shown). Another limitation was the extent of missing data on socioeconomic status prior to July 2006, and on remoteness area prior to July 2005. In order to address this, our primary analysis was restricted to use data from July 2006 on, and admission rate ratios (which used earlier years) were a secondary analysis. The findings were consistent across both the primary and secondary analyses, however, and an additional sensitivity analysis we undertook suggested that the subset we used had not biased the results (Additional file 1).

As genital warts are predominantly managed in primary care or sexual health clinics [19], these admissions data will only represent a fraction of warts cases. Admissions involving a primary diagnosis of genital warts likely represent more serious cases of warts which have not responded to earlier treatment, or where surgical treatment is not as readily available on an outpatient basis. Admissions where warts were a contributing (but not primary) diagnosis were generally for another purpose (for example treatment of cervical abnormalities in women, as previously described in the Methods). Therefore, the absolute admission rates and variation in these by SES and remoteness area could potentially relate to a combination of access and behavioural issues; for example a greater choice of treatment options outside hospitals in major cities. As the main purpose of this analysis was to examine whether the relative reduction (if any) in admission rates varied by SES, these potentially access-related differences are not likely to affect our findings unless there was a change in service usage unrelated to vaccination during the same time period; however this seems unlikely given that no changes were observed in older females.

Australia has had an organised, government-subsidised cervical screening program in place since 1991, and yet, while the program has been successful in reducing both cervical cancer incidence and mortality, socioeconomic and geographic disparities persist in cervical cancer [20]. Lower socioeconomic status is associated with lower participation in cervical screening and higher cervical cancer incidence and mortality [20]. Residing in outer regional areas of Australia is associated with higher cervical cancer mortality compared to more urban areas of Australia [20] (but not incidence, suggesting treatment variation may be a factor) [21]; while residing in remote or very remote regions is associated with both higher incidence and mortality [13]. In contrast, the uptake of school-based HPV vaccination [3] and, as reported here, its impact on genital warts, appears to have been relatively equal across socioeconomic groups including in different remoteness areas. This is potentially due to high school-participation rates [22]; the relative ease of vaccine administration (three doses) compared to repeated cervical cancer screening over many years; comparatively smaller (if any) out of pocket costs; and fewer issues of access (which for example are potentially a factor in poorer cancer survival in more remote areas) [21]. This suggests that the school-based HPV vaccination program in Australia may play an important role in reducing disparities in cervical cancer, which exist even in the context of an organised screening program and publicly-subsidised healthcare more broadly. The finding of relatively equal vaccine uptake in Australia [3, 4] is consistent with data from other countries suggesting that school-based programs result in more equitable uptake across socioeconomic strata [23–26], implying our findings on impact may also have relevance for other settings. It is therefore very important to continue to monitor both HPV vaccine uptake and impact in subgroups to ensure that the results observed to date continue. It will also be useful to assess the impact of HPV vaccination on cervical abnormalities by socioeconomic status and remoteness area to ascertain whether these findings for genital warts are also observed in cervical cancer precursors; however as records of cervical abnormalities on screening registers only include women who attend for screening and screening attendance varies by SES [13], this approach will have some limitations. Therefore monitoring of genital warts in population subgroups is likely to continue to be useful, and will additionally offer the opportunity to examine vaccine impact in subgroups of males, who have been included in the HPV vaccination program since 2013.

Conclusions

The relative reduction in genital warts since the implementation of the NHVP in Australia appears similar in young females across different levels of disadvantage, including within and outside major cities. The impact of the program appears to have been relatively equal, both for females predominantly vaccinated at school and in the community, and also in terms of its indirect protection of males. Routinely-collected hospital admissions data on genital warts are an important source of information for ongoing monitoring of the impact of the NHVP in subgroups and in males as, while undoubtedly important in monitoring, data from cervical screening registers will not completely fulfil this role.

Competing interests

BL holds shares in bioCSL, distributor of the HPV vaccine Gardasil in Australia. PM is an investigator on a survey of HPV seroprevalence in Australia that is partly funded by bioCSL. KC is co-principal investigator of an investigator-initiated trial of cytology and primary HPV screening in Australia ('Compass') (NCT02328872), which is conducted and funded by the Victorian Cytology Service (VCS), a government-funded health promotion charity. The VCS have received equipment and a funding contribution for the Compass trial from Roche Molecular Systems and Ventana Inc. USA. However, neither KC nor her institution on her behalf (Cancer Council NSW) receive direct funding from industry for this trial or any other project.

BL and KC receive salary support from the National Health and Medical Research Council Australia. The National Centre for Immunisation Research and Surveillance is supported by the Australian Government Department of Health, the NSW Ministry of Health, and the Children's Hospital at Westmead. The funding sources had no role in the study design, analysis, interpretation of results, writing of the manuscript, or the decision to submit the article for publication.

All other authors report no competing interests.

Authors' contributions

Study conception: MAS, BL, PM. Contributed to study design: All authors. Data analysis: MAS. Interpretation of data: All authors. Drafted the manuscript: MAS. Critically reviewed all drafts of the manuscript: BL, PM, RM, AD, KC. Approved the final version: all authors.

Acknowledgments

We thank Han Wang (National Centre of Immunisation Research and Surveillance) for assistance with data management and coding.

BL and KC receive salary support from the National Health and Medical Research Council Australia (grant number numbers CDF APP1061473 for BL; CDFs APP1007994 and APP1082989 for KC). The National Centre for Immunisation Research and Surveillance is supported by the Australian Government Department of Health, the NSW Ministry of Health, and the Children's Hospital at Westmead. No specific support was received for this study.

Author details

[1]School of Public Health, University of Sydney, Sydney, NSW 2006, Australia. [2]Prince of Wales Clinical School, UNSW Australia, Sydney, NSW 2052, Australia. [3]School of Public Health and Community Medicine, UNSW Australia, Sydney, NSW 2052, Australia. [4]The Sax Institute, Sydney, PO Box K617, Haymarket, NSW 1240, Australia. [5]National Centre for Immunisation Research and Surveillance Children's Hospital, Westmead, Locked Mail Bag 4001, Sydney 2145NSW, Australia. [6]Sydney Medical School, University of Sydney, Sydney, NSW 2006, Australia. [7]Present address: Cancer Research Division, Cancer Council NSW, Kings Cross NSW 1340, PO Box 572, Sydney, NSW 2011, Australia. [8]Present address: School of Public Health and Community Medicine, UNSW Australia, Sydney, NSW 2052, Australia.

References

1. Brotherton JM. How much cervical cancer in Australia is vaccine preventable? A meta-analysis Vaccine. 2008;26(2):250–6.
2. Garland SM, Steben M, Sings HL, James M, Lu S, Railkar R, et al. Natural history of genital warts: analysis of the placebo arm of 2 randomized phase III trials of a quadrivalent human papillomavirus (types 6, 11, 16, and 18) vaccine. J InfectDis. 2009;199(6):805–14.
3. Barbaro B, Brotherton JM. Assessing HPV vaccine coverage in Australia by geography and socioeconomic status: are we protecting those most at risk? Aust N Z J Public Health. 2014;38(5):419–23.
4. Barbaro B, Brotherton JM, Gertig DM. Human papillomavirus vaccination and cervical cancer screening by socioeconomic status. Victoria Med J Aust. 2012;196(7):445.
5. Canfell K, Egger S, Velentzis LS, Brown JD, O'Connell DL, Banks E, et al. Factors related to vaccine uptake by young adult women in the catch-up phase of the National HPV Vaccination Program in Australia: Results from an observational study. Vaccine. 2015;33(20):2387–94.
6. Australian Bureau of Statistics: 3235.0 - Population by Age and Sex, Regions of Australia. Canberra; 2013.
7. Australian Bureau of Statistics: Socio-Economic Indexes for Areas (SEIFA). ABS Catalogue no. 2033.0.55.001. Canberra; 2013.
8. Australian Bureau of Statistics: Socio-Economic Indexes for Areas (SEIFA). ABS Catalogue no. 2039.0.55.001. Canberra; 2008.
9. Australian Bureau of Statistics: 1216.0.15.003 - Australian Standard Geographical Classification (ASGC) Remoteness Area Correspondences, 2006. Canberra; 2011.
10. Australian Bureau of Statistics: ASGC Remoteness Classification: Purpose and Use (Census Paper No. 03/01). Canberra; 2003.
11. Australian Bureau of Statistics: 4102.0 - Australian Social Trends, 2000. Canberra; 2000.
12. Smith MA, Liu B, McIntyre P, Menzies R, Dey A, Canfell K. Fall in genital warts diagnoses in the general and Indigenous Australian population following a national HPV vaccination program: analysis of routinely collected national hospital data. J Infect Dis. 2015;211(1):91–9.
13. Australian Institute of Health and Welfare: Cervical screening in Australia 2011–2012. Cancer series no.82. Cat. no. CAN 79. Canberra: AIHW; 2014.
14. Palefsky JM. Human Papillomavirus-Related Disease in Men: Not Just a Women's Issue. J Adolesc Health. 2010;46(4, Supplement):S12–9.
15. Nyitray AG, da Silva RJ C, Baggio ML, Smith D, Abrahamsen M, Papenfuss M, et al. Six-Month Incidence, Persistence, and Factors Associated With Persistence of Anal Human Papillomavirus in Men: The HPV in Men Study. J Infect Dis. 2011;204(11):1711–22.
16. Niccolai LM, Julian PJ, Meek JI, McBride V, Hadler JL, Sosa LE. Declining rates of high-grade cervical lesions in young women in Connecticut, 2008–2011. Cancer Epidemiol Biomarkers Prev. 2013;22(8):1446–50.
17. Brotherton JML, Liu B, Donovan B, Kaldor JM, Saville M. Human papillomavirus (HPV) vaccination coverage in young Australian women is higher than previously estimated: independent estimates from a nationally representative mobile phone survey. Vaccine. 2014;32(5):592–7.
18. Tabrizi SN, Brotherton JM, Kaldor JM, Skinner SR, Liu B, Bateson D, et al. Assessment of herd immunity and cross-protection after a human papillomavirus vaccination programme in Australia: a repeat cross-sectional study. Lancet Infect Dis. 2014;14(10):958–66.
19. Grulich AE, de Visser RO, Badcock PB, Smith AM, Richters J, Rissel C, et al. Knowledge about and experience of sexually transmissible infections in a representative sample of adults: the Second Australian Study of Health and Relationships. Sex Health. 2014;11(5):481–94.
20. Australian Institute of Health and Welfare, Cancer Australia: Gynaecological

cancers in Australia: An overview. Cancer series no. 70. Cat no. CAN 66. Canberra: AIHW; 2012.

21. Jong KE, Smith DP, Yu XQ, O'Connell DL, Goldstein D, Armstrong BK. Remoteness of residence and survival from cancer in New South Wales. Med J Aust. 2004;180(12):618–22.
22. Australian Bureau of Statistics: Schools, Australia, 2013 (cat. no. 4221.0). Canberra: ABS; 2014.
23. Musto R, Siever J, Johnston J, Seidel J, Rose M, McNeil D. Social equity in Human Papillomavirus vaccination: a natural experiment in Calgary Canada. BMC Public Health. 2013;13(1):640.
24. Kumar VM, Whynes DK. Explaining variation in the uptake of HPV vaccination in England. BMC Public Health. 2011;11:172.
25. Fisher H, Audrey S, Mytton JA, Hickman M, Trotter C. Examining inequalities in the uptake of the school-based HPV vaccination programme in England: a retrospective cohort study. J Public Health. 2014;36(1):36–45.
26. Hughes A, Mesher D, White J, Soldan K. Coverage of the English national human papillomavirus (HPV) immunisation programme among 12 to 17 year-old females by area-level deprivation score, England, 2008 to 2011. Euro Surveill. 2014;19(2).

Permissions

All chapters in this book were first published in ID, by BioMed Central; hereby published with permission under the Creative Commons Attribution License or equivalent. Every chapter published in this book has been scrutinized by our experts. Their significance has been extensively debated. The topics covered herein carry significant findings which will fuel the growth of the discipline. They may even be implemented as practical applications or may be referred to as a beginning point for another development.

The contributors of this book come from diverse backgrounds, making this book a truly international effort. This book will bring forth new frontiers with its revolutionizing research information and detailed analysis of the nascent developments around the world.

We would like to thank all the contributing authors for lending their expertise to make the book truly unique. They have played a crucial role in the development of this book. Without their invaluable contributions this book wouldn't have been possible. They have made vital efforts to compile up to date information on the varied aspects of this subject to make this book a valuable addition to the collection of many professionals and students.

This book was conceptualized with the vision of imparting up-to-date information and advanced data in this field. To ensure the same, a matchless editorial board was set up. Every individual on the board went through rigorous rounds of assessment to prove their worth. After which they invested a large part of their time researching and compiling the most relevant data for our readers.

The editorial board has been involved in producing this book since its inception. They have spent rigorous hours researching and exploring the diverse topics which have resulted in the successful publishing of this book. They have passed on their knowledge of decades through this book. To expedite this challenging task, the publisher supported the team at every step. A small team of assistant editors was also appointed to further simplify the editing procedure and attain best results for the readers.

Apart from the editorial board, the designing team has also invested a significant amount of their time in understanding the subject and creating the most relevant covers. They scrutinized every image to scout for the most suitable representation of the subject and create an appropriate cover for the book.

The publishing team has been an ardent support to the editorial, designing and production team. Their endless efforts to recruit the best for this project, has resulted in the accomplishment of this book. They are a veteran in the field of academics and their pool of knowledge is as vast as their experience in printing. Their expertise and guidance has proved useful at every step. Their uncompromising quality standards have made this book an exceptional effort. Their encouragement from time to time has been an inspiration for everyone.

The publisher and the editorial board hope that this book will prove to be a valuable piece of knowledge for researchers, students, practitioners and scholars across the globe.

List of Contributors

Jing-fen Lu, Guo-rong Shen, Qiong Li, Xu Chen, Chun-fang Ma and Tong-hua Zhu
Department of Clinical laboratory, Wujiang First People's Hospital, Suzhou, People's Republic of China

Etienne E. Müller
Centre for HIV and Sexually Transmitted Infections, National Institute for Communicable Diseases, National Health Laboratory Service, Johannesburg, South Africa

Kevin Rebe and Helen Struthers
Anova Health Institute, Johannesburg, South Africa
Anova Health Institute, Cape Town, South Africa
Department of Medicine, Division of Infectious Diseases and HIV Medicine, University of Cape Town, Cape Town, South Africa

Tobias F. Chirwa
Division of Epidemiology and Biostatistics, School of Public Health, University of the Witwatersrand, Johannesburg, South Africa

James McIntyre
Anova Health Institute, Johannesburg, South Africa
Anova Health Institute, Cape Town, South Africa
Division of Epidemiology & Biostatistics, School of Public & Family Medicine, University of Cape Town, Cape Town, South Africa

David A. Lewis
Western Sydney Sexual Health Centre, Western Sydney Local Health District, Parramatta, Australia
Marie Bashir Institute for Infectious Diseases and Biosecurity & Sydney Medical School-Westmead, University of Sydney, Sydney, Australia

Carol Y. Lin
Centers for Disease Control and Prevention, Atlanta, GA, USA

Ling Li
United Arab Emirates University, Al Ain, UAE

Madhav P. Bhatta
Department of Biostatistics, Environmental Health Sciences, and Epidemiology, College of Public Health Kent State University, Kent, OH 44242, USA

Derek C. Johnson
Department of Public Health & Community Medicine, Tufts University School of Medicine, Boston, MA, USA

Mingma Lama and Pema Lhaki
NFCC, International, Kathmandu, Nepal

Shilu Aryal
Family Health Division, Nepal Ministry of Health, Kathmandu, Nepal

Sadeep Shrestha
Department of Epidemiology, School of Public Health, University of Alabama at Birmingham, Birmingham, AL, USA

M. Chantal Umulisa and Maurice Gatera
Ministry of Health of Rwanda, Kigali, Rwanda

Fidele Ngabo
Ministry of Health of Rwanda, Kigali, Rwanda
Université Libre de Bruxelles, Ecole de Santé Publique, Brussels, Belgium

Silvia Franceschi, Iacopo Baussano, Vanessa Tenet and Gary M. Clifford
International Agency for Research on Cancer, 150 cours Albert Thomas, 69372 Lyon Cedex 08, France

Peter J. F. Snijders and Anne M. Uyterlinde
Department of Pathology, VU University Medical Center, De Boelelaan 1117, 1081 HV Amsterdam, The Netherlands

Fulvio Lazzarato
International Agency for Research on Cancer, 150 cours Albert Thomas, 69372 Lyon Cedex 08, France
Unit of Cancer Epidemiology, Department of Medical Sciences, University of Turin, Turin, Italy

Agnes Binagwaho
Ministry of Health of Rwanda, Kigali, Rwanda
Harvard Medical School, Boston, MA, USA
Geisel School of Medicine, Dartmouth, Hanover, USA

George Krashias, Dana Koptides and Christina Christodoulou
Department of Molecular Virology, The Cyprus Institute of Neurology and Genetics, 6 International Airport Avenue, 2370 Nicosia, Cyprus

Birgit Engesæter, Stefan Lönnberg and Mari Nygård
Cancer Registry of Norway, Oslo, Norway

Bianca van Diermen Hidle and Pia Moltu
Department of Pathology, Stavanger University Hospital, Stavanger, Norway

Mona Hansen and Irene Kraus Christiansen
Department of Microbiology and Infection Control, Akershus University Hospital, Lørenskog, Norway

Kjersti Mangseth Staby
Department of Pathology, Haukeland University Hospital, Bergen, Norway

Siri Borchgrevink-Persen
Department of Pathology and Medical Genetics, St. Olavs Hospital, Trondheim University Hospital, Trondheim, Norway

Olav K. Vintermyr
Department of Pathology, Haukeland University Hospital, Bergen, Norway
The Gade Laboratory for Pathology, Department of Clinical Medicine (K1), University of Bergen, Bergen, Norway

Emiel A. M. Janssen
Department of Pathology, Stavanger University Hospital, Stavanger, Norway
Department of Mathematics and Natural Sciences, University of Stavanger, Stavanger, Norway

Philip E. Castle
Albert Einstein College of Medicine, Bronx, NY, USA

Dong Hang, Meiqun Jia, Hongxia Ma, Jing Zhou, Yin Yin and Guangfu Jin
Department of Epidemiology and Biostatistics, School of Public Health, Nanjing Medical University, Nanjing 211166, China

Ni Li, Min Dai, Xiaoshuang Feng, Zhangyan Lyu, Jian Yin and Hong Cui
Program Office for Cancer Screening in Urban China, National Cancer Centre/Cancer Hospital, Chinese Academy of Medical Sciences and Peking Union Medical College, Beijing 100021, China

Zhibin Hu and Hongbing Shen
Department of Epidemiology and Biostatistics, School of Public Health, Nanjing Medical University, Nanjing 211166, China
State Key Laboratory of Reproductive Medicine, Nanjing Medical University, Nanjing 211166, China

Kai Zhang
Department of Cancer Prevention, National Cancer Centre/Cancer Hospital, Chinese Academy of Medical Sciences and Peking Union Medical College, Beijing 100021, China

Samantha E. Rudolph
UC Berkeley-UCSF Joint Medical Program, Berkeley, CA, USA

Jorge Salmerón
Unidad de Investigación Epidemiológica y en Servicios de Salud, Instituto Mexicano del Seguro Social, Cuernavaca, Morelos, México

Paula Ramírez and Berenice Rivera
Unidad de Investigación Epidemiológica y en Servicios de Salud, Instituto Mexicano del Seguro Social, Cuernavaca, Morelos, México
Centro de Investigación en Salud Poblacional, Instituto Nacional de Salud Pública, Avenida Universidad 655, Colonia Sta. María Ahuacatitlán, 62100 Cuernavaca, Morelos, Mexico

Attila Lorincz and Jack Cuzick
Wolfson Institute of Preventive Medicine, Barts and The London School of Medicine, Queen Mary University of London, London, UK

Cosette M. Wheeler and Patti Gravitt
Department of Pathology, University of New Mexico School of Medicine, Albuquerque, NM, USA

Eduardo Lazcano-Ponce, Leticia Torres-Ibarra and Rubí Hernández
Centro de Investigación en Salud Poblacional, Instituto Nacional de Salud Pública, Avenida Universidad 655, Colonia Sta. María Ahuacatitlán, 62100 Cuernavaca, Morelos, Mexico

Leith León-Maldonado
CONACYT, Centro de Investigación en Salud Poblacional, Instituto Nacional de Salud Pública, Cuernavaca, Morelos, México, USA

Eduardo L. Franco
Division of Cancer Epidemiology, McGill University, Montreal, Canada

Natasha O. Moraka
Botswana Harvard AIDS Institute Partnership, Gaborone, Botswana

Pablo Méndez-Hernández
Departamento de Enseñanza, Capacitación e Investigación, Secretaría de Salud de Tlaxcala, Tlaxcala, Tlaxcala, Mexico
Facultad de Ciencias de la Salud, Universidad Autónoma de Tlaxcala, Tlaxcala, Tlaxcala, Mexico

Agnihotram V. Ramanakumar, Mariam El-Zein, Flavia R. Silva and Eduardo L. Franco
Division of Cancer Epidemiology, Department of Oncology, McGill University, Montreal, Canada

Eileen Shaw
Division of Cancer Epidemiology, Department of Oncology, McGill University, Montreal, Canada
Department of Epidemiology, Biostatistics and Occupational Health, McGill University, 546 Pine Avenue West, Montreal, QC H2W 1S6, Canada

Lenice Galan, Maria L. Baggio and Luisa L. Villa
Ludwig Institute for Cancer Research, São Paulo, Brazil
Molecular Biology Laboratory, Centre of Translational Oncology, Instituto do Câncer do Estado de São Paulo, São Paulo, Brazil

Lili Qian, Yu Zhang, Yimin Chen, Ying Yu and Yonglin Liu
Department of Laboratory Medicine, the First Affiliated Hospital of Zhejiang Chinese Medical University, Hangzhou, China

Dawei Cui, Bin Lou and Yu Chen
Department of Laboratory Medicine, Center of Clinical Laboratory, the First Affiliated Hospital, School of Medicine, Zhejiang University, No. 79, Qingchun Road, Hangzhou 310003, China

Catharina J. Alberts and Liza Coyer
Department of Infectious Diseases Research and Prevention, Public Health Service of Amsterdam (GGD), Nieuwe Achtergracht 100, Amsterdam 1018 WT, The Netherlands

Alexandra Kovaleva
Department of Infectious Diseases Research and Prevention, Public Health Service of Amsterdam (GGD), Nieuwe Achtergracht 100, Amsterdam 1018 WT, The Netherlands
AMC Graduate School, Academic Medical Center, Meibergdreef 9, Amsterdam 1105 AZ, The Netherlands

Tim Waterboer and Angelika Michel
German Cancer Research Center (DKFZ), Im Neuenheimer Feld 280, Heidelberg 69120, Germany

Marieke B. Snijder
Department of Public Health, Academic Medical Center, Meibergdreef 9, Amsterdam 1105 AZ, The Netherlands

Wilma Vermeulen
Public Health Laboratory, Public Health Service of Amsterdam (GGD), Nieuwe Achtergracht 100, Amsterdam 1018 WT, The Netherlands

Maria Prins and Maarten Schim van der Loeff
Department of Infectious Diseases Research and Prevention, Public Health Service of Amsterdam (GGD), Nieuwe Achtergracht 100, Amsterdam 1018 WT, The Netherlands
Department of Internal Medicine, Center for Infection and Immunity Amsterdam (CINIMA), Academic Medical Center, Meibergdreef 9, Amsterdam 1105 AZ, The Netherlands

Zulqarnain Baloch, Yuanyue Li, Yue Feng, Li Liu, Binghui Wang, A-mei Zhang and Xueshan Xia
Faculty of Life Science and Technology, Kunming University of Science and Technology, Kunming 650500, China
The Research Center for Molecular Medicine, Kunming 650500, China

Tao Yuan, Yanqing Liu, Wenlin Tai and Xiaomei Wu
The First Hospital in Yunnan province, Kunming 650034, China

Lei Zhang, Qingqing Bi, Hua Deng, Juan Chen and Xiaofeng Mu
Department of Laboratory Medicine, Qingdao Central Hospital, Second Affiliated H ospital of Qingdao University, Siliunan Road #127, Qingdao 266042, China

Jing Xu
Department of Pathology, Qingdao Central Hospital, Qingdao, China

Meilian Zhang
Clinical Laboratory, Qingdao Cancer Hospital, Qingdao, China

Sylvia Taylor
GSK Vaccines, 20, Avenue Fleming, Parc de la Noire Epine, B-1300 Wavre, Belgium

Eveline Bunge and Marina Bakker
Pallas Health Research and Consultancy BV, Rotterdam, The Netherlands

Xavier Castellsagué
Cancer Epidemiology Research Program, Catalan Institute of Oncology (ICO), IDIBELL, L'Hospitalet de Llobregat, Catalonia, Spain
CIBER Epidemiología y Salud Pública (CIBERESP), Barcelona, Spain

Takeo Nakayama
Department of Health Informatics, Kyoto University School of Public Health, Kyoto, Japan

Xiuting Mo
Department of Health Informatics, Kyoto University School of Public Health, Kyoto, Japan

Ruoyan Gai Tobe and Rintaro Mori
Department of Health Policy, National Center for Child Health and Development, Okura 2-10-1, Setagaya-ku, Tokyo 157-8535, Japan

Lijie Wang
Department of Gynecology, Qilu Hospital of Shandong University, Jinan, China

Xianchen Liu
College of Pharmacy, The University of Tennessee Health Science Center, Memphis, TN, USA

Bin Wu
Medical Decision and Economic Group, Department of Pharmacy, Ren Ji Hospital affiliated with Medical School of Shanghai Jiao tong University, Shanghai, China

Chie Nagata
Department of Education for Clinical Research, National Centre for Child Health and Development, Tokyo, Japan

Na Zuo, Can He, Jing Yang, Mengfei Xu, Caiyun Ge, Ziye Song and Hongbing Cai
Department of Gynecological Oncology, Zhongnan Hospital of Wuhan University, Hubei Cancer Clinical Study Center, Hubei Key laboratory of Tumor Biological Behaviors, Wuhan 430071, People's Republic of China

Huiwen Luo
Nanjing Drum Tower Hospital affiliated Medical School of Nanjing University, Nanjing, China

Niresh Thapa
Department of Gynecological Oncology, Zhongnan Hospital of Wuhan University, Hubei Cancer Clinical Study Center, Hubei Key laboratory of Tumor Biological Behaviors, Wuhan 430071, People's Republic of China
Karnali Academy of Health Sciences, Jumla, Nepal

Muna Maharjan
Zhongnan Hospital of Wuhan University, HOPE School of Nursing, Wuhan, Hubei, China

Girishma Shrestha
Patan Hospital, Patan Academy of Health Sciences, Patan, Nepal

Narayani Maharjan
Department of Clinical Laboratory Science, Zhongnan Hospital of Wuhan University, Wuhan, Hubei, China

Marcia A. Petrini
Faculty of Nursing, Chiang Mai University, Chiang Mai, Thailand

Zhangyan Lyu, Xiaoshuang Feng, Ni Li, Luopei Wei, Yuheng Chen, Wenjing Yang and Min Dai
Program Office for Cancer Screening in Urban China, National Cancer Center / Cancer Hospital, Chinese Academy of Medical Sciences and Peking Union Medical College, No.17 Panjiayuannanli, Chaoyang District, Beijing 100021, China

Wei Zhao and Bing Yao
Reproductive Medical Center, Jinling Hospital, Nanjing 210029, China

Dong Hang
Department of Epidemiology and Biostatistics, Jiangsu Key Lab of Cancer Biomarkers, Prevention and Treatment, Collaborative Innovation Center For Cancer Personalized Medicine, School of Public Health, Nanjing Medical University, Nanjing 211166, China

Hongxia Ma, Zhibin Hu and Hongbing Shen
Department of Epidemiology and Biostatistics, Jiangsu Key Lab of Cancer Biomarkers, Prevention and Treatment, Collaborative Innovation Center For Cancer Personalized Medicine, School of Public Health, Nanjing Medical University, Nanjing 211166, China
State Key Laboratory of Reproductive Medicine, Nanjing Medical University, Nanjing 211166, China

Kai Zhang
Department of Cancer Prevention, National Cancer Center / Cancer Hospital, Chinese Academy of Medical Sciences and Peking Union Medical College, Beijing 100021, China

Andrew Ndlovu and Ishmael Kasvosve
Department of Medical Laboratory Sciences, Faculty of Health Sciences, University of Botswana, Private Bag UB072, 4775 Notwane Rd., Gaborone, Botswana

Patricia S. Rantshabeng
Department of Medical Laboratory Sciences, Faculty of Health Sciences, University of Botswana, 4775 Notwane Rd., Gaborone, Botswana
Department of Pathology, Faculty of Medicine, University of Botswana, Gaborone, Botswana

Sikhulile Moyo, Iain J. MacLeod and Simani Gaseitsiwe
Harvard T. H. Chan School of Public Health, Department of Immunology and Infectious Diseases, Boston, MA, USA
Botswana Harvard AIDS Institute Partnership, Gaborone, Botswana

Pingsen Zhao, Sudong Liu, Jingyuan Hou, Lifang Lin, Ruiqiang Weng and Luxian Su
Clinical Core Laboratory, Meizhou People's Hospital (Huangtang Hospital), Meizhou Hospital Affiliated to Sun Yat-sen University, Meizhou 514031, People's Republic of China
Center for Precision Medicine, Meizhou People's Hospital (Huangtang Hospital), Meizhou Hospital Affiliated to Sun Yat-sen University, Meizhou 514031, People's Republic of China Guangdong Provincial Engineering and Technology Research Center for Molecular Diagnostics of Cardiovascular Diseases, Meizhou 514031, People's Republic of China
Meizhou Municipal Engineering and Technology Research Center for Molecular Diagnostics of Cardiovascular Diseases, Meizhou 514031, People's Republic of China

Johannes Horn
Helmholtz Centre for Infection Research, Inhoffenstr. 7, 38124 Braunschweig, Germany

Zhixiong Zhong
Center for Precision Medicine, Meizhou People's Hospital (Huangtang Hospital), Meizhou Hospital Affiliated to Sun Yat-sen University, Meizhou 514031, People's Republic of China Guangdong Provincial Engineering and Technology Research Center for Molecular Diagnostics of Cardiovascular Diseases, Meizhou 514031, People's Republic of China
Meizhou Municipal Engineering and Technology Research Center for Molecular Diagnostics of Cardiovascular Diseases, Meizhou 514031, People's Republic of China

Nanxiang Lei, Tao Hou and Haikun Yang
Department of Gynaecology, Meizhou People's Hospital (Huangtang Hospital), Meizhou Hospital Affiliated to Sun Yat-sen University, Meizhou 514031, People's Republic of China

Kathrin Thöne
Leibniz-Institute for Prevention Research and Epidemiology - BIPS, Achterstr.30, 28359 Bremen, Germany
Hubertus Wald Tumor Center, University Cancer Center Hamburg (UCCH)/ University Medical Centerm Hamburg-Eppendorf (UKE), Martinistr.52, 20246 Hamburg, Germany

Rafael Mikolajczyk
Helmholtz Centre for Infection Research, Inhoffenstr. 7, 38124 Braunschweig, Germany
Hannover Medical School, Carl-Neuberg-Str. 1, 30625 Hannover, Germany
Institute for Medical Epidemiology, Biometrics, and Informatics, Medical Faculty of the Martin-Luther University Halle-Wittenberg, 06112 Halle (Saale), Germany

Mette Tranberg and Berit Andersen
Department of Public Health Programmes, Randers Regional Hospital, Skovlyvej 15, 8930 Randers NØ, Denmark
Department of Clinical Medicine, Aarhus University, Palle Juul-Jensens Boulevard 82, 8200 Aarhus N, Denmark

Jørgen Skov Jensen
Research Unit for Reproductive Microbiology, Statens Serum Institut, Artillerivej 5, 2300 Copenhagen S, Denmark

Bodil Hammer Bech
Section for Epidemiology, Department of Public Health, Aarhus University, Bartholins Allé 2, 8000 Aarhus C, Denmark

Jan Blaakær
Department of Obstetrics and Gynecology, Odense University Hospital, Sdr. Boulevard 29, 5000 Odense C, Denmark
Department of Clinical Medicine, University of Southern Denmark, J.B. Winslows Vej 25, 5000 Odense C, Denmark

Hans Svanholm
Department of Pathology, Randers Regional Hospital, Østervangsvej 48, 8930 Randers NØ, Denmark

Karen Canfell and Megan A. Smith
School of Public Health, University of Sydney, Sydney, NSW 2006, Australia
Prince of Wales Clinical School, UNSW Australia, Sydney, NSW 2052, Australia
Cancer Research Division, Cancer Council NSW, Kings Cross NSW 1340, Sydney, NSW 2011, Australia

Bette Liu
School of Public Health and Community Medicine, UNSW Australia, Sydney, NSW 2052, Australia
The Sax Institute, Sydney, Haymarket, NSW 1240, Australia

Peter McIntyre and Aditi Dey
National Centre for Immunisation Research and Surveillance Children's Hospital, Westmead, Sydney 2145NSW, Australia

Robert Menzies
National Centre for Immunisation Research and Surveillance Children's Hospital, Westmead, Locked Mail Bag 4001, Sydney 2145NSW, Australia
Sydney Medical School, University of Sydney, Sydney, NSW 2006, Australia
School of Public Health and Community Medicine, UNSW Australia, Sydney, NSW 2052, Australia

Index